NURSING

Solved Question Papers for BSc Nursing—2nd Year (2019–2014)

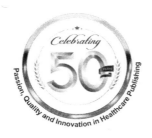

NURSING
Solved Question Papers for BSc Nursing—2nd Year (2019–2014)

(As per INC Syllabus)

Fourth Edition

I Clement
Doctorate of Philosophy in Nursing (PhD)
MSc Nursing (Medical Surgical Nursing)
MA (Sociology) MSc (Psychology)
MBA in Education
MA Child Care and Education
MA (Education) MPhil in Education
Postgraduate in Hospital Administration
PhD Guide, Examiner, Thesis Evaluator
Rajiv Gandhi University of Health Sciences
Bengaluru, Karnataka, India

Principal and Professor
Department of Medical Surgical Nursing
Columbia College of Nursing
Bengaluru, Karnataka, India

Former Principal
VSS College of Nursing
Bengaluru, Karnataka, India

Chief Editor for Nursing Journals
Editorial Chief for Various International Nursing Journals

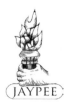

JAYPEE BROTHERS MEDICAL PUBLISHERS
The Health Sciences Publisher
New Delhi | London

Jaypee Brothers Medical Publishers (P) Ltd

Headquarters
Jaypee Brothers Medical Publishers (P) Ltd
4838/24, Ansari Road, Daryaganj
New Delhi 110 002, India
Phone: +91-11-43574357
Fax: +91-11-43574314
Email: jaypee@jaypeebrothers.com

Overseas Office
J.P. Medical Ltd
83 Victoria Street, London
SW1H 0HW (UK)
Phone: +44 20 3170 8910
Fax: +44 (0)20 3008 6180
Email: info@jpmedpub.com

Website: www.jaypeebrothers.com
Website: www.jaypeedigital.com

© 2020, Jaypee Brothers Medical Publishers

The views and opinions expressed in this book are solely those of the original contributor(s)/author(s) and do not necessarily represent those of editor(s) of the book.

All rights reserved. No part of this publication may be reproduced, stored or transmitted in any form or by any means, electronic, mechanical, photocopying, recording or otherwise, without the prior permission in writing of the publishers.

All brand names and product names used in this book are trade names, service marks, trademarks or registered trademarks of their respective owners. The publisher is not associated with any product or vendor mentioned in this book.

Medical knowledge and practice change constantly. This book is designed to provide accurate, authoritative information about the subject matter in question. However, readers are advised to check the most current information available on procedures included and check information from the manufacturer of each product to be administered, to verify the recommended dose, formula, method and duration of administration, adverse effects and contraindications. It is the responsibility of the practitioner to take all appropriate safety precautions. Neither the publisher nor the author(s)/editor(s) assume any liability for any injury and/or damage to persons or property arising from or related to use of material in this book.

This book is sold on the understanding that the publisher is not engaged in providing professional medical services. If such advice or services are required, the services of a competent medical professional should be sought.

Every effort has been made where necessary to contact holders of copyright to obtain permission to reproduce copyright material. If any have been inadvertently overlooked, the publisher will be pleased to make the necessary arrangements at the first opportunity. The **CD/DVD-ROM** (if any) provided in the sealed envelope with this book is complimentary and free of cost. **Not meant for sale.**

Inquiries for bulk sales may be solicited at: jaypee@jaypeebrothers.com

Nursing: Solved Question Papers for BSc Nursing—2nd Year (2019–2014)

First Edition: 2010
Second Edition: 2013
Third Edition: 2017
Fourth Edition: **2020**

ISBN: 978-93-89587-14-2

Printed at Nutech Print Services - India

Preface to the Fourth Edition

It gives me immense pleasure to complete this fourth edition of BSc nursing second year solved question bank, first of all I would like to thank my Lord Almighty for his powerful blessings that had helped me to complete this task in time, this question bank has the contents framed in lucid English with adequate tables and diagrams for better understanding of the subjects. This question bank has all the second year subjects, such as pharmacology, pathology and genetics, sociology, medical-surgical nursing, communication and education technology and community health nursing, these subjects are framed based on the syllabus recommended by Indian Nursing Council. This question bank covers six years 2014-2019 solved question papers, the students whoever reads this solved question bank are sure to get good marks in their exams. I wish all the best for all the students.

I Clement

Preface to the First Edition

Examination is an art; it requires organization of content, presentation and rich of knowledge. Presentation is a skill; it cannot be learned in one day, and it requires constant and continuous practice to achieve the highest score. Students have knowledge about the subject, but they are unable to put it on the paper in a proper way. This book will guide the students to prepare and write in an organized way.

This book has been prepared with comprehensive approach, which will be very useful to 2nd year BSc Nursing Students as an essential ready-reference tool.

This book contains fully-solved (2009–2000) questions and answers in all the subjects of 2nd year BSc Nursing. The questions and answers are prepared as per Rajiv Gandhi University of Health Sciences (RGUHS) curriculum based on Indian Nursing Council (INC) regulations.

I Clement

Contents

PHARMACOLOGY, PATHOLOGY AND GENETICS

Paper *2019* *1*
Paper *2018* *16*
Paper *2017* *37*
Paper *2016* *55*
Paper *2015* *82*
Paper *2014* *106*

SOCIOLOGY

Paper *2019* *135*
Paper *2018* *147*
Paper *2017* *161*
Paper *2016* *175*
Paper *2015* *199*
Paper *2014* *215*

COMMUNITY HEALTH NURSING

Paper *2019* *231*
Paper *2018* *244*
Paper *2017* *258*
Paper *2016* *272*
Paper *2015* *293*
Paper *2014* *311*

MEDICAL SURGICAL NURSING

Paper *2019* *325*
Paper *2018* *343*
Paper *2017* *357*
Paper *2016* *376*
Paper *2015* *397*
Paper *2014* *425*

COMMUNICATION AND EDUCATIONAL TECHNOLOGY

Paper *2019* *445*
Paper *2018* *459*
Paper *2017* *478*
Paper *2016* *488*
Paper *2015* *512*
Paper *2014* *536*

Pharmacology, Pathology and Genetics

2019

Pharmacology, Pathology and Genetics

PHARMACOLOGY

LONG ESSAYS

1. Enumerate general anesthetics; write the pharmacological actions, uses and adverse effects of halothane.
2. Classify the drugs used in tuberculosis, mention the therapeutic uses and adverse effects of streptomycine.

SHORT ESSAYS

3. Potassium-sparing diuretics.
4. Bronchodilators.
5. Uses of beta-blockers.
6. Tetracycline.
7. Chlorpromazine.

SHORT ANSWERS

8. Mention one therapeutic use (clinical condition) and one important adverse effect of adrenaline.
9. Mention one therapeutic use (clinical condition) and one important adverse effect of sodium valparic acid.
10. Mention one therapeutic use (clinical condition) and one important adverse effect of sodium metronidazole.
11. Mention one therapeutic use (clinical condition) and one important adverse effect of heparin.

PATHOLOGY AND GENETICS

LONG ESSAYS

1. What is wound healing? Describe the stages and factors affecting wound healing.
2. Describe the etiopathology and complications of tuberculosis.

SHORT ESSAYS

3. Peptic ulcer.
4. Blood grouping.
5. Seman analysis.
6. Differentiate Benign and malignant tumors.

SHORT ANSWERS

7. What is trisomy? and give two examples.
8. What is infertility?
9. Goals of human genome project.
10. Define chromosomal aberrations.
11. Name any three clinical features huntington's disease.
12. Define genetic counseling and two steps taken during the process.

PHARMACOLOGY

LONG ESSAYS

1. Enumerate general anesthetics; write the pharmacological actions, uses and adverse effects of halothane.

General anesthetics are medicines that render a patient reversibly unconscious and unresponsive in order to allow surgeons to operate on that patient. General anesthetics are normally administered intravenously or by inhalation by a specialist doctor called an anesthetist who also monitors the patient's vital signs (breathing, heart rate, blood pressure, temperature) during the procedure. While under general anesthesia, a patient is unable to feel pain and will likely wake with some short-term amnesia.

Drugs that can be used intravenously to produce anesthesia or sedation, the most common are:
1. Barbiturates: Amobarbital (trade name: Amytal), methohexital (trade name: Brevital)
2. Thiamylal (trade name: Surital)
3. Benzodiazepines: Diazepam, lorazepam, midazolam
4. Etomidate
5. Ketamine
6. Propofol.

Pharmacological Actions, Uses and Adverse Effects of Halothane

Halothane is a general inhalation anesthetic used for induction and maintenance of general anesthesia. It reduces the blood pressure and frequently decreases the pulse rate and depresses respiration. It induces muscle relaxation and reduces pains sensitivity by altering tissue excitability. It does so by decreasing the extent of gap junction mediated cell-cell coupling and altering the activity of the channels that underlie the action potential.

Mechanism of action: Halothane causes general anesthesia due to its actions on multiple ion channels which ultimately depresses nerve conduction, breathing, cardiac contractility. Its immobilizing effects have been attributed to its binding to potassium channels in cholinergic neurons. Halothane's effect are also likely due to binding to NMDA and calcium channels, causing hyperpolarization.

Indications: Fluothane (halothane, USP) is indicated for the induction and maintenance of general anesthesia.

Dosage and administration: Fluothane (halothane) may be administered by the nonrebreathing technique, partial rebreathing, or closed technique. The induction dose varies from patient to patient but is usually within the range of 0.5–3%. The maintenance dose varies from 0.5% to 1.5%.

Serious side effects of fluothane (halothane) include:
1. Abnormal heart rhythm
2. Decreased lung function
3. Decreased oxygen in the tissues or blood
4. Hepatitis
5. Kidney damage
6. Malignant hyperthermia
7. Problems with circulation
8. Yellowing of skin or eyes (jaundice).

2. Classify the drugs used in tuberculosis, mention the therapeutic uses and adverse effects of streptomycine.

The antitubercular drugs are used in different combinations in different circumstances. For example, some anti-TB drugs, the first-line drugs, are only used for the treatment of new patients who are very unlikely to have resistance to any of the TB drugs. There are other TB drugs, the second-line drugs that are only used for the treatment of drug-resistant TB.

Classification of Anti-TB Drugs

First-line drugs for tuberculosis: • Isoniazid • Refampicin • Ethambutol • Pyrizanamide • Streptomycin	Third-line durgs for tuberculosis: • Rifabutin • Macrolides like clarythromycin • Linezolid • Thioacetazone • Vitamin D • Thioridazone
Second-line drugs: • Amikacin, kanamycin • Capreomycin • Ciprofloxacin, levofloxacin, moxifloxacin • Ethionamide, prothionamide • Cycloserine • Para-aminosalicylic acid	

First-line TB drugs: The first-line TB drugs are:
1. Isoniazid (H/Inh)
2. Rifampicin (R/Rif) (in the United States rifampicin is called rifampin)
3. Pyrazinamide (Z/Pza)
4. Ethambutol (E/Emb).

These are the antitubercular drugs that generally have the greatest activity against TB bacteria. This medicine for TB is particularly used for someone with active TB disease who has not had TB drug treatment before.

Side effects of TB drugs: The side effects of TB drugs depends on the exact combination of drugs that are being taken. The side effects can range from mild to severe. One drug with a particularly severe side effect is streptomycin. This drug can cause people to become deaf and it should be avoided if at all possible. It should only be used for the treatment of drug-resistant TB when no other drug is available.

Therapeutic Uses and Adverse Effects of Streptomycin

Streptomycin is an antibiotic **used** to treat a number of bacterial infections. This includes tuberculosis, *Mycobacterium avium* complex, endocarditis, brucellosis, *Burkholderia* infection, plague, tularemia, and rat bite fever. Streptomycin is an aminoglycoside antibiotic used with other medications to treat active tuberculosis (TB) infection if you cannot take other drugs for TB or if you have a type of TB that cannot be treated with other drugs (drug-resistant TB).

Uses of Streptomycin
1. Tuberculosis
2. Tularemia
3. Bacterial endocarditis
4. Bacterial meningitis
5. Plague.

Common Side Effects of Streptomycin Include:
1. Nausea
2. Vomiting
3. Stomach upset
4. Loss appetite
5. Spinning sensation (vertigo)
6. Injection site reactions (pain, irritation, and redness)
7. Tingling or prickling sensation in the face
8. Rash
9. Fever
10. Hives, and
11. Swelling (edema).

SHORT ESSAYS

3. Potassium-sparing diuretics.

Potassium-sparing diuretics are diuretic drugs that do not promote the secretion of potassium into the urine. They are used as adjunctive therapy, together with other drugs, in the treatment of hypertension and management of congestive heart failure.

	Potassium-sparing	
Trade Name	**Agent**	**Hydrochlorothiazide**
Aldactazide	Spironolactone 25 mg	50 mg
Aldactone	Spironolaztone 25, 50, or 100 mg	...
Dyazide	Triamterene 37.5 mg	25 mg
Dyrenium	Triamterene 50 or 100 mg	...
Inspra	Eplerenone 25, 50 or 100 mg	...
Maxzide	Triamterene 75 mg	50 mg
Maxzide-25 mg	Triamterene 37.5 mg	25 mg
Midamor	Amiloride 5 mg	...
Moduretic	Amiloride 5 mg	50 mg

Medical uses: Potassium-sparing diuretics are generally used in combination with other diuretic drugs (e.g. loop diuretics) that would otherwise tend to decrease the potassium levels to potentially dangerous low levels (hypokalemia). The combination therefore helps maintain a normal reference range for potassium.

Mechanism of action: The potassium-sparing diuretics are competitive antagonists that either compete with aldosterone for intracellular cytoplasmic receptor sites, or directly block sodium channels. The former prevents the production of proteins that are normally synthesized in reaction to aldosterone. These mediator proteins are not produced, and so stimulation of sodium-potassium exchange sites in the collection tubule does not occur. This prevents sodium reabsorption and potassium and hydrogen ion secretion in the late distal tubule and collecting duct of a nephron in the kidneys.

Adverse effects: On their own this group of drugs may raise potassium levels beyond the normal range, termed hyperkalemia which risks potentially fatal arrhythmias.

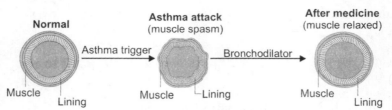

Fig. 1: Effects of bronchodilator.

4. Bronchodilators.

Bronchodilators are medications that open (dilate) the airways (bronchial tubes) of the lung by relaxing bronchial muscles and allow people who have difficulty breathing to breath better. Bronchodilators are used for treating: Asthma chronic obstructive pulmonary disease (COPD). Allergic reactions (Fig. 1).

Bronchodilators' mechanism of action: includes targeting the beta-2 receptor, which is a G-protein coupled receptor, in the lung airways. When the beta-2 receptor is activated, the smooth muscle of the airway relaxes. Subsequently, the patient experiences better airflow for a period.

Types of bronchodilator:

The three types of bronchodilators used for treating asthma are: (1) beta-adrenergic bronchodilators; (2) anticholinergic bronchodilators; and (3) xanthine derivatives.
  1. **Beta-adrenergic bronchodilators** dilate bronchial airways by relaxing the muscles that surround the airways. Beta-adrenergic bronchodilators are beta-2 agonists. These medications stimulate beta-2 receptors on the smooth muscle cells that line the airways, causing these muscle cells to relax, thus opening airways.
  2. **Anticholinergic bronchodilators** block the effect of acetylcholine on airways and nasal passages. Acetylcholine is a chemical that nerves use to communicate with muscle cells. In asthma, cholinergic nerves going to the lungs cause narrowing of the airways by stimulating muscles surrounding the airways to contract. The "anticholinergic" effect of anticholinergic bronchodilators blocks the effect of cholinergic nerves, causing the muscles to relax and airways to dilate.
  3. **Xanthine derivatives** open airways by relaxing the smooth muscles in the walls of the airways and they also suppress the response of the airways to stimuli. The mechanism of action of xanthines is not fully understood. Xanthine derivatives may dilate bronchi by blocking the action of phosphodiesterase (PDE) enzymes which ultimately leads to increased concentration of chemicals that dilate bronchial airways.

5. Uses of beta-blockers.

Beta-blockers are medicines that work by temporarily stopping or reducing the body's natural 'fight-or-flight' responses.

Beta-blockers are used to treat the following:
 1. Angina, or chest pain
 2. Heart failure
 3. Hypertension, or high blood pressure
 4. Atrial fibrillation, or irregular heartbeat
 5. Myocardial infarction, or heart attack.

Functions:
  1. Beta-blockers block the hormones adrenaline and noradrenaline in the sympathetic nervous system.

2. The sympathetic nervous system is part of the autonomic nervous system. It activities the fight or flight responses.
3. Adrenaline and noradrenaline prepare the muscles in the body for exertion. This is a crucial part of responding to danger.
4. Overexposure to these hormones can be harmful. Too much adrenaline can lead to rapid heartbeat, high blood pressure, excessive sweating, anxiety, and palpitations.
5. Blocking the release of these hormones blockers decrease the oxygen demand and reduce stress on the heart.
6. This lowers the force of the contractions of the heart muscles, and blood vessels in the heart, brain, and the rest of the body.
7. Beta-blockers also obstruct the production of angiotensin II, a hormone produced by the kidneys.
8. Reducing the amount of angiotensin relaxes and widens the blood vessels, easing the flow of blood through the vessels.

Uses:

Less commonly, they may be used for migraines, glaucoma, overactive thyroid, tremors, and anxiety.

1. **Glaucoma**: The high pressure within the eyeball is reduced using beta-blocker eye drops. The medication lowers the production of fluid inside the eyeball.
2. **Anxiety:** Beta-blockers block the effects of stress hormones. As a result, they can also reduce the physical symptoms of anxiety such as trembling and sweating. A person experiencing persistent anxiety, however, may also need additional treatment, such as counseling.
3. **Hyperactive thyroid and tremor:** Beta-blockers can reduce symptoms, such as tremor and slow the heart rate of patients with an overactive thyroid.

6. Tetracycline. *(See Q.2, 2015)*

7. Chlorpromazine. *(See Q.5, 2014)*

SHORT ANSWERS

8. Mention one therapeutic use (clinical condition) and one important adverse effect of adrenaline.

Uses: This medication is used in emergencies to treat very serious allergic reactions to insect stings/bites, foods, drugs, or other substances. Epinephrine acts quickly to improve breathing, stimulate the heart, raise a dropping blood pressure, reverse hives, and reduce swelling of the face, lips, and throat.

Common adverse reactions to systemically administered epinephrine include anxiety, apprehensiveness, restlessness, tremor, weakness, dizziness, sweating, palpitations, pallor, nausea and vomiting, headache, and respiratory difficulties.

9. Mention one therapeutic use (clinical condition) and one important adverse effects of sodium valparic acid.

Uses: This medication is used to treat seizure disorders, mental/mood conditions (such as manic phase of bipolar disorders, and to prevent migraine headaches). It works by restoring the balance of certain natural substances (neurotransmitters) in the brain.

Adverse effects: Diarrhea, dizziness, drowsiness, hair loss, blurred/double vision, change in menstrual periods, ringing in the ears, shakiness (tremor), unsteadiness, weight changes may occur. If any of these effects persist or worsen, tell your doctor or pharmacist promptly.

10. Mention one therapeutic use (clinical condition) and one important adverse effects of sodium metronidazole.

Uses: Metronidazole is an antibiotic that is used to treat a wide variety of infections. It may also be used to prevent infection after bowel surgery. It works by stopping the growth of certain bacteria and parasites.

Side Effects: Dizziness, headache, stomach upset, nausea, vomiting, loss of appetite, diarrhea, constipation, or metallic taste in the mouth may occur. If any of these effects last or get worse, tell your doctor or pharmacist promptly. This medication may cause your urine to turn darker in color. This effect is harmless and will disappear when the medication is stopped.

11. Mention one therapeutic use (clinical condition) and one important adverse effects of heparin.

Indications of Heparin
Heparin sodium injection is indicated for:
1. Anticoagulant therapy in prophylaxis and treatment of venous thrombosis and its extension; (In a low-dose regimen) for prevention of postoperative deep venous thrombosis and pulmonary embolism in patients undergoing major abdomino-thoracic surgery or who for other reasons are at risk of developing thromboembolic disease;
2. Prophylaxis and treatment of pulmonary embolism;
3. Atrial fibrillation with embolization;
4. Diagnosis and treatment of acute and chronic consumption coagulopathies (disseminated intravascular coagulation);
5. Prevention of clotting in arterial and heart surgery;
6. Prophylaxis and treatment of peripheral arterial embolism;
7. As an anticoagulant in blood transfusions, extracorporeal circulation, and dialysis procedures and in blood sample.

Adverse Effects of Heparin
Hypersensitivity: Patients with documented hypersensitivity to heparin should be given the drug only in clearly life-threatening situations.

Hemorrhage: Hemorrhage can occur at virtually any site in patients receiving heparin. An unexplained fall in hematocrit, fall in blood pressure, or any other unexplained symptom should lead to serious consideration of a hemorrhagic event

PATHOLOGY AND GENETICS

LONG ESSAYS

1. What is wound healing? Describe the stages and factors affecting wound healing.

The verb form of the word "wound" means to injure or to damage. In short, a wound is a cut or break in the continuity of a tissue.

Classification of Wounds

A wound is a break in the skin or mucous membrane or other body structure resulting from physical means. It may be superficial affecting only the surface structures, or severe involving blood vessels, muscles, nerves, fascia, tendons, ligaments or bones.

Wounds may be classified in a variety of ways: Classification according to continuity of surface covering.

Open wounds: These are wounds involving a break in skin or mucous membrane. Their cause is trauma by sharp object or blow, e.g. surgical incision, vein puncture and gunshot wounds.

Closed wounds: These are wounds in volving no break in skin integrity. Their causes are twisting, straining, bone fracture or tear of visceral organ wounds.

Classification According to Cause

1. **Intentional:** Examples of such wounds are surgical incised wounds, stab.
2. **Accidental wounds:** Such wounds occur under unexpected conditions, e.g. traumatic injury, and knife wound.

Classification According to Type of Injury

1. Abrasion is a superficial wound produced by friction or scraping.
2. Laceration is tearing of tissues which occurs with irregular wound edges, e.g. from animal bites, machinery cut or tissues cut by broken glass.
3. Contusion is a closed wound caused by a blow to body by some blunt object. It is characterized by swelling, discoloration and pain.
4. Puncture (stab) is a wound made with a pointed object, such as nail, wire or bullet that pierces deeper tissues, leaving only a small opening on the surface.
5. Penetrating wound occurs as a result of an instrument, passing through skin or mucous membrane, to deeper tissues and entering a body cavity or organ.
6. Perforating wound is caused by an instrument that both enters and emerges from a body cavity or organ. A gunshot wound may be perforating or penetrating.

Classification According to the Activity of Invading

Microorganisms

1. A clean wound: It is one containing no pathogenic organisms, e.g. closed surgical wounds. The wound heals without infection.

2. **Clean contaminated wound:** It is made under aseptic conditions but it involves a body cavity that normally harbors microorganisms.
3. **Contaminated wound:** It is a wound in which the potential for infection is relatively great, such as in open, traumatic accidental wound, in which break occurs in asepsis.
4. **Infected wound:** Bacterial organism is present in the wound which presents signs of infection, inflammation, purulent drainage, or skin separation.
5. **Colonized wound:** It is around containing multiple microorganisms, e.g. pressure sore.

Factors that Impair Wound Healing

1. Aging alters all phases of wound healing. In young age, wound healing is better
2. Malnutrition
3. Obesity
4. Inadequate blood supply and impaired oxygenation to the affected area

The factors influencing wound healing is categorized into local and systemic factors which are summarized in the Table 1.

Table 1: Categorization of factors influencing wound healing into local and systemic factors.

Systemic factors	Local factors
Age—healing delayed in elderly	Location of wound
Malnutrition	Nature of tissue
Deficiency of methionine and cysteine	Type of size of wound
Vitamin C deficiency	Status of mobility of the site of wound
Deficiency of zinc	Vascularity of the site
Defects in functioning of leukocytes	Presence of infection
Diabetes mellitus	Presence of foreign body

2. Describe the etiopathology and complications of tuberculosis.

Tuberculosis (TB) is a potentially serious infectious disease that mainly affects the lungs. The bacteria that cause tuberculosis are spread from one person to another through tiny droplets released into the air via coughs and sneezes.

Pathophysiology of tuberculosis:

Inhalation of bacilli (A), containment in a granuloma (B), and breakdown of the granuloma in less immunocompetent individuals (C). In patients infected with M tuberculosis, droplets can be coughed up from the bronchus and infect other persons.

Complications:

Without treatment, tuberculosis can be fatal. Untreated active disease typically affects your lungs, but it can spread to other parts of your body through your bloodstream. Examples of tuberculosis complications include:

1. **Spinal pain:** Back pain and stiffness are common complications of tuberculosis.
2. **Joint damage:.** Tuberculosis arthritis usually affects the hips and knees.

3. **Swelling of the membranes that cover your brain (meningitis):** This can cause a lasting or intermittent headache that occurs for weeks. Mental changes also are possible.
4. **Liver or kidney problems:** Your liver and kidneys help filter waste and impurities from your bloodstream. These functions become impaired if the liver or kidneys are affected by tuberculosis.
5. **Heart disorders:** Rarely, tuberculosis can infect the tissues that surround your heart, causing inflammation and fluid collections that may interfere with your heart's ability to pump effectively. This condition, called cardiac tamponade, can be fatal.

SHORT ESSAYS

3. Peptic ulcer. (See Q. 2, 2015)

4. Blood grouping.

There are four main blood groups (types of blood)—A, B, AB and O. Your blood group is determined by the genes you inherit from your parents. Each group can be either RhD positive or RhD negative which means in total there are eight main blood groups (Fig. 2).

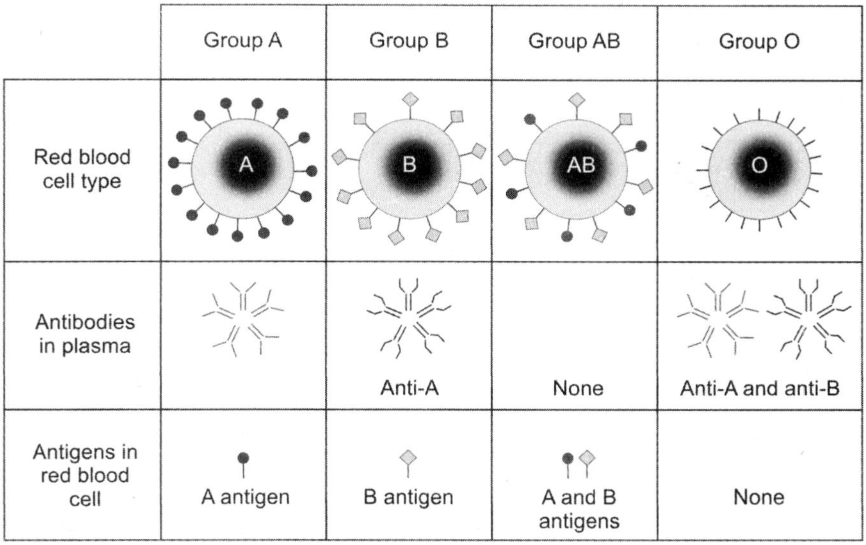

	Group A	Group B	Group AB	Group O
Red blood cell type	A	B	AB	O
Antibodies in plasma		Anti-A	None	Anti-A and anti-B
Antigens in red blood cell	A antigen	B antigen	A and B antigens	None

Fig. 2: Types of blood groups.

The ABO System

There are four main blood groups defined by the ABO system:
1. **Blood group A**—has A antigens on the red blood cells with anti-B antibodies in the plasma
2. **Blood group B**—has B antigens with anti-A antibodies in the plasma
3. **Blood group O**—has no antigens, but both anti-A and anti-B antibodies in the plasma
4. **Blood group AB**—has both A and B antigens, but no antibodies.

The Rh system:
Red blood cells sometimes have another antigen, a protein known as the RhD antigen. If this is present, your blood group is RhD positive. If it is absent, your blood group is RhD negative. This means you can be one of eight blood groups:
1. A RhD positive (A+)
2. A RhD negative (A-)
3. B RhD positive (B+)
4. B RhD negative (B-)
5. O RhD positive (O+)
6. O RhD negative (O-)
7. AB RhD positive (AB+)
8. AB RhD negative (AB-)

5. Seman analysis.

A semen analysis (plural: Semen analyses), also called "seminogram" evaluates certain characteristics of a male's semen and the sperm contained therein. It is done to help evaluate male fertility, whether for those seeking pregnancy or verifying the success of vasectomy.

Parameter	Lower reference limit
Semen volume (mL)	1.5
Sperm concentration (10^6/mL)	15
Total sperm number (10^6/ejaculate)	39
Progressive motility (PR, %)	32
Total motiligy (PR + NP, %)	40
Vitality (live sperms, %)	58
Sperm morphology (NF, %)	4
pH	>/=7.2
Leucocyte (10^6/mL)	<1
MAR/Immunobead test (%)	<50

A semen analysis is used to determine whether a man might be infertile—unable to get a woman pregnant. The semen analysis consists of a series of tests that evaluate the quality and quantity of the sperm as well as the semen, the fluid that contains them. The test may be used, in conjunction with other infertility tests, help to determine the cause of a couple's inability to get pregnant (conceive) and help to guide decisions about infertility treatment.

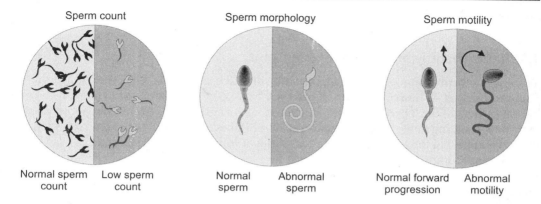

The semen analysis also can be used to determine whether sperm are present in semen after a man has had a vasectomy, a surgical procedure that prevents sperm from being released within the ejaculate. This surgery is considered a permanent method of birth control (99.9%) when performed successfully.

6. Differentiate Benign and malignant tumors. (See Q.1, 2015)

Benign tumors tend to remain localized and usually do not pose a threat to one's health. Whereas a malignant tumor consists of renegade cells that do not respond to the body's genetic controls on growth and division.

Benign tumors	Malignant tumors
Slowly growing mass	Rapidly growing mass
Regular surface, capsulated, not attached to deep structures	Irregular surfaces, non-capsulated attached to deep structures
Noninvasive to another organ or tissues	Invasive to other organs
No spread or metastasis	Spread and metastasis
Well differentiated	Poorly differentiated, moderately or well differentiated
No recurrence after surgery	Recurrence after surgery
No bleeding in cut surfaces	Bleeding from cut surfaces is common
Named by adding suffix—oma	Named by adding suffix sarcoma or carcinoma
Slight pressure effect on the neighboring organ	Remarkable pressure effect on neighboring tissue

SHORT ANSWERS

7. What is trisomy and give two examples.

Trisomy is a form of aneuploidy, an abnormality in which an organism has the wrong number of chromosomes. In humans, a normal baby will have 46 chromosomes in 23 pairs, with each parent contributing 23 chromosomes. When trisomy occurs, one of the chromosomes has an extra pair, resulting in 47 chromosomes instead of 46. The results of this extra data can vary, but tend to manifest in the form of birth defects, some of which can be quite severe.

The most common cause of trisomy is a problem in the duplication of chromosomes to create egg and sperm cells. Somewhere along the way, a chromosome duplicates itself twice, creating a full pair. When the egg or sperm cell joins with its counterpart, the extra chromosome is taken along, creating a set of three where should be two. In some cases, a chromosome only duplicates partially, leading to partial trisomy.

Some of the more well-known forms of trisomy are trisomies 13, 18, and 21. Trisomy 13 is also known as Patau syndrome, after the doctor who identified it. Patau syndrome is characterized by physical and mental defects, with heart defects being very common. Trisomy 18 is known as Edward's syndrome, and it is accompanied by severe mental and physical problems; most patients do not survive beyond a year. Trisomy 21 is Down's syndrome, a condition which is often accompanied by severe mental disabilities

8. What is infertility?

Infertility is the inability of a couple to become pregnant (regardless of cause) after 1 year of unprotected sexual intercourse (using no birth control methods). Infertility affects men and women equally. Most infertility cases are treated with medication or surgery.

Infertility occurs when something in this pattern does not happen. The problem could be with the woman (female infertility), with the man (male infertility), or with both. Unknown factors cause infertility 10% of the time. For infertility with an unknown cause, all findings from standard tests may be normal. The actual cause of infertility may not be detected because the problem may be with the egg or sperm itself or with the embryo and its inability to implant.

9. Goals of human genome project.

The human genome project (HGP) is an international scientific research project with a primary goal of determining the sequence of chemical base pairs which make up DNA, and of identifying and mapping the approximately 20,000–25,000 genes of the human genome from both a physical and functional standpoint.

While the objective of the Human Genome Project is to understand the genetic makeup of the human species, the project has also focused on several other nonhuman organisms, such as *E. coli*, the fruit fly, and the laboratory mouse. It remains one of the largest single investigative projects in modern science.

The Human Genome Project originally aimed to map the nucleotides contained in a human haploid reference genome (more than three billion). Several groups have announced efforts to extend this to diploid human genomes including the International HapMap Project, applied biosystems, Perlegen, Illumina, J Craig Venter Institute, personal genome project, personal genome project, and Roche-454.

The "genome" of any given individual (except for identical twins and cloned organisms) is unique; mapping "the human genome" involves sequencing multiple variations of each gene. The project did not study the entire DNA found in human cells; some heterochromatic areas (about 8% of the total genome) remain unsequenced.

10. Define chromosomal aberrations.

Chromosome aberrations are departures from the normal set of chromosomes either for an individual or from a species. They can refer to changes in the number of sets of chromosomes (ploidy), changes in the number of individual chromosomes (somy), or changes in appearance of individual chromosomes through mutation-induced rearrangements. They can be associated with genetic disorders or with species differences.

11. Name any three clinical features Huntington's disease.

Huntington's disease (HD) is the most common monogenic neurodegenerative disease and the genetic dementia in the developed world. With autosomal dominant inheritance, typically mid-life onset, and unrelenting progressive motor, cognitive and psychiatric symptoms over 15-20 years, its impact on patients and their families is devastating. The causative genetic mutation is an expanded CAG trinucleotide repeat in the gene encoding the Huntingtin protein, which leads to a prolonged polyglutamine stretch at the N-terminus of the protein.

Some common early symptoms:
1. Slight changes in coordination, affecting balance or making you more clumsy
2. Fidgety movements that you can not control
3. Slowing or stiffness
4. Trouble thinking through problems
5. Depression or irritability.

12. Define genetic counseling and two steps taken during the process.

Genetic counseling: An educational counseling process for individuals and families who have a genetic disease or may be at risk for a disease to facilitate informed decision-making.

Genetic counseling is a communication process which involves providing information about the consequences of the disorder, the chance of developing or passing on the disorder for a given person, and ways to prevent or treat the disorder. This involves several steps:
1. Raise awareness
2. Organize the campaign
3. Find sponsors
4. Educate yourself
5. Lobby campaign
6. Prepare for hearing
7. Follow-up

Genetic counseling is the process through which knowledge about the genetic aspects of illnesses is shared by trained professionals with those who are at an increased risk or either having a heritable disorder or of passing it on to their unborn offspring. A genetic counselor provides information on the inheritance of illnesses and their recurrence risks; addresses the concerns of patients, their families, and their healthcare providers supports patients and their families dealing with these illnesses.

2018

Pharmacology, Pathology and Genetics

PHARMACOLOGY

LONG ESSAYS
1. Classify pencillins; describe the mechanism of action, uses and adverse effects of amoxicillin.
2. Enumerate corticosteroids; describe the uses, adverse effects and contraindications of prednisolone.

SHORT ESSAYS
3. Sublingual route of drug administration.
4. Loop diuretics.
5. Preanesthetic medications.
6. Metronidazole.
7. Lignocaine.

SHORT ANSWERS
8. Amikacin.
9. Methotrexate.
10. Heparine.
11. Atropine.

PATHOLOGY AND GENETICS

LONG ESSAYS
1. Discuss cutaneous wound healing by first intention, mention local and systemic factors that influence wound healing, enumerate the complications of the same.
2. Discuss the etiology and pathogenesis of rheumatic heart disease.

SHORT ESSAYS
3. Describe Benign prostate hyperplasia.
4. Explain the etiology and pathogenesis of bronchogenic carcinoma.

5. Describe the acute pyogenic meningitis.
6. Explain about infective endocarditis.

SHORT ANSWERS

7. Define infertility.
8. Define karyotyping.
9. What is mutation?
10. Factors responsible for chromosomal aberration.
11. Clinical features of turners syndrome.
12. Name the various procedures of prenatal diagnosis.

PHARMACOLOY

LONG ESSAYS

1. Classify pencillins; describe the mechanism of action, uses and adverse effects of amoxicillin.

Penicillin is derived from fungi named *Penicillium*. They are a group of beta-lactam antibiotics, which are used in the treatment or prevention of bacterial infections originated by susceptible, particularly gram-positive organisms. They are usually bactericidal in action.

Classification of Penicillin

Based upon penicillin's ability to execute or destroy bacterium and effectiveness (ranging from limited to extensive), they can be classified into following four classes:

1. *Natural penicillins (penicillin V, penicillin G, benzathine, procaine penicillin):*

In the penicillin family, antibiotics of natural penicillin class were the first innovative agents, which were launched for clinical purposes. The original structure of penicillin-G is the basis of natural penicillins. Antibiotics from this particular class of penicillin are mainly useful against gram (+) strains of staphylococci and streptococci and a few gram (-) bacteria (for example, meningococcus). Additionally, you need to know that penicillin V is not only useful for anaerobic coverage in patients who are suffering infections of oral cavity, but also it is considered as the agent of choice for treating streptococcal pharyngitis.

2. *Penicillinase-resistant penicillins (oxacillin, dicloxacillin, cloxacillin, methicillin, nafcillin):*

The first drug of this class was methicillin. After that, one by one oxacillin, nafcillin, cloxacillin and dicloxacillin were added in this class. Penicillins of this class do not possess broad spectrum activity as compared to previous class of penicillin. Particularly, the antimicrobial efficacy of penicillinase-resistant penicillins are aimed straightly against penicillinase-creating strains of gram (+) cocci, more specifically against staphylococcal species. For this reason, these penicillins are often called as antistaphylococcal penicillins.

3. *Aminopenicillins (amoxicillin, bacampicillin, ampicillin):*

The aminopenicillins were the first class of penicillins, which were discovered as active agents against several gram (-) bacteria (e.g. *H. influenzae* and *E. coli*). This class of penicillins have acid resistant properties, and for this reason they are available in oral dosage forms. Orally administered drugs (amoxicillin, bacampicillin and ampicillin) of this class are usually used in several mild infections, including sinusitis, tonsillitis, otitis media, bronchitis, bacterial diarrhea and UTIs. In addition, you need to know that for the otitis media treatment, amoxicillin is considered as the drug of choice.

4. *Extended spectrum penicillins:*

Extended spectrum penicillins are also called as antipseudomonal penicillins. They include both acylaminopenicillins (mezlocillin, piperacillin, and azlocillin) and alpha-carboxypenicillins (ticarcillin and carbenicillin). The antibiotics of this class penicillin have similar spectrum of antibacterial activity as compared to aminopenicillins. However, these penicillins have an additional antibacterial activity against many organisms (gram-negative) of the enterobacteriaceae family including several strains of *Pseudomonas aeruginosa*. The antibiotics of this class may be administered alone or in combination with aminoglycosides. In addition, you need to know that like the aminopenicillins, drugs of this class are also vulnerable to inactivation by beta-lactamases.

Penicillin Mechanism

Penicillin is a widely used antibiotic prescribed to treat staphylococci and streptococci bacterial infections. Penicillin belongs to the beta-lactam family of antibiotics, the members of which use a similar mechanism of action to inhibit bacterial cell growth that eventually kills the bacteria.

Bacteria cells are surrounded by a protective envelope called the cell wall. One of the primary components of the bacterial cell wall is peptidoglycan, a structural macromolecule with a net-like composition that provides rigidity and support to the outer cell wall. In order to form the cell wall, a single peptidoglycan chain is cross-linked to other peptidoglycan chains through the action of the enzyme DD-transpeptidase [also called a penicillin binding protein—(PBP)]. Throughout a bacterial lifecycle, the cell wall (and thus the peptidoglycan crosslinks) is continuously remodeled in order to accommodate for repeated cycles of cell growth and replication.

Penicillins and other antibiotics in the beta-lactam family contain a characteristic four-membered beta-lactam ring. Penicillin kills bacteria through binding of the beta-lactam ring to DD-transpeptidase, inhibiting its cross-linking activity and preventing new cell wall formation. Without a cell wall, a bacterial cell is vulnerable to outside water and molecular pressures, and quickly dies. Since human cells do not contain a cell wall, penicillin treatment results in bacterial cell death without affecting human cells.

Gram-positive bacteria have thick cell walls containing high levels of peptidoglycan, while gram-negative bacteria are characterized by thinner cell walls with low levels of peptidoglycan. The cell walls of gram-negative bacteria are surrounded by a lipopolysaccharide (LPS) layer than prevents antibiotic entry into the cell. Therefore, penicillin is most effective against gram-positive bacteria where DD-transpeptidase activity is highest.

Amoxicillin

The main function of antibiotic is to completely suppress the bacterial growth in the human body. When bacteria enter human body, they treat the body as a host ground and starts multiplying. This causes various infections and diseases. Depending upon the seriousness of the disease or the infection, a licensed medical practitioner prescribes an antibiotic. Amoxicillin is used to treat many different types of infections caused by bacteria, such as ear infections, bladder infections, pneumonia, gonorrhea, and *E. coli* or *Salmonella* infection. Amoxicillin is also sometimes used together with another antibiotic called clarithromycin (biaxin) to treat stomach ulcers caused by *Helicobacter pylori* infection. This combination is sometimes used with a stomach acid reducer called lansoprazole (prevacid).

Mechanism of action: More effective against gram-negative bacteria due to enhanced ability to penetrate outer membrane of gram-negative bacteria.

Uses: Commonly given to treat urinary tract infections, sinusitis, otitis, and lower respiratory tract infections.

Untoward effects: Hypersensitivity like other penicillins.

Pharmacokinetics: Oral absorption better than ampicillin.

Dose: 0.25–0.5 g TID given orally; pediatric dose 20–40 mg/kg/d in 3 doses given orally.

2. Enumerate corticosteroids; describe the uses, adverse effects and contraindications of prednisolone.

Steroids released from the adrenal cortex. Corticosteroids include both mineral corticoids and glucocorticoids. Mineral corticoids maintain salt and fluid balance in the body, while glucocorticoids have metabolic and anti-inflammatory effects and are important mediators of the stress response.

Classifications

By chemical structure: In general, corticosteroids are grouped into four classes based on chemical structure. Allergic reactions to one member of a class typically indicate an intolerance of all members of the class. This is known as the "Coopman classification", after S Coopman, who defined this classification in 1989. The highlighted steroids are often used in the screening of allergies to topical steroids.

Group A—hydrocortisone type: Hydrocortisone, hydrocortisone acetate, cortisone acetate tixocortol, pivalate, prednisolone, methylprednisolone, and prednisone (short-to medium-acting glucocorticoids).

Group B—acetonides (and related substances): Triamcinolone acetonide, triamcinolone alcohol, mometasone, amcinonide, budesonide, desonide, and halcinonide.

Group C—betamethasone type: Betamethasone, betamethasone sodium phosphate, dexamethasone sodium phosphate and fluocortolone.

Group D—esters

Group D1—halogenated (less labile): Hydrocortisone-17-valerate, alclometasone dipropionate, betamethasone valerate, betamethasone dipropionate, prednicarbate, clobetasone-17-butyrate, clobetasol-17-propionate, fluocortolone caproate, fluocortolone pivalate and fluprednidene acetate.

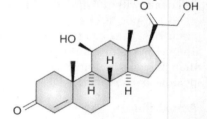

Group D2—labile prodrug esters: Hydrocortisone-17-butyrate, 17-aceponate, 17-buteprate, and prednicarbate.

Pharmacological Effects

Corticosteroids are key regulators of whole body homeostasis that provide an organism with the capacity to resist environmental changes and invasion of foreign substances. The effects of corticosteroids are widespread including profound alterations in carbohydrate, protein, and lipid metabolism, and the modulation of electrolyte and water balance. Corticosteroids affect all of the major systems of the body, including cardiovascular, musculoskeletal, nervous, and immune systems, and play critical roles in fetal development including the maturation of the fetal lung. Because so many systems are sensitive to corticosteroid levels, tight regulatory control is exerted on the system. The direct effects of corticosteroids are sometimes difficult to separate from their complex relationship with other hormones, in part due to the permissive action of low levels of corticosteroid on the effectiveness of other hormones including catecholamines and glucagon. Nevertheless, the effects of corticosteroids can be classified into two general categories: Glucocorticoid (intermediary metabolism, inflammation, immunity, wound healing, myocardial, and muscle integrity) and mineralocorticoid (salt, water, and mineral metabolism). Although the following section discusses the separate effects of glucocorticoids and mineral corticoids, it must be emphasized that natural steroids possess both glucocorticoid and mineral corticoid activity to some extent. The ratio between the two activities ranges from all glucocorticoid and almost no mineral corticoid activity (cortisol) to all mineral corticoid and almost no glucocorticoid activity (aldosterone).

Side Effects of Short-term Course

If systemic steroids have been prescribed for month or less, side effects are rarely serious. However the following problems may arise particularly when higher doses are taken:

1. Sleep disturbance
2. Increased appetite
3. Weight gain
4. Psychological effects including increased or decreased energy.

Rare but more worrisome side effects of a short course of corticosteroids include: Mania, psychosis, and delirium, depression with suicidal intent, heart failure, peptic ulceration, diabetes and aseptic necrosis of the hip. The risk increases with increasing dose.

Adverse Reactions

1. Systemic absorption of topical corticosteroids has produced reversible HPA axis suppression, Cushing's syndrome, hyperglycemia, and glycosuria.
2. Conditions that augment systemic absorption include application of more potent steroids, use over large surface areas, prolonged use, addition of occlusive dressings, and patient's age.
3. Perform appropriate clinical and laboratory tests if a topical corticosteroid is used for long periods or over large areas of the body.

SHORT ESSAYS

3. Sublingual route of drug administration.

Definition: Sublingual and buccal medication administration are two different ways of giving medication by mouth. Sublingual administration involves placing a drug under your tongue to dissolve and absorb into your blood through the tissue there. Buccal administration involves placing a drug between the gums and cheek, where it also dissolves and is absorbed into your blood. Both sublingual and buccal drugs come in tablets, films, or sprays.

Advantages

Sublingual or buccal forms of drugs have their advantages. Because the medication absorbs quickly, these types of administration can be important during emergencies when you need the drug to work right away, such as during a heart attack.

Further, these drugs do not go through the digestive system, so they are not metabolized through your liver. This means you may be able to take a lower dose and still get the same results.

Another advantage is that you do not have to swallow the drug. Drugs that are absorbed under the tongue or between the cheek and gum can be easier to take for people who have problems swallowing pills.

Disadvantages

On the other hand, sublingual and buccal drugs also have some disadvantages. Eating, drinking, or smoking, can affect how the drug is absorbed and how well it works. Also, these forms do not work for drugs that need to be processed slowly by your system, such as extended-release formulations. Any open sores in your mouth can also become irritated by the medication.

4. Loop diuretics.

Diuretics are medicines that increase urine flow (cause diuresis). Loop diuretics are a powerful type of diuretic that work by inhibiting the sodium-potassium-chloride ($Na^+/K^+/2Cl$) co-transporter in the thick ascending loop of Henle (hence the name loop diuretic), which is located in the kidneys. This reduces or abolishes sodium, chloride, and potassium reabsorption leading to increased loss of sodium, chloride, and potassium into the nephron (the functional unit of a kidney). As a result, water is also drawn into the nephron and urine volume increases. Loop diuretics also reduce the reabsorption of calcium and magnesium.

Loop diuretics are often used to treat heart failure. Examples of these drugs include:
- Torsemide (demadex)
- Furosemide (lasix)
- Bumetanide

Loop diuretics are diuretics that act at the ascending limb of the loop of Henle in the kidney. They are primarily used in medicine to treat hypertension and edema often due to congestive heart failure or chronic kidney disease.

The more common side effects of diuretics include:
- Too little potassium in the blood
- Too much potassium in the blood (for potassium-sparing **diuretics**)
- Low sodium levels
- Headache
- Dizziness
- Thirst
- Increased blood sugar
- Muscle cramps.

5. Preanesthetic medications.

Preanesthetic medications, such as tranquilizers and sedatives are not recommended with the exception of anticholinergic drugs, because single injection anesthesia techniques have been developed that minimize the handling stress and eliminate the discomfort associated with multiple injections. Serum and tissue atropine esterases found in many rabbits and rats render atropine sulfate ineffective, therefore, subcutaneous (SC) administration of glycopyrrolate (Robinul, AH Robins Company, Richmond, VA), a quaternary ammonium parasympatholytic, should be given to reduce salivary and bronchial secretions and prevent vagal bradycardia.

Preanesthetic Medications

Aims
1. Relief of anxiety
2. Amnesia for pre/postoperative events
3. Supplement analgesic action so less anesthetic needed
4. Decrease secretions and vagal stimulation by anesthetics
5. Antiemetic effect even postoperatively
6. Decrease acidity.0

Class	Drug	Use	Adverse effects
Opioids	Morphine Meperidine	1. Anxiety 2. Pre/postoperative analgesia 3. Smooth induction and reduction in dose of anesthetic	1. Asthma 2. Delay recovery 3. Biliary spasm (because morphine causes contraction of sphincter of Oddi àbiliary spasm) 4. Urinary retention

Contd...

Contd...

Class	Drug	Use	Adverse effects
Sedatives	Diazepam Lorazepam	1. Sedation and smooth induction 2. Respiratory depression—less common 3. No vomiting, minor surgical and endoscopic procedures with either fentanyl or meperidine	
	Midazolam	Midazolam = potent and short-acting drug suitable for preoperative anesthesia	
	Promethazine	1. Sedative 2. Antiemetic 3. Anticholinergic (minimal respiratory depression)	
Anticholinergics		1. Prevent vagal 2. Bradycardia (occur reflexly due to surgical procedures)	Laryngeal spasm precipitated by respiratory secretions
	Hyoscine (derivatives of atropine)	1. Antiemetic 2. Produces amnesia	
	Glycopyrrolate (derivatives of atropine)	1. Local anesthetic atropine substitute 2. Antisecretory 3. Antibradycardic drug	
H_2 blockers		1. Patients undergoing prolonged operations 2. C-sections 3. Obese 4. At risk of gastric regurgitation 5. At risk of aspiration pneumonia	
	Ranitidine Ramotidine	1. Night before and morning prior to surgery 2. Prevent chances of regurgitation/stress ulcers	
PPI	Omeprazole	Same as H_2 blocker	
Antiemetics	Metoclopramide Ondansetron	1. Reduce chance of aspiration 2. Control postanesthetic nausea and vomiting 3. Metoclopramide—increase tone of lower esophageal sphincter 4. Ondansetron = 5-HT3 blocker used in cancer patients	

6. Metronidazole.

Metronidazole is an antibiotic that is used to treat a wide variety of infections. It works by stopping the growth of certain bacteria and parasites. This antibiotic treats only certain bacterial and parasitic infections. It will not work for viral infections (such as common cold, flu).

Mechanism of Action

It inhibits nucleic acid synthesis by disrupting the DNA of microbial cells. This function only occurs when metronidazole is partially reduced, and because this reduction usually happens only in anaerobic bacteria and protozoans, it has relatively little effect upon human cells or aerobic bacteria.

Uses
1. Metronidazole is an antibiotic that is used to treat a wide variety of infections. It works by stopping the growth of certain bacteria and parasites.
2. This antibiotic treats only certain bacterial and parasitic infections. It will not work for viral infections (such as common cold, flu). Using any antibiotic when it is not needed can cause it to not work for future infections.
3. Metronidazole may also be used with other medications to treat certain stomach/intestinal ulcers caused by a bacteria (*H. pylori*).

Common metronidazole side effects may include:
1. Nausea, vomiting, loss of appetite, stomach pain
2. Diarrhea, constipation
3. Headache
4. Unpleasant metallic taste
5. Rash, itching
6. Vaginal itching or discharge
7. Mouth sores, or
8. Swollen, red, or "hairy" tongue.

7. Lignocaine.

Indications

For local or regional anesthesia by infiltration; for regional intravenous anesthesia and nerve blocks, such as major plexus blocks and epidural anesthesia. Treatment or prophylaxis of life-threatening ventricular arrhythmias including those associated with myocardial infarction, general anesthesia in patients predisposed to ventricular arrhythmias, digitalis intoxication, or following resuscitation from cardiac arrest.
1. Anesthesia
2. Pain and irritation
3. Hemorrhoids
4. Postherpetic neuralgia
5. Cardiac arrhythmia
6. Gastrointestinal tract examination
7. Labor pain and discomfort
8. Nerve block to relieve pain.

Adverse effects

Reactions to lignocaine hydrochloride are similar in character to those observed with other local anaesthetics. Adverse experiences are, in general, dose-related and may result from high plasma levels or from a hypersensitivity, idiosyncrasy or diminished tolerance.

Contraindications

Known history of allergy or hypersensitivity to lignocaine or other amide-type local anesthetics, such as prilocaine, mepivacaine or bupivacaine. Stokes-Adams syndrome or severe degrees of sinoatrial, atrioventricular or intraventricular block. Lignocaine suppresses ventricular pacemaker activity and the result may be ventricular arrhythmias including in those undergoing epidural anesthesia. Serious diseases of the CNS or of the spinal cord, such as meningitis, spinal fluid block, cranial or spinal hemorrhage, tumors, poliomyelitis, syphilis, tuberculosis or metastatic lesions of the spinal cord. Patients with myasthenia gravis, severe shock, or impaired cardiac conduction. Local anesthetic techniques must not be used when there is inflammation and/or sepsis in the region of the proposed injection and in the presence of septicemia. Epidural and spinal anesthesia in patients with uncorrected hypotension and in patients with coagulation disorders or receiving anticoagulation treatment.

SHORT ANSWERS

8. Amikacin.

Amikacin injection is used to treat certain serious infections that are caused by bacteria, such as meningitis (infection of the membranes that surround the brain and spinal cord) and infections of the blood, abdomen (stomach area), lungs, skin, bones, joints, and urinary tract.

Uses: This medication is used to prevent or treat a wide variety of bacterial infections. Amikacin belongs to a class of drugs known as aminoglycoside antibiotics. It works by stopping the growth of bacteria.

Side effects: Nausea, vomiting, stomach upset, or loss of appetite may occur. Pain/irritation/redness at the injection site may rarely occur. If any of these effects persist or worsen, tell your doctor or pharmacist promptly.

9. Methotrexate.

Methotrexate is one of the most effective and widely used medications for treating rheumatoid arthritis (RA) and other inflammatory types of arthritis. It is also one of the safest arthritis drugs, insist rheumatologists, despite a common misconception among many patients and even some primary care physicians that methotrexate is highly toxic.

Uses

Methotrexate is used to treat certain types of cancer or to control severe psoriasis or rheumatoid arthritis that has not responded to other treatments. It may also be used to control juvenile rheumatoid arthritis. Methotrexate belongs to a class of drugs known as antimetabolites.

Side Effects

Nausea, vomiting, stomach pain, drowsiness, or dizziness may occur. If any of these effects persist or worsen, tell your doctor or pharmacist promptly. Temporary hair loss may occur. Normal hair growth should return after treatment has ended.

10. Heparin.

Heparin is a heterogenous group of straight-chain anionic mucopolysaccharides, called glycosaminoglycans having anticoagulant properties. Although others may be present, the main sugars occurring in heparin are: (1) α-L-iduronic acid 2-sulfate, (2) 2-deoxy-2-sulfaminoα-D-glucose 6-sulfate, (3) β-D-glucuronic acid, (4) 2-acetamido-2-deoxy-α-D-glucose, and (5) α-L-iduronic acid.

Indications of Heparin

Heparin sodium injection is indicated for:
1. Anticoagulant therapy in prophylaxis and treatment of venous thrombosis and its extension; (In a low-dose regimen) for prevention of postoperative deep venous thrombosis and pulmonary embolism in patients undergoing major abdomino-thoracic surgery or who for other reasons are at risk of developing thromboembolic disease;
2. Prophylaxis and treatment of pulmonary embolism;
3. Atrial fibrillation with embolization;
4. Diagnosis and treatment of acute and chronic consumption coagulopathies (disseminated intravascular coagulation);
5. Prevention of clotting in arterial and heart surgery;
6. Prophylaxis and treatment of peripheral arterial embolism;
7. As an anticoagulant in blood transfusions, extracorporeal circulation, and dialysis procedures and in blood sample.

Contraindications
1. Heparin sodium should not be used in patients:
2. With severe thrombocytopenia;
3. In whom suitable blood coagulation tests—for example the whole-blood clotting time, partial thromboplastin time, etc.—cannot be performed at appropriate intervals (this contraindication refers to full-dose heparin; there is usually no need to monitor coagulation parameters in patients receiving low-dose heparin); PPG-2013.indd 93 10/22/2016 4:52:20 PM

Warning: Heparin is not intended for intramuscular use.

Hypersensitivity: Patients with documented hypersensitivity to heparin should be given the drug only in clearly life-threatening situations.

Hemorrhage: Hemorrhage can occur at virtually any site in patients receiving heparin. An unexplained fall in hematocrit, fall in blood pressure, or any other unexplained symptom should lead to serious consideration of a hemorrhagic event.

Cardiovascular: Subacute bacterial endocarditis. Severe hypertension.

Surgical: During and immediately following (a) spinal tap or spinal anesthesia or (b) major surgery, especially involving the brain, spinal cord, or eye.

Hematologic: Conditions associated with increased bleeding tendencies, such as hemophilia, thrombocytopenia, and some vascular purpuras.

Gastrointestinal: Ulcerative lesions and continuous tube drainage of the stomach or small intestine.

Other: Menstruation, liver disease with impaired hemostasis

11. Atropine.

It is used to treat some poisonings. In surgery, it is used to lower secretions, such as saliva. It is used to treat muscle spasms of the gastrointestinal (GI) tract, gallbladder system, or urinary system. It is used when the heart is not beating.

PATHOLOGY AND GENETICS

LONG ESSAYS

1. Discuss cutaneous wound healing by first intention, mention local and systemic factors that influence wound healing, enumerate the complications of the same.

First intention, also termed primary healing, is the healing that occurs when a clean laceration or a surgical incision is closed primarily with sutures, Steri-Strips, or skin adhesive (Fig. 1).

Healing by First Intention (Primary Union):
Healing of a wound which has the following characteristics:
1. Clean and uninfected—surgically incised
2. Without much loss of cells and tissue
3. Edges of wound are approximated by surgical sutures

Hemostatic or Inflammatory Phase
This phase starts immediately and lasts 2-5 days. Tissue damage releases chemical mediators called cytokines [e.g. transforming growth factor -beta (TGF-beta) interleukin-1β which initiate a complex interrelated process that causes hemostasis and begins the healing process]

Sequence of Events
- Initial hemorrhage—wound is filled with blood which clots, seals the wound against dehydration and infection.
- Acute inflammatory response—polymorphs replaced by macrophages by 3rd day

Phase	Cellular and biophysiologic events
Hemostasis	1. Vascular constriction 2. Platelet aggregation, degranulation, and fibrin formation (thrombus)
Inflammation	1. Neutrophil infiltration 2. Monocyte infiltration and differentiation to macrophage 3. Lymphocyte infiltration
Proliferation	1. Re-epithelialization 2. Angiogenesis 3. Collagen synthesis 4. ECM formation
Remodeling	1. Collagen remodeling 2. Vascular maturation and regression

Epithelial Changes
- Basal cells of epidermis start proliferating and migrating towards incisional space.
- Wound is covered by a layer of epithelium in 48 hours.
- Epidermal cells separate the underlying viable dermis from the overlying necrotic material, forming scab—by 5th day, a multilayered new epidermis is formed.

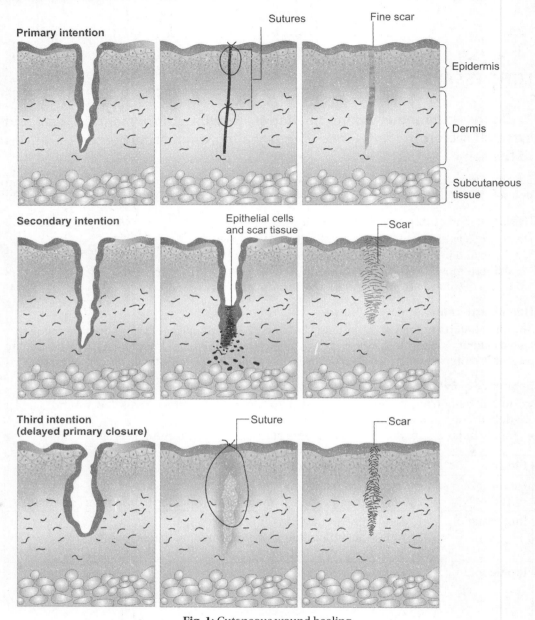

Fig. 1: Cutaneous wound healing.

Organization
- By 3rd day, fibroblasts also invade the wound area.
- By 5th day, new collagen fibrils start forming which dominate till healing is completed.
- In 4 weeks, the scar tissue with scanty cellular and vascular elements is formed.

Local Factors Affecting Wound Healing
- Infection
- Poor blood supply

- Foreign bodies including sutures interfere with healing
- Movement delays wound healing
- Exposure to ionizing radiation delays
- Exposure to ultraviolet light facilitates healing
- Type, size and location of injury.

Systemic Factors Affecting Wound Healing

Systemic factors:
- Age—wound healing rapid in young and slow in aged and debilitated people
- Nutrition—deficiency of protein, vitamin C, zinc delays the wound healing
- Systemic infection delays
- Administration of glucocorticoids
- Uncontrolled diabetics—more prone to develop infections and hence delay in healing.
- Haematologic abnormalities—defect of neutrophil functions, neutropenia and bleeding disorders slow the process of wound healing.

Complications of Wound Healing
- Infection of wound—delays the healing.
- Implantation (epidermal) cyst.
- Pigmentation—rust-like colour due to hemosiderin.
- Deficient scar formation—due to inadequate formation of granulation tissue.
- Incisional hernia—or wound dehiscence.
- Hypertrophied scars and keloid:
  - The scar is excessive, ugly and painful.
  - Excessive formation of collagen may result in keloid formation, tumor-like projection of connective tissue.
- Excessive contraction—Dupuytren's contracture.
- Neoplasia—squamous cell carcinoma in Marjolin's ulcer.

2. Discuss the etiology and pathogenesis of rheumatic heart disease.

Cardiovascular disease is on the rise. In India and other developing countries, rheumatic heart disease (RHD) continues to be a major public health problem and contributes to significant cardiac morbidity and mortality. RHD in the juvenile age group namely juvenile mitral stenosis is a variant which is unique to the Indian subcontinent. Severe valve deformities lead to high morbidity and mortality.

Despite various measures no appreciable decline in prevalence of RHD has been documented. At autopsy, mitral valve was most commonly affected either alone or in combination with aortic and tricuspid valves. Both functional and organic involvement of tricuspid valve was documented. It has been convincingly demonstrated that molecular mimicry between *Streptococcus pyogenes* antigen and human proteins lead to autoimmune reactions both humoral and cell mediated causing RF/RHD. Heart tissues namely the valves, left atrial appendage (LAA) and myocardium reveal variable amounts of infiltration by lymphocytes.

Significant endocarditis and valvulitis is observed in these cases. CD4$^+$ T cells are most likely the ultimate effectors of chronic valve lesions in RHD. They can recognize streptococcal M5 protein peptides and produce various inflammatory cytokines, such as TNF-alpha, IFN-gamma, IL-10, IL-4 which could be responsible for progressive fibrotic valvular lesions. Cardiac myosin has been defined as a putative autoantigen recognized by autoantibodies of RF patients. Cross reactivity between cardiac myosin and group A beta hemolytic streptococcal M protein has been adequately demonstrated.

Cardiac myosin has been shown to produce myocarditis in rats and mice. Valvulitis/ endocarditis have been observed in excised LAA, cardiac valves and in hearts at autopsy from cases of RHD. The disease predominantly affects the valvular endocardium culminating in crippling valve deformities. Endocardial infiltrate and their migration into the valve substance has been elegantly demonstrated in rats and mice.

Immune responses against cardiac myosin lead to valvular heart disease and infiltration of the heart by streptococcal M protein reactive T lymphocytes. Mitral valves showed various degrees of calcification. An interesting observation is the nature of calcification in diseased/ distorted valves in RHD. Recent studies indicate that calcification is not merely an inactive, "dystrophic" process but involves a regulated inflammatory process associated with expression of osteoblast markers and neoangiogenesis.

Increased plasma osteopontin levels correlated with severity of mitral valve calcification. Further evidence of inflammation is supported by high levels of advanced oxidation protein products and high sensitive C-reactive protein in plasma detected in patients with RHD. Presence of inflammatory cells and increased expression of several cytokines in cases of "end stage" RHD reflects a possible subclinical, ongoing insult/injury to some unrecognized antigenic stimulus by beta hemolytic streptococcal antigens that have sensitized/primed the various target tissues and which further culminate in permanent valve deformities.

Complications

Rheumatic heart disease is permanent damage to the heart caused by the inflammation of rheumatic fever. Problems are most common with the valve between the two left chambers of the heart (mitral valve), but the other valves may be affected. The damage may result in one of the following conditions:

1. **Valve stenosis:** This condition is a narrowing of the valve which results in decreased blood flow.
2. **Valve regurgitation:** This condition is a leak in the valve which allows blood to flow in the wrong direction.
3. **Damage to heart muscle:** The inflammation associated with rheumatic fever can weaken the heart muscle, resulting in poor pumping function.
4. **Damage to the mitral valve**, other heart valves or other heart tissues can cause problems with the heart later in life. Resulting conditions may include.
5. **Atrial fibrillation**, an irregular and chaotic beating of the upper chambers of the heart (atria).
6. **Heart failure**, an inability of the heart to pump enough blood to the body.

SHORT ESSAYS

3. Describe Benign prostate hyperplasia.

A common, noncancerous enlargement of the prostate gland. The enlarged prostate may compress the urinary tube (urethra) which courses through the center of the prostate, impeding the flow of urine from the bladder through the urethra to the outside.

Symptoms

The severity of symptoms in people who have prostate gland enlargement varies, but symptoms tend to gradually worsen over time. Common signs and symptoms of BPH include:

1. Frequent or urgent need to urinate
2. Increased frequency of urination at night (nocturia)
3. Difficulty starting urination

4. Weak urine stream or a stream that stops and starts
5. Dribbling at the end of urination
6. Inability to completely empty the bladder.

Less common signs and symptoms include:
1. Urinary tract infection
2. Inability to urinate
3. Blood in the urine.

Complications

Medical tests: A healthcare provider may refer men to a urologist—a doctor who specializes in urinary problems and the male reproductive system—though the healthcare provider most often diagnoses Benign prostatic hyperplasia on the basis of symptoms and a digital rectal exam. A urologist uses medical tests to help diagnose lower urinary tract problems related to Benign prostatic hyperplasia and recommend treatment. Medical tests may include:
- Urinalysis
- A prostate-specific antigen (PSA) blood test
- Urodynamic tests
- Cystoscopy
- Transrectal ultrasound
- Biopsy.

Complications of an enlarged prostate can include:

Sudden inability to urinate (urinary retention): You might need to have a tube (catheter) inserted into your bladder to drain the urine. Some men with an enlarged prostate need surgery to relieve urinary retention.

Urinary tract infections (UTIs): Inability to fully empty the bladder can increase the risk of infection in your urinary tract. If UTIs occur frequently, you might need surgery to remove part of the prostate.

Bladder stones: These are generally caused by an inability to completely empty the bladder. Bladder stones can cause infection, bladder irritation, blood in the urine and obstruction of urine flow.

Bladder damage: A bladder that has not emptied completely can stretch and weaken over time. As a result, the muscular wall of the bladder no longer contracts properly, making it harder to fully empty your bladder.

Kidney damage: Pressure in the bladder from urinary retention can directly damage the kidneys or allow bladder infections to reach the kidneys.

4. Explain the etiology and pathogenesis of bronchogenic carcinoma.

Definition: Bronchogenic carcinoma is a malignant neoplasm of the lung arising from the epithelium of the bronchus or bronchiole.

Pathophysiology
1. Bronchogenic carcinoma tends to form an intraluminal mass which may partially or completely obstruct the bronchus. The neoplasm also may compress or invade local structures, such as aorta, esophagus, superior vena cava or cervical sympathetic chain.
2. Bronchogenic carcinoma may present with a variety clinical manifestations but the major findings are cough, weight loss, chest pain and dyspnea. These neoplasms also have the

capacity to secrete hormones or hormone-like substances which have a variety of clinical effects.

Types: There are 2 main types of bronchogenic carcinoma:
1. **Small cell lung cancer:** Small cell lung cancer is named for the appearance of the cells under a microscope (small cells. This type of cancer is present in approximately 15% of people with lung cancer.
2. **Non-small cell lung cancer:** Non-small cell lung cancer accounts for most bronchogenic carcinomas (around 80%) and is further broken down into lung adenocarcinoma, squamous cell carcinoma of lungs and large cell cancer.

Symptoms
Using the older definition of bronchogenic carcinoma, symptoms are often related to the growth of cancer in the large airways.
1. Coughing up blood
2. Recurrent pneumonia due to obstruction of the airways by a tumor
3. Persistent cough.

At the current time, lung adenocarcinoma is the most common form of lung cancer, accounting for 40–50% of cases. These tumors tend to grow in the periphery of the lungs, rather than in the central airways like the bronchi, and for that reason, the typical symptoms noted above may be absent. The early symptoms of lung adenocarcinoma may instead be signs, such as:
1. Unexplained weight loss
2. Fatigue
3. Shortness of breath, especially with exercise

Treatments
The treatments your doctor recommends will depend on several factors including the type and stage of lung cancer you are diagnosed with. It is important to learn about your diagnosis, as studies suggest that people who are actively involved in their lung cancer care have better outcomes. Treatments may include lung cancer surgery, chemotherapy, targeted therapies, radiation therapy and immunotherapy.

5. Describe the acute pyogenic meningitis.

Meningitis is an inflammation of the membranes (meninges) surrounding your brain and spinal cord. The swelling from meningitis typically triggers symptoms, such as headache, fever and a stiff neck.

Symptoms
Early meningitis symptoms may mimic the flu (influenza). Symptoms may develop over several hours or over a few days.

Possible signs and symptoms in anyone older than the age of 2 include:
1. Sudden high fever
2. Stiff neck
3. Severe headache that seems different than normal
4. Headache with nausea or vomiting
5. Confusion or difficulty concentrating
6. Seizures

7. Sleepiness or difficulty waking
8. Sensitivity to light
9. No appetite or thirst
10. Skin rash (sometimes, such as in meningococcal meningitis).

Bacterial meningitis

Bacteria that enter the bloodstream and travel to the brain and spinal cord cause acute bacterial meningitis. But it can also occur when bacteria directly invade the meninges. This may be caused by an ear or sinus infection, a skull fracture, or, rarely, after some surgeries.
Several strains of bacteria can cause acute bacterial meningitis, most commonly:

Streptococcus pneumoniae (pneumococcus): This bacterium is the most common cause of bacterial meningitis in infants, young children and adults in the United States. It more commonly causes pneumonia or ear or sinus infections. A vaccine can help prevent this infection.

Neisseria meningitidis (meningococcus): This bacterium is another leading cause of bacterial meningitis. These bacteria commonly cause an upper respiratory infection but can cause meningococcal meningitis when they enter the bloodstream. This is a highly contagious infection that affects mainly teenagers and young adults. It may cause local epidemics in college dormitories, boarding schools and military bases. A vaccine can help prevent infection.

Haemophilus influenzae (haemophilus): Haemophilus influenzae type b (Hib) bacterium was once the leading cause of bacterial meningitis in children. But new Hib vaccines have greatly reduced the number of cases of this type of meningitis.

Listeria monocytogenes (listeria): These bacteria can be found in unpasteurized cheeses, hot dogs and lunchmeats. Pregnant women, newborns, older adults and people with weakened immune systems are most susceptible. Listeria can cross the placental barrier, and infections in late pregnancy may be fatal to the baby.

Treatment

Antibiotics: These are usually given intravenously.

Corticosteroids: These may be given if inflammation is causing pressure in the brain, but studies show conflicting results.

Acetaminophen, or paracetamol: Together with cool sponge baths, cooling pads, fluids, and room ventilation, these reduce fever.

Anticonvulsants: If the patient has seizures, an anticonvulsant, such as phenobarbital or dilantin may be used.

Oxygen therapy: Oxygen will be administered to assist with breathing.

Fluids: Intravenous fluids can prevent dehydration, especially if the patient is vomiting or cannot drink.

Sedatives: These will calm the patient if they are irritable or restless.

6. Explain about infective endocarditis.

Infective endocarditis (IE) is defined as an infection of the endocardial surface of the heart, which may include one or more heart valves, the mural endocardium, or a septal defect. Its intracardiac effects include severe valvular insufficiency which may lead to intractable congestive heart failure and myocardial abscesses. If left untreated, IE is almost inevitably fatal.

Pathology

Acute infective endocarditis generally is caused by *Staphylococcus*, *Pneumococcus*, or *Gonococcus* bacteria or by fungi. This form of endocarditis develops rapidly, with fever, malaise, and other signs of systemic infection coupled with abnormal cardiac function and even acute heart failure.

Pathophysiology

- Experimental evidence indicates that 2 factors are needed to establish endocardial infection:
    1. Endothelial denudation over valve cusp with platelet deposition (thrombus)
    2. Episode of bacteremia
- Endothelial damage can be due to aberrant jet streams and turbulent flow in the setting of diseased cardiac valves and septal defects or direct trauma from intravascular devices.
- A platelet/fibrin clot is formed over the exposed underlying extracellular matrix as the reparative process ensues.
- If transient bacteremia occurs before a protective layer of endothelium forms, colonization of the fibrin may develop and progress to an infected vegetation.
- Organism proliferates within the thrombus, forming infective vegetations which elicits inflammatory response resulting in erosion or perforation of the valve cusps leading to valvular aneurysms, perforations and incompetence, damage to the conduction pathway (if in the septal area), or rupture of a sinus of Valsalva (if in the aortic area).
- Prolonged antibiotic treatment is needed to sterilize the vegetations.
- Endocarditis on a prosthetic valve usually begins in the valve ring and may protrude into the valve orifice causing obstruction and regurgitation.
- Annular abscesses around the sewing ring of the valve are common, leading to dehiscence of sutures and paraprosthetic leaks.
- Organisms which can bind via receptors to fibronectin, other subendothelial components or to platelets are the most virulent.
- Healing process depends on the degree of valve damage in the initial acute phase.
- Over time, vegetation decreases in size and organizes as a fibrous nodule which may calcify.
- Cusp fibrosis leads to cusp thickening and retraction.

Symptoms: Endocarditis may develop slowly or suddenly, depending on what germs are causing the infection and whether you have any underlying heart problems. Endocarditis signs and symptoms can vary from person to person.

Common signs and symptoms of endocarditis include:

- Flu-like symptoms, such as fever and chills
- A new or changed heart murmur which is the heart sounds made by blood rushing through your heart
- Fatigue
- Aching joints and muscles
- Night sweats
- Shortness of breath
- Chest pain when you breathe
- Swelling in your feet, legs or abdomen.

Complications: In endocarditis, clumps of bacteria and cell fragments form in your heart at the site of the infection. These clumps, called vegetations, can break loose and travel to your brain, lungs, abdominal organs, kidneys or limbs.

As a result, endocarditis can cause several major complications including:
- Heart problems, such as heart murmur, heart valve damage and heart failure
- Stroke
- Seizure
- Loss of the ability to move part of all of your body (paralysis)
- Pockets of collected pus (abscesses) that develop in the heart, brain, lungs and other organs
- Pulmonary embolism—an infected vegetation that travels to the lungs and blocks a lung artery
- Kidney damage
- Enlarged spleen.

SHORT ANSWERS

7. Define infertility.

Infertility: Diminished or absent ability to conceive and bear offspring. A couple is considered to be experiencing infertility if conception has not occurred after 12 months of sexual activity without the use of contraception. Infertility can have many causes and may be related to factors in the male, female, or both. Treatments can include medications and assisted reproductive technologies.

8. Define karyotyping.

Karyotype: A standard arrangement of the chromosome complement prepared for chromosome analysis. A normal female karyotype would include each of the 22 pairs of autosomes (nonsex chromosomes), arranged in numeric order together with the two X chromosomes.

9. What is mutation?

A mutation is a change that occurs in our DNA sequence, either due to mistakes when the DNA is copied or as the result of environmental factors, such as UV light and cigarette smoke.
A **mutation** occurs when a DNA gene is damaged or changed in such a way as to alter the genetic message carried by that gene.
A **mutagen** is an agent of substance that can bring about a permanent alteration to the physical composition of a *DNA* gene such that the genetic message is changed.
Once the gene has been damaged or changed the mRNA transcribed from that gene will now carry an altered message.

10. Factors responsible for chromosomal aberration.

Chromosomal abnormalities occur when there is a defect in a chromosome, or in the arrangement of the genetic material on the chromosome. Very often, chromosome abnormalities give rise to specific physical symptoms, however, the severity of these can vary from individual to individual. Abnormalities can be in the form of additional material which may be attached to a chromosome, or where part or a whole chromosome is missing, or even in defective formation of a chromosome. Any increases or decreases in chromosomal material interfere with normal development and function. These occur due to a loss or genetic material, or a rearrangement in the location of the genetic material. They include: Deletions, duplications, inversions, ring formations, and translocations. Deletions: A portion of the chromosome is missing or deleted.

11. Clinical features of Turner syndrome

Symptoms of Turner syndrome are:
1. Short stature and nonfunctioning ovaries which causes infertility
2. Some women may also have extra skin on the neck (webbed neck)
3. Puffiness or swelling (lymphedema) of the hands and feet
4. Skeletal abnormalities
5. Heart defects
6. High blood pressure
7. Kidney problems.

12. Name the various procedures of prenatal diagnosis.

The most common screening procedures are routine ultrasounds, blood tests, and blood pressure measurement. Common diagnosis procedures include amniocentesis and chorionic villus sampling.

First trimester screening tests can begin as early as 10 weeks. These usually involve blood tests and an ultrasound. They test your baby's overall development and check to see if your baby is at risk for genetic conditions, such as Down syndrome. They also check your baby for heart defects, cystic fibrosis, and other developmental problems.

Second trimester screening tests occur between 14 and 18 weeks. They can involve a blood test, which tests whether a mother is at risk for having a child with Down syndrome or neural tube defects as well as an ultrasound.

2017

Pharmacology, Pathology and Genetics

PHARMACOLOY

LONG ESSAYS

1. Enumerate the various routes of drug administration with suitable examples, discuss the merits and demerits of intravenous route.
2. Classify opioid analgesics, discuss the therapeutic uses, adverse effects and contraindications of morphine.

SHORT ESSAYS

3. Name four anticholnesterases and its therapeutic uses.
4. Preanesthetic medications.
5. Uses and adverse effects of insulin.
6. Antiemetics.
7. Anticoagulants.

SHORT ANSWERS

8. Define an antiseptic, give two examples.
9. Name four reserve antituberclosis drugs.
10. Name four viral vaccines.
11. Name four drugs useful in hypersensitive emergencies.

PATHOLOGY AND GENETICS

LONG ESSAYS

1. Define thrombosis; explain its causes and mechanism of formation in intravascular thrombosis.
2. How do tumors spread in the body, explain differences between Bengin and malignant neoplasams?

SHORT ESSAYS

3. Describe wound healing.
4. Explain etiopathology of renal calculi.
5. Describe lung abscess.
6. How will you collect urine for routine examination culture, biological tests?

SHORT ANSWERS

7. Mention any four structural aberrations.
8. List out any four causes of congenital anomalies.
9. Types of neural tube defects.
10. Define mutation.
11. Define eugenics.
12. Mention four ethical issues in the role of nurse in genetic counseling.

PHARMACOLOY

LONG ESSAYS

1. Enumerate the various routes of drug administration with suitable examples; discuss the merits and demerits of intravenous route.

(See Q.1, 2016)

2. Classify opioid analgesics, discuss the therapeutic uses, adverse effects and contraindications of morphine.

Analgesics are drugs designed specifically to relieve pain. ... Some products combine acetaminophen with an opioid analgesic for added relief. How do they work? Opioid (also called narcotic) analgesics work by binding to receptors on cells mainly in the brain, spinal cord and gastrointestinal system (Flowchart 1).

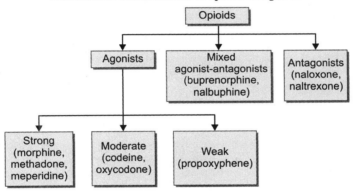

Flowchart 1: Classifications of upload analgesics.

Classify Opioid Analgesics

The opioid analgesics and related drugs are derived from several chemical subgroups and may be classified in several ways:

1. **Spectrum of clinical uses:** Opioid drugs can be subdivided on the basis of their major therapeutic uses (e.g. analgesics, antitussives, and antidiarrheal drugs).
2. **Strength of analgesia:** On the basis of their relative abilities to relieve pain, the analgesic opioids may be classified as strong, moderate, and weak agonists. Partial agonists are opioids that exert less analgesia than morphine, the prototype of a strong analgesic, or full agonist.
3. **Ratio of agonist to antagonist effects:** Opioid drugs may be classified as agonists (full or partial receptor activators), antagonists (receptor blockers), or mixed agonist-antagonists, which are capable of activating one opioid receptor subtype and blocking another subtype.

Morphine

Indications

1. Severe pain (the 20 mg/mL oral solution concentration should only be used in opioid-tolerant patients).

2. Pain severe enough to require daily around-the-clock, long-term opioid treatment and for which alternative treatment options are inadequate (extended-release).
3. Pulmonary edema.
4. Pain associated with MI.

Action: Binds to opiate receptors in the CNS. Alters the perception of and response to painful stimuli while producing generalized CNS depression.

Therapeutic effect(s): Decrease in severity of pain. Addition of naltrexone in *Embeda* product is designed to prevent abuse or misuse by altering the formulation. Naltrexone has no effect unless the capsule is crushed or chewed.

Contraindications/Precautions

Contraindicated in:
1. Hypersensitivity
2. Some products contain tartrazine, bisulfites, or alcohol and should be avoided in patients with known hypersensitivity
3. Acute, mild, intermittent, or postoperative pain (extended/sustained-release)
4. Significant respiratory depression (extended-release)
5. Acute or severe bronchial asthma (extended-release)
6. Paralytic ileus (extended-release).

Use Cautiously in:
1. Head trauma
2. ↑ intracranial pressure
3. Severe renal, hepatic, or pulmonary disease
4. Hypothyroidism
5. Seizure disorder
6. Adrenal insufficiency
7. History of substance abuse
8. Undiagnosed abdominal pain
9. Prostatic hyperplasia
10. Patients undergoing procedures that rapidly ↓ pain (cordotomy, radiation); long-acting agents should be discontinued 24 hours before and replaced with short-acting agents

Adverse Effects:

Central nervous systgem (CNS): Confusion, sedation, dizziness, dysphoria, euphoria, floating feeling, hallucinations, headache, unusual dreams

Ear, nose and throat (ENT): Blurred vision, diplopia, miosis

Respiratory: Respiratory depression

Cerebovascular (CV): Hypotension, bradycardia

Endoscopic: Adrenal insufficiency

SHORT ESSAYS

3. Name four anticholinesterases and its therapeutic uses.

Anticholinesterase drugs that are used more widely in the clinic are those that inhibit acetylcholinesterase in the brain. The most useful application of such agents is in the treatment of Alzheimer disease, in which reduced transmission of acetylcholine contributes to the neuropathology of the disease.

Uses: Anticholinesterases are a class of drugs that decrease breakdown of acetylcholine (a chemical messenger in the brain) and can be used in conditions whereby there is an apparent lack of this messenger transmission, such as in Alzheimer's disease (Flowchart 2).

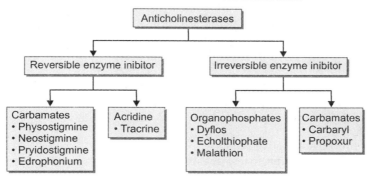

Flowchart 2: Anticholinesterases and its uses.

Members of this class include: Reminyl (galantamine), aricept (donepezil) and exelon (rivastigmine) are used in the treatment of mild to moderately severe dementia. It helps to slow down the progression of dementia and improve alertness to reduce carer burden. They do not change the underlying disease. Studies have shown continued benefit for up to 4 years.

Anticholinesterases

1. Reminyl (galantamine)
2. Aricept (donepezil)
3. Neostigmine (neostigmine)
4. Mestinon (pyridostigmine)
5. Elexon (rivastigmine)

Mechanism of Action

The cognitive dysfunction (memory, attention, learning) in dementia of the Alzheimer type is related to a significant reduction in acetylcholine (a chemical messenger in the brain) transmission. Reminyl (galantamine), aricept (Donepezil) and exelon (rivastigmine) work by inhibiting an enzyme called acetylcholinesterase. By blocking this enzyme the breakdown of acetylcholine, released by the remaining healthy brain cells, is slowed down leaving more chemical messengers available to support normal brain function. In addition, Reminyl (galantamine) also increases the action of acetylcholine on another receptor site called nicotinic receptors. This has been associated with improved cognitive function.

Precautions When Taking Anticholinesterases

Care should be taken when using these medications in patients with:
1. Asthma and chronic obstructive airways disease—may increase shortness of breath.
2. Cardiac conduction abnormalities—anticholinesterases can slow the heart.
3. Peptic ulcer—because of their pharmacological action, cholinesterase inhibitors may be expected to increase gastric acid secretion.
4. Severe renal impairment—may require individual dose titration.

4. Preanesthetic medications.

Preanesthetic medications, such as tranquilizers and sedatives are not recommended with the exception of anticholinergic drugs because single injection anesthesia techniques have been developed that minimize the handling stress and eliminate the discomfort associated with multiple injections. Serum and tissue atropine esterases found in many rabbits and rats render atropine sulfate ineffective, therefore, subcutaneous (SC) administration of glycopyrrolate (Robinul, AH Robins Company, Richmond, VA), a quaternary ammonium parasympatholytic, should be given to reduce salivary and bronchial secretions and prevent vagal bradycardia.

Preanesthetic Medications

Aims
1. Relief of anxiety
2. Amnesia for pre/postoperative events
3. Supplement analgesic action so less anesthetic needed
4. Decrease secretions and vagal stimulation by anesthetics
5. Antiemetic effect even postoperatively
6. Decrease acidity.

Class	Drugs	Uses	Adverse effects
Opioids	Morphine Meperidine	1. Anxiety 2. Pre/postoperative analgesia 3. Smooth induction and reduction in dose of anesthetic	1. Asthma 2. Delay recovery 3. Biliary spasm (because morphine causes contraction of sphincter of Oddi àbiliary spasm) 4. Urinary retention
Sedatives	Diazepam Lorazepam	1. Sedation and smooth induction 2. Respiratory depression—less common 3. No vomiting, minor surgical and endoscopic procedures with either fentanyl or meperidine	

Contd...

Contd...

Class	Drugs	Uses	Adverse effects
	Midazolam	Midazolam = potent and short-acting drug suitable for preoperative anesthesia	
	Promethazine	1. Sedative 2. Antiemetic 3. Anticholinergic (minimal respiratory depression)	
Anticholinergics		1. Prevent vagal 2. Bradycardia (occur reflexly due to surgical procedures)	Laryngeal spasm precipitated by respiratory secretions
	Hyoscine (derivatives of atropine)	1. Antiemetic 2. Produces amnesia	
	Glycopyrrolate (derivatives of atropine)	1. Local anesthetic atropine substitute 2. Antisecretory 3. Antibradycardic drug	
H2 blockers		1. Patients undergoing prolonged operations 2. C-sections 3. Obese 4. At risk of gastric regurgitation 5. At risk of aspiration pneumonia	
	Ranitidine Ramotidine	1. Night before and morning prior to surgery 2. Prevent chances of regurgitation/stress ulcers	
PPI	Omeprazole	Same as H2 blocker	
Antiemetics	Metoclopramide Ondansetron	1. Reduce chance of aspiration 2. Control postanesthetic nausea and vomiting 3. Metoclopramide—increase tone of lower esophageal sphincter 4. Ondansetron = 5-HT3 blocker used in cancer patients	

5. Uses and adverse effects of insulin.

Insulin is a hormone that is responsible for allowing glucose in the blood to enter cells, providing them with the energy to function. A lack of effective insulin plays a key role in the development of diabetes.

Uses: Insulin is a hormone made by the pancreas that allows your body to use sugar (glucose) from carbohydrates in the food that you eat for energy or to store glucose for future use. Insulin helps keeps your blood sugar level from getting too high (hyperglycemia) or too low (hypoglycemia).

Types of insulin: A person can take different types of insulin based on how long they need the effects of the supplementary hormone to last.

People categorize these types based on several different factors:
1. Speed of onset, or how quickly a person taking insulin can expect the effects to start.
2. Peak, or the speed at which the insulin reaches its greatest impact
3. Duration, or the time it takes for the insulin to wear off
4. Concentration, which in the United States is 100 units per milliliter (U-100)
5. The route of delivery, or whether the insulin requires injection under the skin, into a vein, or into the lungs by inhalation.

People most often deliver insulin into the subcutaneous tissue, or the fatty tissue located near the surface of the skin.

Fast-acting insulin: The body absorbs this type into the bloodstream from the subcutaneous tissue extremely quickly.

People use fast-acting insulin to correct hyperglycemia, or high blood sugar, as well as control blood sugar spikes after eating.

This type includes:
- **Rapid-acting insulin analogs:** These take between 5 and 15 minutes to have an effect. However, the size of the dose impacts the duration of the effect. Assuming that rapid-acting insulin analogs last for 4 hours is a safe general rule.
- **Regular human insulin:** The onset of regular human insulin is between 30 minutes and an hour, and its effects on blood sugar last around 8 hours. A larger dose speeds up the onset but also delay the peak effect of regular human insulin.

Intermediate-acting insulin: This type enters the bloodstream at a slower rate but has a longer-lasting effect. It is most effective at managing blood sugar overnight as well as between meals.

Options for intermediate-acting insulin include:
- **Neutral protamin Hagedorn (NPH) human insulin:** This takes between 1 and 2 hours to onset, and reaches its peak within 4–6 hours. It can last over 12 hours in some cases. A very small dose will bring forward the peak effect, and a high dose will increase the time NPH takes to reach its peak and the overall duration of its effect.
- **Premixed insulin:** This is a mixture of NPH with a fast-acting insulin, and its effects are a combination of the intermediate and rapid-acting insulins.

Long-acting insulin: While long-acting insulin is slow to reach the bloodstream and has a relatively low peak, it has a stabilizing "plateau" effect on blood sugar that can last for most of the day.

It is useful overnight between meals and during fasts.

Long-acting insulin analogs are the only available type, and these have an onset of between 1.5 and 2 hours. While different brands have different durations, they range between 12 and 24 hours in total.

Adverse effects of insulin: Hypoglycemias are the main problem especially in intensified treatment. Excessive doses, insufficient calory uptake, or physical exertion are possible triggers.
Early symptoms: Hunger, restlessness, sweating or vertigo, unsteadiness and thought disorders. Specialists do not agree if human insulin hinders the timely recognition of severe hypoglycemias more often than animal insulins.

Considerable weight gain is often observed under the intensified treatment. Generalized hypersensitive reactions also occur with human insulin. A lipodystrophy can occur at the site of injection. Transient visual disturbances are possible after readjustments.

6. Antiemetics.

An antiemetic is a drug that is effective against vomiting and nausea. Antiemetics are typically used to treat motion sickness and the side effects of opioid analgesics, general anesthetics, and chemotherapy directed against cancer.

> **Antiemetics**
> **Classifications:**
> 1. **Anticholinergics:** *Hyoscine, dicyclomine*
> 2. **H1 antihistaminics:** *Promethazine, diphenhydramine, cyclizine, meclozine, cinnarizine*
> 3. **Neuroleptics:** *Chlorpromiazine, prochlorperazine, haloperidol, etc.*
> 4. **Prokinetic drugs:** *Metoclopramide, domperidone, cisapride, mosapride*
> 5. **5HT1-antagonists:** *Ondansetron, granisetron, dolasetron*
> 6. **Adjuvant antiemetics:** *Corticosteroids, benzodiazeplnes, cannabinoids*

Antiemetic drugs are types of chemicals that help ease symptoms of nausea or vomiting. Antiemetic drugs may also be used to treat nausea and vomiting caused by other medications, frequent motion sickness, infections, or stomach flu.

Antiemetic drugs help to block specific neurotransmitters in the body. These neurotransmitters trigger impulses, such as nausea and vomiting, so blocking the impulses will help shut them down.

Feeling nauseated might seem like a simple reaction in the body, but it is a complex process. Because of this, there is a range of antiemetic drugs, each of which is designed to work in different situations.

Common side effects of each drug type include:
- Antihistamines: Sleepiness, dry mouth, and dry nasal passages
- Bismuth-subsalicylate: Dark, blackish stools and changes in tongue color
- Cannabinoids: Altered state of perception and dizziness.

Corticosteroids: Additional symptoms of indigestion, increased appetite or thirst, and acne. Dopamine receptor blockers: Fatigue, constipation, ringing in the ears, dry mouth, restlessness, and muscle spasms.

NK1 receptor blockers: Dry mouth, reduced urine volume, and heartburn

Serotonin receptor blockers: Fatigue, dry mouth, and constipation

Complications: While antiemetic drugs can help people to live without the bothersome symptoms of nausea and vomiting, some complications can occur.

Symptoms that should be addressed by a doctor include:
1. Muscle weakness, spasms, or convulsions
2. Changes in heartbeat, such as palpitations or rapid heartbeat
3. Hearing loss
4. Worsening of nausea or vomiting, even while taking medications
5. Slurred speech

6. Psychological problems, such as hallucinations or confusion
7. Drowsiness that interferes with daily life.

7. Anticoagulants.

Anticoagulants are medicines that help prevent blood clots. They are given to people at a high-risk of getting clots, to reduce their chances of developing serious conditions, such as strokes and heart attacks.

Anticlotting physiology: The goal of coagulation is fibrin formation. Activation of the coagulation cascade leads to the production of thrombin (FIIa). Thrombin then converts fibrinogen (FI) to fibrin. Physiological anticoagulation mechanisms act to reduce thrombin production or reduce the effects of thrombin.

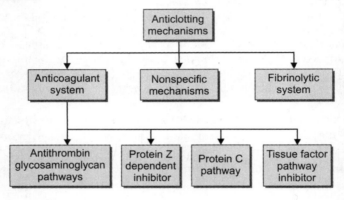

Types of anticoagulants: The most commonly prescribed anticoagulant is warfarin.
Newer types of anticoagulants are also available and are becoming increasingly common. These include:
1. Rivaroxaban (Xarelto)
2. Dabigatran (Pradaxa)
3. Apixaban (Eliquis)
4. Edoxaban

Warfarin and the newer alternatives are taken as tablets or capsules. There is also an anticoagulant called heparin that can be given by injection.

Uses

Anticoagulants are also sometimes used to treat blood clots, such as DVT or a pulmonary embolism, by stopping the clot getting bigger while your body slowly reabsorbs it. How long you will need to take anticoagulants for will depend on why they are needed?

Side Effects of Anticoagulants

Like all medicines, there is a risk of experiencing side effects while taking anticoagulants.

The main side effect is that you can bleed too easily which can cause problem, such as:
1. Passing blood in urine
2. Passing blood when you poo or having black poo
3. Severe bruising
4. Prolonged nosebleeds
5. Bleeding gums

6. Vomiting blood or coughing up blood
7. Heavy periods in women.

SHORT ANSWERS

8. Define an antiseptic, give two examples.

Antiseptic is defined as a substance used to eliminate germs. An example of an antiseptic is hydrogen peroxide.

Some commonly used antiseptics are hydrogen peroxide, alcohol, boric acid, iodine, formaldehyde, and hexachlorophene.

9. Name four reserve antituberclosis drugs.

First line TB drugs
- Isoniazid (H/Inh)
- Rifampicin (R/Rif) (In the United States rifampicin is called rifampin)
- Pyrazinamide (Z/Pza)
- Ethambutol (E/Emb).

10. Name four viral vaccines.

- Chickenpox vaccine
- DTaP immunization (vaccine)
- Hepatitis A vaccine
- Hepatitis B vaccine
- Hib vaccine
- HPV vaccine
- Influenza vaccine
- Meningococcal vaccine.

11. Name four drugs useful in hypersensitive emergencies.

There are many classes of antihypertensives which lower blood pressure by different means. Among the most important and most widely used medications are thiazide diuretics, calcium channel blockers, ACE inhibitors, angiotensin II receptor antagonists (ARBs), and beta-blockers.

PATHOLOGY AND GENETICS

LONG ESSAYS

1. Define thrombosis; explain its causes and mechanism of formation in intravascular thrombosis.

Thrombosis: The formation or presence of a blood clot in a blood vessel. The vessel may be any vein or artery as, for example, in a deep vein thrombosis or a coronary (artery) thrombosis. The clot itself is termed a thrombus. If the clot breaks loose and travels through the bloodstream, it is a thromboembolism. Thrombosis, thrombus, and the prefix thrombo—all come from the Greek thrombos meaning a lump or clump, or a curd or clot of milk.

Types of Thrombi

Two different types of thrombus can form which differ in composition and appearance:
1. Arterial thrombus—typically composed of platelet aggregates (white thrombus)
2. Venous thrombus—largely consists of fibrin and red blood cells (red thrombus).

Propagation of the Platelet Thrombus

In short, thrombus formation is a dynamic process in which some platelets adhere to and others separate from the developing thrombus, and in which shear, flow, turbulence, and the number of platelets in the circulation greatly influence the architecture of the clot.

How thrombi develop? A thrombus can block the flow of blood through a vein or artery.
- If it detaches from the vessel wall and lodges in the lungs or other vital organs, it can become a life-threatening embolus
- The coagulation system depends on a delicate balance between:
  - Natural coagulant and anticoagulant factors
  - The coagulation and fibrinolytic system
- A pathological thrombus forms when there is an imbalance in the blood coagulation system leading to a number of serious health conditions including heart attacks and cardioembolic stroke in patients with AF, and VTE
- VTE can manifest as DVT and/or PE—two distinct but related aspects of the same disease.

Causes

Clotting occurs due to a series of chemical reactions between blood cells known as platelets and proteins called clotting factors. When a person is in good health, the body regulates the clotting process according to its needs. However, a clot can form more easily when a person:
1. Uses tobacco
2. Has high cholesterol
3. Has obesity or is overweight
4. Has cancer
5. Has diabetes
6. Is stressed
7. Has an inactive lifestyle.

Some of these factors also increase the risk of artherosclerosis, a condition wherein fatty plaque deposits line the blood vessels and clog them.

2. How do tumors spread in the body? Explain differences between Bengin and malignant neoplasams.

How do tumors spread in the body?

The place where a cancer starts in the body is called the primary cancer or primary site. Cells from the primary site may break away and spread to other parts of the body. These escaped cells can then grow and form other tumors which are known as secondary cancers or metastases.

Cancer cells can spread to other parts of the body through the bloodstream or lymphatic system. There they can start to grow into new tumors. Cancers are named according to where they first started developing. For example, if you have bowel cancer that has spread to the liver, it is called bowel cancer with liver metastases or secondaries. It is not called liver cancer. This is because the cancerous cells in the liver are actually cancerous bowel cells. They are not liver cells that have become cancerous.

Spread through the blood circulation: When the cancer cells go into small blood vessels they can then get into the bloodstream. They are called circulating tumor cells (or CTCs). The circulating blood sweeps the cancer cells along until they get stuck somewhere. Usually they get stuck in a very small blood vessel, such as a capillary.

Spread through the lymphatic system: The lymphatic system is a network of tubes and glands in the body that filters body fluid and fights infection. It also traps damaged or harmful cells, such as cancer cells. Cancer cells can go into the small lymph vessels close to the primary tumor and travel into nearby lymph glands. In the lymph glands, the cancer cells may be destroyed but some may survive and grow to form tumors in one or more lymph nodes. Doctors call this lymph node spread.

Micrometastases: Micrometastases are areas of cancer spread (metastases) that are too small to see. Some areas of cancer are too small to show up on any type of scan. For a few types of cancer, blood tests can detect certain proteins released by the cancer cells. These may give a sign that there are metastases in the body that are too small to show up on a scan. But for most cancers, there is no blood test that can say whether a cancer has spread or not.

SHORT ESSAYS

3. Describe wound healing.

The stages of wound healing proceed in an organized way and follow four processes: Hemostasis, inflammation, proliferation and maturation. Although the stages of wound healing are linear, wounds can progress backward or forward depending on internal and external patient conditions. The four stages of wound healing are (Fig. 2):

1. Hemostasis phase:

Hemostasis is the process of the wound being closed by clotting. Hemostasis starts when blood leaks out of the body. The first step of hemostasis is when blood vessels constrict to restrict the blood flow. Next, platelets stick together in order to seal the break in the wall of the blood vessel. Finally, coagulation occurs and reinforces the platelet plug with threads of fibrin which are like a molecular binding agent. The hemostasis stage of wound healing happens very quickly. The platelets adhere to the subendothelium surface within seconds of the rupture of a blood vessel's epithelial wall. After that, the first fibrin strands begin to adhere in about 60 seconds. As the fibrin mesh begins, the blood is transformed from liquid to gel through procoagulants and the release of prothrombin. The formation of a thrombus or clot keeps the platelets and blood cells trapped in the wound area. The thrombus is generally important in the stages of wound healing but becomes a problem if it detaches from the vessel wall and goes through the circulatory system, possibly causing a stroke, pulmonary embolism or heart attack.

2. Inflammatory phase:

Inflammation is the second stage of wound healing and begins right after the injury when the injured blood vessels leak transudate (made of water, salt, and protein) causing localized swelling. Inflammation both controls bleeding and prevents infection. The fluid engorgement allows healing and repair cells to move to the site of the wound. During the inflammatory phase, damaged cells, pathogens, and bacteria are removed from the wound area. These white blood cells, growth factors, nutrients and enzymes create the swelling, heat, pain and redness commonly seen during this stage of wound healing. Inflammation is a natural part of the wound healing process and only problematic if prolonged or excessive.

3. Proliferative phase:

The proliferative phase of wound healing is when the wound is rebuilt with new tissue made up of collagen and extracellular matrix. In the proliferative phase, the wound contracts as new tissues are built. In addition, a new network of blood vessels must be constructed so that the granulation tissue can be healthy and receive sufficient oxygen and nutrients. Myofibroblasts cause the wound to contract by gripping the wound edges and pulling them together using a mechanism similar to that of smooth muscle cells. In healthy stages of wound healing, granulation tissue is pink or red and uneven in texture. Moreover, healthy granulation tissue does not bleed easily. Dark granulation tissue can be a sign of infection, ischemia, or poor perfusion. In the final phase of the proliferative stage of wound healing, epithelial cells resurface the injury. It is important to remember that epithelialization happens faster when wounds are kept moist and hydrated. Generally, when occlusive or semiocclusive dressings are applied within 48 hours after injury, they will maintain correct tissue humidity to optimize epithelialization.

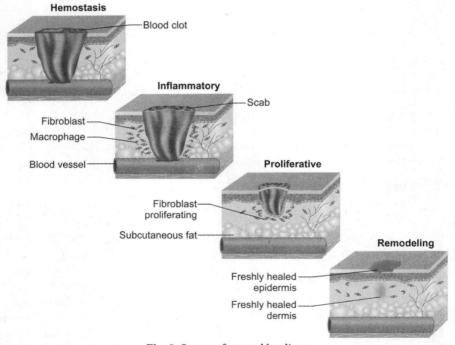

Fig. 2: Stages of wound healing.

4. Maturation phase:

Also called the remodeling stage of wound healing, the maturation phase is when collagen is remodeled from type III to type I and the wound fully closes. The cells that had been used to repair the wound but which are no longer needed are removed by apoptosis, or programed cell death. When collagen is laid down during the proliferative phase, it is disorganized and the wound is thick. During the maturation phase, collagen is aligned along tension lines and water is reabsorbed so the collagen fibers can lie closer together and cross-link. Cross-linking of collagen reduces scar thickness and also makes the skin area of the wound stronger. Generally, remodeling begins about 21 days after an injury and can continue for a year or more. Even with cross-linking, healed wound areas continue to be weaker than uninjured skin, generally only having 80% of the tensile strength of unwounded skin.

4. Explain etiopathology of renal calculi.

Kidney stones (renal lithiasis, nephrolithiasis) are hard deposits made of minerals and salts that form inside your kidneys. Urinary tract stone disease is likely caused by supersaturation of the urine by stone-forming constituents, including calcium, oxalate, and uric acid. Crystals or foreign bodies can act as nidi, upon which ions from the supersaturated urine form microscopic crystalline structures. The resulting calculi give rise to symptoms when they become impacted within the ureter as they pass toward the urinary bladder. The overwhelming majority of renal calculi contain calcium. Uric acid calculi and crystals of uric acid with or without other contaminating ions comprise the bulk of the remaining minority.

5. Describe lung abscess.

Lung abscess is a type of liquefactive necrosis of the lung tissue and formation of cavities (more than 2 cm) containing necrotic debris or fluid caused by microbial infection. This pus-filled cavity is often caused by aspiration which may occur during anesthesia, sedation, or unconsciousness from injury.

Lung abscess is defined as necrosis of the pulmonary tissue and formation of cavities containing necrotic debris or fluid caused by microbial infection. The formation of multiple small (<2 cm) abscesses is occasionally referred to as necrotizing pneumonia or lung gangrene. Both lung abscess and necrotizing pneumonia are manifestations of a similar pathologic process. Failure to recognize and treat lung abscess is associated with poor clinical outcome.

Symptoms of a lung abscess: The most noticeable symptom of a lung abscess is a productive cough. The contents that are coughed up may be bloody or pus-like with a foul odor.

Other symptoms include:
1. Bad breath
2. Fever of 101°F or higher
3. Chest pain
4. Shortness of breath
5. Sweating or night sweats
6. Weight loss
7. Fatigue.

Lung abscess treatment: The primary treatment for a lung abscess is antibiotics. Long-term use of medication might be necessary for up to 6 months. Lifestyle changes, such as not smoking and drinking more fluids may also be suggested. In some cases, more invasive procedures or surgery may be necessary. A tube can be inserted into the lungs to drain pus from the abscess, or a surgical procedure may be required to remove infected or damaged lung tissue.

6. How will you collect urine for routine examination culture, biological tests?

Urine specimen and culture: A urinalysis (UA), also known as routine and microscopy (R&M), is the physical, chemical, and microscopic examination of urine. It involves a number of tests to detect and measure various compounds that pass through the urine. It has been a useful tool of diagnosis since the earliest days of medicine. The color, density, and odor of urine can reveal much about the state of health of an individual.

Procedure
1. Instruct the patient to use the cotton ball or towelette to clean urethral area thoroughly to prevent external bacteria from entering the specimen.
2. Let the patient void into the container.
3. Label the specimen container with patient identifying information, and send to the lab immediately. A delay in examining the specimen may cause a false result when bacterial determinations are to be made.
4. Wash your hands and instruct the patient to do it as well.
5. Note that the sample was collected.

Midstream "Clean-Catch" Urine Specimen
Midstream "clean-catch" urine collection is the most common method of obtaining urine specimens from adults particularly men. This method allows a specimen which is not contaminated from external sources to be obtained without catheterization. It is important to follow the "clean-catch" protocol in order to have accurate results from an uncontaminated sample.

Purpose
The clean-catch urine method is used to prevent germs from the penis or vagina from getting into a urine sample. It is a method of collecting a urine sample for various tests including urinalysis, cytology, and urine culture.

Supplies and Equipment
- Sterile specimen cup
- Zephiran, a soap solution, or three antiseptic towelettes
- Three cotton balls (to use with zephiran or soap solution)
- Laboratory request form.

Preparations
Explain to the patient that this kind of urine collection involves first voiding approximately one-half of the urine into the toilet, urinal, or bedpan, then collecting a portion of midstream urine in a sterile container, and allowing the rest to be pass into the toilet. Discuss that this is done to detect the presence or absence of infecting organisms and therefore, must be free from contaminating matter that may be present on the external genital areas.

Procedure
For female patients:
1. Wash hands with soap and water.
2. Instruct the patient to clean perineal area with towelettes or cotton balls.
3. Tell the patient to separate folds of urinary opening with thumb and forefinger and clean inside with towelettes or cotton balls using downward strokes only; keep labia separated during urination.
4. Instruct the patient to void a small amount of urine into the toilet to rinse out the urethra, void the midstream urine into the specimen cup, and the last of the stream into the toilet. The midstream urine is considered to be bladder and kidney washings; the portion that the physician wants tested.
5. Fill out the laboratory request form completely, label the specimen container with patient identifying information, and send to the lab immediately. A delay in examining the specimen may cause a false result when bacterial determinations are to be made.

6. Wash your hands and instruct the patient to do it as well.
7. Note that the specimen was collected. Record any difficulties the patient had or if the urine had an abnormal appearance.

For male patients:
1. Wash hands with soap and water.
2. Instruct the patient to completely retract foreskin and cleanse penis with towelettes or cotton balls.
3. Instruct the patient to void a small amount of urine into the toilet to rinse out the urethra, void the midstream urine into the specimen cup, and the last of the stream into the toilet. The midstream urine is considered to be bladder and kidney washings; the portion that the physician wants tested.
4. Fill out the laboratory request form completely, label the specimen container with patient identifying information, and send to the lab immediately. A delay in examining the specimen may cause a false result when bacterial determinations are to be made.
5. Wash your hands and instruct the patient to do it as well.
6. Note that the specimen was collected. Record any difficulties the patient had or if the urine had an abnormal appearance.

SHORT ANSWERS

7. Mention any four structural aberrations.

Structural aberrations: They include: Deletions, duplications, inversions, ring formations, and translocations. Known disorders include Wolf-Hirschhorn syndrome which is caused by partial deletion of the short arm of chromosome 4; and Jacobsen syndrome, also called the terminal 11q deletion disorder.

8. List out any four causes of congenital anomalies.

Genetic or inherited causes include:
1. **Chromosomal defects:** Caused by too few or too many chromosomes, or problems in the structure of the chromosomes, such as Down syndrome and extra copy of chromosome 21 and sex chromosome abnormalities.
2. **Dominant inheritance:** When one parent (who may or may not have the disease) passes along a single faulty gene, such as achondroplasia and Marfan syndrome.
3. **Recessive inheritance:** When both parents, who do not have the disease, pass along the gene for the disease to the child, such as cystic fibrosis and Tay Sachs.

9. Types of neural tube defects.

Neural tube defects are birth defects of the brain, spine, or spinal cord. They happen in the first month of pregnancy, often before a woman even knows that she is pregnant. The two most common neural tube defects are spina bifida and anencephaly. In spina bifida, the fetal spinal column does not close completely. There is usually nerve damage that causes at least some paralysis of the legs. In anencephaly, most of the brain and skull do not develop. Babies with anencephaly are usually either stillborn or die shortly after birth. Another type of defect, Chiari malformation causes the brain tissue to extend into the spinal canal.

10. Define mutation.

Mutation: A permanent change, a structural alteration, in the DNA or RNA. In humans and many other organisms, mutations occur in DNA. However, in retroviruses like HIV, mutations occur in RNA which is the genetic material of retroviruses.

In most cases, such changes are neutral and have no effect or they are deleterious and cause harm, but occasionally a mutation can improve an organism's chance of surviving and of passing the beneficial change on to its descendants. Mutations are the necessary raw material of evolution. Mutations can be caused by many factors including environmental insults, such as radiation and mutagenic chemicals. Mutations are sometimes attributed to random chance events.

11. Define eugenics.

Eugenics: A pseudoscience with the stated aim of improving the genetic constitution of the human species by selective breeding. Eugenics is from a Greek word meaning 'normal genes.' The use of Albert Einstein's sperm to conceive a child by artificial insemination would represent an attempt at positive eugenics. The Nazis notoriously engaged in negative eugenics by genocide in World War II. It is important to note that no experiment in eugenics has ever been shown to result in measurable improvements in human health.

12. Mention four ethical issues in the role of nurse in genetic counseling.

Genetic counseling is provided in places where genetic tests are carried out. The process involves pretest counseling as well as post-test counseling to enable the individuals to face the situation and take appropriate decisions with the right frame of mind. Major ethical principles which govern the attitudes and actions of counselors include: Respect for patient autonomy, nonmaleficence, beneficence, or taking action to help benefit others and prevent harm, both physical and mental, and justice which requires that services be distributed fairly to those in need. Other moral issues include veracity, the duty to disclose information or to be truthful, and respect for patient confidentiality. Nondirective counseling, a hallmark of this profession, is in accordance with the principle of individual autonomy.

2016

Pharmacology, Pathology and Genetics

PHARMACOLOGY

LONG ESSAYS

1. Mention the different routes of drug administration with suitable examples. Write the advantages and disadvantages of intravenous route.
2. Classify various local anesthetic drugs. Write briefly about the pharmacology of lignocaine.

SHORT ESSAYS

3. Uses and adverse effects of adrenaline.
4. Radioactive iodine.
5. Pethidine.
6. Nitrates.
7. Succinylcholine.

SHORT ANSWERS

8. Mention one therapeutic use (clinical condition) and one important adverse effect of **streptomycin**.
9. Mention one therapeutic use (clinical condition) and one important adverse effect of **metoclopramide**.
10. Mention one therapeutic use (clinical condition) and one important adverse effect of **salbutamol**.
11. Mention one therapeutic use (clinical condition) and one important adverse effect of **ramipril**.

PATHOLOGY AND GENETICS

LONG ESSAYS

1. Define **inflammation.** Briefly describe the vascular changes in acute inflammation.
2. Define **cirrhosis of liver**. Mention the types and describe etiology and morphology of micronodular cirrhosis.

SHORT ESSAYS

3. Describe chemotaxis.
4. Explain lymphatic edema.
5. Describe dry gangrene.
6. Describe callus.

SHORT ESSAYS

7. Define karyotype.
8. Characteristics of autosomal recessive inheritance.
9. Effect of deficiency of **vitamin A and D** on fetal growth.
10. Name the **adverse effects of four commonly used drugs** on fetal growth and development.
11. Name the **noninvasive techniques** used for parental diagnosis.
12. Define **anencephaly.**

PHARMACOLOGY

LONG ESSAYS

1. Mention the different routes of drug administration with suitable examples. Write the advantages and disadvantages of intravenous route.

Drugs can be administered by many routes. The goal is to deliver the drug to the target organ or tissue, so it can exert its therapeutic effect. The nurse can deliver drugs by a number of routes. An understanding of possible methods to deliver a drug is required as part of using the drug for therapeutic benefit.

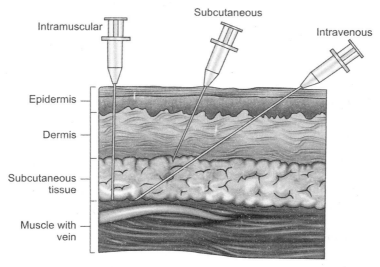

Routes of Administration

The route of a drug depends on its properties, desired effect, and the patient's physical and mental condition.

I. **Oral routes:**
1. Oral administration
2. Sublingual administration
3. Buccal administration.

II. **Parenteral routes:**
1. Subcutaneous
2. Intradermal
3. Intramuscular
4. Intravenous
5. Intrathecal
6. Intraosseous
7. Intraperitoneal
8. Intrapleural.

III. **Topical administration:** In this, drugs are applied to skin and mucous membrane.

Applications to Skin
1. By painting to skin
2. By spreading it over an area
3. Applying moist dressings
4. Soaking body parts in a solution
5. Giving medicated baths.

Route for Administration Time Until Effect
1. Intravenous—30–60 seconds
2. Intraosseous—30–60 seconds
3. Endotracheal—2–3 minutes
4. Inhalation—2–3 minutes
5. Sublingual—3–5 minutes
6. Intramuscular—10–20 minutes
7. Subcutaneous—15–30 minutes
8. Rectal—5–30 minutes
9. Ingestion—30–90 minutes
10. Transdermal (topical) variable (minutes to hours).

Routes of Drug Administration

Enteral

Enteral preparations are meant for administration into GI tract orally by nasogastric tube, gastrostomy tube, or intestinal tube. Absorption through GI tract is undependable for the following reasons: Liquids absorb more rapidly than solids. Absorption often diminished due to presence of food, and increased due to absence of food. Absorption is rapid in small intestine. Increased motility of ten decreases time available for absorption. When administered sublingually absorption takes place within 3–5 minutes.

Parenteral

Parenteral preparations are administered as: Intramuscular (TM) injections that are effective within 10–15 minutes, intravenous (IV) route of administration that has immediate effect (often given by continuous infusion system), subcutaneous (SC) injections that are effective within 10–15 minutes (often by insulin pumps), intradermal (ID) injection, epidural, intrathecal, intra-articular, intraosseous, intraperitoneal and intrapleural (administered often by access devices, such as mediports, port-a-caths, and Hickmans) administration. Poor circulation, shock, trauma, and edema may slow down absorption, in such situations massage and application of local heat increases drug absorption.

Topical

Topical administration through body surface parts, such as: Cornea, mucous membrane (e.g. rectal absorption, vaginal applications, buccal administration, nasal drops, sublingual medications, and eye and ear ointments), and skin (transdermal delivery system), e.g. creams, gels and ointments.

Local applications, such as lidocaine and epinephrine can have adverse systemic effects, whereas the systemic effect of local administration of a drug, such as nitroglycerine paste or patch will have beneficial effect in case of angina. Local application to damaged skin enhances systemic absorption.

Dense vascularity of vagina usually enhance drug absorption, similarly large vascular surface in the rectum facilitate rapid absorption of drugs, such as acetylsalicylic acid within 10–15 minutes.

Fecal matter in the sigmoid colon and hemorrhoids results in incomplete absorption of drug administered rectally.

Inhalants

Inhalants are systemically absorbed through the lungs, e.g. oxygen administration by nasal cannula and mask, inhalation of aerosols, and administration of general anesthesia. The large surface area of lungs (alveoli) enhances absorption and results can be expected within 2–3 minutes.

Injection

It is defined as the forcing of fluid into a cavity, a blood vessel, or body tissue through a hollow tube or needle.

Purposes of Injections

1. To get a rapid systemic effect of the drug.
2. To give drug when other routes are undesirable.
3. To obtain local effect at the site of injection.
4. To restore blood volume.
5. To give nourishment.

Advantages of Parenteral Injection

1. Rapidity and efficiency of absorption from the injection site when systemic action is desired.
2. Certainty of the amount absorbed is greater.
3. Medicines will not be destroyed by the digestive system and it will not irritate the digestive system.
4. Easy to administer to unconscious and critically ill patients.
5. Localization of medication at a specific site in the body, e.g. kidney dialysis.

Disadvantages of Parenteral Injections

1. Aseptic technique must be maintained during the preparation and administration of the drug.
2. Injection may be painful and cause infection at the site of injection.
3. It is possible for the needle to break off in the tissues.
4. An irritating or slowly absorbed drug may cause tissue necrosis, skin slough abscess and persistent pain.
5. Injury to nerve or vital structures.
6. It can easily cause anaphylaxis and adverse reactions, if care is not taken.
7. Psychic trauma.
8. Errors in administration of medicine.
9. Air embolism.
10. Pyrogenic reaction.
11. Serum hepatitis.
12. Circulatory overload.

Drugs and Fluids Commonly Injected

1. Hormones, minerals, vitamins and fluids.
2. Antibiotics, antitoxins, toxoids and vaccines.
3. Narcotics, sedatives, anesthetetics.

Administration of IV Medications

- Use of gloves and sterile techniques is mandatory while administering IV medications.

- Before starting infusion flush IV line and all ports with normal saline.
- Watch for signs of thrombophlebitis (inflammation of vein: Symptoms are redness, warmth, and pain), extravasation (leaking of fluid into the surrounding tissue: symptoms are edema, coolness, and decreased IV flow), and fluid overload (manifested as tachycardia, tachypnea, and pulmonary edema).
- Medication should never be pushed through the difficult or clogged IV line.
- Check the accuracy of flow.
- Peripheral site for IV should be rotated every 72 hours.
- Do not use filters for IV administration of insulin, nitroglycerine, amphotericin B, alteplase recombinant, lipids and total parenteral nutrition.
- Needle insertion site and IV cannula must be properly viewed at all times, for those reasons never tape them.

Golden Rules of Giving Injections

1. **Administer the right drug:** To prevent mistakes, take time to check the name and spelling of each drug you administer against the patient's medicine card. Check a drug, at least, twice before giving it. First, when you remove it from the stock cupboard and, second time, before administering it to the patient. Avoid distractions. If you are unfamiliar with the ordered drug, learn about the drug from the pharmacist and the doctor. When in doubt, clear the doubt from the doctor.
2. **Administer the drug to the right patient:** Make sure that the name of the patient is correct before you give the medicines. Check the name, diagnosis, and IP number. Adopt as a practice to confirm the right patient each time you administer the drug. Never leave a drug at the patient's bedside.
3. **Administer the right dose:** You must check and double check the drug dose ordered against the dose you are about to give. Be especially careful when you are administering toxic medications, such as antineoplastic drugs. With these, the margin between a therapeutic and a potentially lethal dose is slim. Use an infusion pump as indicated and monitor the patient closely especially after an initial or loading dose is given or any time a dose is increased.
4. **Administer the drug by the right route:** The parenteral route demands more vigilance. Parenteral drugs act so rapidly that a medication error may be very harmful—even fatal. If the order does not special route, call the doctor immediately for a clarification.
5. **Administer the drug at the right time:** Therapeutic blood levels of many drugs depend on consistent, regular administration times. Never give a drug more than half-an-hour before or after the scheduled time, without checking with the doctor. A hospital drug policy manual is one way to prevent errors associated with administration times. Make sure you coordinate drug administration with the laboratory schedule.
6. **Educate your patient about the drug he is receiving:** Take advantage of every opportunity to teach your patient and his family about his prescribed medication. Stress the need for consistent and timely administration. Make sure they understand the importance of taking the medications for the entire prescribed course. Many patients, who begin to feel better after the first few doses, stop taking the drug.
7. **Take patient's complete drug history:** It is necessary to know all the drugs your patient has been receiving and all the help he wants. By doing this you ensure his safety. The risk of adverse drug reactions and interactions, of course, rises with the number of drugs being taken.
8. **Find out if the patient has any drug allergies:** No drug is completely safe. Any drug may cause an unpredictable reaction producing many different adverse effects—some

appearing immediately, others developing over a period of time. Stay alert as you assess your patient's reaction to any drug you give him. Warn him that he should avoid drugs that have caused even a mild allergic response.

9. **Document each drug you administer:** Never document a drug before administering it, but document you must after it is administered.

2. Classify various local anesthetic drugs. Write briefly about the pharmacology of lignocaine.

An anesthetic drug (which can be given as a shot, spray, or ointment) numbs only a small, specific area of the body (for example, a foot, hand, or patch of skin). With local anesthesia, a person is awake or sedated, depending on what is needed. Local anesthesia lasts for a short period of time and is often used for minor outpatient procedures (when patients come in for surgery and can go home that same day). For someone having outpatient surgery in a clinic or doctor's office (such as the dentist or dermatologist), this is probably the type of anesthetic used. The medicine used can numb the area during the procedure and for a short time afterwards to help control postsurgery discomfort.

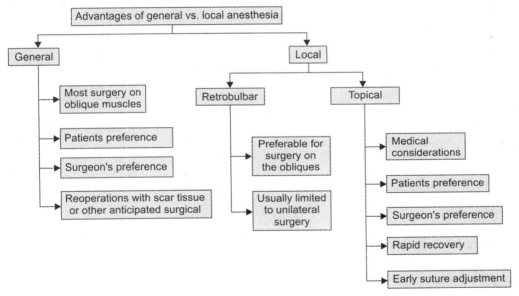

Chemical Structure

The basic chemical structure of a local anesthetic molecule consists of 3 parts:
1. Lipophilic group—an aromatic group, usually an unsaturated benzene ring.
2. Intermediate bond—a hydrocarbon connecting chain, either an ester (-CO-) or amide (-HNC-) linkage. The intermediate bond determines the classification of local anesthetic.
3. Hydrophilic group—a tertiary amine and proton acceptor.

Classifications

There are basically 2 classes of local anesthetics, the aminoamides (amide-ethers) and aminoesters (amine-esters). Some of these are available in many different formulations including topical sprays, patches, ointments and injections. Duration of action depends on the agent and formulation chosen. Compounds with local anesthetic properties may be classified according to their action upon the nerve membrane. Four classes of agent are recognized: A. Compounds acting at the exterior of the sodium channels; B. Compounds acting at the axoplasmic part of the sodium channels; C. Compounds acting through a physicochemical mechanism; BC. Compounds acting by a combination of B and C mechanisms. The chemical basis for these different mechanisms is discussed.

XYLOCAINE

Lignocaine (Lidocaine hydrochloride, Xylocaine)

Infiltration, nerve block and topical anesthesia. It is more potent than procaine. Onset of action is quick. It possesses high degree of penetration. For infiltration anesthesia into 2% is used. Duration is longer and depth is more than procaine. It is less toxic. It has surface anesthetic action also.

Side effects: Myocardial depression, hypotension, drowsiness instead of excitement, tremor, respiratory arrest.

Uses

Infiltration, topical and block anesthesia, arrhythmia, myocardial infarction (IV drip).

Pharmacokinetics

1. Initially distributes rapidly into a smaller "central compartment" that includes the heart, lung, liver, kidney and brain when given IV.
2. Lidocaine then distributes into peripheral tissues (e.g. skeletal muscle and fat) with a time course having a half life of 8 minutes.
3. Lidocaine's total volume of distribution is 1.1 L/kg (77 liters in a 70 kg patient)
4. Loading doses cannot be given as a single bolus because toxicity will occur due to high drug levels achieved in the central compartment.
5. Elimination half life from the body is 90–110 minutes.
6. The time to achieve 90% of the steady-state drug level with continuous dosing is 3.3 elimination half-lives (e.g. 5 hours for lidocaine).
7. CHF: reduces lidocaine clearance due to poor liver perfusion, typically requiring a 1/2 reduction of infusion rates to maintain the same steady state plasma level.
8. Liver disease can also reduce lidocaine clearance.

Untoward effects

These are related to overdose that includes lightheadedness, tinnitus, metallic taste, blurred vision, numbness, twitching, convulsions, and hypotension.

SHORT ESSAYS

3. Uses and adverse effects of adrenaline.

Adrenalin® (epinephrine, USP) Injection is a clear, colorless, sterile solution containing 1 mg/mL (1:1,000) epinephrine in a 3 mL clear glass vial. Each 1 mL of Adrenalin® solution contains 1 mg epinephrine, 9.0 mg sodium chloride, 1.0 mg sodium metabisulfite, hydrochloric acid to adjust pH, and water for injection. The pH range is 2.2–5.0.

Therapeutic Uses

Epinephrine is used to control hemorrhage from minor cuts, but it is not effective when a vein or artery is involved. It relieves nasal congestion by vasoconstriction for a short duration. It is used in conjunction with local anesthetics to prolong their action and to lessen the possibility of hemorrhage.

Epinephrine is valuable in treating bronchial asthma, as an injection or by inhalation. It is also used frequently to relieve such allergic disorders as urticaria, serum reactions, and anaphylactic shock, for which epinephrine is the most often used drug. Certainheart failures can be corrected by injecting epinephrine directly into the heart. However, epinephrine is not of much value in the treatment of hemorrhagic.

Cardiogenic or traumatic shock or circulatory collapse, and it may be harmful.

Action and Uses

Ephedrine occurs naturally in various plants. This drug is very similar to epinephrine in its action. The administration of ephedrine results in vasoconstriction and stimulation of the heart that produces an elevation of blood pressure. Although this effect upon the blood pressure is not as great as that produced by the administration of epinephrine, it lasts seven to 10 times as long. The use of ephedrine produces relaxation of bronchial muscles that is less prominent than that obtained with epinephrine, but is sustained for a much longer time.

4. Radioactive iodine.

Radioactive iodine (commonly called radioiodine) is a form of iodine chemically identical to nonradioactive iodine. Therefore, the thyroid gland, which takes up iodine to make thyroid hormone, cannot distinguish between the two. However, the nucleus of a radioactive iodine molecule has excess energy and gives off radiation that can have effects on the cells in which it is concentrated.

Radioactive iodine treatment of hyperthyroidism makes use of the thyroid glands natural need for iodine to make thyroid hormone. The thyroid is the only part of the body that collects and retains iodine. In hyperthyroidism, the thyroid cells are overstimulated and make larger amounts of thyroid hormone. The excess amount of hormones is secreted into the blood, and produces the symptoms of hyperthyroidism. When radioiodine is given, the thyroid gland cannot tell if the iodine is radioactive or not, and collects it in the normal way in proportion to the activity of the thyroid. Radioiodine thus accumulates in the cells that make thyroid hormone and remains there long enough to radiate the gland and to slow thyroid production. Radioiodine that is not retained by the thyroid gland is secreted rapidly by the body (within 2 or 3 days), primarily through the kidneys into the urine.

5. Pethidine.

Pethidine, an opioid used to control pain, is sold under the brand name Demerol. Not as popular as it once was, pethidine can be a useful medication, but it also can cause serious side effects. Pethidine consists of an active ingredient known as pethidine hydrochloride. This agent belongs to a group of medicine known as narcotic analgesics (opioid pain-relievers). Pethidine acts on specific opioid receptors in the brain, blocking the delivery of pain messages. In doing so, pethidine decreases the brain's awareness of the pain, thus providing pain relief.

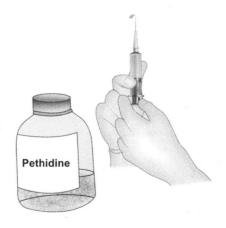

Pethidine consists of an active ingredient known as pethidine hydrochloride. This agent belongs to a group of medicine known as narcotic analgesics (opioid pain-relievers). Pethidine acts on specific opioid receptors in the brain, blocking the delivery of pain messages. In doing so, pethidine decreases the brain's awareness of the pain, thus providing pain relief.

Side Effects

Constipation, nausea, vomiting, headache, drowsiness, confusion, rash or skin irritation, dry mouth, dizziness, fatigue or weakness, small pupils, sweating, increased feelings of well-being, changes in urination, hallucinations, blushing of the face, low blood pressure and feeling cold are all side effects of pethidine.

Other Medications

Drowsiness is a common side effect of pethidine. This side effect will be increased when pethidine is combined with alcohol, antipsychotics, barbiturates, benzodiazepines, anti-epileptics, morphine, codeine, antihistamines, sleeping pills and antidepressants.

Pregnancy: Pethidine is sometimes given to pregnant women during labor to relieve pain. However, this can cause side effects in the baby, such as trouble breathing and drowsiness. Pethidine can also diminish a baby's sucking reflex, making nursing difficult.

Allergic reactions: Allergic reactions to pethidine include swelling of the throat, mouth, lips and tongue, hives or a rash and difficulty breathing. These side effects should be brought to the attention of a doctor.

Severe Side Effects

Fainting, chest pain, difficulty breathing, irregular heartbeat, moodiness, numbness of the limbs, tremor, vision changes, severe dizziness and headache are all considered serious side effects of pethidine. Anyone experiencing these side effects should consult a medical professional.

Nurse Responsibility

1. Check for the written and fully signed order of the registered medical practioner in administering pethidine for the patient.
2. Check the six rights of medication administration.
3. Double check with another registered nurse for accurate dosage and site.
4. Document the patient condition including vital signs and levels of consciousness before administration.
5. Always administer the drug in presence of another registered nurse.
6. Monitor vital signs and pain level 15 minutes after pethidine administration.
7. Check for all possible side effects and complications of the drug.
8. Document in the drug chart and nurses record.
9. Information supervisor or registered medical officer in case of any abnormal drug reactions and document it.
10. Enter in the ward stock book the total number of pethidine remaining.

6. Nitrates.

Oral nitrates: Oral nitrates have a longer-lasting effect than sublingual NTG, and are equally effective in controlling angina on a chronic basis. Oral nitrates are available in two forms: Isosorbide dinitrate (ISDN) and isosorbide-5-mononitrate (5-ISMN).

Isosorbide Dinitrate

Isosoribide dinitrate, often taken two or three times per day, begins acting within 15–30 minutes and lasts for 3 to 6 hours. ISDN allows you to exercise for upto 8 hours. The body tends to develop a tolerance (decreased sensitivity) to ISDN when it is used continuously over 24 hours, but a carefully planned dose schedule may prevent this problem.

Isosorbide-5-mononitrate

5-ISMN usually begins acting within 30 minutes and its effects last 6–8 hours. The body tends to develop a tolerance (decreased sensitivity) to ISMN when it is used continuously over 24 hours. A carefully planned dose schedule and use of extended release forms of ISMN may prevent this problem. The extended release form of ISMN is taken only once per day.

Transdermal Nitroglycerin

Transdermal NTG (NTG patch) is a convenient type of long-lasting nitrate treatment. These patches deliver a constant dose of NTG. Transdermal NTG begins acting within 30 minutes and its effects last for 8–14 hours. Wearing a patch continuously leads to tolerance, so patches must be removed each day to allow for a "nitrate-free" interval. Since most people experience angina with activity, the patch is usually applied in the morning and removed in the evening. In contrast, people who have nocturnal (night-time) angina should apply the patches at night and remove them in the morning.

Nitrates and Tolerance

Continuous nitrate treatment leads to tolerance of the drug within 24–48 hours; at this time, normal doses of nitrates are no longer effective. Tolerance is a problem with long-acting nitrates (oral and transdermal nitrates), which is why a nitrate-free interval is necessary. Nitrate tolerance does not usually develop with sublingual NTG.

The best way to avoid tolerance is to use long-acting nitrates intermittently, by scheduling 8–12 hour nitrate-free breaks, frequently done during periods of sleep. Some people notice that angina worsens during this nitrate-free period, which is a phenomenon called rebound angina. This can be treated by increasing the dose of other drugs. Several medications and antioxidant vitamins are being evaluated for their ability to prevent nitrate tolerance; however, they are still investigational and they are not yet widely available.

Timing of Nitrates

People who have stress or exertional angina (angina during activity or exercise) are usually advised to take nitrates during the day, whereas people with nighttime angina or heart failure are usually advised to take nitrates in the evening. Nitrates may alleviate certain nighttime symptoms of heart failure, such as shortness of breath when lying down or waking up breathless in the middle of the night.

Side Effects

The most common side effects of nitrates are headache, lightheadedness, flushing, and an increase in heart rate. Elderly people are often susceptible to lightheadedness and should be especially careful in hot weather. Alcohol may also worsen dizziness and lightheadedness.

Nitrates can also cause a decrease in blood pressure and may cause some people to faint (especially when other medications that lower blood pressure are being used or the patient is dehydrated). Paradoxically, nitrates can worsen angina in some people. These side effects tend to improve over time, but it is still important to discuss any side effects you are having with your healthcare provider. The combination of nitrates and medications for erectile dysfunction (e.g. Viagra®, Cialis®, Levitra®) is particularly hazardous. Erectile dysfunction medications **must be avoided** while taking a nitrate medication (short or long-acting). If you take nitrates and are considering treatment for erectile dysfunction, speak with your healthcare provider.

7. Succinylcholine.

Relaxing muscles during surgery or when using a breathing machine (ventilator). It is also used to induce anesthesia or when a tube must be inserted in the windpipe. It may also be used for other conditions as determined by your doctor. Succinylcholine is a depolarizing muscle relaxant. It works by keeping muscles from contracting, which causes paralysis of the muscles in the face and those used to breathe and move.

Mechanism of Action

Depolarizing drugs are agonists at ACh receptors. Succinylcholine is the only depolarizing NMBD in clinical use. It is effectively two ACh molecules joined through the acetate methyl groups. The two quaternary ammonium radicals bind to the two α-subunits of one nicotinic receptor, and depolarization occurs.

Side Effects

The following additional adverse reactions have been reported: cardiac arrest, malignant hyperthermia, arrhythmias, bradycardia, tachycardia, hypertension, hypotension, hyperkalemia, prolonged respiratory depression or apnea, increased intraocular pressure, muscle fasciculation, jaw rigidity, postoperative muscle pain,

Contraindications

It is also contraindicated in patients after the acute phase of injury following major burns, multiple trauma, extensive denervation of skeletal muscle, or upper motor neuron injury, because succinylcholine administered to such individuals may result in severe hyperkalemia which may result in cardiac arrest.

Adverse Effects

The following additional adverse reactions have been reported: Cardiac arrest, malignant hyperthermia, arrhythmias, bradycardia, tachycardia, hypertension, hypotension, hyperkalemia, prolonged respiratory depression or apnea, increased intraocular pressure, muscle fasciculation, jaw rigidity, postoperative muscle pain.

SHORT ANSWERS

8. Mention one therapeutic use (clinical condition) and one important adverse effect of streptomycin.

Streptomycin is an aminoglycoside antibiotic used with other medications to treat active tuberculosis (TB) infection if you cannot take other drugs for TB or if you have a type of TB that cannot be treated with other drugs (drug-resistant TB). Common side effects of streptomycin include nausea, vomiting, stomach upset, loss of appetite, spinning sensation (vertigo), injection site reactions (pain, irritation, and redness), tingling or prickling sensation in the face, rash, fever, hives, and swelling (edema).

Therapeutic Uses

Streptomycin is an antibiotic (antimycobacterial) drug, the first of a class of drugs called aminoglycosides to be discovered, and it was the first effective treatment for tuberculosis. It is derived from the actinobacterium *Streptomyces griseus*. Streptomycin is a bactericidal antibiotic.

Adverse Effects

Common side effects of streptomycin have included vestibular toxicity (nausea, vomiting, vertigo), paresthesia of the face, rash, fever, urticaria, angioneurotic edema, and eosinophilia. Side effects may be more likely and more severe in patients with underlying renal insufficiency.

9. Mention one therapeutic use (clinical condition) and one important adverse effect of metoclopramide.

Metoclopramide increases muscle contractions in the upper digestive tract. This speeds up the rate at which the stomach empties into the intestines. Metoclopramide is used short-term to treat heartburn caused by gastroesophageal reflux in people who have used other medications without relief of symptoms. Metoclopramide is also used to treat slow gastric emptying in people with diabetes (also called diabetic gastroparesis), which can cause nausea, vomiting, heartburn, loss of appetite, and a feeling of fullness after meals.

Therapeutic Uses

It works by increasing the movements or contractions of the stomach and intestines. It relieves symptoms such as nausea, vomiting, heartburn, a feeling of fullness after meals, and loss of appetite. Metoclopramide is also used to treat heartburn for patients with gastroesophageal reflux disease (GERD).

Adverse effects: Reglan is available in the generic form as metoclopramide. Common side effects of Reglan are decreased energy, diarrhea, dizziness, drowsiness, headache, nausea, vomiting, restlessness, malaise, trouble sleeping (insomnia), breast tenderness or swelling, changes in your menstrual periods, or urinating more than usual.

10. Mention one therapeutic use (clinical condition) and one important adverse effect of salbutamol.

Salbutamol is a short-acting, selective beta 2-adrenergic receptor agonist used in the treatment of asthma and COPD. It is 29 times more selective for beta 2 receptors than beta1 receptors giving it higher specificity for pulmonary beta receptors versus beta 1-adrenergic receptors located in the heart. Salbutamol is formulated as a racemic mixture of the R- and S-isomers. The R-isomer has 150 times greater affinity for the beta 2-receptor than the S-isomer and the S-isomer has been associated with toxicity. This lead to the development of levalbuterol, the single R-isomer of salbutamol. However, the high cost of levalbuterol compared to salbutamol has deterred wide-spread use of this enantiomerically pure version of the drug. Salbutamol is generally used for acute episodes of bronchospasm caused by bronchial asthma, chronic bronchitis and other chronic bronchopulmonary disorders, such as chronic obstructive pulmonary disorder (COPD). It is also used prophylactically for exercise-induced asthma.

Salbutamol Uses

Salbutamol is used to treat a number of problems.

It is a member of the class of drugs called short-acting beta-2 agonists and is sometimes called albuterol.

In general, this drug is used for the relief of asthma symptoms as it produces rapid, short-term dilation of the airways (termed bronchodilation), but it can also be used to delay delivery in women undergoing premature labor.

Benefits of being on this drug can include short-term symptoms relief of asthma and other conditions similar to asthma such as chest tightness, wheezing and coughing, the prevention of asthma symptoms brought on by exercise or by an unavoidable exposure to a known allergen, and the temporary delay in the delivery of premature babies. Symptomatic treatment of asthma attacks and symptoms relief of conditions associated with reversible airways obstruction.

Prevention of bronchospasm (tightening of the wind pipe causing difficulty in breathing) which can be brought on by exercise or by an unavoidable exposure to a known allergen.

11. Mention one therapeutic use (clinical condition) and one important adverse effect of ramipril.

Ramipril (Altace) is an ACE inhibitor. ACE stands for angiotensin converting enzyme. Ramipril are used to treat high blood pressure (hypertension) or congestive heart failure, and to improve survival after a heart attack. Ramipril (Altace) is an ACE inhibitor. ACE stands for angiotensin converting enzyme. Ramipril is used to treat high blood pressure (hypertension) or congestive heart failure, and to improve survival after a heart attack. Ramipril may also be used for purposes not listed in this medication guide.

Adverse Effects

High potassium level (slow heart rate, weak pulse, muscle weakness, tingly feeling; dry mouth, thirst, confusion, swelling, and urinating less than usual or not at all; pale skin, dark colored urine, easy bruising or bleeding; jaundice (yellowing of the skin or eyes).

The acute inflammatory response—vascular changes: When tissue is first injured, the small blood vessels in the damaged area constrict momentarily, a process called vasoconstriction. Following this transient event, which is believed to be of little importance to the inflammatory response, the blood vessels dilate (vasodilatation), increasing blood flow into the area. Vasodilatation may last from 15 minutes to several hours. Next, the walls of the blood vessels, which normally allow only water and salts to pass through easily, become more permeable. Protein-rich fluid, called exudate, is now able to exit into the tissues.

Substances in the exudate include clotting factors, which help prevent the spread of infectious agents throughout the body. Other proteins include antibodies that help destroy invading microorganisms. As fluid and other substances leak out of the blood vessels, blood flow becomes more sluggish and white blood cells begin to fall out of the axial stream in the center of the vessel to flow nearer the vessel wall. The white blood cells then adhere to the blood vessel wall, the first step in their emigration into the extravascular space of the tissue.

PATHOLOGY AND GENETICS

LONG ESSAYS

1. Define inflammation. Briefly describe the vascular changes in acute inflammation.

The word **inflammation** comes from the Latin *"inflammo"*, meaning *"I set alight, I ignite"*. Inflammation is part of the body's immune response. Initially, it is beneficial when, for example, your knee sustains a blow and tissues need care and protection. However, sometimes inflammation can cause further inflammation; it can become self-perpetuating. More inflammation is created in response to the existing inflammation.

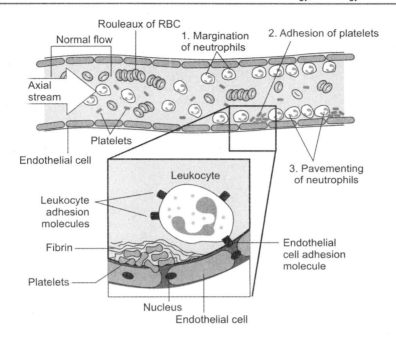

Acute inflammation is the early (almost immediate) response of a tissue to injury. It is nonspecific and may be evoked by any injury short of one that is immediately lethal. Acute inflammation may be regarded as the first line of defense against injury and is characterized by changes in the microcirculation: Exudation of fluid and emigration of leukocytes from blood vessels to the area of injury. Acute inflammation is typically of short duration, occurring before the immune response becomes established, and it is aimed primarily at removing the injurious agent. Until the late 18th century, acute inflammation was regarded as a disease. John Hunter (1728–1793, London surgeon and anatomist) was the first to realize that acute inflammation was a response to injury that was generally beneficial to the host: "But if inflammation develops, regardless of the cause, still it is an effort whose purpose is to restore the parts to their natural functions." Clinically, acute inflammation is characterized by 5 cardinal signs: **rubor** (redness), **calor** (increased heat), **tumor** (swelling), **dolor** (pain), and **functio laesa** (loss of function). The first four were described by Celsus (ca 30 BC–38 AD); the fifth was a later addition by Virchow in the nineteenth century. Redness and heat are due to increased blood flow to the inflamed area; swelling is due to accumulation of fluid; pain is due to release of chemicals that stimulate nerve endings; and loss of function is due to a combination of factors. These signs are manifested when acute inflammation occurs on the surface of the body, but not all of them will be apparent in acute inflammation of internal organs. Pain occurs only when there are appropriate sensory nerve endings in the inflamed site—for example, acute inflammation of the lung (pneumonia) does not cause pain unless the inflammation involves the parietal pleura, where there are pain-sensitive nerve endings. The increased heat of inflamed skin is due to the entry of a large amount of blood at body core temperature into the normally cooler skin. When inflammation occurs internally—where tissue is normally at body core temperature—no increase in heat is apparent.

Etiology

Physical agents—extreme temperatures, electric shock, radiation, mechanical injures, etc.
Chemical agents—products of metabolism, acids, alkalis, drugs, tissue necrosis
Biological agents—microorganisms (bacteria, viruses, fungi), parasites (helmints, insects), immune cells and complexes.

Classification

According to the course
- Acute
- Subacute
- Chronic.

According to the predominant phase
- Alterative
- Exudative
- Proliferative (productive).

According to the causative factors
- Trivial
- Specific.

Acute Inflammation

1. Lasts from several days up to several months.
2. In the focus of inflammation—neutrophils, intravascular platelet activation.
3. Exudative inflammation and rarely observed productive (viruses).

Subacute Inflammation

1. Lasts from several weeks up to several months.
2. In the focus of inflammation—neutrophils, lymphocytes, plasmocytes, macrophages (approximately in equal proportions).
3. Exudative—productive inflammation.

Chronic Inflammation

1. Lasts from a few months up to tens of years.
2. Alternating exacerbations and remissions.
3. In the focus of inflammation—mononuclear cells (lymphocytes, plasmocytes, and macrophages), in case of exacerbations neutrophils are added.
4. Productive inflammation, during exacerbations an exudative reaction is added.

Acute Inflammatory Response

Inflammation is a common response to tissue injury or infection. Acute inflammation develops quickly and resolves within days, whereas chronic inflammation can last for months or years, usually because of the persistence of the initiating factor. The histological appearance of acute inflammation is quite different from chronic inflammation and the distinctive features can point to the initiating agent. For example, an infection of the skin with *Staphylococcus aureus* usually produces an acute inflammatory response, whereas infection with *Mycobacterium leprae* (leprosy) typically produces persistent infection and chronic inflammation.

There are three main components of inflammation:
1. An increase in the blood supply to the affected area, caused by dilation of arterioles supplying the area.

2. An increase in the permeability of capillaries, which allows larger serum molecules such as antibodies to enter the tissue.
3. Migration of leukocytes from the blood into the tissues—the cells cross the endothelial cells, which line the venules, and then move out into the tissue. This process is mediated by signalling molecules called chemokines, which are bound to the endothelial surface.

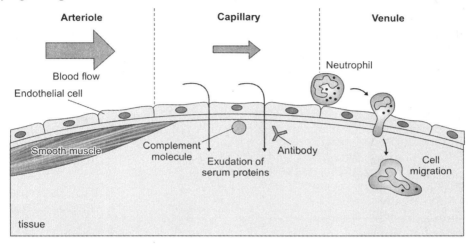

Figure: The three main features of inflammation are controlled at different places in the vasculature. The diagram shows a longitudinal section through an arteriole, capillary and venule. Smooth muscle in the arterioles controls blood flow into the site of inflammation. Exudation of serum molecules occurs in capillaries as endothelial cells retract in response to inflammatory mediators. This allows antibodies and molecules of the complement system to enter the site of inflammation. Migration of leukocytes takes place in venules, partly because the shear force is lowest in venules and partly because signalling molecules are present on the endothelium of the venules which attract leukocytes at this point. All of these processes bring the defense systems of the body to the affected area. The blood contains a number of proteins that stop bleeding, help clear infection and induce repair or regeneration of the tissues. It also contains different types of leukocyte (white blood cells), each of which has evolved to deal with different types of infection. One of the key histological differences between acute and chronic inflammation is seen in the sets of leukocytes that are present in the tissues. In acute inflammation polymorphonuclear neutrophils usually predominate, whereas macrophages and lymphocytes predominate in chronic inflammation. Eosinophils are often prevalent in sites of helminth infections. Hence, the characteristics of inflammation are determined both by the tissue in which it occurs and by the initiating agent and its persistence.

2. Define cirrhosis of liver. Mention the types and describe etiology and morphology of micronodular cirrhosis.

Cirrhosis is the 12th leading cause of death in the United States, according to the National Institute of Diabetes and Digestive and Kidney Diseases. Because of chronic damage to the liver, scar tissue slowly replaces normal functioning liver tissue, progressively diminishing blood flow through the liver. As the normal liver tissue is lost, nutrients, hormones, drugs, and poisons are not processed effectively by the liver. In addition, protein production and other substances produced by the liver are inhibited.

Causes Cirrhosis
The most common cause of cirrhosis is alcohol abuse. Other causes include:
1. Hepatitis and other viruses.

2. Use of certain drugs.
3. Chemical exposure.
4. Bile duct obstruction.
5. Autoimmune diseases.
6. Obstruction of outflow of blood from the liver (for example, Budd-Chiari syndrome).
7. Heart and blood vessel disturbances.
8. Alpha1-antitrypsin deficiency.
9. High blood galactose levels.
10. High blood tyrosine levels at birth.
11. Glycogen storage disease.
12. Cystic fibrosis.
13. Diabetes.
14. Malnutrition.
15. Hereditary accumulation of too much copper (Wilson disease) or iron (hemochromatosis).

In addition to a complete medical history and physical examination, diagnostic procedures for cirrhosis may include:

Diagnostic Evaluation

1. **Laboratory tests.**
2. **Liver function tests:** A series of special blood tests that can determine if the liver is functioning properly.
3. **Liver biopsy:** A procedure in which tissue samples from the liver are removed (with a needle or during surgery) for examination under a microscope.
4. **Cholangiography:** X-ray examination of the bile ducts using an intravenous (IV) dye (contrast).
5. **Computed tomography scan (CT or CAT scan):** A diagnostic imaging procedure using a combination of X-rays and computer technology to produce horizontal, or axial, images (often called slices) of the body. A CT scan shows detailed images of any part of the body including the bones, muscles, fat, and organs. CT scans are more detailed than general X-rays.
6. **Ultrasound (also called sonography):** A diagnostic imaging technique, which uses high-frequency sound waves and a computer to create images of blood vessels, tissues, and organs. Ultrasounds are used to view internal organs of the abdomen, such as the liver, spleen, and kidneys and to assess blood flow through various vessels.

Pathogenesis of Alcoholic Liver Diseases

The pathogenesis of liver disease associated with alcohol ingestion is incompletely understood. What is known is that some patients who chronically abuse alcohol develop liver disease, primarily because the liver metabolizes the majority of ingested ethanol. Furthermore, the metabolism of ethanol is required for hepatic injury to occur, although variations in ethanol metabolism do not completely explain the variable susceptibility to alcoholic liver disease.

This topic review will focus on three issues related to the development of alcoholic liver disease:
- The basic aspects of alcohol metabolism
- The mechanisms that may be responsible for the development of hepatic disease
- The factors that determine the frequency with which alcohol abuse leads to liver disease
- The different pathologic types of alcoholic liver disease are discussed separately.

SHORT ESSAYS

3. Describe chemotaxis.

During chemotaxis, cells move in response to chemical signals. The action of neutrophils is just one example of how the body uses chemotaxis to respond to an infection. Aside from the cells that are already in position in the tissues (such as the fixed tissue macrophages and mast cells, neutrophils) are the first responders to inflammation.

Chemotaxis refers to the unidirectional movement of a cell in response to a chemical gradient. Leukocytes move from a low to a high concentration of chemoattractant. In the absence of a gradient, chemotactic factors increase the random motion of leukocytes. This has been termed chemokinesis. The directed migration, or chemotaxis, of immune cells is an essential feature of the immune system. It is necessary for the development and homeostatic trafficking of immune cells and for orchestrating the juxtaposition of immune cells and antigen necessary to generate long-lasting antigen specific immunity. Chemotaxis also plays an essential role in the recruitment of leukocytes into sites of inflammation and infection.

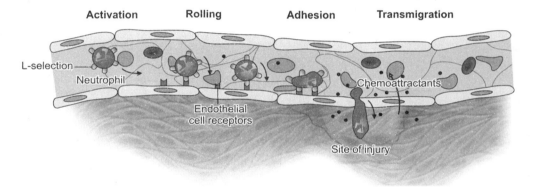

4. Explain lymphatic edema.

Lymphatic edema or lymphatic obstruction is a chronic (long-term) condition in which excess fluid (lymph) collects in tissues causing edema (swelling). Lymphedema can be very debilitating. In short, lymphedema is edema due to lymphatic fluid; a blockage of the lymphatic system. The lymphatic system is an important part of our immune and circulatory systems.

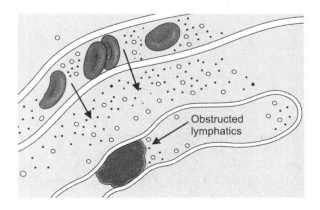

Lymphedema commonly affects one of the arms or legs. In some cases, both arms and both legs may be affected. Some patients may experience swelling in the head, genitals or chest. It is often a consequence of surgically removing the lymph nodes in the armpit (axilla) or groin, or their damage caused by radiography. The normal drainage of lymphatic fluid is faulty. Lymphedema can also be caused by a tumor which presses on lymphatic vessels.

Symptoms of Lymphedema

People with lymphedema in their arm or leg may experience the following symptoms:
1. Swelling that begins in the arm or leg.
2. A heavy feeling in the arm or leg.
3. Weakness or decreased flexibility.
4. Rings, watches, or clothes that become too tight.
5. Discomfort or pain.
6. Tight, shiny, warm, or red skin.

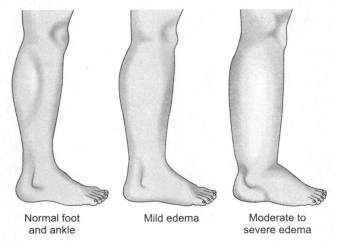

Normal foot and ankle   Mild edema   Moderate to severe edema

7. Skin that does not indent at all when pressed, or hardened skin.
8. Thicker skin.
9. Skin that may look like an orange peel (swollen with small indentations).
10. Small warts or blisters that leak clear fluid.

Symptoms of head and neck lymphedema include:
1. Swelling of the eyes, face, lips, neck, or area below the chin.
2. Discomfort or tightness in any of the affected areas.
3. Difficulty moving the neck, jaw, or shoulders.
4. Scarring (fibrosis) of the neck and facial skin.
5. Decreased vision because of swollen eyelids.
6. Difficulty swallowing, speaking, or breathing.
7. Drooling or loss of food from the mouth while eating.
8. Nasal congestion or long-lasting middle ear pain, if swelling is severe.

Symptoms of lymphedema may begin very gradually and are not always easy to detect. Sometimes, the only symptoms may be heaviness or aching in an arm or leg. But sometimes, lymphedema may begin more suddenly. If you develop any symptoms of lymphedema, talk with your doctor as soon as possible. You will need to learn how to manage them, so they do not get worse. Because swelling may be a sign of cancer, it is also important to see your doctor to be sure the cancer has not come back.

Causes of Lymphedema

Lymphedema is usually a predictable long-term side effect of some cancer treatments. The most common causes of lymphedema in cancer survivors include:
1. Surgery in which lymph nodes were removed. For example, surgery for breast cancer often involves the removal of one or more nearby lymph nodes to check for cancer. And this can cause lymphedema to develop in the arm.
2. Radiation therapy or other causes of inflammation or scarring in the lymph nodes and vessels.
3. Blockage of the lymph nodes and/or vessels by the cancer.

The risk of lymphedema increases with the number of lymph nodes and vessels removed or damaged during cancer treatment or biopsies. Sometimes, lymphedema is not related to cancer or its treatment. For instance, a bacterial or fungal infection or another disease involving the lymphatic system may cause this problem.

Stages of Lymphedema

Doctors describe lymphedema according to its stage, from mild to severe:

Stage 0: Swelling is not yet visible even though damage to the lymphatic system has already occurred. Most people do not have any symptoms at this stage. And it may exist months or even years before swelling occurs.

Stage I: The skin indents when it is pressed, and there is no visible evidence of scarring. Elevating the affected limb often helps reduce the swelling.

Stage II: The skin does not indent when it is pressed, and there is moderate to severe scarring. Elevating the affected limb does not help the swelling.

Stage III: The skin has hardened, the affected body part has swollen in size and volume, and the skin has changed texture. Stage III lymphedema is permanent.

Managing and Treating Lymphedema

Relieving side effects is an important part of cancer care and treatment. This is called symptom management or palliative care. Talk with a member of your healthcare team about any lymphedema symptoms you experience, so you can begin treatment as soon as possible. This should include any new symptoms or a change in symptoms. Treatments for lymphedema are designed to reduce swelling, prevent it from getting worse, prevent infection, improve the appearance of the affected body part, and improve the person's ability to function. Although treatment is able to control lymphedema, there is currently no cure. You may want to ask your doctor to recommend a certified lymphedema therapist (CLT). A CLT is a health professional who specializes in managing lymphedema. The therapist can assess your condition and develop a treatment plan which may include:

Manual Lymphatic Drainage

Manual lymphatic drainage (MLD) is a specialized technique that involves a type of gentle skin massage to help blocked lymphatic fluid drain properly into the bloodstream. This may help reduce swelling. For best results, you should begin MLD treatments as close to the start of lymphedema as possible. A member of your healthcare team can refer you to a CLT trained in this technique.

Exercise

Exercising usually improves the flow of the lymphatic system and strengthens muscles. A lymphedema therapist can show you specific exercises that will improve your range of motion. Ask your doctor or therapist when you can start exercising and which exercises are right for you.

Compression

Nonelastic bandages and compression garments, such as elastic sleeves, place gentle pressure on the affected area. This helps prevent fluid from refilling and swelling after decongestive therapy (see below). There are several options depending on the location of the lymphedema. All compression devices apply the most pressure farthest from the center of the body and less pressure closer to the center of the body. Compression garments must fit properly and be replaced every 3–6 months.

Complete Decongestive Therapy

Complete Decongestive Therapy (CDT), also known as complex decongestive therapy, combines skin care, manual lymphatic drainage, exercise, and compression. A doctor who specializes in lymphedema or a CLT should perform CDT. The therapist will also teach you how to perform the necessary techniques yourself at home and will tell you how often to do them. Ask your doctor for a referral.

Skin Care

Because lymphedema can increase the risk of infection, it is important to keep the affected area clean, moisturized, and healthy. Apply moisturizer each day to prevent chapped skin. Avoid cuts, burns, needle sticks, or other injury to the affected area. If you shave, use an electric razor to reduce the chance of cutting the skin. When you are outside, wear a broad-spectrum sunscreen that protects against both UVA and UVB radiation and has a sun protection factor (SPF) of at least 30. If you do cut or burn yourself, wash the injured area with soap and water and use an antibiotic cream as directed by your doctor or nurse.

Elevation

Keeping an affected limb elevated often helps reduce swelling and encourages fluid drainage through the lymphatic system. However, it is often not practical to maintain an elevated position for a long time.

Low-level Laser Treatments

A small number of clinical trials have found that low-level laser treatments (LLLTs) could provide some relief of lymphedema after removal of the breast, particularly in the arms.

Medications

The doctor may prescribe antibiotics to treat infections or drugs to relieve pain when necessary.

Physical Therapy

If you have trouble in swallowing or other issues that result from lymphedema of the head and neck, you may need physical therapy.

5. Describe dry gangrene.

Gangrene may be caused by a variety of chronic diseases and post-traumatic, postsurgical, and spontaneous causes. There are three major types of gangrene: Dry, moist, and gas (a type of moist gangrene). Dry gangrene is a condition that results when one or more arteries become obstructed. In this type of gangrene, the tissue slowly dies, due to receiving little or no blood supply, but does not become infected. The affected area becomes cold and black, begins to dry out and wither, and eventually drops off over a period of weeks or months. Dry gangrene is most common in persons with advanced blockages of the arteries (arteriosclerosis) resulting from diabetes.

Areas of either dry or moist gangrene are initially characterized by a red line on the skin that marks the border of the affected tissues. As tissues begin to die, dry gangrene may cause some pain in the early stages or may go unnoticed especially in the elderly or in those individuals with diminished sensation to the affected area. Initially, the area becomes cold, numb, and pale before later changing in color to brown, then black. This dead tissue will gradually separate from the healthy tissue and fall off.

Diagnosis
A diagnosis of gangrene will be based on a combination of the patient history, a physical examination, and the results of blood and other laboratory tests. A physician will look for a history of recent trauma, surgery, cancer, or chronic disease. Blood tests will be used to determine whether infection is present and determine the extent to which an infection has spread. A sample of drainage from a wound, or obtained through surgical exploration may be cultured with oxygen (aerobic) and without oxygen (anaerobic) to identify the microorganism causing the infection and to aid in determining which antibiotic will be most effective. The sample obtained from a person with gangrene will contain few, if any, white blood cells and when stained (with gram stain) and examined under the microscope will show the presence of purple (gram-positive), rod-shaped bacteria.

Treatment
Gas gangrene is a medical emergency because of the threat of the infection rapidly spreading via the bloodstream and infecting vital organs. It requires immediate surgery and administration of antibiotics. Areas of dry gangrene that remain free from infection (aseptic) in the extremities are most often left to wither and fall off. Treatments applied to the wound externally (topically) are generally not effective without adequate blood supply to support wound healing. Assessment by a vascular surgeon along with X-rays to determine blood supply and circulation to the affected area can help determine whether surgical intervention would be beneficial.

6. Describe callus.

Calluses occur most often on the heels and balls of the feet, the knees, and the palms of the hands. However, they can develop on any part of the body that is subject to repeated pressure or irritation. Calluses are usually more than an inch wide-larger than corns. They generally do not hurt unless pressure is applied.

Types of Calluses
A plantar callus, a callus that occurs on the sole of the foot, has a white center. Hereditary calluses develop where there is no apparent friction, run in families, and occur most often in children.

Causes and Symptoms
Corns and calluses form to prevent injury to skin that is repeatedly pinched, rubbed, or irritated. The most common causes are:
1. Shoes that are too tight or too loose, or have very high heels.
2. Tight socks or stockings.
3. Deformed toes.
4. Walking down a long hill, or standing or walking on a hard surface for a long time.
5. Jobs or hobbies that cause steady or recurring pressure on the same spot can also cause calluses.

Symptoms include hard growths on the skin in response to direct pressure. Corns may be extremely sore and surrounded by inflamed, swollen skin.

Diagnosis

Corns can be recognized on sight. A family physician or podiatrist may scrape skin off what seems to be a callus, but may actually be a wart. If the lesion is a wart, it will bleed. A callus will not bleed, but will reveal another layer of dead skin.

Treatment

Corns and calluses do not usually require medical attention unless the person who has them has **diabetes mellitus,** poor circulation, or other problems that make self-care difficult. Treatment should begin as soon as an abnormality appears. The first step is to identify and eliminate the source of pressure. Placing moleskin pads over corns can relieve pressure, and large wads of cotton, lamb's wool, or moleskin can cushion calluses.

Using hydrocortisone creams or soaking feet in a solution of Epsom salts and very warm water for at least 5 minutes a day before rubbing the area with a pumice stone will remove part or all of some calluses. Rubbing corns just makes them hurt more.

Applying petroleum jelly or lanolin-enriched hand lotion helps keep skin soft, but corn-removing ointments that contain acid can damage healthy skin. They should never be used by pregnant women or by people who are diabetic or who have poor circulation.

It is important to see a doctor if the skin of a corn or callus is cut, because it may become infected. If a corn discharges pus or clear fluid, it is infected. A family physician, podiatrist, or orthopedist may:
1. Remove (debride) affected layers of skin.
2. Prescribe oral **antibiotics** to eliminate infection.
3. Drain pus from infected corns.
4. Inject cortisone into the affected area to decrease pain or inflammation.
5. Perform surgery to correct toe deformities or remove bits of bone.

SHORT ANSWERS

7. Define karyotype.

Turner syndrome, also known as Ullrich-Turner syndrome and monosomy X, was first described by Henry Turner in 1938 (Turner, 1938). However, it was not until 1959 that the chromosomal basis for the condition was first reported (Ford et al., 1959). Turner syndrome is a sex chromosomal abnormality typically involving the presence of one X chromosome and the complete absence of a second sex chromosome. This condition has a karyotype of 45,X.

Karyotypes commonly associated with Turner syndrome	
Karyotype	Description
45,X	Monosomy X
45,X/46,XX	Monosomy X mosaic with normal female sex chromosome complement
46,X,i(Xq)	Isochromosome X
46,X,del(X)	Deletion chromosome X
46,X,r(X)	Ring chromosome X
45,X/47,XXX	Monosomy X mosaic with triple X chromosome complement

8. Characteristics of autosomal recessive inheritance.

Autosomal recessive is one of several ways that a trait, disorder, or disease can be passed down through families. An autosomal recessive disorder means two copies of an abnormal gene must be present in order for the disease or trait to develop. Inheriting a specific disease, condition, or trait depends on the type of chromosome that is affected (autosomal or sex chromosome). It also depends on whether the trait is dominant or recessive. A mutation in a gene on one of the first 22 nonsex chromosomes can lead to an autosomal disorder. Genes come in pairs. One gene in each pair comes from the mother, and the other gene comes from the father. Recessive inheritance means both genes in a pair must be abnormal to cause disease. People with only one defective gene in the pair are called carriers. However, they can pass the abnormal gene to their children.

Key Features of Autosomal Recessive Inheritance
1. **Two mutated copies** of a gene are necessary to cause the condition.
2. Males and females are usually affected equally.
3. There is **horizontal transmission** (usually siblings in the same generation are affected).
4. Consanguinity from GHR is more likely to be present.
5. De novo mutations are rare and parents are usually **unaffected carriers**.
6. Conditions typically have an early onset with a more severe phenotype.

9. Effect of deficiency of vitamin A and D on fetal growth.

Pregnancy is a period of rapid growth and cell differentiation, both for the mother and the fetus she carries. Consequently, it is a period when both are very susceptible to alterations in dietary supply, especially of nutrients which are marginal under normal circumstances. Inappropriate nutrition leads not only to an increased risk of death in utero, but also to alterations in birth weight and functional changes in the neonatal organs. These changes can have far-reaching consequences. For example, babies who are small at birth are at an increased risk of cardiovascular disease and diabetes as adults, while animals who are born to zinc deficient mothers have a compromised immune system.

The underlying mechanisms relate to nutrition effects on gene expression in the fetus. There is an argument, therefore, for supplementation in the diet, in order to avoid the consequences of deficiency during pregnancy.

Vitamin A

Retinoids are essential for growth, development and reproduction with demonstrated roles in vision, embryogenesis, spermatogenesis, skin development and in the maintenance of differentiated epithelial cells. Vitamin A is the parent compound of biologically active retinoids, such as retinaldehyde (or retinal), the active element of visual pigment, and retinoic acid, an intracellular messenger which modulates cellular differentiation. In many areas of the world, vitamin A intakes are below recommended daily levels due either to limited and seasonal availability of foods rich in retinol or its precursor beta-carotene, lack of nutritional awareness or inappropriate dietary choices. The World Health Organization estimates that upto 50% of pregnant women have daily intakes below defined minimum levels. Worryingly, 51% of pregnant women in rural Nepal suffer from night blindness.

Vitamin A deficiency during pregnancy has been associated with increased vertical transmission of the human immunodeficiency virus-7 and has particularly serious effects on fetal lung development. Damage caused to the lungs by such deficiency can be irreversible, affecting lung function throughout adult life.

Vitamin D

In addition to the factors associated with inadequate vitamin status described above, lack of exposure to sunlight and excess clothing can predispose individuals to vitamin D deficiency. Maternal serum parathyroid hormone levels at term are inversely related to neonatal crown heel length, suggesting that vitamin D deficiency affects fetal growth through an effect on maternal calcium homeostasis. In a study comparing bone mineral content and calcium status of summer born and winter born babies, Namgung observed that babies born between January and March had a higher bone mineral content, lower serum osteocalcin and higher serum calcium than babies born between July and September. These data suggest that the vitamin D status of the mother 6 months prior to parturition affects the calcium status of her offspring.

10. Name the adverse effects of four commonly used drugs on fetal growth and development.

In general, however, using drugs during pregnancy can result in the following:
1. Miscarriage.
2. Stillbirth.
3. Small size.
4. Low-birth weight.
5. Premature birth.
6. Birth defects.
7. Sudden infant death syndrome.
8. Drug dependency in the baby.

Some of the specific consequences of drug use during pregnancy
1. Low-birth weight places an infant at a higher risk for illness, intellectual disability, and even death.
2. Premature birth increases the risk of lung, eye, and learning problems in the infant.
3. Birth defects that often occur due to drug use include seizure, stroke, intellectual and learning disabilities.
4. Fetuses can become dependent on the drug(s) the mother is using and may experience withdrawal symptoms after delivery.

11. Name the noninvasive techniques used for parental diagnosis.

Prenatal diagnosis employs a variety of techniques to determine the health and condition of an unborn fetus. Without knowledge gained by prenatal diagnosis, there could be an untoward outcome for the fetus or the mother or both. Congenital anomalies account for 20–25% of perinatal deaths. Specifically, prenatal diagnosis is helpful for:
1. Managing the remaining weeks of the pregnancy.
2. Determining the outcome of the pregnancy.
3. Planning for possible complications with the birth process.
4. Planning for problems that may occur in the newborn infant.
5. Deciding whether to continue the pregnancy.
6. Finding conditions that may affect future pregnancies.

There are a variety of noninvasive and invasive techniques available for prenatal diagnosis. Each of them can be applied only during specific time periods during the pregnancy for greatest utility. The techniques employed for prenatal diagnosis include:
1. Ultrasonography.
2. Amniocentesis.
3. Chorionic villus sampling.
4. Fetal blood cells in maternal blood.
5. Maternal serum alpha-fetoprotein.
6. Maternal serum beta-hCG.
7. Maternal serum estriol.

12. Define anencephaly.

Anencephaly is a condition that prevents the normal development of the brain and the bones of the skull. This condition results when a structure called the neural tube fails to close during the first few weeks of embryonic development. The neural tube is a layer of cells that ultimately develops into the brain and spinal cord. Because anencephaly is caused by abnormalities of the neural tube, it is classified as a neural tube defect. Because the neural tube fails to close properly, the developing brain and spinal cord are exposed to the amniotic fluid that surrounds the fetus in the womb. This exposure causes the nervous system tissue to break down (degenerate). As a result, people with anencephaly are missing large parts of the brain called the cerebrum and cerebellum. These brain regions are necessary for thinking, hearing, vision, emotion, and coordinating movement. The bones of the skull are also missing or incompletely formed. Because these nervous system abnormalities are so severe, almost all babies with anencephaly die before birth or within a few hours or days after birth.

2015

Pharmacology, Pathology and Genetics

PHARMACOLOGY

LONG ESSAYS

1. Classify **antiepileptic agents**; mention the pharmacological action, adverse effects and uses of sodium valproate.
2. Enumerate **tetracycline** preparations; mention the mechanism of action, antimicrobial spectrum, adverse effect and uses of doxycycline.

SHORT ESSAYS

3. Zero order kinetics and first order kinetics.
4. Prazosin.
5. Ketamine.
6. Cough suppressants.
7. Prepare 500 mL of 5% DNS solution, mention its uses.

SHORT ANSWERS

8. Aspirin—therapeutic use and important adverse effect.
9. Atenolol—therapeutic use and important adverse effect.
10. Chloroquine—therapeutic use and important adverse effect.
11. Amlodipine—therapeutic use and important adverse effect.

PATHOLOGY

LONG ESSAYS

1. Discuss the differences between Benign and malignant tumors.
2. Discuss etiology, morphology and complications of peptic ulcer.

SHORT ESSAYS

3. Enumerate about aneurisms.
4. Describe bone healing.

5. Describe hemoglobin estimation.
6. Explain the etiopathogenesis of primary tuberculosis.

GENETICS

SHORT ANSWERS
1. Mention any four prenatal diagnostic tests.
2. Role of nurse in genetic counseling.
3. Structure of the chromosome.
4. Define karyotyping.
5. List any five autosomal abnormalities.
6. Define infertility.

PHARMACOLOGY

LONG ESSAYS

1. Classify antiepileptic agents; mention the pharmacological action, adverse effects and uses of sodium valproate.

Anticonvulsants (also commonly known as **antiepileptic** drugs or as antiseizure drugs) are a diverse group of pharmacological agents used in the treatment of epileptic seizures. A variety of the anticonvulsant drugs including carbamazepine, phenytoin, primidone, phenobarbital, clonazepam, valproic acid, and ethosuximide are available for use in the treatment of patients with seizure disorders. These anticonvulsants vary in their efficacy against experimental seizures in animals and against seizures in humans. The mechanistic basis for this variability in anticonvulsant drug action remains uncertain, but numerous mechanisms of action have been proposed (Fig. 1).

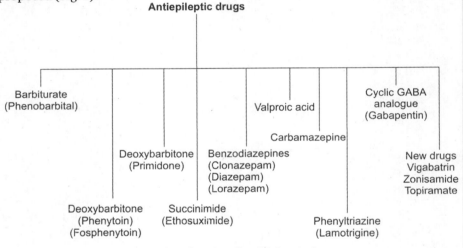

Fig. 1: Classification of antiepileptic drugs.

Sodium Valproate

Sodium valproate (valproate) was first marketed as an anticonvulsant almost 50 years ago in France. Its indications have expanded and it is now the most prescribed antiepileptic drug worldwide. However, it has many potential adverse effects.

Pharmacology

Valproate is available in tablet (immediate-release or enteric coated), syrup and intravenous formulations. There is no single mechanism of action that can explain valproate's broad effects on neuronal tissue. Its pharmacological effects include:
1. Increased gamma-aminobutyric acid transmission.
2. Reduced release of excitatory amino acids.
3. Blockade of voltage-gated sodium channels.
4. Modulation of dopaminergic and serotonergic transmission.

When fasting, oral valproate is rapidly absorbed and reaches peak plasma concentrations within 4 hours (immediate-release formulation)–7 hours (enteric coated formulation). It is highly plasma protein bound and has a half-life of 8–20 hours in most patients, but this may occasionally be much longer, for example, in renal impairment or overdose. The relationship between dose, plasma concentration and therapeutic effect is not well understood.

Valproate is almost completely metabolized in the liver mainly by glucuronidation. It then undergoes further metabolism with oxidation which is complex and involves several cytochrome P450 enzyme systems. It has multiple metabolites which may contribute to both its efficacy and toxicity. There are many potential drug interactions.

Indications

Although, there is clinical experience with valproate in epilepsy, some of its other accepted indications, such as migraine prophylaxis have not been approved by the Therapeutic Goods Administration.

Epilepsy

Valproate is a broad spectrum antiepileptic drug and is used to treat either generalized or focal seizures. It is recommended in Australian and International Clinical Practice guidelines. There is evidence that it is more effective than lamotrigine or topiramate in treating:
1. Idiopathic generalized epilepsy syndromes
2. Seizures that are difficult to classify.

Some authors have expressed concern that there remains a dearth of well-designed, properly conducted, randomized controlled trials for adults with generalized seizures/epilepsy syndromes and for children in general.

Bipolar Disorder

Valproate was first used for the maintenance treatment of bipolar disorder in Europe in 1966. Over the past two decades, there has been a dramatic rise in its use for this condition. However, the authors of a recent Cochrane review said that, in view of the lack of clear findings in their review and the limited available evidence, conclusions regarding the efficacy and acceptability of valproate compared to placebo or lithium cannot be made with any degree of confidence. Longer-term and larger sample size randomized controlled trials are required to better assess the clinical utility of valproate in the maintenance therapy of bipolar disorder.

Neuropathic Pain

Valproate use should be reserved for cases of neuropathic pain where other proven treatment options have failed, are not available, or are not tolerated.

Migraine

Preventative therapy for migraine is often undertaken if patients have more than one attack per month. First-line drugs for migraine prophylaxis include amitriptyline, propranolol and pizotifen. A systematic review found that valproate is also effective in reducing migraine frequency and is reasonably well tolerated.

Adverse Effects

Common adverse effects of valproate include nausea, upper abdominal cramps, abnormal liver function, weight gain and diarrhea. Neurological adverse effects, such as tremor, fatigue, sedation, confusion and dizziness are often observed. Other potential adverse effects include alopecia, reduced bone density, thrombocytopenia, anemia, leukopenia and hyperammonemia. There are several cutaneous adverse effects of valproate. They include pruritus, urticaria, erythema multiforme, toxic epidermal necrolysis, Stevens-Johnson syndrome, and drug reaction with eosinophilia and systemic symptoms (DRESS).

Contraindications and Precautions

Valproate should be avoided in patients with liver disease or a family history of liver disease. Although uncommon, patients with a urea cycle disorder or porphyria should also avoid valproate. Renal failure can impair protein binding and lead to the accumulation of metabolites, so a lower dose may be required in patients with impaired renal function. Routine laboratory studies should be performed before commencing therapy, but regular monitoring is not required for most patients. The onset of lethargy, vomiting or ataxia is an indication to measure serum ammonia to exclude hyperammonemic encephalopathy. Spontaneous bruising or bleeding may occur and necessitates clinical review and investigation. Such patients may have developed thrombocytopenia or altered platelet function.

2. Enumerate tetracycline preparations; mention the mechanism of action, antimicrobial spectrum, adverse effect and uses of doxycycline.

Tetracyclines are broad, spectrum bacteriostatic. They bind to bacterial 30S ribosomal subunit and block attachment of aminoacyl-tRNA to A site: Thereby inhibit protein synthesis. Bacterium slowly develops resistance to tetracycline by blocking its entry into the bacterial cells or start pumping it out. Cross-resistance between tetracycline and chloramphenicol is noticed. With the exception of doxycycline, other tetracyclines are excreted through kidneys.

Doxycyclines enter bile in significant quantities and also secreted in milk. Drugs that induce cytochrome-P450 enhance the rate of tetracycline metabolism.

Uses

To treat infections caused by gram-positive and gram-negative bacteria, aerobic and anaerobic bacteria, and Lyme arthritis. Commonly used drugs: Oxytetracycline (terramycine), doxycycline (vibramycin), and minocycline (minocin).

Untoward Effects

1. Hepatotoxicity, nephrotoxicity, and photosensitivity.
2. Get deposited in bones and teeth and cause permanent discoloration of teeth.
3. Minocycline is known to cause vestibular toxicity.
4. Tetracyclines are the most common antibiotics known to cause marked suppression of intestinal flora. Pseudomembranous enterocolitis is the most serious complication.

Doxycycline

Doxycycline is a tetracycline antibiotic. It fights bacteria in the body. Doxycycline is used to treat many different bacterial infections, such as acne, urinary tract infections, intestinal infections, eye infections, gonorrhea, chlamydia, periodontitis (gum disease), and others. Doxycycline is also used to treat blemishes, bumps, and acne-like lesions caused by rosacea. It will not treat facial redness caused by rosacea. Some forms of doxycycline are used to prevent malaria, to treat anthrax, or to treat infections caused by mites, ticks, or lice.

Uses

Doxycycline is used to treat bacterial infections including pneumonia and other respiratory tract infections; Lyme disease; acne; infections of skin, genital, and urinary systems; and anthrax (after inhalational exposure). It is also used to prevent malaria. Doxycycline is in a class of medications called tetracycline antibiotics. It works by preventing the growth and spread of bacteria. Antibiotics will not work for colds, flu, or other viral infections.

Doxycycline Side Effects
1. Changes in your vision
2. Severe stomach pain, diarrhea that is watery or bloody
3. Fever, swollen glands, body aches, flu symptoms, weakness
4. Skin rash, pale skin, easy bruising or bleeding, severe tingling, numbness, pain, muscle weakness
5. Upper stomach pain (may spread to your back), loss of appetite, dark urine, jaundice (yellowing of the skin or eyes)
6. Chest pain, irregular heart rhythm, feeling short of breath
7. Confusion, nausea and vomiting, swelling, rapid weight gain, little or no urinating
8. New or worsening cough with fever, trouble breathing
9. Increased pressure inside the skull—severe headaches, ringing in your ears, dizziness, nausea, vision problems, pain behind your eyes; or
10. Severe skin reaction—fever, sore throat, swelling in your face or tongue, burning in your eyes, skin pain, followed by a red or purple skin rash that spreads (especially in the face or upper body) and causes blistering and peeling.

Common doxycycline side effects may include:
1. Nausea, vomiting, upset stomach
2. Mild diarrhea
3. Skin rash or itching; or
4. Vaginal itching or discharge.

SHORT ESSAYS

3. Zero order kinetics and first order kinetics.

Zero order
A constant amount of drug is eliminated per unit time. For example, 10 mg of a drug may be eliminated per hour, this rate of elimination is constant and is independent of the total drug concentration in the plasma. **Zero order kinetics** are rare elimination mechanisms are saturable.

Zero-order Elimination Kinetics
The plasma concentration—time profile during the elimination phase is linear. For example, 1.2 mg are eliminated every hour, independently of the drug concentration in the body. Order 0 elimination is rather rare, mostly occurring when the elimination system is saturated. An example is the elimination of ethanol.

First-order Elimination Kinetics
For first-order elimination, the plasma concentration—time profile during the elimination phase shows an exponential decrease in the plot with linear axes and is linear if plotted on a semilogarithmic plot (plasma concentration on logarithmic axis and time on linear axis); for example, 1% of the drug quantity is eliminated per minute. Many drugs are eliminated by first order kinetics. The time course of the decrease of the drug concentration in the plasma can be described by an exponential equation of the form:

The elimination rate constant λ can be calculated by fitting the data points during the elimination phase to a single exponential; yielding in this example a λ of $0.34\ h^{-1}$. An alternative method consists in plotting the logarithm of the drug plasma concentration as a function of time which will yield a straight line. The steepness of this line equals $-\lambda$

With
C = drug concentration
$C(0)$ = extrapolated initial drug concentration
λ = elimination rate constant
t = time

Clinical Implications

In clinical pharmacology, first order kinetics are considered as a linear process, because the rate of elimination is proportional to the drug concentration. This means that the higher the drug concentration, the higher its elimination rate. In other words, the elimination processes are not saturated and can adapt to the needs of the body, to reduce accumulation of the drug. About 95% of the drugs in use at therapeutic concentrations are eliminated by first-order elimination kinetics. A few substances are eliminated by zero-order elimination kinetics, because their elimination process is saturated. Examples are ethanol, phenytoin, salicylates, cisplatin, fluoxetin, omeprazol. Because in a saturated process the elimination rate is no longer proportional to the drug concentration but decreasing at higher concentrations, zero-order kinetics are also called "nonlinear kinetics" in clinical pharmacology.

4. Prazosin.

Treating high blood pressure or Benign prostatic hyperplasia (BPH). It may also be used for other conditions as determined by your doctor. Prazosin is an alpha-blocker. It works by causing the blood vessels and the muscles around the urethra (the tube leading out of the bladder) to relax. This helps to lower blood pressure and to improve urinary symptoms associated with enlargement of the prostate (BPH).

Side Effects

Most common—dizziness, headache, drowsiness, lack of energy, weakness, palpitations and nausea.
Gastrointestinal—vomiting, diarrhea and constipation.
Heart—edema, low blood pressure, difficulty in breathing and fainting.
Central nervous system—unsteadiness, depression and nervousness.
Skin—rash.
Genitourinary—urinary frequency.
Eye and ENT—blurred vision, redness, nosebleed, dry mouth and nasal congestion.

The typical dose is 1 mg, taken two or three times per day. If your blood pressure is still high, your doctor can then increase your dose. The 2 mg and 5 mg capsules would not be used for your starting dose.

The most common side effects of prazosin include dizziness, headache, and drowsiness, lack of energy, weakness, heart palpitations, and nausea.

Dizziness and drowsiness may occur after your first dose of prazosin. Avoid driving or performing any hazardous tasks for the first 24 hours after taking this medicine or when your dose is increased.

5. Ketamine.

Ketamine hydrochloride injection is indicated as the sole anesthetic agent for diagnostic and surgical procedures that do not require skeletal muscle relaxation. Ketamine hydrochloride injection is best suited for short procedures but it can be used with additional doses for longer procedures.

Indications for Ketamine HCl Injection

Sole anesthetic agent for diagnostic and surgical procedures not requiring skeletal muscle relaxation. Induction prior to other general anesthesia. Supplement to low-potency agents (e.g. nitrous oxide).

Adult

Individualize

Pretreat with atropine, scopolamine or other drying agent prior to induction. Give by slow IV over 60 seconds. IV induction—initial range: 1–4.5 mg/kg; usually 2 mg/kg to produce 5–10 minutes surgical anesthesia. Alternatively, 1–2 mg/kg at rate of 0.5 mg/kg/minute may be used. In addition, diazepam 2–5 mg doses given in separate syringe over 60 seconds, may be used. IM induction—initial range: 6.5–13 mg/kg; usually 10 mg/kg to produce 12–25 minutes surgical anesthesia. Maintenance: Repeat as needed in increments of 1/2 to full induction dose; see literature. Supplementary to nitrous oxide/oxygen: Use reduced ketamine dose with diazepam.

Children

Individualize

Usual range: 9–13 mg/kg IM to produce surgical anesthesia within 3–4 minutes following injection with effects lasting 12–25 minutes.

Contraindications

Significant hypertension.

Warnings/Precautions

It is to be administered under the supervision of experienced clinicians, and have resuscitative equipment available. Avoid monotherapy and/or mechanical stimulation in pharynx, larynx or bronchial tree surgery/diagnostic procedures; may require muscle relaxants. Hypertensive or cardiac decompensated; monitor cardiac function. Monitor for psychological manifestations postoperative. Preanesthetic elevated cerebrospinal fluid pressure.

Interactions

Concomitant barbiturates and/or narcotics may prolong recovery time.

Pharmacological Class

NMDA receptor antagonist.

Adverse Reactions

Hyper- or hypotension, bradycardia, arrhythmia, respiratory depression (may be severe; especially with rapid IV or high-doses), apnea, laryngospasms, airway obstruction, diplopia, nystagmus, intraocular pressure, tonic/clonic movements, anorexia, GI upset, anaphylaxis, injection site pain, exanthema, transient erythema, rash; emergence reactions (e.g. pleasant dream-like states, hallucinations, delirium, confusion, excitement, irrational behavior), elevated cerebrospinal fluid pressure.

6. Cough suppressants.

Cough medicines are commonly bought to treat coughs that occur when you have an upper respiratory tract infection (URTI). Cough medicines are often divided into those for a dry cough, and those for a chesty cough. It is thought that cough medicines do not really work.

However, some people feel that they work for them and they are thought to be reasonably safe medicines. Children who are aged 6 years and younger should only be given simple cough mixtures, such as glycerin, honey and lemon. Lots of cough medicines are available to buy from pharmacies or supermarkets. They usually contain one or more of the following:
1. An antitussive (cough suppressant)—for example, dextromethorphan, or pholcodine.
2. An expectorant—for example, guaifenesin, or ipecacuanha.
3. An antihistamine—brompheniramine, chlorphenamine, diphenhydramine, doxylamine, promethazine, or triprolidine.
4. A decongestant—for example, phenylephrine, pseudoephedrine, ephedrine, oxymetazoline, or xylometazoline.

Cough suppressants block, or suppress, the cough reflex. Generally, coughing is a healthy way to clear the airways of mucus, so cough suppressants should only be used for dry, hacking coughs.

Expectorants are substances claimed to make coughing easier while enhancing the production of mucus and phlegm. Two examples are acetylcysteine and guaifenesin. Antitussives, or cough suppressants are substances which suppress the coughing itself. Examples are codeine, pholcodine, dextromethorphan and noscapine.

Symptoms of Overdose
1. Blurred vision
2. Confusion
3. Difficulty in urination
4. Drowsiness or dizziness
5. Nausea or vomiting (severe)
6. Shakiness and unsteady walk
7. Slowed breathing
8. Unusual excitement, nervousness, restlessness, or irritability (severe).

7. Prepare 500 mL of 5% DNS solution, mention its uses.

Dextrose is the name of a simple sugar chemically identical to glucose (blood sugar) that is made from corn. While dextrose is used in baking products as a sweetener, it also has medical purposes. Dextrose is dissolved in solutions that are given intravenously which can be combined with other drugs, or used to increase a person's blood sugar. Dextrose is also available as an oral gel or tablet. Because dextrose is a "simple" sugar, the body can quickly use it for energy.

NaCl:
a. Vehicle/solvent is normal saline—0.9% NaCl solution.
  To prepare 100 mL of normal saline, NaCl required = 0.9 g.
  To prepare 500 mL of normal saline, NaCl required: $500 \times 0.9/100 = 4.5$ g.
b. Dextrose:
  To prepare 100 mL of solution, amount of dextrose = 5 g.
  To prepare 500 mL of solution, amount of dextrose: $500 \times 5/100 = 25$ g.
  Ingredients required = NaCl = 4.5 g.
  Dextrose = 25 g.

Common Dextrose Preparations
Dextrose is used to make several intravenous (IV) preparations or mixtures which are available only at a hospital or medical facility. Examples include:
1. Dextrose injections which are premixed with sterile water, in concentrations from 5 to 70%.

2. Dextrose injections in combination with sodium in several concentrations.
3. Amino acid/dextrose injections which provide nutrition for someone who is unable to eat.

Drug Class and Mechanism

Dextrose monohydrate is sterile intravenous solution for fluid replenishment. Intravenous administration of dextrose solution provides a source of water and glucose (sugar), giving patients fluid and energy.

Preparation

Dextrose 5% is available in water (D5W), normal saline (D5NS), and ½ normal saline (D5 ½ NS). Dextrose is also available in 10%, 20%, 30%, 40%, 50% and 70% concentrated in water.
1. About 5% solution is available in 25 mL, 50 mL, 100 mL, 150 mL, 250 mL, 500 mL, and 1,000 mL plastic containers.
2. About 10% solution is available in 250 mL, 500 mL, and 1,000 mL plastic containers.
3. About 20%, 30%, 40%, and 70% solutions are available 500 mL plastic containers and 50% is available in 1,000 mL plastic containers.

Side Effects of Dextrose

Dextrose should be carefully given to people who have diabetes because they might not be able to process dextrose as quickly as would someone without the condition. Dextrose can increase the blood sugar too much which is known as hyperglycemia.

Symptoms of Hyperglycemia Include
1. Fruity odor on the breath
2. Increasing thirst with no known causes
3. Dry skin
4. Nausea
5. Shortness of breath
6. Stomach upset
7. Unexplained fatigue
8. Urinating frequently
9. Vomiting.

SHORT ANSWERS

8. Aspirin—therapeutic use and important adverse effect.

Aspirin is used to reduce fever and relieve mild to moderate pain from conditions, such as muscle aches, toothaches, common cold, and headaches. It may also be used to reduce pain and swelling in conditions, such as arthritis. **Aspirin** is known as a salicylate and a nonsteroidal anti-inflammatory drug (NSAID).

Adverse Effects

1. Ringing in your ears, confusion, hallucinations, rapid breathing, seizure (convulsions)
2. Severe nausea, vomiting, or stomach pain
3. Bloody or tarry stools, coughing up blood or vomit that looks like coffee grounds
4. Fever lasting longer than 3 days; swelling, or pain lasting longer than 10 days.

Common Aspirin Side Effects May Include
1. Upset stomach, heartburn

2. Drowsiness; or
3. Mild headache.

9. Atenolol—therapeutic use and important adverse effect.

Uses

Atenolol (Tenormin) is in a group of drugs called beta-blockers. Beta-blockers affect the heart and circulation (blood flow through arteries and veins).

Atenolol is used to treat angina (chest pain) and hypertension (high blood pressure). It is also used to treat or prevent heart attack.

Atenolol may also be used for purposes other than those listed in this medication guide.

Atenolol Side Effects

1. Slow or uneven heartbeats
2. Feeling lightheaded, fainting
3. Feeling short of breath, even with mild exertion
4. Swelling of your ankles or feet
5. Nausea, stomach pain, low fever, loss of appetite, dark urine, clay-colored stools, jaundice (yellowing of the skin or eyes)
6. Depression; or cold feeling in your hands and feet.

Less Serious Atenolol Side Effects May Include

1. Decreased sex drive, impotence, or difficulty having an orgasm
2. Sleep problems (insomnia)
3. Tired feeling; or
4. Anxiety, nervousness.

10. Chloroquine—therapeutic use and important adverse effect.

Chloroquine is used to prevent or treat malaria caused by mosquito bites in countries where malaria is common. Malaria parasites can enter the body through these mosquito bites, and then live in body tissues, such as red blood cells or the liver.

Side Effects

Some people taking this medication over long periods of time or at high doses have developed irreversible damage to the retina of the eye. Stop taking chloroquine and call your doctor at once if you have trouble focusing, if you see light streaks or flashes in your vision, or if you notice any swelling or color changes in your eyes.

1. Vision problems, trouble reading or seeing objects, hazy vision
2. Hearing loss or ringing in the ears
3. Seizure (convulsions)
4. Severe muscle weakness, loss of coordination, underactive reflexes
5. Nausea, upper stomach pain, itching, loss of appetite, dark urine, clay-colored stools, jaundice (yellowing of the skin or eyes); or severe skin reaction
6. Fever, sore throat, swelling in your face or tongue, burning in your eyes, skin pain, followed by a red or purple skin rash that spreads (especially in the face or upper body) and causes blistering and peeling.

Other, less serious side effects may be more likely to occur. Continue to take chloroquine and talk to your doctor if you experience:
1. Diarrhea, vomiting, stomach cramps
2. Temporary hair loss, changes in hair color; or
3. Mild muscle weakness.

11. Amlodipine—therapeutic use and important adverse effect

Amlodipine is in a group of drugs called calcium channel blockers. Amlodipine relaxes (widens) blood vessels and improves blood flow. Amlodipine is used to treat high blood pressure (hypertension) or chest pain (angina) and other conditions caused by coronary artery disease.

Uses

Amlodipine is used alone or together with other medicines to treat angina (chest pain) and high blood pressure (hypertension). High blood pressure adds to the workload of the heart and arteries. If it continues for a long time, the heart and arteries may not function properly. This can damage the blood vessels of the brain, heart, and kidneys, resulting in a stroke, heart failure, or kidney failure. High blood pressure may also increase the risk of heart attacks. These problems may be less likely to occur if blood pressure is controlled.

Side Effects

Dizziness, lightheadedness, swelling ankles/feet, nausea, abdominal/stomach pain, or flushing may occur. If any of these **effects** persist or worsen, tell your doctor or pharmacist promptly. To lower your risk of dizziness and lightheadedness, get up slowly when rising from a sitting or lying position.

Warnings and Precautions

Hypotension

Symptomatic hypotension is possible, particularly in patients with severe aortic stenosis. Because of the gradual onset of action, acute hypotension is unlikely.

Increased Angina or Myocardial Infarction

Worsening angina and acute myocardial infarction can develop after starting or increasing the dose of amlodipine particularly in patients with severe obstructive coronary artery disease.

Patients with Hepatic Failure

Because amlodipine is extensively metabolized by the liver and the plasma elimination half-life ($t\frac{1}{2}$) is 56 hours in patients with impaired hepatic function, titrate slowly when administering amlodipine to patients with severe hepatic impairment.

PATHOLOGY

LONG ESSAYS

1. Discuss the differences between Benign and malignant tumors.

Simply, there are two types of tumors—**Benign** or **malignant**. A Benign tumor is not always thought of in the same serious light as malignant tumors. Benign growths usually have little or no clinical effect, however, depending on the location; a Benign tumor can cause a number of signs or symptoms if it presses against important neighboring organs like a gland or nerve. A malignant tumor invades surrounding tissue while growing in size, destroying organs and tissue and may spread to other areas of the body (Fig. 2).

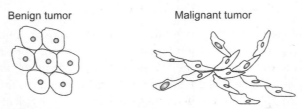

Fig. 2: Difference between Benign and malignant tumors.

The two terms malignant and Benign are medical terms and they are often confused with each other. The fact is that they are poles apart in meaning. Malignant means that the affected cells in the body are cancerous. The tumors which are malignant can attack the tissues lying the surrounding region and spread in the body. On the other hand, Benign tumor means that the tumor is not cancerous. It might grow in size but it will not spread to other parts of the body. Therefore, we can say that malignant tumors love to grow and conquer the surrounding area, while the Benign tumors like to stay.

There is a condition which falls in the middle of Benign and malignant. This means that there are certain tumors which can become malignant but their cells have not started growing abnormally. Some types of moles fall under this category and they are termed as precancerous. So we can say that a precancerous tumor is not really Benign, but it has not attained the aggressiveness to become malignant. Now this kind of precancerous growth will react well to the surgical intrusion but the doctor may want to observe it for some time to see any chances of malignancy, before declaring it completely normal.

1. A Benign tumor does not grow abnormally and is not harmful in the long run.
2. A malignant tumor has cancer cells which are active and grow abnormally.
3. A malignant tumor will require aggressive treatment methods but a Benign tumor becomes fine in one surgical intervention.
4. The tumor which is precancerous can have the potential to be malignant, but its present state is a matter of concern and observation.

Difference between Benign and malignant tumor.

Benign tumor	Malignant tumor
Mobile mass	Fixed or ulcerating mass
Smooth and round with a surrounding fibrous capsule	Irregular shaped with no capsule

Contd...

Contd...

Benign tumor	Malignant tumor
Cells multiply slowly	Cells multiply rapidly
Tumor grows by expanding and pushing away and against surrounding tissue	Tumor grows by invading and destroying surrounding tissue
Mass is mobile. Not attached to surrounding tissue	Mass is fixed. Attached to surrounding tissue and deeply fixed in surrounding tissue
Never spread to other sites (metastasize)	Almost always spreads to other sites if not removed or destroyed
Easier to remove and does not recur after excision	Difficult to remove and recurs after excision

2. Discuss etiology, morphology and complications of peptic ulcer.

Peptic ulcers are sores that develop in the lining of the stomach, lower esophagus, or small intestine (the duodenum), usually as a result of inflammation caused by the bacteria *H. pylori*, as well as from erosion from stomach acids. Peptic ulcers are a fairly common health problem.

There are three types of peptic ulcers:
1. Gastric ulcers: Ulcers that develop inside the stomach.
2. Esophageal ulcers: Ulcers that develop inside the esophagus.
3. Duodenal ulcers: Ulcers that develop in the upper section of the small intestines called the duodenum.

Causes of Peptic Ulcer
Different factors can cause the lining of the stomach, the esophagus, and the small intestine to break down. These include:
1. *Helicobacter pylori* (*H. pylori*): A bacteria that can cause a stomach infection and inflammation.
2. Frequent use of aspirin, ibuprofen, and other anti-inflammatory drugs (risk associated with this behavior increases in women and people over the age of 60).
3. Smoking.
4. Drinking too much alcohol.
5. Radiation therapy.
6. Stomach cancer.

Symptoms of Peptic Ulcer
The most common symptom of a peptic ulcer is burning abdominal pain that extends from the navel to the chest which can range from mild to severe. In some cases, the pain may wake you up at night. Small peptic ulcers may not produce any symptoms in the early phases.

Other common signs of a peptic ulcer include:
1. Changes in appetite
2. Nausea
3. Bloody or dark stools (melena)
4. Unexplained weight loss
5. Indigestion
6. Vomiting
7. Chest pain.

Pathogenesis

The two most important causative factors for the development of peptic ulcer include:
1. *Helicobacter pylori* infection and
2. Mucosal exposure to gastric acid and pepsin. Other factors which cause injury to the mucosa include consumption of aspirin and NSAIDs, cigarette smoking, alcohol consumption and duodenal gastric reflux.

There are certain mucosal defensive forces which prevent the development of peptic ulcers. These include:
1. Surface mucus secretion
2. Bicarbonate secretion in the mucus
3. Epithelial regenerative capacity and
4. Elaboration of prostaglandins.

An imbalance between the mucosal defensive forces and damaging factors are responsible for the development of peptic ulcer.

Gross Morphology

The ulcers are round, sharply demarcated punched out craters approximately 2–4 cm in diameter. The location is on the anterior and posterior wall of the first part of the duodenum and the lesser curvature of the stomach. The margins of the ulcer are edematous and the surrounding mucosal folds may radiate like spokes of a wheel. The ulcer base is clean due to peptic digestion of the necrotic tissue.

Microscopy

Four zones are identified on microscopy:
1. The base comprising of a thin layer of necrotic debris
2. Zone of active nonspecific inflammatory infiltrate
3. Granulation tissue and
4. Fibrous, collagenous scar.

Healing occurs by proliferation of the granulation tissue and re-epithelialization from the margins of the ulcer.

Clinical Features

The patients present with a burning or boring type of epigastric pain especially 1–3 hours after meals. The pain is relieved by alkalis. Other symptoms include nausea, bloating, belching and loss of weight.

Complications

1. Bleeding is the most common complication and is life-threatening.
2. Perforation of the wall of the stomach duodenum.
3. Rare complications include obstruction and malignant transformation.

SHORT ESSAYS

3. Enumerate about aneurysms.

An aneurysm occurs when an artery's wall weakens and causes an abnormally large bulge. This bulge can rupture and cause internal bleeding. Although an aneurysm can occur in any part of your body, they are most common in the: Brain, aorta, legs, spleen.

An abdominal aortic aneurysm occurs when the large blood vessel (the aorta) that supplies blood to the abdomen, pelvis and legs becomes abnormally large or balloons outward. This type of aneurysm is most often found in men over age 60 who have at least one or more risk factor, including emphysema, family history, high blood pressure, high cholesterol, obesity and smoking.

Causes of Aneurism

Although, the exact cause of an aneurysm is unclear, certain factors contribute to the condition. For example, damaged tissue in the arteries can play a role. The arteries can be harmed by blockages, such as fatty deposits. These deposits can trigger the heart to pump harder than necessary to push blood past the fatty buildup. This stress can damage the arteries because of the increased pressure.

Atherosclerotic Disease

It can also lead to an aneurysm. People with atherosclerotic disease have a form of plaque buildup in their arteries. This buildup is due to a hard substance called plaque that damages the arteries and prevents blood from flowing freely.

High Blood Pressure

High blood pressure may also cause an aneurysm. The force of your blood as it travels through your blood vessels is measured by how much pressure it places on your artery walls. If the pressure increases above a normal rate, it may enlarge or weaken the blood vessels. Blood pressure for an adult is considered normal at or below 120/80 mm Hg, or millimeters of mercury. A significantly higher blood pressure can increase the risk for heart, blood vessel, and circulation problems. Higher than normal blood pressure does not necessarily put you at risk for an aneurysm.

Types of Aneurism

An aneurysm may occur anywhere in your body, but the most common locations of aneurysms are (Fig. 3):

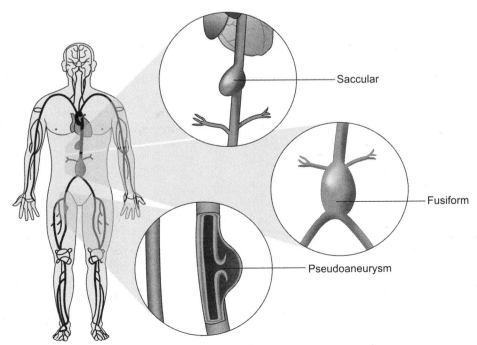

Fig. 3: Types of aneurysm.

Aorta

The aorta is the largest blood vessel in the body. It begins at the left ventricle of the heart and travels down the abdomen where it splits off into both legs. The aorta is a common site for arterial aneurysms.
1. Aneurysms in the chest cavity are called thoracic aortic aneurysms.
2. Abdominal aortic aneurysms are the most common type. In rare cases, both the chest and abdomen can be affected by arterial damage.

Brain

Aneurysms in the brain can be any size. These often form in the blood vessels that lie deep within the brain. They also may not present any symptoms or signs. You may not even know you have an aneurysm. Aneurysms of this type may cause bleeding in as many as 3% of people.

Symptoms

Symptoms of an aneurysm vary with each type and location. It is important to know that aneurysms that occur in the body or brain generally do not present signs or symptoms until they rupture. Aneurysms that occur near the surface of the body may show signs of swelling and pain. A large mass may also develop. The symptoms of ruptured aneurysms anywhere in the body can include:
1. Bleeding
2. Increased heart rate
3. Pain
4. Feeling dizzy or lightheaded.

Treatment

Treatment typically depends on the location and type of aneurysm. For example, a weak area of a vessel in your chest and abdomen may require a type of surgery called an endovascular stent graft. This minimally invasive procedure may be chosen over traditional open surgery because it involves repairing and reinforcing damaged blood vessels. The procedure also reduces the chance of infection, scarring, and other problems. Other treatments can include medications that treat high blood pressure and high cholesterol. Certain types of beta-blockers may also be prescribed to lower blood pressure. Lowering blood pressure may keep aneurysm from rupturing.

4. Describe bone healing.

Bone healing, or **fracture healing**, is a proliferative physiological process in which the body facilitates the repair of a bone fracture. Generally, bone fracture treatment consists of a doctor reducing (pushing) dislocated bones back into place via relocation with or without anesthetic, stabilizing their position, and then waiting for the bone's natural healing process to occur.

Physiological Process of Bone Healing

In the process of fracture healing, several phases of recovery facilitate the proliferation and protection of the areas surrounding fractures and dislocations. The length of the process depends on the extent of the injury, and usual margins of 2–3 weeks are given for the reparation of most upper bodily fractures; anywhere above 4 weeks given for lower bodily injury. The process of the entire regeneration of the bone can depend on the angle of dislocation or fracture. While the bone formation usually spans the entire duration of the healing process, in some instances, bone marrow within the fracture has healed 2 or fewer weeks before the final remodeling phase.

While immobilization and surgery may facilitate healing, a fracture ultimately heals through physiological processes. The healing process is mainly determined by the periosteum (the connective tissue membrane covering the bone). The periosteum is one source of precursor cells which develop into chondroblasts and osteoblasts that are essential to the healing of bone. The bone marrow (when present), endosteum, small blood vessels, and fibroblasts are other sources of precursor cells.

Stages of Bone Healing (Fig. 4)
1. A hematoma is formed.
2. Acute inflammation of the injured area, marrow cavity and surrounding soft tissues occurs. Blood vessels from the periosteum invade where normal blood supply has been interrupted, organizing it into a granulation tissue. Cellular proliferation begins throughout the affected bone within 24 hours of injury, after a few days, it is confined to the fracture area.
3. Formation of a primary callus. During the first month after injury a fibrocartilaginous callus is formed. The dead bone is resorbed and immature woven bone appears. The size of the callus is affected by the immobility of the fracture site; the smaller the amount of movement, the smaller the callus.
4. Woven bone is gradually replaced by lamellar bone, and the fracture is united by this bony secondary callus.
5. The final phase is remodeling where the shape of the bone is gradually returned to normal. This may take several years.

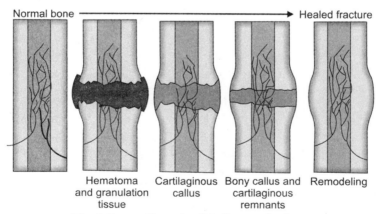

Fig. 4: Types of bone healing/fracture healing.

5. Describe hemoglobin estimation.

Principle
Anticoagulated blood is added to the 0.1 N HCl and kept for 5-7 minutes to form acid hematin. The color of this acid hematin should be matched with the solution, present in the calibration tube. Distilled water is added to the acid hematin until the color matches and the final reading is directly noted from the graduation in the calibration tube. (Please note that 100% on the scale corresponds to 14.5–15 g%).

Requirements
Sahli's hemoglobinometer, hydrochloric acid, distilled water.

Procedure

Place N/10 HCl in diluting tube up to the mark 20. Take blood in the hemoglobin pipette up to 20 cu mm mark and blow it into diluting tube and rinse well. After 10 minutes add distilled water in drops and mix the tube until it has exactly the same color as the comparison standards. Note the reading which indicates the percentage of hemoglobin.

Results

The Hb estimation of the given sample is ..... g/100 mL of blood/.....g/dL of blood/.....g%.

Precautions

1. Pipetting of blood should be done cautiously.
2. Mix the blood properly with HCl by using stirrer.
3. Match the color cautiously.

6. Explain the etiopathogenesis of primary tuberculosis.

Phagocytosis of tubercle bacilli by antigen-presenting cells in human lung alveoli initiates a complex infection process by *Mycobacterium tuberculosis* and a potentially protective immune response by the host (Fig. 5).

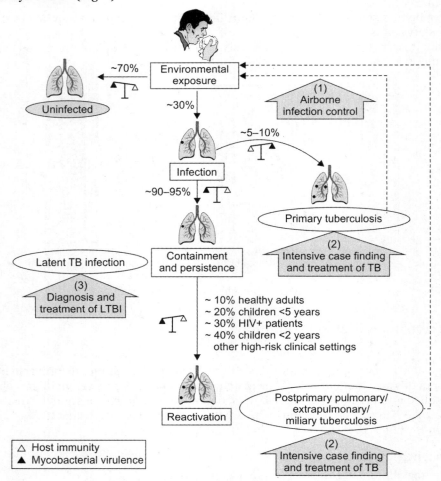

Fig. 5: Etiopathogenesis of primary tuberculosis.

M. tuberculosis has devoted a large part of its genome towards functions that allow it to successfully establish latent or progressive infection in the majority of infected individuals. The failure of immune-mediated clearance is due to multiple strategies adopted by *M. tuberculosis* that blunt the microbicidal mechanisms of infected immune cells and formation of distinct granulomatous lesions that differ in their ability to support or suppress the persistence of viable *M. tuberculosis*.

GENETICS

SHORT ANSWERS

1. Mention any four prenatal diagnostic tests.

Prenatal testing is used to identify women at risk of having a child with genetic disorders. This includes prenatal screening, prenatal and preimplantation diagnosis. Prenatal screening is performed using different testing procedures maternal serum testing, ultrasound, and molecular testing, etc. If screening results reveals abnormality then advance prenatal testing is carried out using techniques, such as amniocentesis, chorionic villus sampling (CVS), condrocentesis to investigate genetic condition of the fetus. These tests satisfactorily detect all trisomies, many chromosomal disorders and almost 100% Mendelian disorders. Another important role of prenatal testing is to help couple to plan pregnancy in advance if they have a known family history of genetic disorders for example, in case of phenylketonuria or 21-hydroxylase deficiency couples will not opt to terminate the affected pregnancy. Hence, a careful assessment for determining severity of genetic disorders is inevitable especially for some diseases causing still birth or early death in childhood.

Indications for Prenatal Testing

Prenatal testing is generally offered to:
1. Women at advanced child-bearing age, i.e. above 35 years.
2. Women inheriting serious genetic disorder, such as chromosomal translocation, congenital abnormalities and are at high-risk of transmitting the disease to the fetus.
3. Women or couple exposed to mutagens or radiations.

Types of Prenatal Testing

Prenatal diagnosis employs variety of techniques to determine the well-being of developing fetus. They are broadly classified as— 1. Invasive, 2. Noninvasive.
1. **Amniocentesis:** Amniocentesis is the most widely used invasive procedure preferably performed between 15–16 weeks of gestation. Since amniotic fluid contains fetal cells, it constitute good source for detecting fetal abnormalities, such as neural tube defect, Down's syndrome or 21-hydroxylase deficiencies. As the fluid contains fewer cells it required in vitro culture for 8–10 days before conducting biochemical tests.
2. **Chorionic villus sampling:** Chorionic villus sampling is an important invasive prenatal diagnostic technique commonly used to derive fetal material via transcervical or transabdominal route. Both the methods are performed following ultrasonography with constant vigilance on fetal viability. The main advantage of CVS over amniocentesis is the earlier procedure timing; it can be performed as early as 10–12 weeks of gestation.
3. **Cordocentesis:** Cordocentesis also referred as fetal blood sampling process allows rapid detection of fetal abnormalities particularly in the second or third trimester of pregnancy. Since the test provides direct access to the fetal blood, it helps monitor the pathological and physiological changes occurring in developing fetus.

2. Role of nurse in genetic counseling.

Genetic counselors are health professionals with specialized graduate degrees and experience in the areas of medical genetics and counseling. Most enter the field from a variety of disciplines including biology, genetics, nursing, psychology, public health, and social work. Genetic counselors work as members of a healthcare team providing information and support to families who have members with birth defects or genetic disorders and to families who may be at risk for a variety of inherited conditions. They identify families at risk, investigate the problem present in the family, interpret information about the disorder, analyze inheritance patterns and risks of recurrence, and review available options with the family.

Genetic counselors also provide supportive counseling to families, serve as patient advocates, and refer individuals and families to community or state support services. They serve as educators and resource people for other healthcare professionals and for the general public. Some counselors also work in administrative capacities. Many engage in research activities related to the field of medical genetics and genetic counseling.

Career Opportunities

Genetic counseling is a growing field that offers opportunities in a variety of areas. Among the possibilities are:
1. **Clinical:** Working with patients and families in hospitals, private practice, or on a consulting basis. Genetic counselors may specialize in genetic counseling in the prenatal, pediatric, cancer-risk, adult, cardiovascular, hematology, and neurogenetics setting.
2. **Commercial:** Working with biotech companies which design, sell, and administer genetic tests.
3. **Diagnostic laboratories:** Working as a liaison between the diagnostic laboratory and referring physicians and their patients.
4. **Education and public policy:** Teaching and advising companies, students, and lawmakers.
5. **Research:** Working as a study coordinator for research projects involved in genetics.

Steps in Genetic Counseling

Although specific procedures vary among testing centers, genetic testing for Huntington's disease generally involves several sessions that take place over the period of at least 1 month.

Step 1: Pretest genetic counseling:

A genetic counselor provides the individual who is considering testing with basic background knowledge about genetics, the inheritance of HD, and the testing procedure. These preliminary sessions ensure that the individual understands the clinical and psychological implications of genetic testing and is prepared to receive the test results.

Step 2: Neurological examination:

The purpose of this clinical phase is to determine whether the at risk individual is already showing symptoms of HD. A neurologist tests body movement, reflexes, eye movement, hearing, and balance. Brain imaging scans may also be used to check for the characteristic changes in brain structure caused by HD. These clinical observations are combined with an extensive family medical history in order to yield the diagnosis. If an individual is found to be symptomatic, he/she can either continue with the genetic testing process to confirm the diagnosis, or withdraw from genetic testing.

What is the difference between testing for HD and diagnosing HD?

Genetic testing shows whether or not an individual carries the HD allele, a mutated version of the *Huntington* gene. A positive test result indicates that the HD allele is present and that the individual will eventually develop Huntington's disease. However, the genetic test is not sufficient to diagnostic HD because it does not show whether the clinical symptoms are already being expressed. This information can only be obtained through the neurological examination discussed above, which is the definitive means of diagnosing or establishing the onset of HD.

Step 3: Psychological/psychiatric interview:
In this phase, a mental health professional assesses the mental and emotional state of the individual considering testing and provides counseling support services.

Generally, there is a time interval between the preliminary sessions and the actual genetic test. This waiting period provides the individual with sufficient time to consider the implications of genetic testing and reach a final decision.

3. Structure of the chromosome.

In the nucleus of each cell, the DNA molecule is packaged into thread-like structures called chromosomes. Each chromosome is made up of DNA tightly coiled many times around proteins called histones that support its structure. Chromosomes are not visible in the cell's nucleus not even under a microscope—when the cell is not dividing. However, the DNA that makes up chromosomes becomes more tightly packed during cell division and is then visible under a microscope. Most of what researchers know about chromosomes was learned by observing chromosomes during cell division.

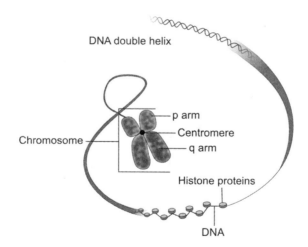

Fig. 6: Structure of chromosome.

Each chromosome has a constriction point called the centromere which divides the chromosome into two sections, or "arms." The short arm of the chromosome is labeled the "p arm." The long arm of the chromosome is labeled the "q arm." The location of the centromere on each chromosome gives the chromosome its characteristic shape, and can be used to help describe the location of specific genes (Fig. 6).

4. Define karyotyping.

Karyotyping is a test to examine chromosomes in a sample of cells. This test can help identify genetic problems as the cause of a disorder or disease. Most living things have **chromosomes**

or units of genetic information in their cells. The number and appearance of chromosomes vary among species. A **karyotype** is the number, size, and shape of chromosomes in an organism. To determine the karyotype of an organism, scientists must follow these steps:
1. Collect a cell from an individual.
2. Induce the cell to divide.
3. Stop cell division in metaphase when chromosomes are easiest to see.
4. Stain the chromosomes to make them visible.
5. View the cell under a microscope.

5. List any five autosomal abnormalities.

1. Klinefelter syndrome.
2. Turner syndrome.
3. Patau syndrome.
4. Chromosome abnormalities.
5. Down syndrome.

6. Define infertility.

Infertility refers to an inability to conceive after having regular unprotected sex. Infertility can also refer to the biological inability of an individual to contribute to conception, or to a female who cannot carry a pregnancy to full-term. Infertility means you cannot get pregnant (conceive).

There are two types of infertility:
1. Primary infertility refers to couples who have not become pregnant after at least 1 year having sex without using birth control methods.
2. Secondary infertility refers to couples who have been able to get pregnant at least once, but now is unable.

Female Infertility

Female infertility may occur when:
1. A fertilized egg or embryo does not survive once it attaches to the lining of the womb (uterus)
2. The fertilized egg does not attach to the lining of the uterus
3. The eggs cannot move from the ovaries to the womb
4. The ovaries have problems producing eggs

Female infertility may be caused by:
5. Autoimmune disorders, such as antiphospholipid syndrome (APS)
6. Birth defects that affect the reproductive tract
7. Cancer or tumor
8. Clotting disorders
9. Diabetes
10. Drinking too much alcohol
11. Exercising too much
12. Eating disorders or poor nutrition
13. Growths (such as fibroids or polyps) in the uterus and cervix
14. Medicines, such as chemotherapy drugs
15. Hormone imbalances
16. Obesity
17. Older age

18. Pelvic infection or pelvic inflammatory disease (PID)
19. Scarring from sexually transmitted infection, abdominal surgery or endometriosis
20. Smoking
21. Surgery to prevent pregnancy (tubal ligation) or failure of tubal ligation reversal (reanastomosis)
22. Thyroid disease.

Male Infertility

Male infertility may be due to:
1. Decreased number of sperm
2. Blockage that prevents the sperm from being released
3. Defects in the sperm.

Male infertility can be caused by:
1. Birth defects
2. Cancer treatments, including chemotherapy and radiation
3. Exposure to high heat for prolonged periods
4. Heavy use of alcohol, marijuana, or cocaine
5. Medicines, such as cimetidine, spironolactone, and nitrofurantoin
6. Obesity
7. Older age
8. Scarring from sexually transmitted infections, injury, or surgery
9. Smoking
10. Toxins in the environment
11. Vasectomy or failure of vasectomy reversal

Healthy couples under age 30 who have sex regularly will have a 25–30% per month chance of getting pregnant each month. A woman is most fertile in her early 20s. The chance a woman can get pregnant drops greatly after age 35 (and especially after age 40). The age when fertility starts to decline varies from woman-to-woman. Infertility problems and miscarriage rates increase significantly after 35 years of age. There are now options for early egg retrieval and storage for women in their 20's. This will help ensure a successful pregnancy if childbearing is delayed until after age 35. This is an expensive option, but for women who know they will need to delay childbearing, it may be worth considering.

Treatment

Treatment depends on the cause of infertility. It may involve:
1. Education and counseling about the condition
2. Fertility treatments, such as intrauterine insemination (IUI) and in vitro fertilization (IVF)
3. Medicines to treat infections and clotting disorders
4. Medicines that help the growth and release of eggs from the ovaries. Couples can increase the chances of becoming pregnant each month by having sex at least every 3 days before and during ovulation. Ovulation occurs about 2 weeks before the next menstrual cycle (period) starts. Therefore, if a woman gets her period every 28 days the couple should have sex at least every 3 days between the 10th and 18th day after her period starts.

Having sex before ovulation occurs is especially helpful:
1. Sperm can live inside a woman's body for at least 3 days
2. However, a woman's egg can only be fertilized by the sperm for a few hours after it is released
3. Women who are under or overweight, may increase their chances of becoming pregnant by getting to a healthier weight.

2014

Pharmacology, Pathology and Genetics

PHARMACOLOGY

LONG ESSAYS

1. Classify **antihypertensive drugs**, write the mechanism of action, therapeutic uses and adverse effects of calcium channel blocker.
2. Mention the drugs used in the treatment of **bronchial asthma**, add a note on beta antagonists.

SHORT ESSAYS

3. Drugs used in the treatment of **AIDS**.
4. Uses and adverse effects of **anticholinergic drugs**.
5. Chlorpromazine's.
6. Uses of **glucocorticoids**.
7. Beta-lactamase inhibitors.

SHORT ANSWERS

8. Mention one therapeutic use (clinical condition) and one important adverse effects of furosemide.
9. Mention one therapeutic use (clinical condition) and one important adverse effects of clopidogrel.
10. Mention one therapeutic use (clinical condition) and one important adverse effects of phenytoin sodium.
11. Mention one therapeutic use (clinical condition) and one important adverse effects of omeprazole.

PATHOLOGY

LONG ESSAYS

1. Define cirrhosis of liver, explain etiopathogenesis of cirrhosis of liver.
2. Describe pathology and complications of peptic ulcer.

SHORT ESSAYS

3. Inflammation.
4. Pneumonia.
5. Urine culture and sensitivity.
6. Breast cancer.

GENETICS

SHORT ANSWERS

7. Isochromosome.
8. Mention four characteristics of sex-linked recessive inheritance.
9. Mention four prenatal diagnostic tests.
10. Genetic counseling.
11. Mention any four causes of congenital anomalies.
12. Phenylketonuria.

PHARMACOLOGY

LONG ESSAYS

1. Classify antihypertensive drugs, write the mechanism of action, therapeutic uses and adverse effects of calcium channel blocker.

Hypertension refers to the prolonged and persistent elevation of blood pressure above the normal range. If not treated properly, hypertension can cause severe complications, such as stroke, coronary heart disease and kidney failure. Patients with hypertension must take antihypertensive drugs on a long-term basis. Although such drugs cannot give a radical cure, they can prevent heart failure, kidney failure and acute stroke induced by hypertension and delay the development of atherosclerosis by controlling the blood pressure. Generally speaking, antihypertensive drugs must be taken for life.

Classification of the Antihypertensive Drugs

I. Diuretics

Diuretics are still used as initial drugs of choice for mild hypertension in the majority of cases. They can be used alone, or in combination with other classes of antihypertensive drugs.

Methyldopa: Trimethaphan is a short-acting ganglion blocking agent. The blocking action is exerted at the postsynaptic cholinergic receptor in autonomic ganglia. This competitive antagonism is short-lived.

Guanethidine: After propranolol many beta-blockers have been introduced. All beta-blockers share the common property of being competitive inhibitors of catecholamines.

II. Antihypertensive Alpha-adrenoceptor Blocker

Prazosin: Prazosin acts by a competitive postsynaptic alpha 1-adrenoceptor blockade. It does not block the presynaptic inhibitory effects which allow reflex action to overcome the postural hypotension usual with alpha-blockade.

Doxazosin: Terazosin is a long-acting selective alpha 1-adrenoceptor blocker. It reduces TPR, and has little effect on the heart rate. Terazosin may be used alone or with a diuretic in patients with mild to moderate hypertension.

Phenoxybenzamine: Labetalol has an alpha blocking action, with a nonspecific beta and beta-adrenoceptor blocking action. On oral administration the ratio of alpha to beta blockade is about 1:3.

Hydralazine: Minoxidil dilates arteriolar resistance vessels with minimal effects on venous capacitance vessels. It reduces calcium uptake through the cell membrane, thereby reducing arteriolar tone and lowering peripheral vascular resistance.

Diazoxide: Sodium nitroprusside is a short-term hypotensive agent. It reduces TPR by a direct action on blood vessels and may be used in the treatment of hypertensive crisis.

Verapamil: Verapamil is a calcium blocker used in the chronic management of angina pectoris; and in the control of supraventricular arrhythmias. Verapamil is also useful in the control of mild to moderate hypertension.

III. Antihypertensive Angiotensin II Receptor Blockers

Losartan is a recently introduced blocker of the AT1 receptor. It has no effect on bradykinin metabolism, and therefore a more selective blocker.

IV. Angiotensin Effects than the ACE Inhibitors

Pinacidil is a potent vasodilator, and is the first antihypertensive drug classified as a potassium channel opener, although, it is likely that minoxidil and diazoxide also lower BP by this mechanism.

Side Effects of the Antihypertensive Drugs

Side effects of antihypertensive drugs vary with individual drugs. Common side effects include the following temporary reactions:
1. Headache, weakness or fatigue
2. Dizziness upon rising quickly from a sitting or lying position
3. Numbness or sharp pain in fingers or toes
4. Cold hands and feet
5. Dry eyes, mouth and throat
6. Nightmares or sleeping difficulties.

Advice on Medication

The following should be borne in mind when taking antihypertensive drugs:
1. Learn the name and dosage of the drugs you are taking.
2. Take the drugs regularly as instructed by your doctor in order to have effective control of hypertension. Keep on taking the drugs even if your conditions improve.
3. Do not stop medication without your doctor's instruction. Take your medicines at the same fixed time every day as far as possible. If you miss a dose, take it as soon as possible unless it is almost time for the next scheduled dose. In that case, skip the missed dose and take the next dose as directed. Do not take double doses.
4. The drugs should not be taken with alcoholic drinks to avoid dizziness or fainting.
5. If you have to take other drugs as well, such as cough syrup, drugs for common cold and anticough medicines, you should consult your doctor first to avoid affecting the efficacy of the antihypertensive drugs. You may bring along your medical history or labeled drug bags for your doctor's reference during follow-up consultation.
6. Do not put different drugs in the same bottle. Each drug should be put into its original labeled container.
7. The stock of drugs should be sufficient for several days' use. Do not wait till the last minute to fill the prescription.

Life Adaptations

People with hypertension should take note of the following in their daily lives:
1. Quit smoking
2. Reduce salt intake. Eat less preserving and processed food such as sausages, pickles and potato chips
3. Drink less caffeinated beverages like strong tea, coffee and coke
4. Do moderate exercise regularly
5. Keep optimal body weight
6. Learn self-relaxation because anxiety, loss of temper and overstrain all give rises to increased blood pressure.

Angiotensin Converting Enzyme Inhibitors

Angiotensin converting enzyme inhibitors (ACE inhibitors) used in the management of mild to moderate hypertension. They lower the BP in both renovascular hypertension and essential hypertension.

Mechanism of Action

Causes a fall in BP by arteriolar dilatation without affecting cardiac output. Inhibits conversion of angiotensin I to angiotensin II.

Decreases aldosterone secretion and compete with angiotensin II to block its effect. Examples: Captopril, enalapril, lisinopril and perindopril. The magnitude of fall in BP is sodium dependent; if sodium levels are low the fall in BP is significant.

Drug interactions: NSAIDs attenuate the hypotensive action potassium—sparing diuretics can cause hyperkalemia.

Contraindications

To be avoided in bilateral renal artery disease, pregnancy, high salt intake, patients on high dose diuretic therapy, and dry cough.

Untoward Effects

Severe hypotension, palpitation, tachycardia, chest pain, severe proteinuria (associated with renal hypertension), hyperkalemia (serum potassium of more than 5 mEq/L), and hypermagnesemia.

Nursing Implications

1. Rebound hypertension can occur if medication is stopped abruptly.
2. Monitor blood counts and serum potassium levels.
3. Educate patient to have BP and pulse checked every day, and report to physician if blood pressure is more than 140/90 mm Hg, or pulse rate of more than 100 beats/mm.
4. Advise to take nitroglycerine immediately and go to emergency room if chest pain occurs.

2. Mention the drugs used in the treatment of bronchial asthma, add a note on beta antagonists.

Prevention and long-term control are key in stopping asthma attacks before them start. Treatment usually involves learning to recognize your triggers, taking steps to avoid them and tracking your breathing to make sure your daily asthma medications are keeping symptoms under control. In case of an asthma flare-up, you may need to use a quick-relief inhaler, such as albuterol.

Medications

The right medications for you depend on a number of things—your age, symptoms, asthma triggers and what works best to keep your asthma under control. Preventive, long-term control medications reduce the inflammation in your airways that leads to symptoms. Quick-relief inhalers (bronchodilators) quickly open swollen airways that are limiting breathing. In some cases, allergy medications are necessary.

Long-term asthma control medications, generally taken daily, are the cornerstone of asthma treatment. These medications keep asthma under control on a day-to-day basis and make it less likely you will have an asthma attack. Types of long-term control medications include:

Inhaled corticosteroids: These anti-inflammatory drugs include fluticasone (flonase, flovent HFA), budesonide (pulmicort flexhaler, rhinocort), flunisolide (aerospan HFA), ciclesonide (alvesco, omnaris, zetonna), beclomethasone (qnasl, qvar), mometasone (asmanex) and fluticasone furoate (arnuity ellipta). You may need to use these medications for several days to weeks before they reach their maximum benefit. Unlike oral corticosteroids, these corticosteroid medications have a relatively low risk of side effects and are generally safe for long-term use.

Leukotriene modifiers: These oral medications—including montelukast (singulair), zafirlukast (accolate) and zileuton (zyflo)—help relieve asthma symptoms for up to 24 hours. In rare cases, these medications have been linked to psychological reactions, such as agitation, aggression, hallucinations, depression and suicidal thinking. Seek medical advice right away for any unusual reaction.

Long-acting beta agonists: These inhaled medications which include salmeterol (serevent) and formoterol (foradil, perforomist), open the airways. Some research shows that they may increase the risk of a severe asthma attack, so take them only in combination with an inhaled corticosteroid. And because these drugs can mask asthma deterioration, do not use them for an acute asthma attack.

Combination inhalers: These medications, such as fluticasone-salmeterol (advair diskus), budesonide-formoterol (symbicort) and formoterol-mometasone (dulera) contain a long-acting beta agonist along with a corticosteroid. Because these combination inhalers contain long-acting beta agonists, they may increase your risk of having a severe asthma attack.

Theophylline: Theophylline (Theo-24, elixophyllin, others) is a daily pill that helps keep the airways open (bronchodilator) by relaxing the muscles around the airways. It is not used as often now as in past years.

Quick-relief (rescue) medications are used as needed for rapid, short-term symptom relief during an asthma attack or before exercise if your doctor recommends it. Types of quick-relief medications include:

Short-acting beta agonists: These inhaled quick-relief bronchodilators act within minutes to rapidly ease symptoms during an asthma attack. They include albuterol (proAir HFA, ventolin HFA, others) and levalbuterol (xopenex). Short-acting beta agonists can be taken using a portable, hand-held inhaler or a nebulizer—a machine that converts asthma medications to a fine mist, so that they can be inhaled through a face mask or a mouthpiece.

Ipratropium (atrovent): Like other bronchodilators, ipratropium acts quickly to immediately relax your airways, making it easier to breathe. Ipratropium is mostly used for emphysema and chronic bronchitis, but it is sometimes used to treat asthma attacks.

Oral and intravenous corticosteroids: These medications which include prednisone and methylprednisolone, relieve airway inflammation caused by severe asthma. They can cause serious side effects when used long-term, so they are used.

Allergy medications may help if your asthma is triggered or worsened by allergies. These include:

Allergy shots (immunotherapy): Overtime, allergy shots gradually reduce your immune system reaction to specific allergens. You generally receive shots once a week for a few months, then once a month for a period of 3–5 years.

Omalizumab (xolair): This medicatio, given as an injection every 2–4 weeks, is epecifically for people who have allergies and severe asthma. It acts by altering the immune system.

Bronchial thermoplasty: This treatment which is not widely available nor right for everyone is used for severe asthma that does not improve with inhaled corticosteroids or other long-term asthma medications. Generally, over the span of three outpatient visits, bronchial thermoplasty heats the insides of the airways in the lungs with an electrode, reducing the smooth muscle inside the airways. This limits the ability of the airways to tighten, making breathing easier and possibly reducing asthma attacks.

Beta Antagonists

Beta-blockers block beta-adrenergic substances, such as epinephrine (adrenaline) in the autonomic nervous system (involuntary nervous system). They slow down the heartbeat, decrease the force of the contractions of the heart muscles, and reduce blood vessel contraction in the heart, brain, as well as the rest of the body. Doctors may prescribe beta-blockers for patients with tachycardias (rapid heart rates). They help patients with angina by lowering the amount of oxygen the heart muscles require. Angina pectoris occurs when the heart requires more oxygen than it is getting.

Indications

Beta-blockers block the release of noradrenaline in parts of the body. Noradrenaline is released by the nerves when they are stimulated—it is a chemical that conveys messages to other parts of the body including muscles, blood vessels and the heart.

1. **Heart problems**—for a patient with heart problems beta-blockers can reduce the workload for the heart; so that it does not have to work so hard to supply all parts of the body with oxygen-rich blood. For people with angina, heart failure, or after a heart attack, reducing the heart's workload is crucial. Beta-blockers can also block the stimulation of the heart form electrical impulses—they can control irregular heartbeats—thus lowering the activity of the heart and slowing down the heart rate.
2. **Hypertension**—beta-blockers lower blood pressure by slowing down the heart rate, as well as reducing the force of the heart. Blood still gets to all parts of the body, but at reduced pressure.
3. **Glaucoma**—pressure within the eyeball is reduced with beta-blocker eye drops. The medication lowers the production of fluid inside the eyeball (aqueous humor).

Side Effects of Beta-blockers

The most common side effects of beta-blockers are:
1. Cold feet
2. Cold hands
3. Diarrhea
4. Fatigue
5. Nausea
6. Very slow heartbeat.

The following less common side effects are also possible:
1. Sleeping difficulties and disturbances
2. Bad dreams (nightmares)
3. Erectile dysfunction (male inability to achieve or sustain an erection during sex).

Driving

Some patients may experience dizziness or fatigue; in such cases they should not drive. However, this is rare.

Beta-blocker Interactions with other Drugs

Drug interaction is the extra effects of two different medicines can have on the body when taken together—effects beyond their primary purposes. Beta-blockers can interact with the following medications:

1. **Antipsychotics**—these medications are commonly prescribed for patients with bipolar disorder or schizophrenia. When taken with some beta-blockers the risk of arrhythmias is greater.
2. **Clonidine**—a medication prescribed for either patients with hypertension (high blood pressure) or migraines. A patient who is taking both clonidine and beta-blockers and then

suddenly stops taking clonidine has a greater risk of experiencing a sudden and sharp rise in blood pressure (rebound hypertension).
3. **Digoxin**—prescribed for patients with congestive heart failure and certain cardiac arrhythmias. When taken with beta-blockers, there is a higher risk of slow heart rate (bradycardia).
4. **Diltiazem**—a medication that dilates blood vessels, prescribed for patients with angina pectoris or hypertension. When taken with beta-blockers, there is a higher risk of slow heart rate (bradycardia).
5. **Drugs to control high blood pressure (antihypertensives)**—when taken with beta-blockers the patient may experience hypotension (a serious drop in blood pressure).
6. **Drugs to control irregular heartbeats (antiarrhythmics)**—when taken with beta-blockers the risk of impaired function of the heart (myocardial depression) is greater, as is the risk of irregular heartbeats (arrhythmias).
7. **Mefloquine**—a drug for the treatment of malaria resistant to chloroquine phosphate. When taken with beta-blockers the result may be bradycardia.
8. **Nifedipine**—this drug reduces calcium ions available to heart and smooth muscle, used in the treatment of angina pectoris. When taken with beta-blockers, there is a higher risk of hypotension (low blood pressure).
9. **Nisoldipine**—a calcium channel blocker used in the treatment of high blood pressure (hypertension). When taken with beta-blockers there is a higher risk of hypotension (low blood pressure).
10. **Verapamil**—used in the treatment of hypertension, angina pectoris, and certain cardiac arrhythmias. When taken with beta-blockers, there is a higher risk of hypotension (low blood pressure).

SHORT ESSAYS

3. Drugs used in the treatment of AIDS.

HIV infection starts when the virus is transmitted through contact with infected body fluids, such as blood, semen, or breast milk. HIV targets the immune system and invades white bloods cells called T helper cells. These are cells that fight infection. By entering your body's cells, the virus hides from your immune system. After the virus invades these cells, it replicates inside of them. Then the cells explode. They release many viral cells that go on to invade other normal cells. This process destroys your immune system's ability to fight infections and generally keeps your body from working well.

Multiclass Combination Drugs
Combination drugs combine medications from different groups into one drug form. You take these medications once per day. Each person's dosage is different. These drugs include:
1. Efavirenz/emtricitabine/tenofovir disoproxil fumarate (atripla).
2. Emtricitabine/rilpivirine/tenofovir disoproxil fumarate (complera).
3. Elvitegravir/cobicistat/emtricitabine/tenofovir disoproxil fumarate (stribild).
4. Abacavir/dolutegravir/lamivudine (triumeq).

Nucleoside/Nucleotide Reverse Transcriptase Inhibitors (NRTIs)
They work by interrupting the life cycle of HIV as it tries to copy itself. These drugs also have other actions that prevent HIV from replicating in your body. NRTI drugs include:

1. Abacavir (ziagen).
2. Efavirenz/emtricitabine/tenofovir disoproxil fumarate (atripla).
3. Lamivudine/zidovudine (combivir).
4. Emtricitabine/rilpivirine/tenofovir disoproxil fumarate (complera).
5. Emtricitabine (emtriva).
6. Lamivudine (epivir).
7. Abacavir/lamivudine (epzicom).
8. Zidovudine (retrovir).
9. Abacavir/lamivudine/zidovudine (trizivir).
10. Emtricitabine/tenofovir disoproxil fumarate (truvada).
11. Didanosine (videx).
12. Didanosine extended release (videx EC).
13. Tenofovir disoproxil fumarate (viread).
14. Stavudine (zerit).

Non-nucleoside Reverse Transcriptase Inhibitors (NNRTIs)

These drugs work in the same way as NRTIs. They stop the virus from replicating itself in your body. These drugs include:
1. Rilpivirine (edurant)
2. Etravirine (intelence)
3. Delavirdine mesylate (rescriptor)
4. Efavirenz (sustiva)
5. Nevirapine (viramune)
6. Nevirapine extended-release (viramune XR).

Protease Inhibitors

Protease inhibitors work by binding to protease. This is a protein that HIV needs to replicate in the body. When protease cannot do its job, the virus cannot complete the process that makes new copies. This reduces the number of viruses that can infect more cell.

Entry Inhibitors (Including Fusion Inhibitors)

Entry inhibitors are another class of HIV medications. HIV needs a host T cell in order to make copies of itself. These drugs block the virus from entering a host T cell. This prevents the virus from replicating itself. These drugs also prevent the destruction of targeted cells. This action helps your immune system work better. An example of an entry inhibitor includes: Enfuvirtide (fuzeon) which comes in an injectable form.

Integrase Inhibitors

Integrase inhibitors are a class of drugs that stop the action of integrase. This is a viral enzyme that HIV uses to infect CD4+ T cells. These drugs include:
1. Raltegravir (isentress).
2. Dolutegravir (tivicay).
3. Elvitegravir (vitekta).

Chemokine coreceptor antagonists (CCR5 antagonists): CCR5 antagonists prevent the spread of HIV. These drugs block infection in one of two molecules found on the surface of each body cell. Because it only affects one molecule, this drug is usually used with other medications for full HIV treatment. An example of this type of drug includes: Maraviroc (selzentry).

Cytochrome P4503A (CYP3A) inhibitors: CYP3A is an enzyme that protects liver and gastrointestinal (GI) health. HIV can destroy this enzyme leading to problems with your liver and GI tract. CYP3A inhibitors protect these enzymes to keep you healthy. These drugs affect your liver and come with the risk of jaundice. This may cause yellowing of your skin and the whites of your eyes. An example of this type of drug includes: Cobicistat (tybost).

Immune-based Therapies

Because HIV affects your immune system, researchers are studying ways that drugs can help boost immunity. Certain immune-based treatments have been successful in some people. Like some protease inhibitors, these drugs are used off-label for HIV. They are used along with other HIV medications. An example of an immune-based therapy includes: Hydrochloroquine sulfate (plaquenil), which is a drug approved to treat autoimmune diseases, such as lupus and rheumatoid arthritis.

4. Uses and adverse effects of anticholinergic drugs.

Anticholinergics are a class of drugs that block the action of the neurotransmitter acetylcholine in the brain. They are used to treat diseases like asthma, incontinence, gastrointestinal cramps, and muscular spasms. They are also prescribed for depression and sleep disorders. The drugs help to block involuntary movements of the muscles associated with these diseases. They also balance the production of dopamine and acetylcholine in the body. Anticholinergics can also be used to treat certain types of toxic poisoning, and are sometimes used as an aid to anesthesia.

Anticholinergics are used to treat a variety of conditions. These include:
1. Gastrointestinal disorders, such as diarrhea, overactive bladder, and incontinence
2. Asthma
3. Chronic obstructive pulmonary disease (COPD)
4. Insomnia
5. Dizziness and motion sickness
6. Poisoning caused by toxins, such as organophosphates or muscarine
7. Hypertension (high blood pressure)
8. Symptoms of Parkinson's disease.

Side Effects Depend on Dose

You may or may not experience any side effects. Check with your healthcare professional if side effects continue or become bothersome or severe. Side effects of anticholinergics may include:
1. Dry mouth
2. Blurred vision
3. Constipation
4. Drowsiness
5. Sedation
6. Hallucinations
7. Memory impairment
8. Difficulty urinating
9. Confusion
10. Delirium
11. Decreased sweating
12. Decreased saliva.

Signs of an overdose include:
1. Dizziness
2. Severe drowsiness
3. Fever
4. Severe hallucinations
5. Confusion
6. Trouble breathing
7. Clumsiness and slurred speech
8. Fast heartbeat
9. Flushing and warmth of the skin.

An overdose of certain anticholinergics or taking them with alcohol can result in unconsciousness or even death. Seek emergency help immediately if you or someone you know may have taken an overdose.

5. Chlorpromazine's.

Chlorpromazine is used to treat the symptoms of schizophrenia (a mental illness that causes disturbed or unusual thinking, loss of interest in life, and strong or inappropriate emotions) and other psychotic disorders (conditions that cause difficulty in telling the difference between things or ideas that are real and things or ideas that are not real) and to treat the symptoms of mania (frenzied, abnormally excited mood) in people who have bipolar disorder (manic depressive disorder; a condition that causes episodes of mania, episodes of depression, and other abnormal moods). Chlorpromazine is also used to treat severe behavior problems, such as explosive, aggressive behavior and hyperactivity in children 1–12 years of age. Chlorpromazine is also used to control nausea and vomiting, to relieve hiccups that have lasted 1 month or longer, and to relieve restlessness and nervousness that may occur just before surgery. Chlorpromazine is also used to treat acute intermittent porphyria (condition in which certain natural substances build up in the body and cause stomach pain, changes in thinking and behavior, and other symptoms). Chlorpromazine is also used along with other medications to treat tetanus (a serious infection that may cause tightening of the muscles, especially the jaw muscle). Chlorpromazine is in a class of medications called conventional antipsychotics. It works by changing the activity of certain natural substances in the brain and other parts of the body.

Pharmacokinetics

Chlorpromazine is readily absorbed from the gastrointestinal tract, however its bioavailability is variable due to considerable first pass metabolism by the liver. Liquid concentrates may have greater bioavailability than tablets. Food does not appear to affect bioavailability consistently. IM administration bypasses much of the first pass effect and higher plasma concentrations are achieved. The onset of action after IM administration is usually 15–30 minutes and after oral administration 30–60 minutes. Rectally administered chlorpromazine usually takes longer to act than oral.

Chlorpromazine is highly bound to plasma proteins (>90%), principally albumin. It is not dialysable. It is distributed widely throughout the body; crossing the blood-brain barrier, the placenta and is distributed into milk. Volume of distribution is about 20 L/kg.

Chlorpromazine is metabolized extensively and at least 12 different metabolites are known. Less than 1% is excreted unchanged. Most metabolites are excreted in the urine as unconjugated or conjugated forms. The terminal half-life of chlorpromazine is variable at approximately 30 hours.

Indications

The management of psychotic disorders including manifestations of manic depressive illness, manic phase and severe behavioral problems in children; nausea and vomiting due to stimulation of the chemoreceptor trigger zone.

Contraindications

Comatose or depressed states due to CNS depressants; blood dyscrasias; bone marrow depression; liver damage. Hypersensitivity to chlorpromazine. Cross allergenicity with other phenothiazines may occur.

It should be avoided in children or adolescents with signs or symptoms suggestive of Reye's syndrome. Its antiemetic effect may mask the signs and its CNS effect may be confused with the signs of Reye's syndrome or other encephalopathies.

Precautions

1. Phenothiazines should be used with caution in patients with cardiovascular disease. Chlorpromazine is an alpha-adrenergic blocking agent and increased pulse rate and transient hypotension have both been reported in some patients receiving these drugs.
2. Hypotension, which is typically orthostatic, may occur especially in elderly and in alcoholic patients. This effect may be additive with other agents that cause a lowering of blood pressure. If chlorpromazine should cause severe hypotension, most patients will respond to cautious expansion of the intravascular volume with sodium chloride. If vasopressor drugs are needed, the drugs of choice are alpha-receptor agonists, such as phenylephrine or methoxamine.
3. Chlorpromazine has direct negative inotropic action. It prolongs PR and QT intervals, blunts the T wave and depresses the S-T segment. These changes appear to be reversible and related to disturbance in repolarization. Give phenothiazines cautiously to patients with heart disease.
4. Most reported cases of agranulocytosis associated with the administration of phenothiazine derivatives have occurred between the fourth and tenth week of treatment. Therefore, observe patients on prolonged therapy with particular care during that time for the appearance of such signs as sore throat, fever and weakness. If these symptoms appear, discontinue the drug and perform WBC and differential counts.
5. Chlorpromazine should be used with caution in patients who have impaired liver function or alcoholic liver disease. CNS depression may be potentiated.
6. If bilirubinemia or icterus occurs, discontinue the drug and perform liver function tests.
7. Phenothiazines have been associated with retinopathy. Discontinue chlorpromazine if retinal changes are observed. Regular ophthalmologic exams are recommended.
8. Use chlorpromazine cautiously in patients with a history of seizures since the drug tends to lower the seizure threshold.
9. The anticholinergic action of chlorpromazine may be a factor in some cases of intestinal pseudo-obstruction.
10. Chlorpromazine may mask signs of overdosage of toxic drugs and may obscure conditions, such as intestinal obstruction and brain tumor.

6. Uses of glucocorticoids.

A: Arthritis, acute respiratory distress syndrome (ARDS), aspiration pneumonia, allergic reaction, adrenal-pituitary axis function testing, autoimmune (hemolytic anemia, multiple scierosis (MS), idiopathic thrombocytopenic purpura).

B: Bronchial asthma (acute exacerbation, severe chronic asthma, status asthmaticus), Bell's palsy.
C: Collagen diseases (SLE, PAN, nephrotic syndrome, glomerulonephritis), cerebral edema, cysticercosis, cancer (ALL, Hodgkin's and other lymphoma, breast carcinoma, secondary hypercalcemia).
D: Dermatologic (pemphigus vulgaris, exfoliative dermatitis, Stevens-Johnson syndrome).
E: Eye disease (allergic conjunctivitis, iritis, keratitis, retinitis, optic neuritis, uveitis).
G: Graft rejection.
I: Intestinal disease (UC, CD, celiac disease), infection (sepsis).

7. Beta-lactamase inhibitors.

Beta-lactamase inhibitors block the activity of beta-lactamase enzymes. Some species of bacteria produce beta-lactamase enzymes which cleave the beta-lactam group in antibiotics, such as penicillin, that have a beta-lactam ring in their structure. A drug may be classified by the chemical type of the active ingredient or by the way it is used to treat a particular condition. Each drug can be classified into one or more drug classes. In doing so the beta-lactamase enzyme inactivates the antibiotic and becomes resistant to that antibiotic. To avoid development of resistance, beta-lactamase inhibitors are administered with the beta-lactam antibiotics, so the action of beta-lactamase is inhibited. This tends to widen the spectrum of antibacterial activity.

SHORT ANSWERS

8. Mention one therapeutic use (clinical condition) and one important adverse effects of furosemide.

Furosemide (Lasix)

It is a potent, prompt diuretic causing massive changes in fluid balance. Onset of action is in 20 minutes and duration is 4 hours.

It blocks reabsorption of sodium in ascending loop of Henle. It impairs normal process of urinary concentration and decreases renal vascular resistance leading to increased renal flow.

Urinary sodium loss may be as high as 40% of filtered amount. Loss of potassium is less while there is greater excretion of chloride than thiazides. There is no change in the pH of the urine with diuresis in both acidotic and alkalotic states. The action is more rapid and shorter than thiazide.

Uses

Severe edema, pulmonary edema, cerebral edema and also to induce diuresis in barbiturate poisoning. It can reduce blood volume in heart failure. High dose is useful in incipient acute renal failure.

Dose

About 40–80 mg oral, 25–50 mg IV.

Side Effects

Fatigue, dizziness, muscle cramp, orthostatic hypotension, temporary loss of hearing. It can precipitate hepatic coma.

Improper use can cause serious electrolyte and water disturbance. Hypokalemia, hypochloremic alkalosis, hyperuricemia, hypovolemia can also occur.

9. Mention one therapeutic use (clinical condition) and one important adverse effects of clopidogrel.

Reducing the risk of stroke, heart attack, or death in patients who have already had a heart attack or stroke, have other circulatory problems caused by narrowing and hardening of the arteries, or have certain other heart problems (e.g. unstable angina). It also may be used for other conditions as determined by your doctor. Clopidogrel is a platelet aggregation inhibitor. It works by slowing or stopping platelets from sticking to blood vessel walls or injured tissues.

Warning

Increases the risk of bleeding; discontinue 5 days prior to surgery if an antiplatelet effect is not desired. Avoid lapses in therapy; if therapy must be temporarily discontinued, restart as soon as possible. Premature discontinuation may increase risk of CV events. Thrombotic thrombocytopenic purpura (TTP) reported. Hypersensitivity (e.g. rash, angioedema, hematologic reaction) reported including in patients with a history of hypersensitivity or hematologic reaction to other thienopyridines.

Contraindications

Active pathological bleeding (e.g. peptic ulcer, intracranial hemorrhage), hypersensitivity (e.g. anaphylaxis) to clopidogrel or any component of the product.

Side Effects

Heart—swelling, high blood pressure, inflammation of blood vessels.
Central nervous system—headache, dizziness, depression, confusion.
Skin—rash, itching, severe allergic reactions (severe rash, itching, swelling, severe dizziness, trouble breathing) Stevens-Johnson syndrome, toxic epidermal necrolysis.
Eye and ENT—bleeding in retina, conjunctiva.
Gastrointestinal—abdominal pain, diarrhea, stomach upset, nausea, inflammation of colon (including ulcerative or lymphocytic), inflammation of pancreas, mouth ulcer, taste disorders.
Genitourinary—urinary tract infection, kidney disease, increased creatinine levels.
Blood—bruising, nose bleeds, anemia, bleeding (including intracranial, GI, and retroperitoneal hemorrhage), and decrease in platelets.
Liver—abnormality in liver enzymes, inflammation of liver.
Metabolic—increase in cholesterol.
Musculoskeletal—muscle pain, back pain, muscle weakness.
Respiratory—upper respiratory tract infection, difficulty in breathing, inflammation of bronchus, stuffy nose, coughing.
Miscellaneous—accidental injury, chest pain, influenza-like symptoms, fatigue, fainting, hypersensitivity reactions, serum sickness, bleeding of wounds.

10. Mention one therapeutic use (clinical condition) and one important adverse effects of phenytoin sodium.

Phenytoin sodium is a commonly used antiepileptic. Phenytoin acts to suppress the abnormal brain activity seen in seizure by reducing electrical conductance among brain cells by stabilizing the inactive state of voltage-gated sodium channels. Aside from seizures, it is an option in the treatment of trigeminal neuralgia in the event that carbamazepine or other first-line treatment seems inappropriate.

Uses

Phenytoin is used to prevent and control seizures (also called an anticonvulsant or antiepileptic drug). It works by reducing the spread of seizure activity in the brain. This section contains uses of this drug that are not listed in the approved professional labeling for the drug, but that may be prescribed by your healthcare professional. Use this drug for a condition that is listed in this section only if it has been so prescribed by your healthcare professional. This drug may also be used to treat certain types of irregular heartbeats.

The recommended dose of phenytoin varies according to individual needs. The usual adult dose is 300–400 mg daily taken by mouth in divided doses or a single dose. An increase to 600 mg taken in divided doses may be needed in some cases. The children's dose is based on age and body weight.

Side Effects

- Bleeding, tender, or enlarged gums
- Changes in muscle movements or coordination
- Changes to the gums including bleeding or swelling
- Confusion
- Difficulty sleeping
- Dizziness
- Headache
- Nausea and vomiting
- Slurred speech
- Unusual eye movement.

11. Mention one therapeutic use (clinical condition) and one important adverse effects of omeprazole.

Omeprazole is **used** to treat symptoms of gastroesophageal reflux disease (GERD) and other conditions caused by excess stomach acid. It is also **used** to promote healing of erosive esophagitis (damage to your esophagus caused by stomach acid). Omeprazole is used to reduce the amount of acid in your stomach. It is used to treat gastric or duodenal ulcers, GERD, erosive esophagitis (inflammation in the esophagus), and hypersecretory conditions (conditions where your stomach makes too much acid). This drug is also used to treat stomach infections caused by the bacteria *Helicobacter pylori*. This drug comes in the form of a capsule or liquid suspension you take by mouth. Omeprazole is available as the brand name drug Prilosec. It is also available as a generic drug.

Prescription omeprazole is used alone or with other medications to treat GERD, a condition in which backward flow of acid from the stomach causes heartburn and possible injury of the esophagus (the tube between the throat and stomach). Prescription omeprazole is used to treat the symptoms of GERD, allow the esophagus to heal, and prevent further damage to the esophagus. Prescription omeprazole is also used to treat conditions in which the stomach produces too much acid, such as Zollinger-Ellison syndrome. Prescription omeprazole is also used to treat ulcers (sores in the lining of the stomach or intestine) and it is also used with other medications to treat and prevent the return of ulcers caused by a certain type of bacteria (*H. pylori*). Nonprescription (over-the-counter) omeprazole is used to treat frequent heartburn (heartburn that occurs at least 2 or more days a week). Omeprazole is in a class of medications called proton-pump inhibitors. It works by decreasing the amount of acid made in the stomach.

Adverse Effects

Common **omeprazole side effects** may include: Stomach pain, gas, nausea, vomiting, diarrhea or headache. Omeprazole may cause side effects. Tell your doctor if any of these symptoms are severe or do not go away:
- Constipation
- Gas
- Nausea
- Vomiting
- Headache.

Some side effects can be serious. If you experience any of these symptoms, call your doctor immediately, or get emergency medical help:
- Rash
- Hives
- Itching
- Swelling of the face, throat, tongue, lips, eyes, hands, feet, ankles, or lower legs
- Difficulty breathing or swallowing
- Hoarseness
- Irregular, fast, or pounding heartbeat
- Excessive tiredness
- Dizziness
- Lightheadedness
- Muscle spasms
- Uncontrollable shaking of a part of the body
- Seizures
- Diarrhea with watery stools
- Stomach pain
- Fever.

PATHOLOGY

LONG ESSAYS

1. Define cirrhosis of liver, explain etiopathogenesis of cirrhosis of liver.

Cirrhosis is a type of liver damage where healthy cells are replaced by scar tissue. The liver is unable to perform its vital functions of metabolism, production of proteins including blood clotting factors, and filtering of drugs and toxins. Many people think that only drinking excessive amounts of alcohol causes liver cirrhosis, but there are a number of other ways that the liver can be damaged and lead to cirrhosis. Depending on the cause, cirrhosis can develop over months or years. There is no cure. Treatment aims to halt liver damage, manage the symptoms and reduce the risk of complications, such as diabetes, osteoporosis (brittle bones), liver cancer and liver failure.

Symptoms depend on the severity of the cirrhosis, but may include:
1. Appetite loss
2. Nausea
3. Weight loss
4. General tiredness

5. Spidery red veins on the skin (spider angiomas)
6. Easily bruised skin
7. Yellowing of the skin and eyes (jaundice)
8. Reddened palms (palmar erythema)
9. Itchy skin
10. Hair loss
11. Dark colored urine
12. Fluid retention in the abdomen and legs
13. Internal bleeding presenting as dark-colored stools or vomiting blood
14. Hormone disruptions that could cause a range of problems including testicular atrophy (shrinking) and impotence in males or amenorrhea (no periods) in women
15. Cognitive problems, such as memory loss, confusion or concentration difficulties.

Causes of Liver Cirrhosis

Two of the most common causes of cirrhosis of the liver are long-term excessive alcohol consumption and hepatitis C, but a number of other conditions also lead to liver damage and cirrhosis. Hepatitis B is an important cause of cirrhosis worldwide and increasingly among migrants from endemic areas in Asia, Africa, Pacific Island and Mediterranean countries.

Alcoholic Liver Cirrhosis

Excessive and chronic alcohol consumption is the most common cause of liver cirrhosis. Cirrhosis from drinking alcohol can develop over many years.

It is important to remember that the amount of alcohol that will damage the liver can vary from person-to-person. If a healthy woman drinks the same amount of alcohol as a healthy man, she has a higher risk of cirrhosis. Children are particularly susceptible to damage from alcohol. Some people also have a genetic predisposition to alcohol-related liver injury.

Liver Cirrhosis and Hepatitis

Hepatitis is a general term meaning inflammation of the liver. Viral hepatitis refers to hepatitis caused by a virus like hepatitis B or C virus. Chronic hepatitis C is a common cause of liver cirrhosis. Hepatitis B can also cause cirrhosis. With either of these conditions, you increase your risk of developing cirrhosis if you drink alcohol.

Liver Cirrhosis and Fatty Liver

Nonalcoholic fatty liver disease (NAFLD) is a condition where fat accumulates in the liver. It now affects about 20% of Australians. It is becoming more common in children who are overweight or obese. Fatty liver does not usually cause pain or nausea.

NAFLD is associated with conditions, such as:
1. Obesity—20% of people with obesity have fatty liver disease
2. High blood cholesterol and triglycerides
3. Type 2 diabetes.

NAFLD can lead to inflammation of the liver and the formation of scar tissue, a condition called nonalcoholic steatohepatitis (NASH) which can then lead to cirrhosis of the liver. NASH usually occurs in people who are obese, have diabetes or have high blood cholesterol and triglycerides, so controlling these conditions is recommended.

People with NASH have a higher risk of liver damage if they have hepatitis C. The effect of alcohol is debated, but it is probably not recommended if there is significant liver scarring present.

Liver Cirrhosis from Inherited Conditions

Some inherited conditions damage the liver and this leads to the scarring that can contribute to cirrhosis. These conditions include:
1. **Hemochromatosis**—the body accumulates iron which can damage many organs including the liver.
2. **Wilson's disease**—the tissues of the body accumulate copper.
3. **Galactosemia**—the body is unable to process galactose (a sugar), so it accumulates in the blood and can result in liver damage.
4. **Cystic fibrosis**—mainly affects the lungs, but can also cause scarring of the liver.
5. **Alpha-1 antitrypsin deficiency**—can affect breathing, but can also affect liver function and lead to cirrhosis and liver failure.

Other Causes of Liver Cirrhosis

A number of other medical conditions that result in liver damage can cause cirrhosis including:
1. **Some autoimmune diseases**—cause immune cells to attack and damage the liver. The rare Conditions that can cause liver cirrhosis include autoimmune hepatitis, primary biliary cirrhosis and primary sclerosing cholangitis (inflammation and scarring of the bile ducts).
2. **Exposure to poisons**—can damage the liver because one of the liver's main roles is to remove toxins from the blood. Prolonged exposure to environmental toxins, such as arsenic can damage the liver and lead to cirrhosis.
3. **Schistosomiasis**—a tropical disease caused by a parasitic worm called *Schistosoma*. The worm is passed to humans from snails, and the disease is also known as bilharziasis. Chronic schistosomiasis causes damage to internal organs including the liver.
4. **Certain medication** (such as those used to manage heart arrhythmias)—in rare cases, may cause cirrhosis in susceptible people.
5. **Unknown conditions**—cause cirrhosis in about one-third of cases (called 'cryptogenic cirrhosis'. Some of these are due to nonalcoholic fatty liver disease).

Complications of Liver Cirrhosis

Without medical treatment, cirrhosis of the liver can lead to a range of potentially life-threatening complications including:
1. **Insulin resistance and type 2 diabetes**—a poorly functioning liver stops the body from properly using insulin, the hormone that moves sugar from the blood into the cells.
2. **Osteoporosis (brittle bones)** caused by changes to metabolism of calcium and vitamin D
3. **Primary liver cancer**—the most common type of cancer caused by cirrhosis is hepatocellular carcinoma.
4. **Liver failure**—scar tissue can impair the functioning of normal liver tissue bleeding from blood vessels in the esophagus or upper stomach (esophageal varices).
5. **Increased blood pressure** in veins that take blood to the liver (portal hypertension).
6. **Build-up of fluid within** the abdominal cavity (ascites).
7. Infection of the fluid found within the abdominal cavity (spontaneous bacterial peritonitis)
8. **Damage to the brain and nervous system** caused by toxins that the liver has failed to remove (hepatic encephalopathy).

Diagnosis of Liver Cirrhosis

Tests used to diagnose liver cirrhosis may include:
1. Medical history
2. Physical examination
3. Blood tests including liver function tests

4. Urine tests
5. Imaging studies including ultrasound, computed tomography (CT scan) or magnetic resonance imaging (MRI)
6. Fibroscan—also known as transient elastography, this test uses an ultrasound-based technique that can accurately and noninvasively detect liver cirrhosis. It may replace the need for liver biopsy in some cases. The test takes about ten minutes, is usually performed by a specialist hepatologist and causes no discomfort. It is less accurate in people with obesity issues unless specially designed XL probes are used
7. Liver biopsy—obtaining liver tissue for laboratory examination.

Treatment of Liver Cirrhosis

The cirrhosis of the liver is incurable but, in some cases, treatment can help to reduce the likelihood that the condition will become worse. Options include:
1. Treating the underlying cause of liver damage—for example, treating the underlying hepatitis (B or C) virus infection, removal of blood to lower iron levels in hemochromatosis.
2. Making dietary and lifestyle changes—a nutritious low-fat diet, high-protein diet and exercise can help people to avoid malnutrition.
3. Avoiding alcohol—alcohol damages the liver and harms remaining healthy tissue.
4. Taking certain medication, such as beta-blockers to reduce blood pressure and lower the risk of bleeding, diuretics to remove excess fluid.
5. Avoiding certain medication that can make the symptoms worse, such as nonsteroidal anti-inflammatory drugs (NSAIDs), opiates or sedatives.
6. Having regular medical check-ups—including scans to check for liver cancer.
7. Having regular endoscopic procedures to check whether there are varicose veins within the esophagus or stomach.
8. Having a liver transplant—an option that may be considered in severe cases.

2. Describe pathology and complications of peptic ulcer.

Peptic ulcer occurs in the duodenum and the stomach. They are chronic, solitary lesions seen commonly in the first portion of the duodenum and in the stomach.

Pathogenesis

The two most important causative factors for the development of peptic ulcer include:
1. *Helicobacter pylori* infection and
2. Mucosal exposure to gastric acid and pepsin. Other factors which cause injury to the mucosa include consumption of aspirin and NSAIDs, cigarette smoking, alcohol consumption and duodenal gastric reflux.

There are certain mucosal defensive forces which prevent the development of peptic ulcers. These include:
1. Surface mucus secretion
2. Bicarbonate secretion in the mucus
3. Epithelial regenerative capacity and
4. Elaboration of prostaglandins.

An imbalance between the mucosal defensive forces and damaging factors are responsible for the development of peptic ulcer.

Gross Morphology

The ulcers are round, sharply demarcated punched out craters approximately 2–4 cm in diameter. The location is on the anterior and posterior wall of the first part of the duodenum and the lesser curvature of the stomach. The margins of the ulcer are edematous and the surrounding mucosal folds may radiate like spokes of a wheel. The ulcer base is clean due to peptic digestion of the necrotic tissue.

Microscopy

Four zones are identified on microscopy:
1. The base comprising of a thin layer of necrotic debris.
2. Zone of active nonspecific inflammatory infiltrate.
3. Granulation tissue and
4. Fibrous, collagenous scar.

Healing occurs by proliferation of the granulation tissue and re-epithelialization from the margins of the ulcer.

Clinical Features

The patients present with a burning or boring type of epigastric pain especially 1–3 hours after meals. The pain is relieved by alkalis. Other symptoms include nausea, bloating, belching and loss of weight.

Complications

1. Bleeding is the most common complication and is life-threatening.
2. Perforation of the wall of the stomach duodenum.
3. Rare complications include obstruction and malignant transformation.

SHORT ESSAYS

3. Inflammation (*See* Q.1, 2016)

4. Pneumonia.

Pneumonia is a breathing (respiratory) condition in which there is an infection of the lung. Community-acquired pneumonia is pneumonia in people who have not recently been in the hospital or another healthcare facility (nursing home, rehabilitation facility) (Fig. 1).

Causes, Incidence, and Risk Factors

Pneumonia is a common illness that affects millions of people each year. Bacteria, viruses, and fungi may cause pneumonia.

Bacteria and viruses living in your nose, sinuses, or mouth may spread to your lungs. Pneumonia caused by bacteria tends to be the most serious kind. In adults, bacteria are the most common cause of pneumonia.

The most common pneumonia-causing germ in adults is *Streptococcus pneumoniae* (*Pneumococcus*).

Atypical pneumonia, often called walking pneumonia, is caused by bacteria, such as *Legionella pneumophila, Mycoplasma pneumoniae*, and *Chlamydophila pneumoniae*.

Pneumocystis jiroveci pneumonia is sometimes seen in people whose immune system is not working well.

Many other bacteria can also cause pneumonia. Viruses are also a common cause of pneumonia especially in infants and young children.

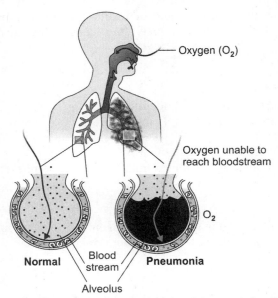

Fig. 1: Difference between normal and diseased alveoli.

Risk factors (conditions that increase your chances of getting pneumonia) include:
1. Cerebral palsy.
2. Chronic lung disease (COPD, bronchiectasis, cystic fibrosis).
3. Cigarette smoking.
4. Difficulty swallowing (due to stroke, dementia, Parkinson's disease, or other neurological conditions).
5. Immune system problem.
6. Impaired consciousness (loss of brain function due to dementia, stroke, or other neurologic conditions).
7. Living in a nursing facility.
8. Other serious illnesses, such as heart disease, liver cirrhosis, or diabetes mellitus.
9. Recent surgery or trauma.
10. Recent cold, laryngitis, or flu.

Symptoms
The most common symptoms of pneumonia are:
1. Cough (with some pneumonias you may cough up greenish or yellow mucus, or even bloody mucus).
2. Fever, which may be mild or high.
3. Shaking chills.
4. Shortness of breath (may only occur when you climb stairs).

Other symptoms include:
1. Confusion, especially in older people
2. Excess sweating and clammy skin
3. Headache
4. Loss of appetite, low energy, and fatigue
5. Sharp or stabbing chest pain that gets worse when you breathe deeply or cough

Signs and Tests
The healthcare provider will likely order a chest X-ray if pneumonia is suspected.
Some patients may need other tests including:
1. Arterial blood gases to see if enough oxygen is getting into your blood from the lungs.
2. Complete blood count (CBC) to check white blood cell count.
3. CT scan of the chest.
4. Gram's stain and culture of your sputum to look for the bacteria or virus that is causing your symptoms.
5. Pleural fluid culture if there is fluid in the space around the lungs.

Treatment
1. Fluids and antibiotics in your veins
2. Oxygen therapy
3. Breathing treatments (possibly).

5. Urine culture and sensitivity.
A urine culture is a laboratory test to check for bacteria or other germs in a urine sample. It can be used to check for a urinary tract infection in adults and children.

Procedure
Most of the time the sample will be collected as a clean catch urine sample in your healthcare provider's office or your home. You will use a special kit to collect the urine. A urine sample can also be taken by inserting a thin rubber tube (catheter) through the urethra into the bladder. This is done by someone in your provider's office or at the hospital. The urine drains into a sterile container, and the catheter is removed. Rarely, your provider may collect a urine sample by inserting a needle through the skin of your lower abdomen into your bladder. The urine is taken to a laboratory to determine which, if any, bacteria or yeast are present in the urine. This takes 24–48 hours.

Abnormal Results
A "positive" or abnormal test is when bacteria or yeast are found in the culture. This likely means that you have a urinary tract infection or bladder infection. Other tests may help your provider know which bacteria or yeast are causing the infection and which antibiotics will best treat it. Sometimes more than one type of bacteria, or only a small amount, may be found in the culture.

6. Breast cancer.
Breast cancer affects one in eight Australian women. It is the most common cancer for Victorian women, with almost 3,700 diagnoses in 2012. Breast cancer can occur at any age, but it is most common in women over the age of 60. Around one quarter of women who are diagnosed with breast cancer are younger than 50. Men can also develop breast cancer, although this is extremely rare. Each year, about 25 men are diagnosed in Victoria. It is treated in the same way as breast cancer in women. There are different types of breast cancer, but they all begin in the milk ducts or the milk lobules (or both) (Fig. 2).

Some breast cancers are found when they are 'in situ'. This means that they have not spread outside the milk duct or lobule where the cancer began. Most breast cancers are found when they are 'invasive'. This means the cancers have grown beyond the duct or lobule, where they began, into other breast tissue, or spread to other parts of the body. Breast cancer that spreads

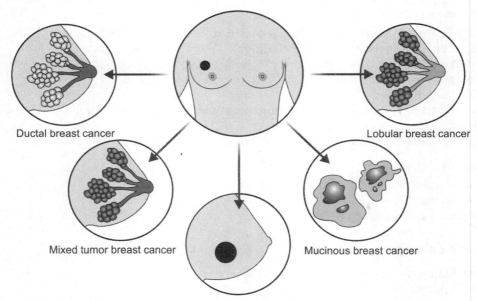

Fig. 2: Types of breast cancer.

out of the breast may spread to lymph nodes in the armpit nearest the breast affected by cancer (axillary lymph nodes). It can also spread to other parts of the body, such as bones, lungs and liver.

Risks and Causes of Breast Cancer

The exact cause of breast cancer is unknown, but factors that seem to increase risk include:
1. Gender—being a woman.
2. Getting older—women over 50 years of age are invited to take part in yearly mammograms to screen for breast cancer (women from the age of 40 are also able to access yearly mammograms).
3. Heredity—having several close family members (mother, sister or daughter) who have had breast cancer.
4. Previous history of breast cancer—women who have had breast cancer have a greater risk of developing it again.
5. Certain breast diseases—some types of breast disease that are found through mammograms indicate an increased risk.

Other Risk Factors for Breast Cancer

Other factors that seem to increase risk include:
1. Not having children or having children after the age of 30.
2. Early age at first period.
3. Later age of natural menopause (55 years or older).
4. Alcohol intake (more than one standard drink per day).
5. Obesity or gaining a lot of weight after menopause.
6. Using the contraceptive pill—the risk is higher while taking the pill and for about ten years after stopping use.
7. Using hormone replacement therapy (HRT)—also known as hormone therapy (HT)—the risk increases the longer you take it, but disappears within about 2 years of stopping use.

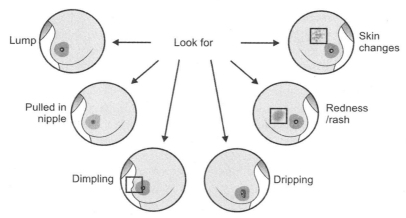

Fig. 3: Inspection and palpation of breast by self-examination

Examination

By regularly checking your breasts, you may be able to recognize changes that could be a sign of breast cancer. Such changes include (Fig. 3):
1. Thickening of the tissue
2. A lump or lumpiness
3. Discharge from the nipple
4. An inverted or 'turned-in nipple' (unless the nipple has always been turned in)
5. Puckering or dimpling of the skin
6. A change in the shape of the breast or nipple
7. A painful area
8. Anything that is not 'usual' for you.

Some of these symptoms can occur without any serious disease being present. Nine out of ten breast changes are not breast cancer. However, just to be sure, your doctor should check any unusual breast change.

Diagnosis of Breast Cancer

Breast changes are investigated through a series of tests organized by your doctor or specialist. Most breast changes are diagnosed as Benign (noncancerous). If your tests show that you may have cancer, your doctor will refer you to a specialist who will advise you about treatment options. Initial tests you may have include:
1. Physical examination—breasts and armpits are examined.
2. Diagnostic mammogram—an X-ray of the breast tissue.
3. Ultrasound—a device that uses soundwaves to scan the breast.

If further tests are required, one or more procedures may be used including:
4. Fine needle aspiration—a very narrow needle is used to withdraw cells from the testing area.
5. Core biopsy—a larger needle is used to take a tissue sample for testing.
6. Open biopsy—surgery is performed under general anesthetic to remove the whole area for testing.
7. Hormone tests—if a cancer is found, it can be checked for special markers called hormone receptors to see if it will respond to hormone treatment.
8. Ductogram (also known as a galactogram) or discharge test—this is for breast cancers that are causing a discharge from the nipple.

Treatment for Breast Cancer

Treatment options for breast cancer include surgery, radiotherapy, and chemotherapy and hormone therapy. Usually, more than one is used. Treatment for breast cancer in men is similar to (and as effective as) the treatment for breast cancer in women.

Surgery Options Include

1. **Breast-conserving surgery**—a small operation removes the cancer and some of the surrounding tissue, and usually some lymph nodes, leaving the bulk of the breast intact.
2. **Mastectomy**—the entire breast is removed along with lymph nodes from the armpit. Extra cancer treatment, such as chemotherapy or radiotherapy is often unnecessary.
3. **Breast reconstruction surgery**—women who have a mastectomy may choose to have reconstruction surgery (at the time of the mastectomy or later). Options include silicone gel or saline-filled implants, or the use of your own muscle and skin to create a breast-like shape. If you do not choose reconstruction, you may use a breast form or prostheses. These are pads that are worn inside your bra. They help to restore balance and are designed to look like a normal breast under clothes. All surgery has some risks. Possible side effects of breast surgery include infection, bleeding, blood clots in the leg (deep vein thrombosis), nerve damage and swelling of the arm. These side effects are not common, but you need to understand the risks.

Other Treatment for Breast Cancer

Depending on the cancer, other treatment options can include:

Radiotherapy—use X-rays (radiation) to kill any remaining cancer cells. Women who have had breast-conserving surgery often have a course of radiotherapy. Side effects can include a short-term reddening of the skin which looks like sunburn, or longer-term thickening of skin.

Chemotherapy—cancer-killing medication is given intravenously (directly into a vein). Chemotherapy can be offered to women with early breast cancer as an extra treatment to surgery, radiotherapy or both. Chemotherapy has side effects that will depend on the type of medication you have, but can include nausea, vomiting and hair loss.

Hormone treatments—many breast cancers are influenced by the sex hormones—estrogen and progesterone. Hormone treatment can reduce the chances of breast cancer developing again.

Biological therapies (also called immunotherapies)—strengthen the immune system to fight cancer. Several types of biological therapies are now used to treat breast cancer. Research is continuing and various types of therapies are being tested in clinical trials.

Complementary and alternative therapies—when used alongside your conventional cancer treatment, some of these therapies can make you feel better and improve quality of life. Others may not be so helpful and in some cases may be harmful. The Cancer Council Victoria booklet called Understanding Complementary Therapies can be a useful resource.

SHORT ANSWERS

7. Isochromosome.

A chromosomal aberration that arises as a result of transverse rather than longitudinal division of the centromere during meiosis; two daughter chromosomes are formed, each lacking one chromosome arm but with the other doubled.

A metacentric chromosome produced during mitosis or meiosis when the centromere splits transversely instead of longitudinally; the arms of such chromosome are equal in length and genetically identical, however, the loci are positioned in reverse sequence in the two arms.

8. Mention four characteristics of sex-linked recessive inheritance.

1. Males are primarily affected. Rarely, females may have symptoms, but carrier females are usually unaffected.
2. A son of a carrier mother has a 50% risk to inherit the mutation and thus have the disorder.
3. There is no male-to-male transmission of the disorder.
4. Affected males transmit the mutation to all daughters who would be carriers, but not to any sons.

9. Mention four prenatal diagnostic tests.

Prenatal diagnostic testing involves testing the fetus before birth (prenatally) to determine whether the fetus has certain abnormalities including certain hereditary or spontaneous genetic disorders. Some of these tests, such as ultrasonography and certain blood tests are often part of routine prenatal care. Ultrasonography and blood tests are safe and sometimes help determine whether more invasive prenatal genetic tests (chorionic villus sampling, amniocentesis, and percutaneous umbilical blood sampling) are needed. Usually, these more invasive tests are done when couples have an increased risk of having a baby with a genetic abnormality (such as a neural tube defect) or a chromosomal abnormality (particularly when the woman is 35 or older). However, many doctors offer this type of testing to all pregnant women, and any pregnant woman can request it. These tests have risks, although very small, particularly for the fetus.

Couples should discuss the risks with their healthcare practitioner and weigh the risks against their need to know. For example, they should think about whether not knowing the results of testing would cause anxiety and whether knowing that an abnormality was not found would be reassuring. They should think about whether they would pursue an abortion if an abnormality was found. If they would not, they should consider whether they still want to know of an abnormality before birth (for example, to prepare psychologically) or whether knowing would only cause distress. For some couples, the risks outweigh the benefits of knowing whether their baby has a chromosomal abnormality, so they choose not to be tested.

10. Genetic counseling.

Genetic counselors are health professionals with specialized graduate degrees and experience in the areas of medical genetics and counseling. Most enter the field from a variety of disciplines, including biology, genetics, nursing, psychology, public health, and social work.

Genetic counselors work as members of a healthcare team, providing information and support to families who have members with birth defects or genetic disorders and to families who may be at risk for a variety of inherited conditions. They identify families at risk, investigate the problem present in the family, interpret information about the disorder, analyze inheritance patterns and risks of recurrence, and review available options with the family.

Genetic counselors also provide supportive counseling to families, serve as patient advocates, and refer individuals and families to community or state support services. They serve as educators and resource people for other healthcare professionals and for the general public. Some counselors also work in administrative capacities. Many engage in research activities related to the field of medical genetics and genetic counseling.

Career Opportunities

Genetic counseling is a growing field that offers opportunities in a variety of areas. Among the possibilities are:
1. **Clinical:** Working with patients and families in hospitals, private practice, or on a consulting basis. Genetic counselors may specialize in genetic counseling in the prenatal, pediatric, cancer-risk, adult, cardiovascular, hematology, and neurogenetics setting.
2. **Commercial:** Working with biotech companies which design, sell, and administer genetic tests.
3. **Diagnostic laboratories:** Working as a liaison between the diagnostic laboratory and referring physicians and their patients.
4. **Education and public policy:** Teaching and advising companies, students, and lawmakers.
5. **Research:** Working as a study coordinator for research projects involved in genetics.

Steps in Genetic Counseling

Although specific procedures vary among testing centers, genetic testing for Huntington's disease generally involves several sessions that take place over the period of at least 1 month.

Step 1: Pretest genetic counseling:

A genetic counselor provides the individual who is considering testing with basic background knowledge about genetics, the inheritance of HD, and the testing procedure. These preliminary sessions ensure that the individual understands the clinical and psychological implications of genetic testing and is prepared to receive the test results.

Step 2: Neurological examination:

The purpose of this clinical phase is to determine whether the at-risk individual is already showing symptoms of HD. A neurologist tests body movement, reflexes, eye movement, hearing, and balance. Brain imaging scans may also be used to check for the characteristic changes in brain structure caused by HD. These clinical observations are combined with an extensive family medical history in order to yield the diagnosis. If an individual is found to be symptomatic, he/she can either continue with the genetic testing process to confirm the diagnosis, or withdraw from genetic testing.

What is the difference between testing for HD and diagnosing HD?

Genetic testing shows whether or not an individual carries the HD allele, a mutated version of the *Huntington* gene. A positive test result indicates that the HD allele is present and that the individual will eventually develop Huntington's disease. However, the genetic test is not sufficient to diagnose HD because it does not show whether the clinical symptoms are already being expressed. This information can only be obtained through the neurological examination discussed above which is the definitive means of diagnosing or establishing the onset of HD.

Step 3: Psychological/psychiatric interview:

In this phase, a mental health professional assesses the mental and emotional state of the individual considering testing and provides counseling support services.

Generally, there is a time interval between the preliminary sessions and the actual genetic test. This waiting period provides the individual with sufficient time to consider the implications of genetic testing and reach a final decision.

11. Mention any four causes of congenital anomalies.

Congenital anomalies are also known as birth defects, congenital disorders or congenital malformations. Congenital anomalies can be defined as structural or functional anomalies (e.g. metabolic disorders) that occur during intrauterine life and can be identified prenatally, at birth or later in life.

Causes and Risk Factors

Although approximately 50% of all congenital anomalies cannot be linked to a specific cause, there are some known causes or risk factors.

Socioeconomic and Demographic Factors

Although low income may be an indirect determinant, congenital anomalies are more frequent among resource-constrained families and countries. It is estimated that about 94% of severe congenital anomalies occur in low and middle-income countries, where women often lack access to sufficient, nutritious food and may have increased exposure to agents or factors, such as infection and alcohol that induce or increase the incidence of abnormal prenatal development. Further, advanced maternal age increases the risk of chromosomal abnormalities including Down syndrome, while young maternal age increases the risk of some congenital anomalies.

Genetic Factors

Consanguinity (when parents are related by blood) increases the prevalence of rare genetic congenital anomalies and nearly doubles the risk for neonatal and childhood death, intellectual disability and other anomalies in first-cousin unions. Some ethnic communities (e.g. Ashkenazi Jews or Finns) have a comparatively high prevalence of rare genetic mutations leading to a higher risk of congenital anomalies.

Infections

Maternal infections, such as syphilis and rubella are a significant cause of congenital anomalies in low and middle-income countries.

Maternal Nutritional Status

Iodine deficiency, folate insufficiency, obesity and diabetes mellitus are linked to some congenital anomalies. For example, folate insufficiency increases the risk of having a baby with a neural tube defect. Also, excessive vitamin A intake may affect the normal development of an embryo or fetus.

Environmental Factors

Maternal exposure to certain pesticides and other chemicals as well as certain medications, alcohol, tobacco, psychoactive drugs and radiation during pregnancy, may increase the risk of having a fetus or neonate affected by congenital anomalies. Working or living near, or in, waste sites, smelters or mines may also be a risk factor especially if the mother is exposed to other environmental risk factors or nutritional deficiencies.

12. Phenylketonuria.

Phenylketonuria (PKU) is a rare genetic condition that causes an amino acid called phenylalanine to build up in the body. Amino acids are the building blocks of protein. Phenylalanine is found in all proteins and some artificial sweeteners. Your body uses an enzyme called phenylalanine hydroxylase to convert phenylalanine into tyrosine, a nonessential amino acid. Your body needs tyrosine to create neurotransmitters, such as epinephrine, norepinephrine, and dopamine. PKU is caused by a defect in the gene that helps create phenylalanine hydroxylase. When this enzyme is missing, the body is unable to break down phenylalanine. This causes a build up of phenylalanine in the body. Early diagnosis and treatment can help relieve symptoms of PKU and prevent brain damage.

PKU is an inherited condition caused by a defect in the *PAH* gene. The *PAH* gene helps create phenylalanine hydroxylase, the enzyme responsible for breaking down phenylalanine. A dangerous buildup of phenylalanine can occur when someone eats high-protein foods, such as eggs and meat. Both parents must pass on a defective version of the *PAH* gene for their child to inherit the disorder. If just one parent passes on an altered gene, the child would not have any symptoms, but they will be a carrier of the gene.

Sociology

2019

Sociology

LONG ESSAYS
1. Define socialization; explain in brief the stages and agencies of socialization.
2. Define family; explain types and functions of family.
3. Define culture; explain the values of culture in health and illness.

SHORT ESSAYS
4. Uses of sociology.
5. Social disorganizations.
6. Characteristics of Indian village.
7. Difference between primary and secondary group.
8. Importance of competition in social life.
9. Population explosion and its effects on health status.
10. Types of social isolation.
11. Forms of accommodation.
12. Juvenile delinquency.

SHORT ANSWERS
13. Race.
14. Urban slums.
15. Formal social control.
16. Hindu marriage act 1955.
17. Customs.
18. Define role and status.
19. Definition of socialization.
20. Crowd.
21. Social groups.
22. HIV/AIDS.

LONG ESSAYS

1. Define socialization; explain in brief the stages and agencies of socialization.

(*See* Q. 18, 2014)

2. Define family; explain types and functions of family.

Man's social life begins with family. It is the most important primary group. It is the oldest social institution known to man. Family is the mother of social institutions. It is the first social environment to which a child is exposed. It is a place where most of the people spend more than one half of their lifetime. Family is the center of our life activities. It gives shape to our personality and provides us inspiration. Family is in the center of the social system. All other system has a close bearing with the family. Family contributes to their strength. Any major change in the family will have repercussions throughout the social system.

Family has regulated the sexual relations to avoid promiscuity, by prescribing customary sex morals. It is a permanent organization which has provided stable family life. It is the shelter where man is fed, clothed, and housed from the beginning. It has upheld and inculcated the traditions and customs of the group. Thus, family is the foundation stone on which the cultural heritage is built. Family as a unit of sociological inquiry is dealt within various ways by sociologists. It is studied as an institution, as an association, as an organization. It is also referred to as a subsystem because it is regarded as one of the parts of the society.

Meaning of Family

The origin of the English word, Family is traced to the Roman word Famulus or to the Latin word Familia meaning a household comprising or servants or workers and of slaves along with other individuals having marriage or blood relations. The word denotes group of procedures consisting of slaves, servants, and members connected by common descent or marriage. Thus originally, family consisted of a man and woman with a child or children and servants. This meaning of family has changed over the years.

Definitions

1. Family is a more or less durable association of husband and wife or without child or of a man or woman alone, with children.

    —MF Nimkoff.

2. Family is a group of persons united by ties of marriage, blood or adaptation consisting a single household interacting and intercommunicating with each other in their respective social roles of husband and wife, father and mother, son and daughter, brother and sister, creating a common culture.

    —Burgess and Locke.

3. Family is the biological social unit composed of husband, wife and children.

    —Eliot and Merrill.

4. Family is a group defined by sex relationship sufficiently precise and enduring to provide for the procreation and upbringing of children.

    —MacIver.

5. Family is a system of patterned expectations defining the proper behavior of persons playing certain roles, enforced both by the incumbents own positive motives for conformity and by the sanction of others.

    —Parsons.

6. Family is a recognized and established usage governing the relations between individuals and groups.

—Ginsberg.

7. Family is a habitual way of living together which have been sanctioned, systematized and established by the authority of communities.

—Ellwood CA.

Modern Family

The modern family is more individualized and democratic where women enjoy a high prestige and position. About hundred years back, the family was more of a community. Today, it has become an association. It has completed the transition from institution to association. The functions of modern family are very limited. The role and status of men and women have very much changed. The economic liberalization of women has resulted in equal status for them. Modern family changed from a production to consumption unit. The changing modern family equation of women in the family has transferred family into a new kind of partnership and created new problem for the family of the present and of the future.

Features of Modern Family

1. The traditional patriarchal family began to crumble after 18th and 19th centuries. The new social, economical and technological forces affected the character of patriarchal family.
2. Industrialization, urbanization process, democratic ideals of liberty and equality, the decline of authoritarian mores have affected the social significance of the family.
3. Women are employed in factories and offices. They are economically independent. The family changed from production to consumption unit. Various home appliances for cooking, baking, washing and the use of readymade food products provide lot of leisure to women.
4. The life partners are selected freely by the youngsters and marriage is based on individual romantic love. Parental control and authority is lessened.
5. The modern family woman is not devoted to man but considered as an equal partner in life with equal rights.
6. Both men and women have ample opportunities for their frequent contact which may lead to laxity of sex relationships resulting in premarital and extramarital relationships.
7. The modern family is a smaller family. It is not a joint family. There is a tendency to have a smaller family and contraceptive are in large use.
8. The modern family is secular in character. There is little religious control. The authority of religion over marriage and divorce has markedly declined.
9. In modern family, physical punishment is rarely given to children. The children themselves decide as to which school will study in, what cloths they will wear, what food will be cooked and to which movie they are to go. It has become a filo-centric family.

Changes in the modern family: In the modern period, the institution of family is undergoing rapid change and modification. The main changes in this connection are shown in Table 1:

Table 1: Changes in the modern family.

Sl. No.	Change in modern family	Description
1.	Reduction in the economic functions of life	In the modern age, many of the economic functions which were previously being performed by the family, are now being performed by the schools, factories, government aid and other associations
2.	Reduction in other activities of family	Many of other functions of the family have now been taken over by other agencies. The work of looking after and bringing up children is now being performed in crèches, children parks, and kindergarten schools and by babysitters. Hospitals undertake the work of delivering children and of treatment. Restaurants prepare food for thousands of families
3.	Increase in family recreation	Modern families have been transformed into centers of recreation with the invention of radio and television, and the advent of indoor games
4.	Laxity in martial and sex relationships	The rigidity traditionally associated with marital and sexual relationships no longer characterizes the modern family
5.	Changes in relationship of men and women	Now that the women have gained equal rights with men, their mutual relationships have undergone many changes. Moreover has correctly written of the modern women, she is no longer the drudge and solve of older days
6.	Increase in importance of children	In the modern family the importance of children has increased. They are now physically maltreated or punished only rarely but are instead taught lovingly. The modern families tend to become filo-centric families
7.	Decrease in importance of blood relationships	In the modern families, there has been a continuous decrease in the importance of blood relationships. The family is now constituted of a husband, a wife and their children
8.	Disorganization of joint family	The modern family is no longer joint. The joint family is rapidly being disorganized
9.	Smaller family	Due to the prolific use of contraceptives and the tendency to regard children as an obstacle in the progress and enjoyment of life, the birth rate is continuously falling and the modern families are becoming smaller
10.	Family disorganization	The process of disorganization is quiet apparent in the modern family. The number of divorces is on the increase. The control which the family exercises over the individual is being lessened
11.	Instability	The modern family is no longer a permanent association. It is precarious and can be rendered violent any time. Marriage has reduced to a mere social contract which it is not difficult to break in the event of even the slightest function

3. Define culture; explain the values of culture in health and illness.

(*See* Q. 1, 2016)

SHORT ESSAYS

4. Uses of sociology. (*See* Q. 6, 2015)

5. Social disorganizations.

Social disorganization is the process opposed to social organization. Social organization, some fundamental concepts' is an orderly relationship of parts. The significance of this orderly arrangement lies in what it does. When the parts of social structure do not perform their functions efficiently and effectively or perform them badly, there occurs an imbalance in society. The social equilibrium is disturbed and society gets out of gear. Emile Durkheim defined social disorganisation as "a state of disequilibrium and a lack of social solidarity or consensus among the members of a society." WI Thomas and Florien Znaniecki conceived of social disorganization as "a decrease of the influence of existing rules of behavior upon individual members of the groups."

According to Mowever, social disorganization is "the process by which the relationships between members of a group are shaken." Stuart A Queen, Walter B Bodenhafer, and Ernest B Harper described social disorganisation in their book 'Social Organization and Disorganisation' as the counterpart of social organization.

Causes of Social Disorganization
1. Division of labor
2. Violation of social rules
3. Cultural lag
4. Natural catastrophes
5. War
6. Maladaptation of inherited nature to culture.

Characteristics of Social Disorganization
The main characteristics of social disorganisation are the following:
1. Conflict of mores and of institutions
2. Transfer of functions from one group to another
3. Individuation
4. Change in the role and status of the individuals.

Symptoms of Social Disorganization
Faris has enumerated the following symptoms of social disorganization:
1. Formalism
2. The decline of sacred elements
3. Individuality of interests and tastes
4. Emphasis on personal freedom and individual rights
5. Hedonistic behavior
6. Population heterogeneity
7. Mutual distrust
8. Unrest phenomena.

6. Characteristics of indian village. (*See* Q. 10, 2015)
7. Difference between primary and secondary group. (*See* Q. 7, 2015)

8. Importance of competition in social life.

Competition is an elementary, universal and impersonal form of social interaction. It is elementary in the sense that it is basic to all other forms of interaction. Each individual is involved in countless ways of which he is generally unaware in a vast web of competitive relationships. This lack of awareness on the part of the competing units gives competition its impersonal character. Of the various concrete expressions, the most obvious is struggle for existence. Every form of life is in constant struggle for life with the impersonal forces of nature that exist everywhere in the natural world.

Definitions: Competition is the struggle for possession of rewards which are in limited supply-money, goods, status, power, love-anything (Horton and Hunt, 1964). It is a process of seeking to obtain a reward by surpassing all rivals.

Importance: Competition is indispensable in social life. It is sociologically significant for the positive and negative effects it produces in social life.

It performs many useful functions in society. Some of the main functions are:
1. It serves the function of allocating scarce rewards among the competitors.
2. It has the additional function of stimulating both individual and group activity in a manner to increase the total productivity of the competitors. It furnishes motivation to excel or to obtain recognition or to achieve reward.
3. It assigns place to each individual in the hierarchical social system. It determines who is to perform what function.
4. It tends to enhance one's ego and helps in satisfying it.
5. It is conducive to progress and welfare of the society. It spurs individuals and groups to exert their best efforts to fulfill their goals.
6. It increases efficiency.

9. Population explosion and its effects on health status.

Population size also reflects mortality, the incidence of death in a country's population. To measure mortality, demographer uses a crude death rate, the number of deaths in a given year for every thousand people in a population. This time, we take the number of deaths in a year divide by the total population and multiply the result by 1,000. The third useful demographic measure is the infant mortality rate, the number of deaths among infants under 1 year of age for each thousand live births in a given year. To compute infant mortality, divide the number of deaths of children under 1 year of age by the number of live births during the same year and multiply the result by 1,000.

Effects of Population Explosion

The growth of population not only affects the people economically but also social, religious living and health conditions also. The problems created by the overpopulation is also called population explosion.

Sl. No.	Methods	Description
1.	Pressure on land	Rapid growth of population increases the pressure on India, has only 2.4% of world's geographical area, but it is 16% of the world's population thus, when compared to other developing countries density of population in India is very high. According to 1991 census, it was 276 people living per square kilometer. The land is almost fixed and does not increase simultaneously with population. Thus growing numbers, density of population goes up, per capita availability of and comes down and available land falls
2.	Unemployment	Employment is another area of serious concern on account of rapid population growth. It is estimated that about 3.3 million unemployed are added every year to existing labor force in India. The society finds it almost impossible to provide employment opportunities to the increasing population. This results in poverty and unemployment. We have already discussed the serious problems which both these social problems create
3.	Poverty	Poverty as a condition of chronic insufficient. It is a condition in which a person is not able to lead a life according to the desirable standard of life. Even after 50 years of independence a major portion of population is found below the poverty line
4.	Housing problem	Shelter or housing in one of the basic needs. As it affects health and character of inmates, abolishing houselessness becomes a serious problem. It is estimated the 25 million people are homeless. It becomes very difficult to provide houses to the ever increasing population with the result that people begin to live in slums and shanties
5.	Food problem	Rapid population growth gives birth to food problems in India is both qualitative and quantitative. About 40–54% of rural population and 41–50% of urban population consume between 2,100 and 2,250 calories per day, which is less than the 2,500 calories, the minimum prescribed to maintain normal health nonavailability of nutritious diet affects the physical and mental health of people
6.	High illiteracy	The number of school going children increases with an increase in population. It has been calculated that for every addition of about 10 crore people in our country, we will require 1.5 lakhs primary and middle schools, 10 thousand higher secondary schools, 50 lakh, primary and middle schools teachers, 1.5 lakhs higher secondary school teachers. The need for educating them puts a heavy pressure on the natural resources

Contd...

Contd...

Sl. No.	Methods	Description
7.	Health problems	Health is a condition of all-round well-being physical, mental, moral and spiritual, so that the members of society can lead a wholesome life. Fertility causes important health problems not only for the society but even for the mother and the child. In India, there is an acute shortage of medical services due to rapid increase of population. Nation finds it almost impossible to provide adequate health facilities to the growing population
8.	Law and order problems	Population explosion creates serious law and order problems because existing agencies which are responsible for maintaining law and order find it impossible to cope with the problem

Other Problems of Population Explosion

1. When nation cannot provide facilities to the growing population, the result is that the getting whatever facilities are available, corrupt means is used. Thus, corruption becomes wide spread in the society.
2. When there is strain on every resource, it becomes difficult to develop talent.
3. It becomes difficult to maintain an even sex ratio which gets disturbed quite frequently, resulting in many social problems.
4. When vast majority lives in shanties than the problem of maintaining moral character arises. Moral usually become low results in many social problems.

10. Types of social isolation.

Social isolation is defined as having little or no contact with other people. It usually lasts for extended periods of time. Social isolation is different from loneliness, in that loneliness is a state of emotion that is felt by individuals who are not satisfied with their social connections. Therefore, a person who is experiencing social isolation does not always experience loneliness, especially in cases where social isolation is voluntary. In addition, loneliness can also be temporary, whereas social isolation can lasts anywhere from a few weeks to years.

Social isolation is an absence of social relationships. It is distinct from solitude which is simply the state of being alone. Social isolation can occur in solitude or in the vicinity of others. Solitude can be chosen or forced, healthy or unhealthy. Social isolation describes an unwanted and often harmful experience. A person may be experiencing social isolation if they:

1. Avoid social interaction due to shame or depression.
2. Spend extended periods of time alone.
3. Experience social anxiety or fears of abandonment at the idea of social interaction.
4. Have only limited or superficial social contact.
5. Develop severe distress and loneliness.

11. Forms of accommodation.

The word accommodation has been used in two senses to indicate a condition of institutional arrangement and to indicate a process. As a condition, accommodation is the fact of equilibrium between individuals and groups. As a process it has to do with the conscious efforts of men to develop such working arrangements among themselves as will suspend conflict and make their relations more tolerable and less wasteful of energy.

Definitions

Reuter and Hart: As a process, accommodation is the sequence of steps by which persons are reconciled to changed conditions of life through the formation of habits and attitudes made necessary by the changed conditions themselves.

MacIver: "The term accommodation refers particularly to the process in which man attains a sense of harmony with his environment."

Forms or Methods of Accommodation

Accommodation is social adaptation that involves the invention or borrowing of devices whereby the one ethnic group develops modes of life, economic and otherwise, that complements or supplements those of the others. It is primarily concerned with the adjustment issuing from the conflict between individuals and RRRRRRRRRRRRRRRRFCVV CVgroups.

1. **Yielding to coercion or admitting one's defeat:** Coercion means the use of force or the threat of force to terminate a conflict. It usually involves parties of unequal strength, the weaker party yields because has been overpowered or because of fear of being overpowered. An armistice or peace treaty following a war is an example of this form of accommodation.
2. **Compromise:** When the combatants are of equal strength neither may be able to prevail over the other, they attain accommodation by agreeing to a compromise. In compromise each party to the dispute makes some concessions and yields to some demand of the other.
3. **Arbitration and conciliation:** Accommodation is also achieved by means of arbitration and conciliation which involve attempts on the part of the third party to bring about an end of the conflict between the contending parties. The labor management conflicts, the conflict between the husband and the wife and sometimes even the political conflicts are resolved through the intervention of an arbitrator or a mediator in whom both the parties have full confidence.
4. **Toleration:** Toleration is the form of accommodation in which there is no settlement of difference but there is only the avoidance of overt conflict. In toleration no concession is made by any of the groups and there is no change in basic policy. It involves acceptance of some state of affairs definitely objectionable; to the accepting group but for some reasons not deemed possible and/or advisable to dispose of in a more conclusive manner.
5. **Conversion:** Conversion involves conviction on the part of one of the contending parties that it has been wrong and its opponent are right. Accordingly it may go over to the other side and identify itself with the new point of view. This process thus consists of the repudiation of one's beliefs or allegiance and the adoption of others. Ordinarily conversion is thought of only in connection with religion but it may also occur in politics, economics and other fields.
6. **Rationalization:** Accommodation through rationalization involves plausible excuses or explanations for one's behavior instead of acknowledging the real defect in one's own self. One thus justifies one's behavior by ascribing his failure to discrimination against him instead of admitting lack of ability.
7. **Superordination and Subordination:** The most common accommodation is the establishment and recognition of the order of superordination and subordination. The organization of any society is essentially the result of such a type of accommodation. In the family the relationships among parents and children are based in terms of superordination and subordination.

12. Juvenile delinquency. *(See Q. 12, 2015)*

SHORT ANSWERS

13. Race. *(See Q. 15, 2015)*

14. Urban slums.

Urban slums are settlements, neighborhoods, or city regions that cannot provide the basic living conditions necessary for its inhabitants, or slum dwellers, to live in a safe and healthy environment. Slum settlement as a household that cannot provide one of the following basic living characteristics:

1. Durable housing of a permanent nature that protects against extreme climate conditions.
2. Sufficient living space which means no more than three people sharing the same room.
3. Easy access to safe water in sufficient amounts at an affordable price.
4. Access to adequate sanitation in the form of a private or public toilet shared by a reasonable number of people.
5. Security of tenure that prevents forced evictions.

15. Formal social control.

Formal social control refers to components of society that are designed for the resocialization of individuals who break formal rules; examples would include prisons and mental health institutions. Some researchers have outlined some of the motivations underlying the formal social control system.

16. Hindu marriage act 1955.

The main purpose of the act was to amend and codify the law relating to marriage among hindu and others. Besides amending and codifying Sastrik law, it introduced separation and divorce, which did not exist in Sastrik Law. This enactment brought uniformity of law for all sections of Hindus. In India there are religion-specific civil codes that separately govern adherents of certain other religions.

This Act applies:

1. to any person who is a Hindu by religion in any of its forms or developments, including a Virashaiva, a Lingayat or a follower of the Brahmo, Prarthana or Arya Samaj;
2. to any person who is a Buddhist, Jain or Sikh by religion; and
3. to any other person domiciled in the territories to which this Act extends who is not a Muslim, Christian, Parsi or Jew by religion, unless it is proved that any such person would not have been governed by the Hindu law or by any custom or usage as part of that law in respect of any of the matters dealt with herein if this Act had not been passed.

17. Customs.

The term "custom" indicates general practices and usages that by common adoption and unvarying habit have come to have the force of law. Custom has been categorized into four types: Conventional custom, general custom, local custom and legal custom. A custom derives its force of law from the tacit consent of the legislature, general adoption by people, and through medium of agreements.

18. Define role and status.

Status is a term used to designate the comparative amounts of prestige, difference or respect accorded to persons who have been assigned different roles in a group or community. The status of a person is high if the role, he is playing, is considered important by the group. If the role is regarded less high, its performer may be accorded lower status. Thus, the status of a person is based on social evaluations.

Definitions
1. Status is the worth of a person as estimated by a group or a class of persons.
   —Secord and Bukman.
2. Status is the rank-order position assigned by a group to a role or to a set of roles.
   —Ogburn and Nimkoff.
3. Status is the social position that determines for its possessor, apart from his personal attribute or social services, a degree of respect, prestige and influence.
   —MacIver.
4. Status is a position in the general institutional system, recognized and supported by the entire society spontaneously evolved rather than deliberately created, rooted in the folkways and mores.
   —Davis.
5. Status defined as a position in social aggregate identified with a pattern of prestige symbols and actions.
   —Martindale and Menachesi.

Role

The word role meant the role on which an actor's part was written. The social system is based on a division of labor in which every person is assigned a specific task. The task performed by an individual makes up the role he is expected to play in the life and community. Since the role is a set of expectations, it, therefore, implies that one role cannot be defined without referring to another. There cannot be a parent without a child, or an employer without an employee. There must be another role doing the expecting. In this sense, roles are but a series of rights and duties that is they represent reciprocal relations among individuals. Holding the status of student, for example, means one will attend classes, complete assignments and more broadly, devote a lot of time to personal enrichment through academic study.

Definitions
1. A role is the function of a status.
   —Young and Mack.
2. Role is a pattern of behavior expected of an individual in a certain group or situation.
   —Lundberg.
3. A role is a set of socially expected and approved behavior patterns, consisting of both duties and privileges, associated with a particular position a group.
   —Ogburn and Nimkoff.
4. Role is the dynamic or the behavior aspect of status.... A role is what an individual does in the status he occupies.
   —Robert Bierstedt.
5. A social role is the expected behavior associated with a social position.
   —Duncan Mitchell.
6. Role defined as behavior expected of someone who holds a particular status.
   —Liton.

19. Definition of socialization.

Socialization is a process by which individuals acquire the knowledge, language, social skills, and value to conform to the norms and roles required for integration into a group or community. It is a combination of both self-imposed (because the individual wants to conform) and externally imposed rules, and the expectations of the others. In an organizational setting, socialization refers to the process through which a new employee 'learns the ropes,' by becoming sensitive to the formal and informal power structure and the explicit and implicit rules of behavior.

20. Crowd. (*See* Q. 16, 2015)

21. Social groups. (*See* Q. 21, 2014)

22. HIV/AIDS. (*See* Q. 24, 2016)

2018

Sociology

LONG ESSAYS

1. a. Define rural community, b. Differentiate between rural community and urban community with their salient features.
2. a. What is social change? b. Explain the various factors that influences social change
3. a. Define family, b. Classify the family, c. Functions of family.

SHORT ESSAYS

4. Scope of sociology in nursing.
5. Differentiate between conflict and competition.
6. Explain the Malthusian theory of population.
7. Explain the forms of marriage.
8. Agencies of socialization.
9. Explain the different types of culture.
10. Theories of caste system.
11. Explain the role of family in socialization.
12. Discuss the major urban problems and their impact on health.

SHORT ANSWERS

13. Folkways.
14. Assimilation.
15. Child abuse.
16. MOB.
17. Polygamy.
18. Health services in a village community.
19. Isolation.
20. Social mobility.
21. In-group and out-group.
22. Race.

LONG ESSAYS

1. a. Define rural community, b. Differentiate between rural community and urban community with their salient features.

Rural sociology is the branch which studies the life of rural people. It is considered with rural society, its social structure, social institutions and their relationships. It studies the life of rural people and analysis their attitudes and beliefs. India is a land of villages; the majority of the people are living in villages. So villages are the significant aspect of Indian society. Indian villages are considered unique and distinct from villages of other countries. Generally, a village refers to a small group of people living permanently in a definite geographic area who depend mainly on farming activities.

Definitions

1. The village is unit of rural society. It is the theater where in the quantum of rural life unfolds itself and functions.
   —AR Desai.

2. The rural community comprises of the constellation of institutions and persons grouped about a small center and sharing common primary interest.
   —Elridge and Merrill.

3. A village as a unit of compact settlement varying in size, smaller than a town.
   —Anthony Giddens.

Difference between rural and urban community.

Sl. No.	Criteria	Rural society	Urban society
1.	Size of population	Rural population is limited	Urban population is large
2.	Environment	Natural environment, more close to nature	Artificial environment and more problems of environmental pollution
3.	Family	Trend of joint family is found	Nuclear family is more common
4.	Occupation	Agriculture and agriculture-based occupations	Industry, trade and different occupations (education, medical, administration, engineering, management, etc.)
5.	Social uniformity	More uniformity found	Heterogeneity and differences are found
6.	Stratification	More based on castes, otherwise stratification is simple	More based on class. Stratification is complex
7.	Mobility	Physical and social mobility are limited	High rate of physical and social mobility
8.	Density of population	Less density	High density

Contd...

Contd...

Sl. No.	Criteria	Rural society	Urban society
9.	Means of recreation	More natural and cultural. Social ridicule is natural	Professional and complex. Media is relatively more powerful
10.	Political awareness	Relatively less, increasing now	Political awareness is more
11.	Marriage and divorce	Marriage is traditional and permanent. Divorce is negligible	Love marriages are also found. Divorce is more common. Marriage institution is in more danger
12.	Condition of social change	Change is less	Changes are fast and more political
13.	Education	Less literacy	Changes are fast and more political
14.	Social problems	Unsociability, child marriage, superstitions, etc. found more	Problems are based on class, economy, power, etc.
15.	Social interaction	Personal and more cordial	Indirect and formal relationship is found more

2. a. What is social change? b. Explain the various factors that influences social change. *(See Q.3, 2014)*

3. a. Define family, b. Classify the family, c. Functions of family.

Man's social life begins with family. It is the most important primary group. It is the oldest social institution known to man. Family is the mother of social institutions. It is the first social environment to which a child is exposed. It is a place where most of the people spend more than one half of their life-time. Family is the center of our life activities. It gives shape to our personality and provides us inspiration. Family is in the center of the social system. All other system has a close bearing with the family. Family contributes to their strength. Any major change in the family will have repercussions throughout the social system.

Family has regulated the sexual relations to avoid promiscuity, by prescribing customary sex morals. It is a permanent organization which has provided stable family life. It is the shelter where man is fed, clothed, and housed from the beginning. It has upheld and inculcated the traditions and customs of the group. Thus, family is the foundation stone on which the cultural heritage is built. Family as a unit of sociological inquiry is dealt with in various ways by sociologists. It is studied as an institution, as an association, as an organization. It is also referred to as a sub-system because it is regarded as one of the parts of the society.

Meaning of Family

The origin of the English word, Family is traced to the Roman word Famulus or to the Latin word Familia meaning a household comprising or servants or workers and of slaves along with other individuals having marriage or blood relations. The word denotes group of procedures, consisting of slaves, servants, and members connected by common descent or marriage. Thus originally, family consisted of a man and woman with a child or children and servants. This meaning of family has changed over the years.

Definitions
1. Family is a more or less durable association of husband and wife or without child or of a man or woman alone, with children.
—MF Nimkoff.
2. Family is a group of persons united by ties of marriage, blood or adaptation consisting a single household interacting and intercommunicating with each other in their respective social roles of husband and wife, father and mother, son and daughter, brother and sister, creating a common culture.
—Burgess and Locke.
3. Family is the biological social unit composed of husband, wife and children.
—Eliot and Merrill.
4. Family is a group defined by sex relationship sufficiently precise and enduring to provide for the procreation and upbringing of children.
—MacIver.
5. Family is a system of patterned expectations defining the proper behavior of persons playing certain roles, enforced both by the incumbents own positive motives for conformity and by the sanction of others.
—Parsons.
6. Family is a recognized and established usage governing the relations between individuals and groups.
—Ginsberg.
7. Family is a habitual way of living together which have been sanctioned, systematized and established by the authority of communities.
—Ellwood CA.

Classifications of Family
Classification of families is generally done on the basis of organization (nuclear and joint), forms of marriage (monogamous or polygamous), authority (matriarchal or patriarchal) and residence etc. Classification of families on different basis are given below:

1. On the Basis of Organization:
In terms of organization families may be of two broad types: the nuclear family and extended/joint family.
1. **Nuclear family:** The nuclear family is a unit composed of husband, wife and their unmarried children. This is the predominant form in modern industrial societies. This type of family is based on companionship between parents and children.
2. **Extended/joint family:** The term extended family is used to indicate the combination of two or more nuclear families based on an extension of the parent-child relationships. In an extended family, a man and his wife live with the families of their married sons and with their unmarried sons and daughters, grand children or great grant children in the paternal or maternal line.

2. On the Basis of Authority:
The family may be either patriarchal or matriarchal on the basis of authority.
1. **Patriarchal family:** Patriarchal family is a type of family in which all authority belongs to the paternal side. In this family, the eldest male or the father is the head of the family. He exercises his authority over the members of the family.

2. **Matriarchal family:** It is a form of family in which authority is centred in the wife or mother. The matriarchal family system implies rule of the family by the mother, not by the father. In this type of family women are entitled to perform religious rites and husband lives in the house of wife.

3. On the Basis of Residence:
In terms of residence, we find following types of families:
1. **Patrilocal family:** When the wife goes to live with the husband's family, it is called the patrilocal family.
2. **Matrilocal family:** When the couple after marriage moves to live with the wife's family, such residence is called matrilocal. The husband has a secondary position in the wife's family where his children live.
3. **Neolocal residence:** When the couple after marriage moves to settle in an independent residence which is neither attached to the bride's family of origin nor bridegroom's family of origin it is called neolocal residence.
4. **Avonculocal family:** In this type of family the married couple moves to the house of the maternal uncle and live with his son after marriage. Avonculocal family is found among the Nayars of Kerala.
5. **Matri-patrilocal family:** In matri-patrilocal family, immediately after marriage the bridegroom moves to the house of the bride and temporarily settles there till the birth of the first child and then comes back to his family of orientation, along with wife and child for permanent settlement. The Chenchuas of Andhra Pradesh live in this type of family.

4. On the Basis of Descent:
On the basis of descent, families may be divided into two types, such as patrilineal and matrilineal.
1. **Patrilineal family:** When descent is traced through the father, it is called patrilineal family. In this type of family inheritance of property takes place along the male line of descent. The ancestry of such family is determined on the basis of male line or the father. A patrilineal family is also patriarchal and patrilocal. This is the common type of family prevalent today.
2. **Matrilineal family:** In this type of family descent is traced along the female line and inheritance of property also takes place along the female line of descent. The Veddas, the North American Indians, some people of Malabar and the Khasi tribe are matrilineal. Generally, the matrilineal families are matriarchal and matrilocal.

Polygamous family: When one man marries several woman or one woman marries several men and constitute the family, it is polygamous family. Again polygamous family is divided into two types, such as polygynous family and polyandrous family.
  a. **Polygynous family:** It is a type of family in which one man has more than one wife at a given time and lives with them and their children together. This kind of family is found among Eskimos, African Negroes and the Muslims, Naga and other tribes of central India.
  b. **Polyandrous family:** In this types of family one wife has more than one husband at given time and she lives with all of them together or each of them in turn. Polyandrous families are found among some Australians, the Sinhalese (Srilankans), the Tibetans, some Eskimos and the Todas of Nilgiri Hills in India.

5. On the Basis of In-group and Out-group Affiliation:
On the basis of in-group and out-group affiliation families may be either endogamous or exogamous.

1. **Endogamous family:** Endogamy is the practice of marrying someone within a group to which one belongs. An endogamous family is one which consists of husband and wife who belong to same group such as caste or tribe.
2. **Exogamous family:** Endogamy means marriage within a group, while exogamy means marriage with someone outside his group. For example a Hindu must marry outside his Kinship group or gotra. When a family is consisted of husband and wife of different groups such as gotra is called exogamous family.

7. On the Basis of Blood-relationship:

Ralph Linton has classified family into two main types namely consanguine and conjugal.
1. **Consanguine family:** The consanguine family is built upon the parent-child relationship (on blood-descent). The family is a descent group through the male line which is firmly vested with authority.
2. **Conjugal family:** The conjugal family is a nucleus of the husband, the wife and their offspring who are surrounded by a fringe of relatives only incidental to the functioning of the family as a unit.

Functions

1. **Satisfaction of sex needs:** The satisfaction of sex desire requires that male and female should live together as husband and wife.
2. **Reproduction:** The task of race perpetuation has always been an important function of the family. A ongoing society must replace its members. It primarily relies on the biological reproduction of its own members.
3. **Sustenance function:** The family provides the daily care and personal protection to its dependant members namely aged, children, etc. The family is an insurance for the individual in times of crisis. Family provides protection and shelter to orphans, widow and her children.
4. **Provision of a home:** Establishment of household life or provision of a home is another essential function of the family. The desire for a home is a powerful instinct for men as well as women
5. **Socialization:** Man is a social animal. But he is not born human or social. He is made social through the process of socialization. Socialization refers to the process through which the growing individual learns the habits, attitudes, values and beliefs of the social group into which he has been born and becomes a person.

Nonessential Functions

The nonessential functions of a family can be the following ones:
1. **Economic functions:** Family serves as an economic unit. The earlier agricultural family was a self-supporting 'business enterprise'. It was producing whatever the family needed.
2. **Property transformation:** The family acts as an agency for holding and transmission of property. Most families accumulate much property, such as land, goods, money and other forms of wealth. The family transmits these property.
3. **Religious function:** Family is a centre for religious training of the children. The children learn various religious virtues from their parents. The religious and moral training of children has always been bound up with the home.
4. **Educative function:** The family provides the bases of all the child's latter formal education learning. Family is the first school of children. The child learns the first letters under the guidance of parents.

5. **Recreational function:** The family provides recreation to its members. The members of the family visit their relations. They enjoy various occasions in the family jointly and derive pleasure. Now recreation is available in clubs and hotels rather than at home.
6. **Wish fulfillment:** The family gives moral and emotional support for the individual member, providing his defence against social isolation and loneliness and satisfying his need for personal happiness and love.

SHORT ESSAYS

4. Scope of sociology in nursing.

The study of sociology helps nurses identify the psycho-social problems of patients, which helps important the quality of treatment. Importance and application of sociology in nursing:
1. Sociology helps understand those forces and pressures which affect patients adversely.
2. Sociology is mainly the study of society, communities and people whereas nursing is a profession which focused on assisting individuals, families, and communities in attaining, maintaining and recovering optimal health and functioning.
3. The scope of sociology is the study of the generic forms of social relationships, behaviors and activities, etc.
4. Sociology helps a nurse understand what makes people "tick" the same way psychology does. The only difference is that sociology does it from a "group" or "community" perspectives.
5. Sociology explores the issues of genders, social classes, stratification, families and economic policies which have impacts on health care and nursing. The information gleaned by even a cursory study in those fields could contribute toward being a kinder and gentler nurse.
6. All of above are important because besides medical knowledge, a nurse really needs to be kind, sympathetic and compassionate

5. Differentiate between conflict and competition.

Conflict and competition are common English words that we all hear and read about in newspapers, magazines, and discussions taking place on television. At first glance, it appears that there is no similarity between conflict and competition as we think of wars and skirmishes when we hear the word conflict, whereas races and all types of sporting events come to our mind we think of competition. However, survival of the fittest theory by Charles Darwin and the very fact that each one of us is different allow for conflict in viewpoints as well as fight for control over limited resources.

Difference between Conflict and Competition:
1. Conflict involves discord and disagreement, whereas competition can take place without any clash or hard feelings.
2. A competition indicates a contest where participants via for the top spot, whereas a conflict indicates a scuffle or a skirmish.
3. Competition is a healthy process that encourages intelligence, innovation, and entrepreneurship whereas conflict crushes all such concepts.
4. In real life, conflict is inevitable because all people are different from one another and different viewpoints lead to conflict.
5. Organizing a competition to choose the best painter, singer, or a player encourages excellence among individuals as participants want to beat others to get top honors.

6. Conflict and competition are two different types of social interaction that are, in addition to cooperation and accommodation.

6. Explain the Malthusian theory of population.

In the strictly Malthusian sense, overpopulation is said to exist in a country when population increases more rapidly than the supply of food and this test should be absolutely reliable a country three-fourth of whose working population are engaged in agriculture. The application of this test leaves us in no doubt about our being overpopulated. Till 1921, cultivation has more than kept peace with the growth of population, after it, cultivation has been lagging behind and the population total has been forging ahead. (While between 1921 and 1951 the area under cultivation hardly increased by 5%). The serious food problem with which country has had to contend all these years is enough to prove that the race between food and population has been badly lost by food.

After Thomas Malthus, the view that human reproduction increases by geometric progression, and thus eventually outstrips the available food supply which increases by arithmetic progression. Famines, therefore, would be an inevitable necessity from time-to-time; the only way of retarding famines are either to voluntarily control reproduction or to kill off people in wars.

Malthusian's summaries:
1. A growing population was good for the economy.
2. A growing population was good for the military.
3. A growing population in a constricted space (city) contributes to increase in mortality rates.
4. A growing population develops division of labor with increasing numbers migrating to the cities.
5. Some consideration should be given to the balance or imbalance between number and resources.
6. Fertility rates tend to be higher in rural areas than in the cities.

7. Explain the forms of marriage. (See Q. 8, 2016)

8. Agencies of socialization.

The human infant comes into the world, as a biological organism with animal needs and impulses. He is slowly moulded by society into a social being. He comes to learn social ways of acting, thinking and feeling. From the very beginning, the individual is taught to respond in socially determined ways. The individual learns the ways of his group or society so well that they become part of his personality. Socialization is based on the learning process. The development of a set of habits, attitudes and traits differentiates us as persons from every other person. It consists of the processes of interaction through which the individual learns the habits, skills, beliefs and standards of judgment that are necessary for his effective participation in social groups and communities.

Agencies of Socialization

There are various agencies responsible for the process of socialization. Personality does not come readymade. They are moulded through the process of socialization. The following agencies are mainly responsible for socialization:
1. **The family:** The process of socialization begins for every one of us in the family. Here the parental and particularly the maternal influence on the child is very great. The intimate

relationship between the mother and child has a great impact on the shaping of child's ability and capacities. The parents are the first persons to introduce to the child the culture of his group. In the family, the child gets both cooperative as well as authoritative socialization.

2. **School and teaching:** The school is the center of learning not only lessons prescribed but also cultural values and patterns. Here the child comes in contact with large number of other children of his own age group, as well as teachers, seniors and juniors, has to learn from textbooks, his habits are moulded often by teachers. They become an ideal for the child and it imitates them is many ways. He learns a lot of new adjustments with regard to food, sleep, time and several other matters. His mind and body develop and become maturer.

3. **Peer groups:** Adolescence brings the youth often into a crisis. His body develops; his interests and attitudes also change to a great extent. New attitudes and values are formed. Heterosexual adjustments are to be made in this stage of life. Further his relationship with the families is to be redefined. All this puts a lot of strain on the individual. Peer group interests develop in a child as he spends a lot of time, in the company of his peers group. The ideals and opinions of the peers are of great importance to the individual. A child may even get into antisocial activities through the influence of the peer groups. Therefore, a lot of precaution is needed in this stage of life.

4. **Religion:** Religion is an important institution which influences in moulding our belief and ways of life. The child sees his parents going to the temple or church and performing religious ceremonies. He listens to religious sermons which may determine his course of life and shape his ideas. Most of the families observe some or other religious practices, which are learnt by children.

5. **The state:** The state is an authoritarian agency. It makes law for the people and lays down the modes of conduct expected of them. The people have compulsorily to obey these laws. If they fail to adjust their behavior in accordance with the laws of the state. State may be punished for such failure. Thus the state also moulds our behavior.

6. **Mass media:** The mass media, in other words are the various forms of communication such as the radio, television, newspaper, magazines, movies and records. They act as influence of newspapers is limited to the educated only while radio, TV, etc. exercises their influence on the entire society. The mass media reinforce the values and norms to make the individuals socialized.

9. Explain the different types of culture.

A culture has four aspects or four types: Material and nonmaterial culture and ideal and real culture. Material culture is related to tangible objects made by man. Buildings, furniture, books are the products of material culture. Nonmaterial culture is related to the abstract things like emotions, attitudes, ideas and beliefs which we feel but cannot verify by observation. Peace, war, cooperation, marriage and lecture are the examples of nonmaterial culture.

1. **Real culture:** Real culture can be observed in our social life. We act upon on culture in our social life is real; its part which the people adopt in their social life is their real one. The whole one is never real because a part of it remains without practice. How far we set upon Islam is our real culture. Being a Muslims, Christian and related to another religion we do not follow Islam, Christianity, etc. fully in our social life. It means the part of religion which we follow is our real culture.

2. **Ideal culture:** The culture which is presented as a pattern or precedent to the people is called ideal. It is the goal of the society. It can never be achieved fully because some part of it remains out of practice. It is explained in textbooks, our leaders' speeches and guidance. The part of

ideal culture practiced in social life is called real culture. Islam is our ideal one. We claim to be true Muslims and this claim is our ideal culture but how far we are Muslims in practice is our real culture. Both the real and ideal cultures are related together and different from each other.

3. **Material culture:** Material culture consists of man-made objects, such as furniture, automobiles, buildings, dams, bridges, roads and in fact, the physical matter converted and used by man. It is closely related with the external, mechanical as well as useful objects. It includes technical and material equipment like railways engines, publication machines, locomotive, radio, etc. It includes our financial institutions, parliaments, insurance policies, etc. and referred to as civilization.

4. **Nonmaterial culture:** The term 'culture' when used in the ordinary sense, means non-material culture'. This term when used in the ordinary sense, means nonmaterial. It is something nonphysical ideas which include values, beliefs, symbols, organization and institutions, etc. Nonmaterial culture includes words we use, the language we speak, our belief held, values we cherish and all the ceremonies observed.

High culture: It is linked with the elite, upper class society, those families and individuals with an ascribed status position. It is often associated with the arts, such as opera, ballet and classical music, sports, such as polo and lacrosse, and leisure pursuits, such as hunting and shooting.

Subculture: It is culture enjoyed by a small group within society. In this sense it is a minority part of majority culture. They have distinct norms and values which make them subsection of society.

Multiculturalism: It it is depicted to be very similar to cultural diversity, other definitions align multiculturalism with different ethnic groups living alongside each other.

Global culture: Globalization is the process by which events in one part of the world come to influence what happens elsewhere in the world. They has become interconnected; socially, politically and economically. A global culture is a key feature of globalization, they emerged due to patterns of migration, trends in international travel and the spread of the media, exposing people to the same images of the same dominant world companies.

10. Theories of caste system.

1. **Traditional theory:** According to this theory, the caste system is of divine origin. It says the caste system is an extension of the varna system, where the 4 varnas originated from the body of Bramha. At the top of the hierarchy were the Brahmins who were mainly teachers and intellectuals and came from Brahma's head. Kshatriyas, or the warriors and rulers, came from his arms. Vaishyas, or the traders, were created from his thighs. At the bottom were the Shudras, who came from Brahma's feet. The mouth signifies its use for preaching, learning, etc. the arms—protections, thighs—to cultivate or business, feet—helps the whole body, so the duty of the Shudras is to serve all the others. The subcastes emerged later due to intermarriages between the 4 varnas. The proponents of this theory cite Purushasukta of Rigveda, Manusmriti, etc. to support their stand.

2. **Racial theory:** The Sanskrit word for caste is varna which means color. The caste stratification of the Indian society had its origin in the chaturvarna system: Brahmins, Kashtriyas, Vaishyas and Shudras. Rig vedic literature stresses very significantly the differences between the Arya and non Aryans (Dasa), not only in their complexion but also in their speech, religious practices, and physical features. The varna system prevalent during the vedic period was mainly based on division of labor and occupation. The three classes: Brahma, Kshatra and Vis are frequently mentioned in the Rig Veda. Brahma and Kshatra represented the poet-priest and the warrior-

chief comprised all the common people. The name of the fourth class, the 'Sudra', occurs only once in the Rig Veda. The Sudra class represented domestic servants.

3. **Political theory:** According to this theory, the caste system is a clever device invented by the Brahmins in order to place themselves on the highest ladder of social hierarchy. Dr Ghurye states, "Caste is a Brahminic child of Indo-Aryan culture cradled in the land of the Ganges and then transferred to other parts of India." The Brahmins even added the concept of spiritual merit of the king, through the priest or purohit in order to get the support of the ruler of the land.

4. **Occupational theory:** Caste hierarchy is according to the occupation. Those professions which were regarded as better and respectable made the persons who performed them superior to those who were engaged in dirty professions. According to Newfield, "Function and function alone is responsible for the origin of caste structure in India." With functional differentiation there came in occupational differentiation and numerous subcastes, such as lohar (blacksmith), chamar (tanner), teli (oil-pressers).

5. **Evolution theory:** According to this theory, the caste system did not come into existence all of a sudden or at a particular date. It is the result of a long process of social evolution.
   1. Hereditary occupations
   2. The desire of the Brahmins to keep themselves pure
   3. The lack of rigid unitary control of the state
   4. The unwillingness of rulers to enforce a uniform standard of law and custom
   5. The 'Karma' and 'Dharma' doctrines also explain the origin of caste system. Whereas the Karma doctrine holds the view that a man is born in a particular caste because of the result of his action in the previous incarnation, the doctrine of Dharma explains that a man who accepts the caste system and the principles of the caste to which he belongs, is living according to Dharma. Confirmation to one's own dharma also remits on one's birth in the rich high caste and violation gives a birth in a lower and poor caste.
   6. Ideas of exclusive family, ancestor worship, and the sacramental meal
   7. Clash of antagonistic cultures particularly of the patriarchal and the matriarchal systems;
   8. Clash of races, cooler prejudices and conquest
   9. Deliberate economic and administrative policies followed by various conquerors
   10. Geographical isolation of the Indian Peninsula
   11. Foreign invasions
   12. Rural social structure.

11. Explain the role of family in socialization.

Individual **socialization** is a lifelong process determined by many factors. Among the social factors that affect individual people in particular are social groups with which a person comes into contact. The most important social group to influence individual's development, however, is the **family**.

There is no better way to start than to talk about the role of family in our social development, as **family** is usually considered to be the most important agent of socialization. As infants, we are completely dependent on others to survive. Our parents, or those who play the parent role, are responsible for teaching us to function and care for ourselves. They along with the rest of our family also teach us about close relationships, group life, and how to share resources. Additionally, they provide us with our first system of values, norms, and beliefs—a system that is usually a reflection of their own social status, religion, ethnic group, and more.

Functioning family environment has in the process of socialization of the individual irreplaceable importance. During socialization one becomes a cultural and social being who acts according to recognized rules directed their behavior towards socially accepted value and meet individually modified roles and expectations. Family provides initial human behavior patterns in an orientation and initial interpersonal relationships. The aim of this study was to find out how individual characteristics of family influence the acquisition of values, rules and roles. As fundamental characteristics of the families, we determined the size and a form of the family.

12. Discuss the major urban problems and their impact on health.

(See Q.6, 2016)

SHORT ANSWERS

13. Folkways.

The literal meaning of the term folkways is way of the folk. Folk means people or group and the ways refers to ways in which a group does things. Thus, these are ways of the folk, i.e. social habit or social expectations that have arisen in the daily life of the group. Folkways are accepted modes of conduct in a society. Every society standards are the result of a long experience achieved in the course of several generations. They are not developed consciously. They include popular habits, conventions; forms of etiquette, fashion, morals, etc., folkway differ from group-to-group. For example, women in India grow their hair long while women in Europe cut it short. Even in dress and in eating habits we notice differences. Folkways are the simplest ways of satisfying the interest of man. They become part of our nature. But we may modify them to meet a change in the conditions of life. Thus folkways concerning religion, property, marriage change slowly.

Definitions
1. The folkways are the recognized or accepted ways of behavior.
—MacIver.
2. Folkways are habitual ways of doing things, which arise out of the adjustment of person and of persons to place.
—Martindale and Manches.
3. Those ways of acting that are common to a society or group and that are handed down from one generation to the next, are known as folkways
—Green.
4. Folkways are defined as behavior patterns of everyday life, which generally arise unconsciously in group-without planned or rational thoughts.
—Gillin and Gillin.
5. Folkways are the typical or habitual beliefs, attitudes and styles of conduct observed within a group or community.
—Lunderberg.
6. The folkways are literally the ways of the folk, that is, social habits of group expectations that have arisen in the daily life of the group.
—Merill.
7. Folkways are simply the customary normal, habitual ways a group does things.
—Horton and Hunt.

14. Assimilation. (See Q. 20, 2015)

15. Child abuse.

Child abuse refers to any emotional, sexual, or physical mistreatment or neglect by an adult in a role of responsibility toward someone who is under 18 years of age.
1. Four types of abuse are neglect and physical, emotional, and sexual abuse.
2. In some countries, using corporal punishment is regarded as child abuse.
3. Signs of abuse can be hard to detect, but being withdrawn, passive, and overly compliant may be an indication.
4. The person who is carrying out the abuse may also need help, for example, a stressed parent.

16. MOB. (See Q. 17, 2016)

17. Polygamy.

Polygamy is defined as a mating system in which an individual has more than one mate simultaneously that can either be male or female. Polygamy is a more general term that encompasses the practice of having multiple mates and should not be confused with the more specific terms of polygyny, having multiple female mates, or polyandry, having multiple male mates.

18. Health services in a village community.

The healthcare infrastructure in rural areas has been developed as a three tier system as follows:

1. **Subcentre:** Most peripheral contact point between Primary Health Care System and Community manned with one HW(F)/ANM and one HW(M).

2. **Primary Health Centre (PHC):** A referral Unit for 6 subcentres 4-6 bedded manned with a medical officer incharge and 14 subordinate paramedical staff

3. **Community Health Centre (CHC):** A 30 bedded hospital/referral unit for 4 PHCs with specialized services.

19. Isolation.

Isolation is a process whereby the individual or a group wills be segregated from others. It is a type of dissociative social process. The great sociologists like Park and Burges considered isolation as opposite to interaction. They defined it as 'A kind of negative interaction". Isolation of the individual is considered to be a negative value. Prolonged isolation is resulted in mental disintegration.

Isolation of an individual is always considered as a negative value. Human being is interdependent. They cannot satisfy their needs and desires without contact with others. The development of culture depends mostly upon contacts between groups. Nevertheless, the partial isolation sometimes helpful to others. If a criminal is not isolated from the group, his presence will be harmful to the other members of the same group.

20. Social mobility. (See Q. 22, 2014)

21. In-group and out-group.

Some of the differences between in-group and out-group are as follows:
1. The groups with which individual identifies himself are his in-group. One's family, one's college are example of his in-group. But out-groups refers to those groups with which individual do not identify himself. These are outside groups. Pakistan is an out-group for Indians.
2. In group members use the term 'we' to express themselves but they use the term 'they' for the members of out-group.
3. Individual is the member of his in-group whereas he is not at all a member of his out-group.
4. In-group based on ethnocentrism. Ethnocentrism is one of the important characteristic of in group. But out-group is not based on ethnocentrism.
5. Similarity in behavior, attitude and opinion is observed among the members of in-group. But they show dissimilar behavior; attitude and opinion towards the members of out-group.
6. In-group members have positive attitude towards their own in-group but they have negative attitudes towards their out group.
7. Members of in-group display cooperation, good-will, mutual help and possess a sense of solidarity, a feeling of brotherhood and readiness to sacrifice themselves for the group. But individual shows a sense of avoidance, dislike, indifference and antagonism towards the members of out-group.
8. In-group is a group to which individual belongs to but all other group to which he does not belongs to are his out-group.
9. Members of in-group feel that their personal welfare is bound up with other members of group but out-group members do not feel so.

22. Race. *(See Q. 15, 2015)*

2017

Sociology

LONG ESSAYS
1. Define sociology; discuss briefly the nature and scope of sociology.
2. List out various social problems in India and briefly explain the causes and remedies of overpopulation.
3. Define social stratification; explain caste system as a form of social stratification.

SHORT ESSAYS
4. Factors favoring and hindering assimilation.
5. Differentiate urban and rural community.
6. Marriage and family problems in India.
7. Voluntary associations.
8. Types of marriage.
9. Joint family system in India.
10. Technology as a factor of social change.
11. Community development programs in India.
12. Rehabilitation of juvenile delinquents.

SHORT ANSWERS
13. Social mobility.
14. Endogamy and exogamy.
15. Cultural lag.
16. Role of religion in social control.
17. Racism.
18. Various forms of conflict.
19. Isolation.
20. Assimilation.
21. Social system.
22. Health consequences of poverty.

LONG ESSAYS

1. Define sociology (*See* Q. 1, 2014); discuss briefly the nature and scope of sociology.

Nature of Sociology

1. Sociology is an independent science. Sociology like any other discipline have its own area of study and not fully dependent on other discipline.
2. Sociology is a social science not a physical science. Social sciences focus on various aspect of human society while physical sciences deal with natural phenomena. Thus sociology is a social science as it deals with man and his social activities.
3. Sociology is a categorical and not a normative discipline. Sociology is value-free. It is only interested in 'what is' and not 'what should be' or 'ought to be'.
4. Sociology is pure science and not an applied science. As a Pure science it is only interested in acquisition of knowledge, it has nothing to do with application of that knowledge. Like Physics is a pure science while engineering is its application.
5. Sociology is relatively an abstract science and not a concrete science. It studies the society in an abstract (Theoretical not physical) way. Like, sociology is not interested in particular families but in family as a social institution that exists in all societies.
6. Sociology is a generalizing science and not a particularizing science. Sociology is not interested in particular events rather it studies events in a general way. Example: History study French Revolution but Sociology will be interested in revolutions in general.
7. Sociology is a general science and not a special social science. Like economy or political science, sociology does not focus on only one aspect of human activity. As it has to deal with society it includes all aspects of human life in a general way.
8. Sociology is both a rational and an empirical science. It studies the social phenomena in scientific way. It is based on reason (logic), observation and experimentation.

Scope of Sociology

It is maintained by some that Sociology studies everything and anything under the sun. This is rather too vague a view about the scope of Sociology. As a matter of fact, sociology has a limited field of enquiry and deals with those problems which are not dealt with by other social sciences.

Specialistic or Formalistic School

Simmel's view: According to Simmel, the distinction between Sociology and other special sciences is that it deals with the same topics as they from a different angle—from the angle of different modes of social relationships.

Social relationships, such as competition, subordination, division of labour etc. are exemplified in different spheres of social life such as economic, the political and even the religious, moral or artistic but the business of Sociology is to disentangle these forms of social relationships and to study them in abstraction.

Synthetic School

The synthetic school wants to make sociology a synthesis of the social sciences or a general science, Durkheim, Hob-house and Sorokin subscribe to this view.

Durkheim's view: According to Durkheim, Sociology has three principal divisions, viz., (i) Social Physiology and (iii) General Sociology. Social morphology is concerned with geographical or territorial basis of the life of people and its relation to types of social organizations and the problems of populations, such as its volume and density, local distribution and the like.

2. List out various social problems in india and briefly explain the causes and remedies of overpopulation.

India is an ancient country and according to some estimates, Indian civilization is about 5,000 years of age. Therefore, it is natural that its society will also be very old and complex. Throughout its long period of history, India has witnessed and received several waves of immigrants, such as Aryans, Muslims, etc. These people brought with themselves their own ethnic varieties and cultures and contributed to India's diversity, richness and vitality. Therefore, Indian society is a complex mix of diverse cultures, people, beliefs and languages which may have come from anywhere but now is a part of this vast country. This complexity and richness gives Indian society a unique appearance of a very vibrant and colorful cultural country.

Major Problems in India

1. Poverty
2. Illiteracy
3. Terrorism
4. Casteism
5. Untouchability
6. Corruption
7. Overpopulation
8. Child marriage
9. Starvation
10. Child labor
11. Gender inequality
12. Dowry
13. Domestic violence against women
14. Sexual violence against women.

Causes and Remedies of Overpopulation

Overpopulation is caused by number of factors. Reduced mortality rate, better medical facilities, depletion of precious resources are few of the causes which results in overpopulation. It is possible for a sparsely populated area to become densely populated if it is not able to sustain life. Growing advances in technology with each coming year has affected humanity in many ways. One of these has been the ability to save lives and create better medical treatment for all. A direct result of this has been increased lifespan and the growth of the population.

Causes of Overpopulation

Decline in the death rate: At the root of overpopulation is the difference between the overall birth rate and death rate in populations. If the number of children born each year equals the number of adults that die, then the population will stabilize. Talking about overpopulation shows that while there are many factors that can increase the death rate for short periods of time, the ones that increase the birth rate do so over a long period of time.

Better medical facilities: Following this came the industrial revolution. Technological advancement was perhaps the biggest reason why the balance has been permanently disturbed. Science was able to produce better means of producing food which allowed families to feed more mouths. Medical science made many discoveries thanks to which they were able to defeat a whole range of diseases. Illnesses that had claimed thousands of lives till now were cured because of the invention of vaccines. Combining the increase in food supply with fewer means of mortality tipped the balance and became the starting point of overpopulation.

More hands to overcome poverty: However, when talking about overpopulation we should understand that there is a psychological component as well. For thousands of years, a very small part of the population had enough money to live in comfort. The rest faced poverty and would give birth to large families to make up for the high infant mortality rate. Families that have been through poverty, natural disasters or are simply in need of more hands to work are a major factor for overpopulation. As compared to earlier times, most of these extra children survive and consume resources that are not sufficient in nature.

Technological advancement in fertility treatment: With latest technological advancement and more discoveries in medical science, it has become possible for couple who are unable to conceive to undergo fertility treatment methods and have their own babies. Today there are effective medicines which can increases the chance of conception and lead to rise in birth rate. Moreover, due to modern techniques pregnancies today are far more safer.

Immigration: Many people prefer to move to developed countries like US, UK, Canada and Australia where best facilities are available in terms of medical, education, security and employment. The end result is that those people settle over there and those places become overcrowded. Difference between the number of people who are leaving the country and the number of people who enter narrows down which leads to more demand for food, clothes, energy and homes. This gives rise to shortage of resources. Though the overall population remains the same, it just affects the density of population making that place simply overcrowded.

Lack of family planning: Most developing nations have large number of people who are illiterate, live below the poverty line and have little or no knowledge about family planning. Getting their children married at an early age increase the chances of producing more kids. Those people are unable to understand the harmful effects of overpopulation and lack of quality education prompts them to avoid family planning measures.

Solutions to Overpopulation

Better education: One of the first measures is to implement policies reflecting social change. Educating the masses helps them understand the need to have one or two children at the most. Similarly, education plays a vital role in understanding latest technologies that are making huge waves in the world of computing. Families that are facing a hard life and choose to have four or five children should be discouraged. Family planning and efficient birth control can help in women making their own reproductive choices. Open dialogue on abortion and voluntary sterilization should be seen when talking about overpopulation.

Making people aware of family planning: As population of this world is growing at a rapid pace, raising awareness among people regarding family planning and letting them know about serious after-effects of overpopulation can help curb population growth. One of the best way is to let them know about various safe sex techniques and contraceptives methods available to avoid any unwanted pregnancy.

Tax benefits or concessions: Government of various countries might have to come with various policies related to tax exemptions to curb overpopulation. One of them might be to waive of certain part of income tax or lowering rates of income tax for those married couples who have single or two children. As we humans are more inclined towards money, this may produce some positive results.

Knowledge of sex education: Imparting sex education to young kids at elementary level should be must. Most parents feel shy in discussing such things with their kids which result in their children going out and look out for such information on internet or discuss it with their peers. Mostly, the information is incomplete which results in sexually active teenagers unaware of contraceptives and embarrassed to seek information about same. It is therefore important for parents and teachers to shed their old inhibitions and make their kids or students aware of solid sex education.

3. Define social stratification (*See* Q. 3, 2011); explain caste system as a form of social stratification.

The caste system in India is primarily associated with Hinduism but also exists among other Indian religious groups. Castes are ranked and named. Membership is achieved by birth. Castes are also endogamous groups. Marriages and relationships between members of different castes, while not actually prohibited, face strong social disapproval and the threat of ostracism or even violence. The castes are hereditary endogamous group with fixed traditional occupations, observing commensal prohibition and social restrictions on interaction. It is believed that there are about 3,000 castes in the country. These castes are grouped as upper castes (like Brahmins, Rajputs, Baniyas, Kayasthas,etc.), intermediate castes (like Ahir, Sunar, Kurmi, etc.) and lower caste (like Dhobi, Nai, etc.). The castes are linked with the four varnas (Brahmins, Kshatriyas, Vaishyas, and Shudras) for determining the status in ritual hierarchy. . Caste system is often portrayed as the ultimate horror, in the media. Thus caste system is going to stay permanently in India and all slogans denouncing the system is a pure and mere eye wash. Caste system although was not sanctioned by Vedas made inroads into the society and got entrenched. With Government policies, further irreparable damage has been done to the society and it would be impossible to eradicate the evil. Vested interests have developed due to various reservations where merit is thrown to winds.

SHORT ESSAYS

4. Factors favoring and hindering assimilation.

Factors that Favors Assimilation

1. **Toleration:** Assimilation is possible only when individuals and groups are tolerant towards the cultural differences of others. Tolerance helps people to come together, to develop contacts towards to participate in common social and cultural activities. When the majority group or the dominant group itself is secure, hospitable and tolerant towards differences, the immigrant groups or minority groups have a greater opportunity to join and to participate in the total community life.

2. **Intimate social relationships:** Assimilation is the final product of social contacts. The relative speed in which it is achieved depends on the nature of the contacts. It takes place naturally and quickly in primary groups, such as family and friendship groups. On the contrary, where contacts are secondary, that is indirect, impersonal and superficial assimilation is slow to take place.

3. **Amalgamation or intermarriage:** A factor which helps complete assimilation is amalgamation which refers to the intermarriage of different groups. Without biological amalgamation complete

assimilation is not possible. Mere intermixture of the groups to a limited degree does not guarantee assimilation. But intermarriage must be accepted in the mores and become a part of the institutional structure, before assimilation exists.

4. **Cultural similarity:** If there are striking similarities between the main constituents of culture of groups assimilation is quick to take place. In America, for example, English speaking protestants are assimilated with greater speed than non-Christians who do not speak English.

5. **Education:** Education is another conducive factor for assimilation. For immigrant people public education has played a prominent role in providing cultural contact. Maurice R. Davis has pointed out in his "World Immigration" that in America the public school has been playing the vital role in the process of Americanising the children of foreign-born parents.

6. **Equal social and economic opportunity:** Public education alone is not enough. People of all groups must have equal access to socioeconomic opportunities. Only then, they can come closer and establish relations among themselves with mutual trust. As it has been observed in the case of America full assimilation is possible only when full participation in social, cultural and economic life is allowed.

Factors Retarding or Hindering Assimilation

1. **Isolation**: Assimilation is possible only when the groups and individuals are in continuous contact with others. Hence isolation is a negation of assimilation. Not only physical isolation but even mental isolation retards assimilation.

2. **Physical or racial differences**: Differences in physical appearance are often used as a means of discrimination. It is easy to keep some people apart on the basis of their skin, color or other physical features. For example, we can see widespread discrimination between the Whites and the Negroes in almost all the places in the world.

3. **Cultural differences**: If there are no common elements in the two cultures, the groups may remain apart socially even though they happen to stay together physically. They may even struggle for supremacy in their intermittent conflicts. Thus, wide cultural differences between groups in customs, religious beliefs, morals, values, languages come in the way of assimilation.

4. **Prejudice as a barrier to assimilation**: Prejudice is the attitude on which segregation depends for its success. As long as the dominant group is prejudiced against a particular group which is kept apart assimilation cannot take place. Prejudice also hampers assimilation between constituent elements within a given society. Prejudice within a community, within a family, or within any group can only contribute to disunity and not to unity.

5. **Dominance and subordination**: Dominance and subordination often come in the way of close intimate contact between groups. If the dominant group does not provide equal chances and opportunities for the minority or immigrant groups, assimilation is very slow to take place. Further, complete assimilation may not take place. Strong feeling of superiority and inferiority associated with dominance and subordination also retard the rate of assimilation.

5. Differentiate rural and urban community.

Difference between Rural and Urban Community

Sl. No.	Criteria	Rural community	Urban community
1.	Size of population	Rural population is limited	Urban population is large
2.	Environment	Natural environment, more close to nature	Artificial environment and more problems of environmental pollution
3.	Family	Trend of joint family is found	Nuclear family is more common
4.	Occupation	Agriculture and agriculture-based occupations	Industry, trade and different occupations (education, medical, administration, engineering, management, etc.)
5.	Social uniformity	More uniformity found	Heterogeneity and differences are found
6.	Stratification	More based on castes, otherwise stratification is simple	More based on class. Stratification is complex
7.	Mobility	Physical and social mobility is limited	High rate of physical and social mobility
8.	Density of population	Less density	High density
9.	Means of recreation	More natural and cultural. Social ridicule is natural	Professional and complex. Media is relatively more powerful
10.	Political awareness	Relatively less, increasing now	Political awareness is more
11.	Marriage and divorce	Marriage is traditional and permanent. Divorce is negligible	Love marriages are also found. Divorce is more common. Marriage institution is in more danger
12.	Condition of social change	Change is less	Changes are fast and more political
13.	Education	Less literacy	Changes are fast and more political
14.	Social problems	Unsociability, child marriage, superstitions, etc. found more	Problems are based on class, economy, power, etc.
15.	Social interaction	Personal and more cordial	Indirect and formal relationship are found more

6. Marriage and family problems in india.

In considering the marriage and family problems in India we have first to consider the status of women in Hindu family. Critics of the Indian family system say that Indian women do not enjoy equal rights with men in the social, political, religious and economic fields; that they are ill-treated and that they cannot claim any share in the family property.

Family Problems in India

Separation: Separation can often be a couple's first step towards trying to improve their relationship although it can also be the first step towards a breakup or divorce.

Divorce: Divorce of your parents may leave you feeling anxious, withdrawn or depressed. These intense feelings may express themselves as shame, anger, grief or poor performance in school. Some kids describe their parents' divorce as the most painful experience of their childhood.

Alcoholic or drug addicted parent: An alcoholic or drug addicted parent can make you sad or anxious. If they are struggling with addiction, they are probably not able to care for you well or give you much attention. This can be very difficult to deal with.

Abused parent: An abused parent's low self-esteem may keep them from seeking help to escape their abusive relationship. They may be anxious and depressed and take it out on you.

Abusive parent: An abusive parent has no right to abuse you. Child abuse is against the law. This includes abuse of any minors (under 18). No parent, step-parent, relative or friend of the family is allowed to abuse you—physically, sexually or emotionally.

Parents who nag or criticize: Parents who nag or criticize can make you frustrated or angry. Sometimes parents have a hard time realizing that you are growing up and becoming more independent. It can help to keep the parents on your side by showing love, appreciation and interest in them and being as pleasant to them as you want them to be to you. Parents want to know you are listening.

Parents who are overprotective: Parents who are overprotective usually make rules because they love you and do not want you to get hurt. Keep them up on the important things going on in your life and introduce them to your friends.

Parents who fight: Parents who fight can be upsetting or disturbing. When they are calm, tell your parents that their fighting bothers you. Try to understand each parent's point of view—do not feel you have to take sides.

Parent's remarriage: A parent's remarriage can be confusing and stressful. It might help to do something nice for your step-parent, to break the ice.

Marriage Problems in India

Marriage is considered to be an institution in India. It is a 'sanskara' or purificatory ceremony obligatory for every Hindu. The Hindu religious books have enjoined marriage as a duty because an unmarried man cannot perform some of the most important religious ceremonies.

Child marriage: The problem of child marriage was very serious in Hindu society till the passing of Sarada Act. The reasons behind the child marriages in Hindu society were religious conservatism, endogamy, sati-custom, the custom of dowry and the joint family. The Hindu marriage act of 1955 has fixed the valid age for marriage of the boys and girls at 18 and

15 respectively. These legal steps could not work immediately because of the widespread conservatism among Hindus, incompleteness of Prohibitive Act and the absence of female education. With the removal of these difficulties in the way of restraint of child marriages, this problem has appreciably diminished in Hindu society.

Widow remarriage: About the condition of widow remarriage in ancient India, AS Aletkar has written, "side by side with Niyoga, the widow remarriage also prevailed in the Vedic society." The custom of widow remarriage, however, disappeared gradually and it was considered to be wrong as early as 200 AD. The restriction of widow remarriage resulted in the increase of immorality among widows, sexual exploitation of child widows, increase of prostitutes and the lowering of general status of women in the Hindu society. Then due to the untiring efforts of Ishwarchandra Vidyasagar the Hindu Widows Remarriage Act was passed in the year of 1856 which declared the legal validity of widow remarriage and laid specific circumstances for its validity.

Dowry: According to Max Radin, "ordinarily dowry is the property which a man receives when he marries, either from his wife or her family." The Websters New International Dictionary has defined dowry as, "the money, goods or estate, which a woman brings to her husband in marriage." In brief, dowry is that money, property or valuables which the bride party has to give to the bride-groom party in exchange of marriage.

7. Voluntary associations.

There are many voluntary and religious organizations which are doing useful work at present and had been doing so in the past. Arya Samaj raised a voice against injustice being done to the untouchables and the women. This organization also started many educational institutions all over the country. Brahmo Samaj raised voice against Sati. Other organizations which need mention are the Servants of India Society, Rama Krishnan Mission, Theosophical Society and Bharat Sewak Samaj. All these organizations have focused the attention of the public and the authorities to the problems which threaten the society. These also created a climate and atmosphere under which people could accept a change without much opposition. In this way, it will be seen that India has been trying to solve her social problems and promote social welfare of the people at all levels and can claim to be a social welfare state.

8. Types of marriage. (*See* Q. 8, 2015)

9. Joint family system in india. (*See* Q. 5, 2016)

10. Technology as a factor of social change. (*See* Q. 9, 2016)

11. Community development programs in india.

The Community Development Programme has been the biggest rural reconstruction scheme undertaken by the government of free India. It has been variously described as the magnac arta of hope and happiness for two-thirds of India's population, the testament of emancipation, the declaration of war on poverty, ignorance, squalor and disease under which millions have been groaning, etc.

Aims: Prof SC Dube has highlighted on two aims of Community Development Programme. They are: (a) achieving substantial agricultural production and considerable progress in the sphere of communication, rural health and rural education and (b) transforming the socioeconomic life of the village through a process of integral cultural change. The aims of the Community

Development Project have been divided into two parts. They are short-term objectives and long-term objectives.

Short-term Objectives:

The short-term objectives are as follows:
1. To increase agricultural production both quantitatively and qualitatively.
2. To solve the problem of rural unemployment.
3. To develop the means of transport and communication in the villages through repairing old roads and constructing new pucka roads.
4. To bring about development in the sphere of primary education, public health and recreation.
5. To assist the villagers to build good and cheap houses with the help of modern plans and new building methods.
6. To set up and encourage cottage industries and indigenous handicrafts.

Long-term Objectives:

The long-term objective of community development projects refers to holistic development of rural life through optimum utilization of physical and human resources. It is further oriented to provide all sorts of facilities available in a Welfare State to the ruralites. Taking care of the social, moral and financial progress of the villagers also comes within the purview of the long-term objectives of community development projects.

The Community Development Programme was inaugurated on October 2, 1952. 55 community projects were launched. The programme launched in 1952 was extended to wider areas at the end of the first five-year plan. Nearly one out of every three villages in India was brought within the orbit of this programme.

The Second five-year plan proposed to bring every village in India under this scheme, 40 % of the area being brought under a more intensive development scheme. The programme was implemented through units of blocks, each community development block comprising generally 100 villages, an area of 400-500 square kms. And a population of 60–70 thousand.

The main items in their programme are:

1. Improvement in farming techniques: The improvements, such as the introduction of better varieties, use of fertilizers, improvement in cropping pattern, improved tools are needed. The object is to make use of the result of scientific research as far as possible.

2. Exploring supplementary avenues of employment: Since farming alone cannot make a farmer prosperous, it is necessary to combine with agriculture some other gainful occupations. This means the development of village and cottage industries.

3. Extension of minor irrigation facilities: It is within the power of villagers to extend irrigation facilities through minor irrigation works. The CD programme gives an important place to this item in their programme.

4. Improvement of transport: For agrarian development good means of transport are must. Accordingly the CD. programme makes a provision for the construction of local roads.

5. Provision of social services: The CD programme makes a provision also for education, health, housing, sanitation, etc. so that the villagers can have a better life and enjoy an increased measure of social welfare.

6. Development of cooperatives and panchayats: For effective implementation of their programme it is necessary that the villagers are organized on democratic lines and there is full participation on their part in the programmes. Thus, cooperatives and Panchayats are encouraged and developed further.

12. Rehabilitation of juvenile delinquents.

Restoration of a juvenile back to the society is very important for the reformation of the child in conflict with the law and to make him/her into a model citizen. The government and non-governmental organizations work together for the rehab of the juvenile. The core concern of the correctional law for juveniles shifted from punishing for the alleged crime to make him grievous of his actions and rehabilitating the juvenile.

Treatment and Rehabilitation of Delinquents:

Delinquency had always been considered as a legal and social problem. So psychologists and psychiatrists did not pay much attention to it until it was considered as a psychological problem. Currently in all the progressive and civilized countries of the world the laws with regard to the juvenile delinquents have been changed. Special courts are established with specially trained magistrates for the trial of the delinquents.

Psychologists, psychiatrists and social workers are always attached to look after their difficulties. In western countries delinquents in small groups are brought up in residential areas and given individual treatment, to have in them the feeling that they are a part and parcel of the society. Thus, they are removed from the aversive environment and allowed to learn about the world of which they are a member.

If such types of delinquents are kept with those who have committed serious crimes, they would in turn learn these from them. So it may aggravate their behavioral problems instead of correcting them.

The teachers of reformatory schools opened for rehabilitating delinquents should act as substitutes of good, warm and understanding parents and help the children to obtain a sense of security and involvement. The school must also develop a number of group activity which will help to change his ego.

The parents must also be helped to develop an insight to the problems of the boy, to have insight to their own behavior as well which has led to the maladjustment in the child.

The society and public should also change their attitude towards delinquency. Society as a whole should give up its fear and hostility against the criminals and delinquents. They should develop a flexible attitude so that proper analysis is made of the conditions leading to delinquency and adequate steps are taken both with respect to the treatment and prevention of delinquency.

SHORT ANSWERS

13. Social mobility. (*See* Q. 22, 2014)

14. Endogamy and exogamy.

Endogamy: Endogamy means marriage within one's own group. The best example for this is caste endogamy. The basic rule followed in caste is to marry within the caste group, that too within the subgroups.

Exogamy: Exogamy means to marry outside the group. It is the process by means of which group ties are expanded. People also believed that to marry within their nearest kin is not a healthy practice. Exogamy is advantageous from the biological point of view. This is beneficial in the reproduction of healthy and intelligent offspring's.

15. Cultural lag. (*See* Q. 16, 2016)

16. Role of religion in social control.

Religion describes the beliefs, values, and practices related to sacred or spiritual concerns. Social theorist Émile Durkheim defined religion as a "unified system of beliefs and practices relative to sacred things". Max Weber believed religion could be a force for social change. Karl Marx viewed religion as a tool used by capitalist societies to perpetuate inequality. Religion is a social institution because it includes beliefs and practices that serve the needs of society. Religion is also an example of a cultural universal because it is found in all societies in one form or another. Functionalism, conflict theory, and interactionism all provide valuable ways for sociologists to understand religion.

17. Racism.

Racism is the belief that a particular race is superior or inferior to another, that a person's social and moral traits are predetermined by his or her inborn biological characteristics. Racial separatism is the belief, most of the time based on racism, that different races should remain segregated and apart from one another.

18. Various forms of conflict. (*See* Q. 8, 2014)

19. Isolation.

Isolation is a process whereby the individual or a group wills be segregated from others. It is a type of dissociative social process. The great sociologists like Park and Burges considered isolation as opposite to interaction. They defined it as "A kind of negative interaction". Isolation of the individual is considered to be a negative value. Prolonged isolation is resulted in mental disintegration.

Isolation of an individual is always considered as a negative value. Human being is interdependent. They cannot satisfy their needs and desires without contact with others. The development of culture depends mostly upon contacts between groups. Nevertheless, the partial isolation sometimes helpful to others. If a criminal is not isolated from the group, his presence will be harmful to the other members of the same group.

20. Assimilation. (*See* Q. 20, 2015)

21. Social system.

A social system basically consists of two or more individuals interacting directly or indirectly in a bounded situation. There may be physical or territorial boundaries, but the fundamental sociological point of reference is that the individuals are oriented, in a whole sense, to a common focus or inter-related foci. Thus, it is appropriate to regard such diverse sets of relationships as small groups, political parties and whole societies as social systems. Social systems are open systems, exchanging information with, frequently acting with reference to other systems. Modern conceptions of the term can be traced to the leading social analysts of the nineteenth century, notably Auguste Comte, Karl Marx, Herbert Spencer and Emile Durkheim; each of whom elaborated in some form or other conceptions of the major units of social systems (mainly societies) and the relationships between such units—even though the expression social system was not a key one. Thus, in Marx's theory, the major units or components of the capitalist societies with which he was principally concerned were socioeconomic classes, and the major relationships between classes involved economic and political power.

22. Health consequences of poverty.

Poverty is that condition in which a person, either because of inadequate income or unwise expenditure, does not maintain a scale of living high enough to provide for his physical and mental efficiency and to enable him and his natural dependents to function usually according to the standards of society of which he is member. —Gillin and Gillin.

"Poverty is a condition of life so degraded by disease, illiteracy, malnutrition and squalor as to deny its victims the basic necessities". —Robert McNamara.

Evil Effects of Poverty
Poverty creates a number of following problems to the society:
1. Poverty causes inadequate diet, high infant mortally, unsanitary living conditions, low life expectancy, sickness, malnutrition.
2. Low rate of education, high rate of illiteracy are the contributions of poverty. Poverty also contributes to high fertility.
3. Poverty creates the problem of unemployment, underemployment and low wages. The poor people are forced to take certain occupations that are harmful to their health.
4. Certain social problems, such as crime, delinquency, child labor, slums, prostitution, beggary, etc. are the consequences of poverty.

Eradication and Control of Poverty
To control and eradicate the poverty, we have to follow the under given suggestions:
1. The disabled persons should be imparted special skills for doing some special jobs.
2. New scientific techniques should be implemented in the agricultural sectors.
3. The cottage, small scale and large scale industries should still be established.
4. The growth of overpopulation should be properly controlled.
5. All the people should be made literate.
6. The wealth should be rationally and proper/distributed.
7. The problems of unemployment and underemployment should be controlled.

Consequences of Poverty
Poverty is a condition of chronic insufficiency, in which a person is not able to lead a life according to the desirable standards of life. Even after so many years of independence a major portion of population is found below the poverty line. Unemployment is another important cause of poverty. Another area of serious concern is the rapid population growth. It is estimated that about 3.3 million unemployed are added every year to existing labor force in India. We have failed to absorb this surplus labor force due to scarcity of production resources. Food problem in India is both quantitative and qualitative. About 40-54% in rural population and 41-50% of the urban population consumes between 2,100 and 2,250 calories per day, which is less than 2,500 calories, the minimum prescribed calories to maintain normal health. Nonavailability of nutritious diet affects the physical and mental health of people.

Poverty in India

In India, poverty is the most important problem. Each year more than 5 million people are added to the growing multitude of the poor. The main cause of poverty is the personal ownership and monopoly of the individual on the land. In cities where land is valuable we find extremes of poverty and richness. Some of the causes of poverty are personal while others are geographical, economic and social incapacity of the individual due to faulty heredity or to the environment, unfavorable physical conditions, such as poor natural resources and maldistribution of the available resources are the main causes of poverty.

In India, people are caught in vicious circle of poverty due to the prevalent sociocultural institutions. In order to fulfill social obligations and observe religious ceremonies people spend extravagantly. With already low income levels and negligible saving the chances of borrowing are great. The level of indebtedness is both the cause and effect of poverty. Poverty is the most obvious problem in India. According to 2003 estimated about 28.6% (308.59 million) population of the country is living below the poverty line.

2016

Sociology

LONG ESSAYS

1. Define culture. Mention the characteristics of culture. Discuss the impact of culture on health and illness.
2. Define social change. Explain the theories of social change.
3. Define caste. Explain the characteristics of caste system.

SHORT ESSAYS

4. Differentiate primary and secondary groups.
5. Merits and demerits of joint family system.
6. Major urban problems and its impact on health.
7. Types of cooperation (with suitable examples).
8. Types of family.
9. Technological factors of social change.
10. "Man is a social animal". Discuss.
11. Types of social system.
12. Write a note on alcoholism.

SHORT ANSWERS

13. Acculturation.
14. Edipal complex.
15. Achieved status.
16. Cultural lag.
17. MOB.
18. Child labor.
19. Health services in rural communities.
20. IRDP.
21. HIV/AIDS.
22. In-group and out-group.

LONG ESSAYS

1. Define culture. Mention the characteristics of culture. Discuss the impact of culture on health and illness.

Culture has been defined in a number of way, some thinkers include in culture all the major social components that bind men together in a society. Culture is that knowledge which a new generation subjectively derives from the previous one. Culture is an essential intergradient of human society. The essential point in regard to culture is that it is acquired by man as a member of society and persists through tradition. These points of acquisition and tradition have been emphasized by Tylor and Redfield in their definitions. The essential factors in this acquisition through tradition are the ability to learn from the group. A man learns his behavior and behavior which is learnt denotes his culture. Singing, talking, dancing and eating belong to the category of culture. Moreover, the behaviors are not his own but are shared by others. They have been transmitted to him by someone, be it his school teacher, his parents or friend.

According to Hames and Joseph (1980)
1. Culture is a group's blueprint for acceptable ways of thinking and behaving.
2. Through culture is universal in man's experience, it is unique for each group (Alfred Weber-culture is unique and civilization is universal).
3. Culture is transmitted from generation to generation.
4. Culture is stable, but continuously adapting.
5. Culture is affected by the environment including such variables as climate, geographical location, food resources and natural resources.
6. Culture does not affect man's basic physiological needs (such as need for food or water) but people from different cultural groups may vary genetically.
7. All cultures have four components in common: Art, forms, language, institutions and technology.

Characteristics of Culture
1. **Culture is an acquired quality: Culture is not innate**—Traits learnt through socialization, habits and thoughts are what are called culture. Man acquires the cultural behavior because he has the capacity of symbolic communication.
2. **Culture is social, not individual:** Every individual takes some part in the transmission and communication of culture, but culture is social rather than individual. It is inclusive of the expectation of the members of groups. Man cannot create or generate culture while existing apart from the group.
3. **Culture is idealistic:** In culture are included those ideal patterns or ideal norms of behavior according to which the members of society attempt to conduct themselves. Society accepts these ideals, norms and patterns.
4. **Culture is communicative:** In this way culture is communicated from one generation to the next. As a result of this, culture is constantly accumulating. The new generation benefits by the experiences of the older generation through the communicability of culture. In this way, culture becomes semitemporary and remains unaffected by the extinction of a group or an individual.
5. **Culture fulfills some needs:** Culture fulfills those ethical and social needs which are ends in themselves. Social habits are included in culture. Habits can be formed of these activities only which tend to fulfill some needs. Without fulfilling these needs culture cannot exist.

6. **Culture has the characteristic of adaptation:** Culture is constantly undergoing change in concurring to the environment and due to this transformation, it is constantly being adapted to external forces but once it is formation, it is constantly being adapted to external forces but once it is developed, the influences of the natural environment begins to decrease. Besides, the various aspects of culture are also undergoing development and some internal adaptation among them consequently being necessitated.
7. **Culture has the quality of becoming integrated:** Cultural possesses an order and a system. Its various parts are integrated with each other and any new element which is introduced is also integrated. Those cultures which are more open to external influences are comparatively more heterogeneous but nevertheless some degree of integration is evident in all cultures.
8. **Culture evolves into more complex forms through division of labor** which develops special skills and increases the independence society's members.
9. **Language is the chief vehicle of culture:** Man lives not only in the present but also in the past and future. This, he is enabled to do because he possesses language which transmits to him what was learnt in the past and enables him to transmit the accumulated wisdom.
10. **Culture is an integrated system**: Culture possesses an order and system. Its various parts are integrated with each other and any new element which is introduced is also integrated.
11. **Culture fulfills some needs**: Culture fulfills those ethical and social needs of the groups which are ends in themselves.

Impact of Culture on Health and Illness

Sociocultural and economic aspects of the community, and their effects on health and illness: Sociocultural factors play a significant role in explaining human action. Human beings cannot exist apart from social order. The survival of human beings depends upon sociocultural and economic needs. The culture of a society determines all aspects of social life. For example, the birth of a child, its growth from childhood to adulthood, its health and its care during illness, the satisfaction of instincts are all determined by sociocultural factors.

In all communities, various norms control the behavior patterns and the social interactions. To check the sexual intercourses, incest taboos are prescribed. The reproductive capacity, though a biological capacity is controlled by sociocultural system. In all societies, we find sex norms like the institution of marriage. Whom to marry and at what age? How many mates one can have? What are the advantages of family life to individuals, to maintain their physical and mental health? How it helps the members in their old age and acts as a means of social security? How it helps the sick? How other problems of health care and economic needs are looked after by the family and other social groups in a community? Family is the basic institution which provides answers to all these problems. Birth and death are two sides of the life. The preservation of life is essential to species. So the maintenance of good health has great cultural value in any society. It is a known fact that a human being is an expensive thing. But life cannot be measured in terms of money, but in happiness. A parent does not hesitate to spend for the well-being of their children and to equip them with all comforts and needs. Health is the foundation of happiness. Health is the main basis of human progress that is why health is considered as wealth.

Good Health of the Members in a Society has Certain Advantages

1. It increases the physical and mental efficiency and happiness
2. It provides bodily comforts
3. A sense of well-being
4. It develops energy
5. It develops alertness and keenness.

Disadvantages or Evil Consequences
1. Sickness brings poverty and suffering
2. Breeds crime
3. Despair or lose all hopes
4. It leads to laziness and lethargy
5. Broken homes
6. Economic loss due to sickness.

To witness the suffering of the sick is hard and to see them die is still harder. Therefore, people are interested in keeping good health and devised various methods of curing the illness and controlling the mortality. The nurses play a vital role in maintaining good health, by serving the sick persons in society.

Sociocultural Practices of Health with Adverse Effects

In ancient societies like Egypt, Babylonia, Jewish, Greek, India and in many Christian societies we find magico-religious theories of illness. For Jews all sickness, all suffering was punishment for violation of Gods law. Such a kind of belief systems are found among Christians and other religious communities of the world. It is also believed that certain diseases are due to the wrath of Gods and Goddesses. What are the remedies for such illness? Prayer, right living, faith, healing, visit to sacred shrines, such as temples, churches, dargas or to take a bath in sacred rivers or ponds.

There are other cultural prescriptions which are irrelevant and irrational to health and life. Sacrifice of animals, human sacrifice, sacrifice of aged, infirm, female infanticide, child sacrifice for ceremonial purposes. In India, the practice of sati system. In some societies cannibalism for ritualistic purposes is practiced. Cannibalism means eating human flesh. A popular 20th century belief is that science particularly medical science replaced religio-magical and superstitions which are irrelevant and injurious to health. But in all communities the medical science cannot fulfill all the functions of religion-magical medicine. Healing cultural and the medical relief both are identified.

2. Define social change. Explain the theories of social change.

Social change is an ever present phenomenon everywhere. An ancient Greek philosopher Heraclitus is an emphatic way hinted at this fact when he said that it is impossible for a man to step into the same river twice. It is impossible, because in the interval of time between the first and the second stepping both the river and man have changed. Neither remains the same. This is the central theme of the Heraclitean philosophy—the reality of change, the impermanent of being, the inconstancy of everything, but change itself. Social change is a reality. Incessant changeability is the inherent nature of human society. It does not mean that society is always as its toes to welcome any kind of society.

Theories of Social Changes

The theories of social change are closely connected with the philosophy of history the theories of social change are generally classified into learners and cyclical theory.

I. Learners Theory

Learner's theory asserts that all aspects of society change continually in a certain direction and they never repeat themselves. These theories assure that there is a cumulative change in social history.

Sl. No.	Contributors	Description
1.	Auguste Comte	Auguste Comte, the founding father of sociology focused his attention on the study of change, development and progress in human society. He divided the study of society into two parts: 1. Social statics and 2. Social dynamics. Comte saw human society and history as a single entity
2.	Spencer	He saw that societies changed from simple to complex form
3.	Hobhouse	He explains social change through mental development and moral ideas
4.	Marx	He traced the historical change through the development of productive forces which changes the relations between classes. He has emphasized the economic conditions and techniques of production have great influence in social activities
5.	Thorstein Veblen	He tries to give a technological explanation of social change by emphasizing that social conditions are directly responsible for technological conditions

II. Cyclical Theory

Cyclical theories are as old as human history. These theories assume that social phenomena recur again and again, exactly as they were before. For example, day and night, the seasons of the year and the birth, growth decay and death of individual organism.

Sl. No.	Contributors	Description
1.	Pareto	He presents the theory of circulation of elites. According to him social change occurs by the struggle between groups for political power. He illustrates the circulation of elites in Rome, but has ignored the development of democratic government in modern times
2.	P Sorokin	He has recognized the cyclic process by making a distinction between three broader types of culture namely ideational, idealist and sensate. These types of culture succeed each other in cycles in the history of societies
3.	Arnold Toynbee	He explains the cyclical character of the growth, arrest and decay of civilization

III. Evolutionary Theory

Evolutionary theories are based on the assumption that societies gradually change from simple beginning into even more complex forms.

Sl. No.	Contributors	Description
1.	LH Morgan	Believed that there were three basic stages in the process, they are savagery, barbarian, and civilization
2.	Charles Darwin's	Theory of organic evolution. Those who were influenced by Darwin's theory of organic evolution applied it to the human society and argued that, societies must have evolved from the too simple and primitive to that of too complex and advanced, such as the Western society

Contd...

Contd...

Sl. No.	Contributors	Description
3.	Herbert Spencer	He argued that society itself is an organism. He said that society has been gradually progressing, towards a better state. He argued that it has evolved from military society to the industrial society
4.	Emile Durkhiem	He advocated that societies have evolved from relatively undifferentiated social structure with minimum of division of labor and with a kind of solidarity called mechanical solidarity to a more differentiated social structure with maximum division of labor given rise to a kind of solidarity called organic solidarity

IV. Conflict Theories or the Deterministic Theories of Social Change

Among contemporary sociologist the deterministic theory of social change is probably the most widely accepted one. According to this view, social change takes place because of certain forces.

Sl. No.	Contributors	Description
1.	Karl Marx	According to his view individuals and groups with opposing interests are bound to be at conflict. Since the two major social classes, that is, the rich and poor, or capitalists and laborers have mutually hostile interests they are at conflict. This conflict repeats itself off and on until capitalism is overthrown by the workers and a socialistic state is created. What is to be stressed here is that Marx and others conflict theorists deem society as basically dynamic and not static?
2.	George Simmel	Conflict is a permanent feature of society and not just a temporary event. It is a process that binds people together by interaction. Further conflict encourages people of similar interests to unite together to achieve their objectives. Continuous conflict in this way keeps society dynamic and ever changing

V. Functional or Dynamic Theories of Social Change

Sl. No.	Contributors	Description
1.	Talcott Parsons	Considers change not as something that disturbs the social equilibrium, but as something that alters the state of equilibrium, so that a qualitatively new equilibrium results. He has started that change may arise from two sources. They may come from outside the society, through contact with other societies. Pearson advocated that of two process that are at work in social change. In simple societies, institutions are undifferentiated, that is, a single institution serves many functions. For example, the family performs reproductive, educational, economic, recreational, socialization and other functions
2.	Robert K Merton	The strain, tension, contribution and discrepancy between the component parts of social structure may lead to change. Thus, in order to accommodate the concept of change within the functional model. He has borrowed concepts from conflict theories of change

3. Define caste. Explain the characteristics of caste system.

The word caste is used in everyday life and we use it to distinguish one person from another. We say that such and such person belongs to a particular caste. In saying it, we generally mean to convey that he is born of parents or is a member of the family said to belong to a particular caste. The word caste is derived from the Spanish word casta which means breed. Caste is a unique social institution of Indian society, originated from Varna system, described in the Vedas.

Caste system has been the predominant form of social stratification in India, and even today, it exerts considerable influence on our lives and social interaction. Caste is social phenomena found in almost all human societies but at nowhere it took such a well-defined and rigid form as it did it India. Caste is an institution most highly developed in India and it has profoundly influenced the life of the Hindus. Place of residence, mode of life, personal association, the type of food which one can eat and from whom one can accept food and water, occupation and the group in which he has to find his mate are determined by his birth.

Social interaction between castes is very strictly limited and intercaste marriages are strictly prohibited. The caste system is always safeguard by social laws and sanctified by religion. The caste system is very conservative and lends great stability to society. It serves to hand over from one generation to another generation skills and secrets of craftsmanship, but it also acts as deterrent to the introduction of new and improved methods of production in industry and agriculture and results in an economy dependent on the interplay of a large number of segregated and sometimes conflicting interests.

Definitions
1. When status is wholly predetermined, so that men are born to their lot in life without any hope of changing it, then class takes the form of caste.
   —MacIver and Page.
2. A caste is a social group having two characteristics: 1. membership is confined to those who are born of members, and include all people born, 2. the members are forbidden by an inexorable social law to marry outside the group.
   —Ketkar.

Features of Caste System
Kingsley Davis has mentioned certain common feature or tendencies which together distinguish Indian caste from other types of groups as follows:
1. The membership in the caste is hereditary.
2. This inherited membership is fixed for life.
3. Choice of marriage partner is strictly endogamous, for it must take place within the caste group.
4. Contact with other groups is further limited by restrictions on touching, associating with, dining with, eating food cooked by outsiders.
5. Consciousness of caste membership is further emphasized by the caste name.
6. The caste is united by a common traditional occupation.
7. The relative prestige of the different castes in any locality is well established and jealously guarded.

Characteristic of Caste System
1. **Caste is innate:** The membership of caste is determined by birth. A person remains the member of the caste into which he is born and his membership does not undergo any change even if change in his status, occupation, education, wealth, etc. takes place.

2. **There are laws concerning food in the caste:** Each individual caste has its own laws which govern the food habits of its members. Generally, there are no restrictions against fruits, milk, butter, dry fruits, etc.
3. **Occupations of most castes are determined:** In Hindu religious tests, the occupations of all Varnas were determined. According to Manu the functions of Brahmin, Kshatriya, Vaishya and the Shudra were definite. In Hindu society even today in most cases, the son of the blacksmith pursues the occupation of his father; the son of a carpenter becomes a carpenter while the son of a shoemaker becomes a shoemaker.
4. **Caste is endogamous:** The members of each of the many castes marry only within their own caste. Brahmin, Kshatriya, Vaishya and Shudra all marry within their respective castes. Westermark considers this to be chief characteristics of the caste. Hindu society does not sanctify intercaste marriage even now.
5. **Caste has laws concerning position and touchability:** The various castes in the Hindu social organization are divided into a hierarchy of ascent and descent one above the order. In this hierarchy, the Brahmins have the highest and the untouchables the lowest position. In Kerala, a Namboodari Brahmin is defined by the touch of a Nayar, but in the case of a member of Thiya caste, a distance of 36 feet must be kept to avoid being defiled and in the case of members of the Pulayan caste, the distance must be 96 feet. The stringent observation of the system of untouchablity has resulted in some low caste of Hindu society being called untouchables who were consequently forbidden to make use of places of worship, cremation grounds, colleges, public roads and hostels, etc. and well disallowed from living.

SHORT ESSAYS

4. Differentiate primary and secondary groups.

Primary Groups

Primary groups are small and intimate groups. Primary groups are very important in the society. They are foundation and nucleus of social structure. The development of the personality of an individual depends upon primary groups. They play a vital role in the socialization process. The primary group helps a person to increase his efficiency.

Secondary Groups

Secondary groups are important to the modern society. A secondary group is one which is large in size, such as a city, nation, party, corporation, international cartel and labor union. Secondary group are also known as special interest groups. Secondary groups are inevitable in modern society. Secondary groups are opposite to the primary groups in all respect.

Characteristics of Primary and Secondary group

Sl. No.	Primary group	Characteristics
1.	Family	Smaller number
2.	Play group	Personal
3.	Traditional	Face-to-face relationship
4.	Neighborhood	Intimacy, informal, spontaneous, general goals, permanency and stability, We-feeling, members are interact with one another as total personalities, not as segmental personalities

Sl. No.	Secondary group	Characteristics
1.	School	Impersonal
2.	Factory	Formal
3.	Army	Utilitarian
4.	City, neighborhood	Specialized goals
5.	Clubs	Focus on skills and interests, not personality. Communication rational and purposeful. Role expectations precisely defined. Members are together for a purpose and not because they like each other

Difference between Primary and Secondary Group

Difference	Primary group	Secondary group
Physical characteristics	Physical proximity, Small size closeness of relations	Absence of physical proximity, large size, limited responsibility, interest based on relations
Mental characteristics	Similarity of objectives	Infirmity
	Relationship end in itself	Absence of intimacy
	Personal relation	Formal or special reasons
	Develops spontaneously	No emotional attachment
	More controlling power	Competition
	Emotional attachment	Artificially made
	Intimacy	Absence of face-to-face relationship
	Face-to-face relation, We-feeling	
	Mental security	
Examples	Family, neighborhood, play group, ward, staff, small community, friendship group, etc.	Military, political party trade union, college, hospital, religion, national, etc.

5. Merits and demerits of joint family system.

Joint family consists of males having a common male ancestor, female offspring not yet married, and women brought into the group by marriage. All of these persons might live in a common household or in several households near to one another. In any case, so long as the joint family holds together, its members are expected to contribute to the support of the whole and to receive from it a share of the total product.

Definitions

1. Joint family as a group of kinds several generations, ruled by a head, in which residence health of property, and whose members are bound to each other by mutual obligations.
—RN Sharma.

2. Joint family is a group of people who generally live under one roof, who eat food cooked at one hearth, who hold property in common and who participate in common family worship and are related to each other as some particular type of kindred.
—Smt Iravathi Karve.

3. The Hindu joint family is a group constituted of known ancestors and adopted sons and relatives related to these sons through marriage.
—Henry Maine.
4. In joint family not only parents and children, brothers and step-brothers live on the common property, but it may sometimes include ascendants and collaterals up to many generations.
—Jolly.
5. We call that household a joint family which has greater generation depth than individual family and the members of which are related to one another by property, income and mutual rights and obligation.
—IP Desai.

Advantages of Joint Family

Sl. No.	Advantages	Description
1.	Economic advantage	The joint family system has proved to be a very advantageous institution from the economic viewpoint. It prevents property from being divided. Land is protected from extreme subdivision and fragmentation. Land, when divided into many small pieces, becomes an uneconomic holding. Besides keeping the land intact, the joint family also assists in economic position. In a joint agriculturist family, the male members do such work as furrowing, sowing, and irritation. Women assist at the harvest. Children graze the cattle and collect fuel and manure. In this way, the cooperation of all the members helps to save money which would otherwise be paid to a laborer
2.	Protection of members	Praising the joint family system Shri Jawaharlal Lal Nehru had said that the system of joint family is insurance for the family members which has carried a guarantee for those who are mentally and physically weak. In times of crisis, the joint family can provide assistance to the children, the old, the insane, the window and the helpless. The joint family is capable of providing much assistance at such times as pregnancy, sickness, etc.
3.	Means of recreation	The joint family is one of the best means of recreation. A stimulating atmosphere is created by cumulative effect of the stammered talking of the children, love between brother and sister, mother's love, the reproach of the elders and the fun and frolic of the other family members. In this way, the joint family also naturally takes over the role of a club
4.	Development of good habits	In this way, the joint family system makes possible the ideal development of the good qualities of man. In the care of elders, the undesirable and antisocial tendencies of the young and checked, they are prevented from staying from their path and they learn to exercise self-control. In the joint family, young men and women learn the lesson of generosity, patience, service, cooperation and obedience

Contd...

Contd...

Sl. No.	Advantages	Description
5.	Cooperation and economy	The joint family fosters cooperation and economy to extent achieved by few, if any, other institutions. A sense of cultural unity and an associational feeling exists among the members. There can be much economy in expenditure since a large saving can be made in the payment of rent and in cooking for a large family unit
6.	Socialism in wealth	According to Jather and Bery, everyone in a joint family earns according to his capabilities but obtains according to his needs and in this way to a large extent achieves the socialistic order. From each according to his ability to each according to his needs

6. Major urban problems and its impact on health.

The term urban is derived from the Latin word Urbanus. Urbanus means a city or a town. Towns and cities of India make up the urban communities with about twenty percent of the population. Compared with other countries India has a much higher rural population, but the urban population increasing rapidly. Town and cities are over crowding and always expanding. In urban areas most of the people have to work in connection with industry, the manufacture, trade, transport of goods and materials. In urban social life relations are for short-time and impersonal. There is no feeling of oneness, and it is a case of each person for himself. There is keen competition. The basis of urban social life is class rather than caste, and social class depends on economic status, some people by working hard, or by other means, may get rich quickly, and move from lower to middle or even upper class.

Urbanism

Urbanism means a way of behavior and thinking. Urbanization refers to certain features like transiency, superficiality, anonymity, impersonal relations, highly mobile and dynamic. This kind of life pattern is extended to rural areas because of vast network of communications. Urbanization is a process of development. It refers to the movement of population from rural to urban areas. It is not merely shifting of people from village to city but also change of work pattern from agriculture to urban type of work like industry, trade, service, etc. according to Anderson, urbanization is a two way process. It involves not only the movement of people from villages to cities, change of occupations but involves basic changes in thinking and behavior of people.

Urban Social Problems

The rapid urbanization and industrialization processes are responsible for the certain social problems. It is said that city is a center of attraction and at the same time it is pathological.

The common social problems are:
1. Overcrowding
2. Road accidents
3. Growth of slums
4. Poverty
5. Antisocial activities
6. Political unrest
7. Failure of people adjusts
8. Prostitution

9. Crime and delinquency
10. Begging
11. Mental illness/conflicts/disease
12. Alcoholism
13. Drug addiction
14. Gambling
15. Smoking.

Common Problems in India

1. **Death and diseases:** In earlier days the cities suffered from different kinds of epidemics. Medical knowledge was meager and healthcare services were not developed. Hygienic measures were primitive and poor. Consequently the death rates and incidence of diseases were higher in cities. In modern city nowadays more and more hospitals have been established. Highly qualified and superspecialty doctors and well-trained paramedical health team involved in superspecialized medical, surgical and rehabilitative care. Still occurrence of death and diseases are present due new existing social and manmade troubles.
2. **Pollution:** Pollution occurs because of big factories, traffic congestion, smoke, excessive dirt, dust and other types of air contamination, many diseases like respiratory problems, asthma, TB, etc. will spread at a higher rate and there is higher mortality rate. Day-by-day pollutions are increasing at the same time controlling measures also carried out by the exports.
3. **Mental diseases:** City life is very busy, excessive noise, glaring, lights of automobiles, economic pressures, create stress and strain. All these create mental tensions and serious problems and leads to mental illness. Isolation is another cause of emotional disturbance such a situation in extreme cases of individuals leads to suicide.
4. **Slums and housing problems:** Since the dawn of industrial revolution man has gravitated to cities in search of economic opportunities. In cities, he can seek remunerative jobs. Cities made the greatest progress in education, trade, commerce. The new migrants may occupy an area near the place of their work and may construct temporary huts or sheds and began to live in such residential areas. The overcrowding of such areas without any basic amenities become slum.
5. **Transportation congestion:** Transport facility in big cities is a major problem. School children find it difficult to go to their schools because of rush. The increasing use of automobiles, make the traffic congestion. They pollute the environment with heavy smoke.
6. **Sanitation:** Cities and towns in India have failed to provide good sanitation facility. Municipalities or cooperation have failed to remove the garbage and clean the drains. The sweepers are not sincerely performing their duties. The spread of slum adds to the filth and uncleanliness. Because unhealthy sanitation, the diseases like diarrhea, diphtheria, malaria, etc. spread among citizens.
7. **Corruption:** Corruption is rampant in government offices and city corporations.
8. **Inadequate water supply and drainage system:** Water management is a serious problem in cities. Most of the cities face the problem of water supply. No city has the facility of supplying water for 24 hours. Many small towns are depending upon tubes wells or tanks through the government's aim are to provide clean water supply to all the city dwellers, it has failed to formulate a national policy. Drainage system in cities is equally bad. Stagnant water can be seen in every city to lack of proper drainage and the overcrowding of houses. Consequently the cities become the breeding places of mosquitoes and cause diseases like malaria, dengue fever, chikungunya, etc.

9. **Poverty:** Poverty is a major social problem in most of the underdeveloped and developing countries. Poverty is less purchasing capacity or poor economy. Poverty is the most important social as well as health problem. Some of the causes of poverty are personal, while others are geographical, economic and social. In capacity of the individual to earn due to faulty heredity, environment, unfavorable physical conditions, such as poor natural resources and misdistribution of the available resources.
10. **Unemployment:** Unemployment in youth both educated and uneducated is a major social problem in India. Most of the unemployment is educated youth. The present system of education is responsible for unemployment.
11. **Crime:** Crime is an act forbidden by law and every crime has a penalty presented by law. Crime is always an antisocial act and thus a social problem. Some people commit crime out of frustration due to poverty, unemployment and coercion by superiors and powerful man but others do it because of a craving for the riches, fame and power like business men, professionals and politicians.

Measures to Solve the Urban Problems

In order to solve the problems of the city, effective measures must be taken. The following measures are suggested:
1. Prevention of migration.
2. To arrest the individual growth in a particular place. Decentralization of industries.
3. Systematic urban planning and development.
4. Effective and corrupt free local self-governance.
5. To improve the infrastructure and to provide better healthy civic amenities.
6. Decentralized administration in which the local people must participate.
7. Organization of free health check-up camps and supply of free medicines to poor people.
8. Establishment of health centers in all thickly populated mohallas. Health education must be given about the use of drinking water, nutrition, community health services must be provided by trained health personnel's.

7. Types of cooperation (with suitable examples).

Cooperation involves individuals or groups working together for the achievement of their individual or collective goals. In its simplest form, cooperation may involve only two people who work together towards a common goal. Two college students working together to complete a laboratory experiment, or two intercity youths working together to protect their 'turf' from violation by outsiders are examples. In these cases, solidarity between the collaborators is encouraged and they share jointly the reward of their cooperation. Again at the level of two-person interactions, the goals towards which the cooperation parties work may be consistent with each other, but they may not be identical or shared. From the college experience again, student and professor may cooperate towards the student's mastery of professor's discipline, but the student may be working to make a good grade while the professor is working to establish or reinforce his/her reputation as a good teacher. If some of their rewards are shared, some also are individual but attainable only through joint effort. The cooperating parties in this case may be either neutral or kindly disposed towards one another but their relationship is not likely to have lasting solidarity. Man cannot associate without cooperating, without working together in the pursuit of like to common interests. It can be divided into five principal types:
1. **Direct cooperation:** Those activities in which people do like things together play together, worship together, labor together in myriad ways. The essential character is that people do in

company, the things which they can also do separately or in isolation. They do them together because it brings social satisfaction.
2. **Indirect cooperation:** Those activities in which people do definitely unlike tasks toward a single end. Here the famous principle of the 'division of labor' is introduced, a principle that is imbedded in the nature of social revealed wherever people combine their difference for mutual satisfaction or for a common end.
3. **Primary cooperation:** It is found in primary groups such as family, neighborhood, friends and so on. Here, there is an identity end. The rewards for which everyone works are shared or meant to be shared, with every other member in the group. Means and goals become one, for cooperation itself is a highly prized value.
4. **Secondary cooperation:** It is the characteristic feature of the modern civilized society and is found mainly in social groups. It is highly formalized and specialized. Each performs his/her task, and thus helps others to perform their tasks, so that he/she can separately enjoy the fruits of his/her cooperation.
5. **Tertiary cooperation:** It may be found between 2 or more political parties, castes, tribes, religions groups, etc. It is often called accommodation. The two groups may cooperate and work together for antagonistic goals. Cooperation is important in the life of an individual that it is difficult for man to survive without it. CH Cooley says that cooperation arises only when men realize that they have a common interest. They have sufficient theme, intelligence and self-control, to seek this interest through united action.

8. Types of family.

Family has regulated the sexual relations to avoid promiscuity, by prescribing customary sex morals. It is a permanent organization, which has provided stable family life. It is the shelter where man is fed, clothed, and housed from the beginning. It has upheld and inculcated the traditions and customs of the group. Thus, family is the foundation stone on which the cultural heritage is built. Family as a unit of sociological inquiry is dealt with in various ways by sociologists. It is studied as an institution, as an association, as an organization. It is also referred to as a subsystem because it is regarded as one of the parts of the society.

Meaning of Family

The origin of the English word, Family is traced to the Roman word Famulus or to the Latin word Familia meaning a household comprising or servants or workers and of slaves along with other individuals having marriage or blood relations. The word denotes group of procedures, consisting of slaves, servants, and members connected by common descent or marriage. Thus originally, family consisted of a man and woman with a child or children and servants. This meaning of family has changed over the years.

Types of Family

Sl. No.	Types	Classification
1.	Basis of authority	1. Patriarchal family—the father is the most powerful and unquestionable authority (supreme authoritarian) 2. Matriarchal family—mother plays dominant role in the family
2.	Basis of residence	1. Matrilocal family—the husband lives in the wife home 2. Patrilocal family—the wife lives in the husband's home 3. Changing residents—husband and wife alternate continuously change between each other's residence

Contd...

Contd...

Sl. No.	Types	Classification
3.	Basis of ancestry	1. Matrilineal family—mother is the basis of ancestry 2. Patrilineal family—father is the basis of ancestry
4.	Basis of marriage	1. Polygamy family—one man marries many women and lives in a family with his wives and children 2. Polyandrous family—woman marries many men and lives in a family with all of them or with each of them 3. Monogamous family—one man marries only one woman and establishes a family
5.	Based on dominance	1. Nuclear family—husband and wife with their offspring live together 2. Joint family—couple with their children family lives together 3. Extended family—husband, wife, children and other dependents like brothers, sister stay together

Essential Characteristics of Family

1. **Permanent relations between husband and wife:** The family is constituted of the husband and wife and their children. Thus, a permanent relation of some kind between man and woman is the main characteristic of the family. Marital relations in different countries may be more or less permanent, but the relations between man and women have some degree of permanency in all cultures.
2. **Permanent sexual relationship:** The family rests on permanent marital relations because one object of it is the establishment of permanent sexual relationship. Without marriage, there can be no family even though there may be sexual relations.
3. **Attachment of blood relations:** Another necessary characteristic of the family is the existence of blood relationship among the members. These blood relationships can be real as well as imaginary. The members of the family are generally the descendants of the same ancestors. The relation between adopted children and their parents is accepted as legal but blood relationship means no more than that among the members of a family there should exist an attachment of the degree of blood relationship.
4. **Financial provisions for the sustenance of the members:** In a family, there is financial provision for the upkeep of its members, senile folk, children, women folk, etc. the earning members of the family arrange for substance of the other members. In this way, the members of the family are enmeshed in the ties of duties and rights. In different cultures, the burden of earning may fall on different members.
5. **Common habitation:** If the members of a family reside at different places, it would be difficult to call them a family in spite of there being blood and other relationships. It is a different matter for a member to leave temporarily or for the entire family to change its habitat but generally all the members of a family live in one residence be it one room or an entire palace, rented or the ancestral home of the family.
6. **Nomenclature:** Among the essential characteristics of the family, it is a distinct nomenclature which serves to identify the family.

In this way, the family is a group of individuals in which men and women have the permanent sex relations of husband and wife, which is distinguished by a name in which there is adequate financial provision for the relations among the members and who live in common habitual.

9. Technological factors of social change.

Social change is an ever present phenomenon everywhere. An ancient Greek philosopher Heraclitus is an emphatic way hinted at this fact when he said that it is impossible for a man to step into the same river twice. It is impossible, because in the interval of time between the first and the second stepping both the river and man have changed. Neither remains the same. This is the central theme of the Heraclitean philosophy—the reality of change, the impermanent of being, the inconstancy of everything, but change itself. Social change is a reality. Incessant changeability is the inherent nature of human society. It does not mean that society is always as its toes to welcome any kind of society.

Definitions
1. Social change is a term used to describe variation or modification of any aspects of social processes, social patterns, social interactions or social organizations.
—Jones.
2. Social change as, any alterations as occur in social organization that is the structure and functions of society.
—Kingsley Davis.
3. Social change is change in the social relationships.
—MacIver.
4. Social change may be defined as modification in ways of doing and thinking of people.
—Jenson.

Technology refers to the body of knowledge about how to adopt to make use of and act upon physical environment and their material resources in order to satisfy human needs. It includes our knowledge and artifacts. Technology is the most important factors of social change in modern times. Every new invention brings along with it a number of changes in social life. Scientific discoveries and inventions are very important for social change. The motorcar, telephone, railway, steam engine, radio, etc. have great impact on the society and its institutions. The radio and television influence entertainment, education, politics, transportation and many other types of activity.

10. "Man is a social animal". Discuss.

Aristotle, the Greek philosopher writes "Man is a social animal. He lives without society is either a beast or God". Thus, man is by nature a social animal. He is born in society lives in society and dies in society. Society is indispensable for man. Man cannot live as man, without society. Isolation from society is regarded as a punishment. Solitary life is unbearable for him. Social life is necessary for man. The instinct for some form of social life is innate in human being. Professor Park says, "Man is not born human but to be made human". Man can be called social animal for the following reasons:

Man is Social by Nature
Human nature is such that it cannot but live in society. Man's nature impels him to live in society. The human child is endowed with some latent capacities. Human qualities like capacity to learn language, enquire and think, play and work, help or harm others, etc. are developed in human society only. These capacities grow through social interaction with others. One cannot develop into a normal person in isolation. There are eminent sociologist like Maciver and others who have cited a number of case studies. These case studies show the fact that man develops human qualities only in society.

i. **The case of Kasper Hauser:** Kasper Hauser, a young German boy, was isolated from all kinds of human contact when he was a small child. He lived in isolation in the forest of Nuremberg till he reached the age of 17. He was brought out form the forest in 1928 and was taken to the city of Nuremberg. It was found that he could neither walk nor talk properly. He simply muttered a few meaningless phrase. He could not distinguish between inanimate and animate objects after his death, the postmortem. Report revealed that his mental development was not normal. In spite of his subsequent education be could never become a normal man.
ii. **The case of Amala and Kamala:** Two Hindu children Amala and Kamala were discovered in a Wolf den in 1928. By then Amala was two years old and Kamala was nearly eight at the time, when they were discovered from the den. Amala died soon after discovery. Kamala continued to live until 1929. It was found that she behaved like a beast and walked like a four-footed animal. She could not speak and growled like a wolf. She was shy of human contact. It was only after careful and sympathetic training that she could learn some social habits like simple speech, eating, dressing and the like.
iii. **The case of Anna:** Recently the case of Anna, an elegits mint American child was studied by some sociologists and psychologists. Anna at the age of 6 months was placed in a room in complete isolation for nearly 5 years. She was discovered in 1938. On the discovery, it was found that she could not walk or speak and was indifferent to people around her. She was given careful training after which she rapidly developed human qualities. She died in 1942. The case of Anna proves that human nature develops only when he is one of many people sharing a common life. These cases prove that human being is social by nature. Human nature develops in man only when he lives in society.

Development of Self

The human infant, at his birth, is not fully aware of his own "self". He develops the idea of self through the interaction with others. Charles H Cooley says that the very idea of "self' or "I" can arise only in relationship with other people. GH Mead says that at first the child performs the role of others with his parents and other persons at home. Then, gradually he takes the role of other persons, such as playmates, friends, etc. in this way self-develops.

Social Heritage Determines Human Personality

Man is social because he depends on social heritage which is a mixture of customs beliefs and ideals, etc. Society preserves social heritage and transmits it from one generation to another. Social heritage molds man's attitudes, beliefs, morals and ideals. It is said that "Man only becomes man among Men". Man is born with some inborn potentialities. It is the social heritage which determines the manner in which his innate potentialities express themselves in society. Emotional development, intellectual maturity is not possible without society. Therefore, society determines our mental equipment's. It shapes our identity, our thought and our emotions.

Necessity Makes a Man Social

Necessity compels man to live in society. Man has a variety of needs. If he leads a cooperative life with his fellow beings in society he can easily get his needs fulfilled. Many of his needs will remain unsatisfied if he does not lead a cooperative life with his fellow beings. The human child is born helpless. Without proper care he cannot develop himself. During infancy he must be provided with nutrition, shelter and affection. It is society which extends protection, attention and opportunities necessary for his survival and growth.

11. Types of social system.

Society is a web of social organizations. In this way, social organization is a system of social relationships. Social relationships are complex. They are composed into numerous small groups. In these groups are individuals. Social system refers to individual actors interacting with each other in accordance with standard cultural norms. The individual who participates in interactive relationships influence the other individuals and groups. Interactions and inter-relationships between different individuals and social groups create a system called social system.

Definitions

1. A social system basically consists of two or more individuals interacting directly or indirectly in a bounded situation.
   —Mitchell Duncan.
2. A social system is defined in terms of two or more social actors engaged in more or less stable interaction within a bounded environment.
   —A dictionary of Sociology.
3. A social system is a set of persons or groups who interact with one another, the set is conceived of as a social unit distinct from the particular persons who composes it.
   —David Popenoe.
4. A social system consists in a plurality of individual actors, interacting with each other in a situation of environment. Who are motived to the optimization of gratification and whose relation to their situation is defined and meditated interms of a system of culturally structured and shared symbols?

Classification/types of social system

Sl. No.	Classifications	Description
1.	Classification by Morgan and other evolutionist	Classifications based on evolution: 1. Savagery social system 2. Barbarian social system 3. Civilized social system
		Classification based on livelihood: 1. Hunting social system 2. Pastoral social system 3. Agricultural social system 4. Industrial social system
2.	Durkheim's classification	Described as two kind of social system: 1. Mechanical social system 2. Organic social system
3.	Sorokin's classification	Classifications based on cultural system: 1. Sensate 2. Ideational 3. Idealistic

12. Write a note on alcoholism.

Alcoholism is a state of excessive consumption of alcohol and getting addicted to it. It is to be understood that taking alcohol once a while or using it for medicinal purposes cannot be said as a social problem, people who start using alcohol for fun or as social drinking, might end up as alcoholics. Alcoholism is a social evil. For social upliftment and community health. Every person should try to avoid alcohol. Alcohol adversely affects liver, eyes and physical and mental activities. This encourages immorality, violence against women, sexual harassment, rape, crime, murder, poverty, etc. in society. Many of the crimes are committed under the influences of alcohol.

Definition

A problem drinker is one if, as a result of drinking, his health is endangered, his peace of mind affected, his home life made unhappy, his business jeopardized and his reputation clouded and drinking has become his routine.

—Durfee.

Causes

1. Drinking as a recreation.
2. Pressure of friends.
3. To link alcohol with social status and serve it in social functions.
4. Tensions in occupations.
5. Ignorance regarding the evil effects of alcohol.
6. Person's weak mentality, coupled with easy availability of alcohol.
7. Tension, failure of love, disappointments and frustrations.
8. Giving importance to scenes of drinking in media, as well as in films.
9. Take help of alcohol to achieve professional or occupational progress.
10. Home environment.
11. Urbanization/industrialization.

Features of Habitual Drinkers

1. Begins to drink from morning.
2. Drinking as means to escape reality.
3. Continuous increase in the amount of alcohol.
4. Social duties affected because of alcoholism.
5. Unusual behavior.
6. Restlessness and become unconscious.
7. Weight loss, nausea, vomiting and pain in abdomen.
8. Liver diseases.
9. Beating family members, criminal tendencies.

Health Hazards of Alcoholism

Drinking is a social evil and every individual should keep himself away from it. Drinks affect the health of the people adversely. With long time use of alcohol tremors, unsteady gait, lusterless eyes and haggard look may be observed. Alcoholics are more susceptible to many diseases especially that of liver. It leads to crimes and lawlessness. Many resort to crime and other anti-social activities. With continuous use of alcohol the delicate mechanism of brain is adversely affected. People lose their efficiency and self-control. Addiction among students adversely affects their studies. Similarly, the efficiency and alertness of the worker also suffers a lot. Alcoholism is a root cause of family unhappiness, tensions and even total disorganization. Drunkards usually waste a lot of money on alcohol and hence the economic life of the family suffers among lower classes. Many spend their whole earning on alcohol and their wives and children are left to starve. The poverty and misery lead to constant quarrels.

Drunkards of the poor class are often violent and abusive; they may beat up their children and wives. Generally alcohol produces psychic dependence of varying degrees from mild to strong. Use of alcohol causes acute and chronic intoxication, cirrhosis of the liver, toxic psychosis, gastritis, cardiomyopathy and peripheral neuropathy. It is also important in suicide and automobile and other accidents. It does a great social damage resulting in family disorganization, crime and loss of productivity.

SHORT ANSWERS

13. Acculturation.

This term is used to describe both the process of contacts between different cultures and also the customs of such contacts. As the process of contact between cultures, acculturation may involve either direct social interaction or exposure to other cultures by means of the mass media of communication.

As the outcome of such contact, acculturation refers to the assimilation by one group of the culture of another which modifies the existing culture and so changes group identity. There may be a tension between old and new cultures which leads to the adapting of the new as well as the old.

14. Edipal complex.

Sigmund Freud's theory of the **Edipus complex** describes the ideas and emotions which exist within the unconscious mind of children concerning their desire to possess their mothers sexually and kill their fathers. Freud believed that this complex occurred in both male and female children, with both sexes wishing to possess their mothers and eliminate the threat of their fathers who they competed with for the attention of their mothers. Freud believed that the edipus complex occurred during what he referred to as the phallic stage of development, the third of the five stages of a child's psychosexual development that Freud identified, which occurs when a child is between the ages of three and six. During this vital stage of a child's psychosexual development, Freud theorized that the child's genitals served as his/her primary source of pleasure, thus it is during this stage that a child begins to become sexual and recognize him/herself as a sexual being.

During this stage, as Freud contended, a child develops for him/herself a distinct sexual identity as a 'boy' or 'girl' and begins to recognize the physical and social differences between men and women. This realization, Freud believed, changes the dynamic between a child and his/her parents. According to Freud's theory, children then direct their developing sexual desire toward their mother and begin to view their fathers as rivals for the mother's attention.

15. Achieved status.

It is a status achieved by an individual through his own efforts with competitive spirit and showing special abilities, knowledge and skill. It also refers to a social position a person assumes voluntarily that reflects personal ability and effort. For examples, many occupational statuses are considered to be achieved status, advocate, doctor, professor, author, etc. Ascribed status is a social position a person receives at birth or assumes involuntarily later life. This status is not based on individual ability, skill effort or accomplishment. This status is obtained on inheritance in the society. Sex and age status are the most obvious and universal. Example of ascribed status includes being a daughter, a Cuban, a teenager, or a widower.

16. Cultural lag.

The concept of cultural lag was first formulated by WF Ogburn in his book "Social change". The existence of cultural lag was also implied in the writings of other sociologists like Summer, Vierkandt, Walls, Spencer and so on. Nevertheless, Ogburn was the first to elaborate the concept of cultural lag and to formulate the hypothesis. It became a favorite subject with many sociologists. Ogburn stressed the role of inventions in the occurring of rapid social change. Ogburn had distinguished between "material culture" and "nonmaterial culture". According to him, the material culture changes rapidly, and the nonmaterial culture lags behind. Lag means being behind. Because the different parts of culture does not change at the same rate a lag occurs between material culture and nonmaterial culture. Ogburn opined that the adoption of material culture may take a considerable length of time.

17. MOB.

MOB is an extremely emotional acting crowd that directs its violence against a specific target. It is disordered crowd especially that has gathered to attack or cause mischief.

Characteristics of MOB are as follows:
1. **Mental homogeneity:** The members of a MOB tend to show a similarity in feelings, thought and action, irrespective of the variation in education, occupation or intelligence. This uniformity of behavior of people of varying degrees of intelligence and education leads to assert that the individual in the crowd loses his 'personality' and he behaves like automation'.
2. **Emotionality:** The heightened emotionality is a characteristic feature of mob behavior. For instance, anger, fear, joy and such other emotions can be expected in the mob behavior. It is this intense emotionality that is responsible for the mob violence.
3. **Irrationality:** The member of a MOB is fickle, intolerant and unreasoning. The MOB will not to think and consider the pros and cons and weigh the evidence. The individual who is overpowered by anger or fear or sense of shame behaves in an irrational way. Violence whether it be by an individual or by a collection of individuals has the same characteristics of heightened emotionality and lowered reasoning.
4. **Diminished sense of responsibility:** The individual behaves in a most irresponsible manner. We find that the normal social controls which inhibit violence and destruction. The infuriated MOB behaves in a irresponsible way, burning valuable property, looting, arson, setting fire, etc.
5. **Sense of power:** Associated with a sense of irresponsibility is the sense of omnipotence in the members of a MOB. They feel that they are capable of doing anything and that no power on earth can stop them. A MOB of students for example, feel that they can do anything to achieve their goals.
6. **Sense of anon unity:** The people in a crowd do not know each other. That is why they feel perfectly confident and behave in the way in which the other members of the crowd behave, Each man feels secure that he will not be detected and punished because there are so many people doing the same act. There is the brutal behavior in the MOB take full advantage of the confusion that is prevailing.

18. Child labor.

Children are the valuable assets of a nation. They need to be protected and well looked after if a country in all spheres of human activity. It is said that "the children are the citizens of tomorrow", "the child is the father of a man" and children are the nation-builders of tomorrow", etc. in India, the condition of child labor is alarming and dissatisfactory. A glance at child labor in India convinces that child labor is underpaid, brutally exploited—physically and mentally deprived of all opportunities. As a result the children fail to develop their full social and economic potentialities, which would enable them to grow as a useful member of the community. This fact perpetuates the cycle of social and economic backwardness among the future generation.

International Labor Organization (ILO) has conducted a worldwide study regarding the involvement of children in different dimensions of work and categorized four forms of child labor:

1. **Domestic nonmonetary work:** With the collapse of rural economy, the disintegration of joint family system and large-scale, industrialization compel children to participate in the collective task of finding nonmonetary work for the sake of the family. For example, looking after elder brothers and sisters, working in the family kitchen, keeping the area clean, washing the clothes of family members in the tender age.
2. **Nondomestic and nonmonetary work:** This type of child laborers are involved in watching crops, gardening and grazing the animal, weeding, hunting and fishing or working along with the parents in their family economic activity.
3. **Wage labor:** Among the working children many are the major wage earners in the family who are always worried about fulfilling the needs of their dependents. Some work for 9–10 hours including night shifts. A considerable number of child labor are employed in factories and in unorganized sectors like brick making, tanning, carpet manufacturing, wool cleaning, mica and shell factories, bangle making, agarbathi making, sericulture, cotton ginning, garages, beedi making, agriculture, domestic work, rag picking, hotels and restaurants, mines and quarries, fireworks, etc.
4. **Bonded labor:** Child labor is inextricably linked to bonded labor. In Andhra Pradesh, 21% of the bonded laborers are below 14 years. In Karnataka, 10.3% and 8.7% in Tamil Nadu belongs to this age group. A study shows that at the time of entering bondage, many laborers are as young as 5 years old. In Odisha, one common way of clearing debt is to sell daughters as maidservants to the creditor.

19. Health services in rural communities.

Some of the goals of the mission are:
1. Reduction in child and maternal mortality.
2. Universal access to public healthcare services along with public services for food and nutrition, sanitation and hygiene.
3. Prevention and control of communicable and noncommunicable diseases including locally endemic diseases.
4. Access to integrated comprehensive primary health care.

Accredited Social Health Activist (ASHA) is Responsible for Creating Awareness on Health including
1. Providing information to the community on nutrition, hygiene and sanitation.
2. Providing information on existing health services and mobilizing and helping the community in accessing health-related services available at health centers.
3. Registering pregnant women and helping poor women to get BPL certification.
4. Counseling women on birth preparedness, safe delivery, breastfeeding, contraception RTI/STI and care of young child.
5. Arranging escort/accompany pregnant women and children requiring treatment/admission to the nearest health center.

6. Promoting universal immunization.
7. Providing primary medical care for minor ailments. Keeping a drug kit containing generic AYUSH and allopathic formulations for common ailments.
8. Promoting construction of household toilets.
9. Facilitating preparation and implementation of the Village Health Plan through anganwadi worker (AWW), auxiliary nurse midwife (ANM), self-help group (SHG) members under the leadership of village health committee.
10. Organizing health day once/twice a month at the anganwadi with the AWW and ANM.
11. ASHA is also a depot holder for essential services like iron folic acid (IFA), oral contreceptive pills (OCP), condoms, oral rehydration solution (ORS), disposable delivery kit (DDK), etc. issued by AWW.

20. IRDP.

Integrated Rural Development Program (IRDP) aims at providing assets and self-employment opportunities for the rural poor. Assistance under IRDP is given to a target group of rural poor belonging to families below poverty line in the form of subsidy by the government and term credit by financial institutions. The target group under IRDP consists of small and marginal farmers, agricultural laborers, rural artisans, scheduled castes and scheduled tribes and socially and economically backward classes having annual income below ₹ 11, 000 defined as poverty-line for the Eighth Plan.

In order to ensure that benefits under the program, the more vulnerable sectors of the society, stipulated that at least 50% of assisted family should be from scheduled castes and ached tribes with corresponding flow of resources. Furthermore, 40% of the coverage should of women beneficiaries and 3% of coverage should be of handicapped persons. The optional strategy of IRDP intended to follow the 'HA hold approach' rather than 'individual approve. The poorest households are identified and the anomic upliftment of these households is soar through a package of activities involving allowing members, with particular attention being given to women. The IRDP is implemented through District Rural Development Agencies (DRDAs) and Level Agencies at the grass roots level. The giving body of DRDAs includes local MP's, MLAs, chairman of Zila Parishads, heads of district development departments, representatives of SCs/and women.

21. HIV/AIDS.

Acquired immunodeficiency syndrome (AIDS) is a virus-borne communicable disease. This fatal disease is caused by human immunodeficiency virus (HIV).

It transmitted through sexually, destroys the antibody producing white blood cells (WBC) which are called T-cells and thus cripples the immune system. The first case of AIDS was discovered at the center of disease control in Atlanta, USA, in the year 1981. The causative organism was discovered in the year 1983.

Major symptoms are:
1. Weight loss.
2. Fever more than 1 month.
3. Diarrhea for more than 1 month.
4. Extrapulmonary TB at more than one site.

Minor Symptoms
1. Persistent cough for more than a month.
2. Itching skin diseases.

3. Thrush in the mouth and throat.
4. Swollen glands.
5. Chronic generalized herpes simplex (a viral disease).

HIV Spread by:
1. The most important reason for spread of AIDS is sexual contact. This includes homosexuality, group sex, sexual intercourse by person infected with AIDS with person of opposite sex, anal sexes which are the main bases for spreading HIV.
2. Transmission by blood—use of infected syringes, needles or instruments. AIDS spread through the blood transfusion.
3. People who take injections of intoxicants drugs.
4. Maternal-fetal transmission—a pregnant mother can transmit infection to the fetus.
5. Using a common razor at the barber's shop or tonsuring at religious places.

HIV does not spread by:
1. Living with or caring for people with HIV/AIDS.
2. Using the same toilets are the infected people.
3. Swimming in pools used by infected persons.
4. Shaking hands, hugging or kissing infected persons.
5. Drinking water from the same glass used by an infected person.
6. By bites of mosquito which has already bitten an infected person.

The HIV/AIDS epidemic is a health problem in which the disease impacts not only on the physical health of individuals, but also on their social identity, making it different from most other fatal diseases. It was first associated with gagmen, drug users and sex worker, individuals, and groups already caring the burden of societal stigmatization. Awareness of HIV infection can create enormous psychological pressures and anxieties that can delay constructive change or worsen illness especially in view of the fear, misunderstanding, and discrimination provoked by the HIV epidemic.

22. In-group and Out-group.

In-group and out-group relationship are very simple and direct. WG Sumner and AG Keller first introduced the concept of in-group and out-group in their work. The Science of Society—there is a sense of solidarity, a feeling of brotherhood, loyalty, sacrifice, etc. in an in-group. But their attitudes towards outsiders are hostility contempt and hatred. In-group and out-group are found in all societies through the interest which they develop vary from society, in India with thousands of tribes, castes, subcastes, religions and races. In-group life, there may be conflict among individuals and also between different groups.

In-groups and out-group are found in all societies through the interests around which they develop vary from society-to-society. The in-group and out-group attitudes are very striking. One has to make adjustments and develop a sense of tolerance and coexistence; otherwise there will be conflicts, tension and disturbances. In-groups and out-groups are important because they affect behavior. From fellow members of an in-group we expect recognition, loyalty and helpfulness. Between them, there is always a considerable degree of sympathy. In their relationships towards each other display cooperation, goodwill, mutual help and respect for one another's right.

2015

Sociology

LONG ESSAYS
1. Define social control and explain the formal and informal means of social control.
2. Define family; explain the essential and nonessential functions of family.
3. Define culture; explain the sociocultural factors in health and disease.

SHORT ESSAYS
4. Technological factors of social change.
5. Achieved status.
6. Uses of sociology.
7. primary and secondary groups.
8. Forms of marriage.
9. Social mobility.
10. Characteristics of Indian village.
11. Problems of modern family.
12. Write a note on juvenile delinquencies.

SHORT ANSWERS
13. Branches of sociology.
14. AIDS.
15. Race.
16. Crowd.
17. Exogamy.
18. Child marriage.
19. Closed system.
20. Assimilation.
21. Crime.
22. Nuclear family.

LONG ESSAYS

1. Define social control and explain the formal and informal means of social control.

Man is a social animal. He lives in groups. Life in a group requires that each member must recognize his duties and obligations to his fellowmen and to his society. Every society has harmony and order. Society, in order to exist and progress, should exercise certain control over its members. Any deviation from the established way is considered dangerous to the welfare of the society. Social control acts as an influence. It may be through public opinion, compulsion, social suggestion, religion, etc. This influence is exercised by group. The group may be family, church, state, school, etc. The influence is exercised for promoting the welfare of the group as a whole.

Definitions
1. Social control refers to the system of devices whereby society brings its members into conformity with the accepted standards of behavior.
   —EA Ross.
2. Social control is the sum total of the processes whereby society or any sub-group within society, secures, conformity to expectation on the part of its constituent units, individuals and groups.
   —Fairchild.
3. Social control is the sum of those methods by which a society tries to influence human behavior to maintain a given order.
   —Manheim.
4. Social control refers to the patterns of pressure which a society exerts to maintain order and established rules.
   —Ogburn and Nimkoff.
5. Social control is collective term used to refer to those processes planned or planned, by which individuals are taught, persuaded or compelled to conform to the usages and life values of groups.
   —JS Roucek.
6. Social control designates those social behavior which influence individuals or groups toward conformity to established or desired norms.
   —GA Lungberg.

Means of Social Control

EA Ross was the first American sociologist to deal at length with social control in a book of that title published in the year 1901.

Sl. No.	Means	Description
1.	Belief	Belief influences man's behavior in society. They are vital for human relations. Beliefs may be true or false
2.	Folkways	Folkways are individual habits later on accepted by the group. They however exercise powerful influence over man's behavior, in society. Some examples are like greeting others when we meet others in the morning

Contd...

Contd...

Sl. No.	Means	Description
2.	Social suggestions	Suggestions may be conscious or unconscious, intentional or unintentional. They are the powerful means of social control
3.	Mores	Mores are important for the welfare of the society. Examples are the need of wearing some cloths to remove nakedness, to be faithful to one's wife or husbands and to love and care for children
4.	Ideologies	They stimulate action. They provide a set of values. They are motivators of social action. They make life meaningful
5.	Customs	Customs are well-established habits of people which been passed down from generation-to-generation. They arise and grow spontaneously and gradually. In customs are included several folkways and mores. Our patterns of marriages and family, worship, religious festivals, rituals, etc. are part of custom. Dowry and bride price have also become custom
6.	Religion	It has a powerful influence on man's behaviors in a group. It is an attitude towards superhuman powers. Religion makes people benevolent characterable and truthful. Religion is found in all human societies, tribal, rural and urban. Religion exerts a powerful control over human behavior. Religion is an important agency of socialization, personality development and social integration. Religion encourages the development of good virtues and ideals like love, sacrifice, honesty, modesty, mercy, forgiveness and social service
7.	Morals	Every society has its own concept of good and evil and the conscience of individuals regarding proper and improper behavior is based on this. All societies have their own moral code. Generally, it is held that religions are the creators, custodians, and promoters of morals, e.g. morals based on Jain, or Hindu religion and morals based on Christian or Muslim religion
8.	Rituals	Ritual is a form of behavior presented by custom, law, rule or religion (Fairchild). Among various primitive peoples, ritual is thought to be particularly pleasing to the gods, and deviations from the established rituals are punished. Rituals include prayers, testimonies, and standing, bowing, kneeling, and clasping the hands, marching, and singing, caring a cross, staff or other insignia. Rituals is considered especially important in church, temples, fraternal, governmental and formal social activities, in admitting new members, in initiation, in induction into office, in introducing members to each other or in the group
9.	Law	The law, enacted by the state, is probably the most important means of social control in modern times. Law is one of the most explicit and concrete forms of social control, though by no means the only or the most influential form
10.	Art and literature	Art is one of the primary social institutions attempting to answer symbolically the riddle of the life (Fairchild). Art and literature may not exert any direct control, but they are important in developing values and public opinion. For example, the role played by the cinema or television in affecting the traditional pattern of life and thought may also be mentioned

Contd...

Contd...

Sl. No.	Means	Description
11.	Humor and satire	Humor and satire can also be used as agencies of social control without creating any tension. In our country, these are often used to releases tension at the time ridicule a person or his action and make him a public example
12.	Education	Education is a process of socialization. Along with knowledge, the values, ideals and morals are imparted in. We aim at molding and changing the behavior of the growing individuals through education
13.	Family	Family is possibly the most effective agency of social control. Through intimate, interpersonal relationships, family exerts tremendous influence on the life of all its members. In early stages, children are under the constant control and care of elders. Family is a group in which every member exerts influence on every other member. The control is natural, unconscious and internal, that is hardly felt by the members
14.	Leadership	Leadership may also be an effective means of social control; any social group has a leader, whether it be a family, playground, tribal, caste, community or state. The ideals, gestures and activities of the leader influence the followers or other members of the group
15.	Social values	Social values are defined as objectives, inanimate or animate, human, artificial or nonmaterial, to which some value for the group has been imputed by group consensus. The value may be positive or negative. Values are so general that they do not specify appropriate ways of thinking, feeling and acting. Examples of the value are democracy, patriotism, nonviolence, and charity
16.	Force or Coercion	When persuasive measures of control become ineffective, force may be used to bring about control. For instance, if a child does not listen to the loving admonition of parents, physical punishments are used

2. Define family; explain the essential and nonessential functions of family.

Man's social life begins with family. It is the most important primary group. It is the oldest social institution known to man. Family is the mother of social institutions. It is the first social environment to which a child is exposed. It is a place where most of the people spend more than one half of their life-time. Family is the center of our life activities. It gives shape to our personality and provides us inspiration. Family is in the center of the social system. All other system has a close bearing with the family. Family contributes to their strength. Any major change in the family will have repercussions throughout the social system. Family has regulated the sexual relations to avoid promiscuity, by prescribing customary sex morals. It is a permanent organization, which has provided stable family life. It is the shelter where man is fed, clothed, and housed from the beginning. It has upheld and inculcated the traditions and customs of the group. Thus, family is the foundation stone on which the cultural heritage is built. Family as a unit of sociological inquiry is dealt with in various ways by sociologists. It is studied as an institution, as an association, as an organization. It is also referred to as a subsystem because it is regarded as one of the parts of the society.

Definitions

1. Family is a more or less durable association of husband and wife or without child or of a man or woman alone, with children.
—MF Nimkoff.

2. Family is a group of persons united by ties of marriage, blood or adaptation consisting a single household interacting and intercommunicating with each other in their respective social roles of husband and wife, father and mother, son and daughter, brother and sister, creating a common culture.
—Burgess and Locke.

3. Family is the biological social unit composed of husband, wife and children.
—Eliot and Merrill.

4. Family is a group defined by sex relationship sufficiently precise and enduring to provide for the procreation and upbringing of children.
—MacIver.

5. Family is a system of patterned expectations defining the proper behavior of persons playing certain roles, enforced both by the incumbents own positive motives for conformity and by the sanction of others.
—Parsons.

Functions of Family

Sl. No.	Means	Description
1.	Psychological function	The psychological function includes affection, sympathy, love, security, attention, and emotional satisfaction of responses. The affectional activities in the family include the care of offspring, sexual relationship, companionship, intimacy and romantic fulfillments
2.	Educational function	Home is the first institution of the child and mother is the first teacher who gives primary care. Child receives the earliest knowledge and experience in the family, which lay foundation for the child's personality and character formation
3.	Protective function	It has to protect the interest of the child. It gives security in all the dimensions of healthy behavior
4.	Recreational function	The family provides entertainment for its members
5.	Religious function	The family has to provide some religious instructions to child to develop thoughts kind hatredness are fulfilling fellow feeling
6.	Cultural function	Family keeps the culture of the society alive. It moulds its members accordingly to the social culture. Family serves as an instrument of cultural continuity of the society. It transmits ideas, ideologies, folkways, mores, customs, traditions, beliefs and values from one generation to another. Thus, it helps to maintain status of family
7.	Social function	To establish status. It is a socializing agency maintains social control. Accumulation and transmission of social heritage and social contract with all members is established

Contd...

Contd...

Sl. No.	Means	Description
8.	Stable satisfaction of sex	Sex drive is powerful in human being. Man is susceptible to sexual stimulation throughout his life. The sex need is irresistible also. It motivates man to seek an established basis for its satisfaction. Family regulates sexual behavior of man by its agent, the marriage
9.	Reproductive and procreation	Reproductive activity is carried on by all lower and higher animals. But it an activity that needs control or regulation. The result of sexual satisfaction is reproduction. The process of reproduction is institutionalized in the family
10.	Provision of home	Family provides the home for its members. The desire for home is strongly felt in men and women. Though children are often born in hospitals, clinics, maternity homes, etc. they are ultimately nurtured and sustained at home. Even the parents who work outside are dependent on their home for comfort, protection and peace
11.	Status ascribing function	The family also performs a pair of functions—status ascription for the individual and societal identification for the individual
12.	Affectional function	Man has his physical, as well as mental needs. He requires the fulfillment of both of these needs. Family is an institution which provides the mental or the emotional satisfaction and security to its individual members. It the family which provides the most intimate and the dearest relationship for all its members
13.	Economic function	The family fulfills the economic needs of its members. This has been the traditional function of family. Previously, the family was an economic unit. Goods were produced in the family. Men used to work in family or in farms for the production of goods. Family members used to work together for this purpose
14.	Governmental function	The role of family in controlling its members is limited to childhood years. In areas of control and administering justice, secondary agencies like the state, laws, regulations and legislations, police, court, etc. are the main agencies

3. Define culture; explain the sociocultural factors in health and disease.

(*See* Q. 1, 2016)

SHORT ESSAYS

4. Technological factors of social change.

(*See* Q. 9, 2016)

5. Achieved status.

(*See* Q. 15, 2016)

6. Uses of sociology.

Sociology improves our understanding of society and increases the power of social action. Knowledge of society, social groups, social institutions, etc. The primary role of medicine comprises diagnosis and treatment the cure process. In contrast the primary role of nursing lies in the care process consisting of caring, comforting and guiding. Nurses plays role in health care profession. Nurses are the key persons who have significant influence over the group members within the society. Nurses have to work for maintenance of healthier lifestyles and high standards of living.

Sociology is closely related to personal and community health. Specialized branches of sociology as medical sociology and hospital sociology have come to existence, which emphasize the importance of sociology in the area of health. Study of sociology is important for nurses due to following:

The Need of Nurses to Study Sociology

Sl. No.	Concepts	Areas
1.	Cultural values	Cultural aspects of health services, health institutions, health problems, health practices prevailing
2.	Prediction	Modes of prediction
3.	Social structure	The nurse needs to know the social structure of the society based on that she can plan the nursing process
4.	Distribution of power	The nurse should provide care to the community effectively by utilizing and distributing their power equally
5.	Political organizations	The nurse needs to know various political organizations existing within the community and nation to help the people to avail healthcare facilities
6.	Mobilization	Mobilization of resources and pattern of their uses within the community in the context of cultural perception and cultural meaning of the health problems

7. Differentiate primary and secondary groups.

(See Q. 4, 2016)

8. Forms of marriage.

Marriage involves the social sanction, generally in the form of civil or religious ceremony, authorizing the persons of opposite sex, to engage in sexual union and other consequent or correlated socioeconomic relations with one another. Marriage is an institution which admits men and women to family life. It is a stable relationship in which a man and a woman are socially permitted to have children implying the right to sexual relations.

Forms of Marriage
1. **Monogamy:** When a male marries with a single female, the marriage is called monogamous type. Monogamy appears to be the most popular form of marriage in all societies. Among Christians monogamy is the rule.

2. **Polygamy:** Polygamy is a type of marriage that permits a man to marry two or more wives at a time. The principle followed in polygany is one husband several wives. Plurality of wives is more frequent and more generally practiced among the pastoral and agriculturalists.
3. **Polyandry:** Polyandry is a type of polygamy. In this kind of marriage a woman is permitted to have two or more husbands at a time. Polyandry is found among the Today's of Nilgiri Hills of Tamil Nadu; the inhabitants of Jaunsar-Bawar in the Siwalik Hills of Uttar Pradesh; the Tibetans and people of Sikkim.
4. **Endogamy:** Endogamy means marriage within one's own group. The best example for this is caste endogamy. The basic rule followed in caste is to marry within the caste group, that too within the subgroups.
5. **Exogamy:** Exogamy means to marry outside the group. It is the process by means of which group ties are expanded. People also believed that to marry within their nearest kin is not a healthy practice. Exogamy is advantageous from the biological point of view. This is beneficial in the reproduction of healthy and intelligent offspring's.
6. **Group marriage:** Two or more women married to the same two or more man, but this arrangement is rare. This type of marriage is found only in polyandrous societies. Group marriage is not a marriage at all but a kind of sexual communism.

Endogamy

Endogamy is the rule that one must marry within one's own caste or other group.
—Folsom.

Forms of Endogamy

1. **Divisional or tribal endogamy:** In which no individual can marry outside own tribe or division.
2. **Caste endogamy:** In which marriage is contracted within the caste.
3. **Class endogamy:** In which, marriage can take place between people of only one class or of a particular status.
4. **Subcaste endogamy:** In which choice for marriage is restricted to the subgroups.
5. **Race endogamy:** In which, one can marry in the race. People of the Veddah race never marry outside the race.
6. **Tribal endogamy:** In this type of endogamy, no one can marry outside his own tribe.

Exogamy

Endogamy is conservative while exogamy is progressive, exogamy is approved from the biological view point.
—Sumner and Keller.

Exogamy means to marry-to-marry outside the group. It is the progress by means of which group ties are expanded. People also believed that to marry within their nearest kin is not a healthy practice.

Forms of Exogamy

1. **Marriage outside gotra:** Among the Brahmins the prevailing practice is to marry outside the gotra. People who marry within the gotra have repent and treat the woman like a sister or mother.
2. **Marriage outside pravar:** Parvar is a kind of religious and spiritual relation. Besides forbidding marriage within the gotra, the Brahmins also forbid marriage between persons belonging to the same pravar. People who utter the name of a common saint at religious functions are believed to belong to the same pravar.

3. **Marriage outside gotras among the Kshatriyas and Vaishyas:** Among Kshatriyas and Vaishyas, it is the gotra of the purohit which is taken into consideration. In these, the ancestry is carried on not through the saint but some follower.
4. **Marriage outside the totem:** In most tribes of India, it is customary to marry outside the totem. Totem is the name given to any specific vegetation or animals with which a tribe believes it has some specific relation.
5. **Village exogamy:** Among many Indian tribes, there is the practice to marry outside side village. This restriction is prevalent in the munda and other tribes of Chota Nagpur of Madhya Pradesh.
6. **Panda exogamy:** In Hindu society, marriage within the panda is prohibited. Panda means common parentage. According to Brahaspati, offspring from five maternal generations and seven paternal generations are sapinda and they cannot intermarry.

Polygamy
1. **Polygamy:** In this one man marries many women. The above mentioned causes are causes of this form of polygamy.
2. **Bigamy:** In this one man marries two women.
3. **Polyandry:** In this one woman marries many men and lives as their wife.
4. **Group marriages:** In this many young men and women are gathered together at some special occasion and married collectively.

Polyandry
Polyandry is the marriage of one woman with several men. It is much less common than polygamy. The practice of polyandry is to be seen in many parts of the world. In India, the tribes, such as Tiyan, Toda, Khasa and Bota of Ladakhi. The Nairs of Kerala were polyandrous previously.
1. **Fraternal polyandry:** In this one woman is regarded as the wife of all brothers who have sexual relations with her. The resulting children are treated as the offspring of the eldest. This practice is found in Punjab, Malabar, Nilgiri, Ladakh, Sikkim and Assam. It also exists in Tibet.
2. **Nonfraternal polyandry:** In this one woman has many husbands with whom she cohabits in turn. It is not necessary that these husbands be brothers. If a child is born then any husbands is elected its social parent by a special ritual. This practice once prevailed among the Nayars of Malabar but is now almost completely defunct.

Polygyny
1. **Sororal polygyny:** It is type of marriage in which the wives are invariably the sisters. It is often called sororate. The Latin word soror stands for sister. When the several sisters are simultaneously or potentially the spouses of the same man, the practice is called sororate.
2. **Nonsororal polygyny:** It is a type of marriage in which the wives are not related as sisters. For social, economic, political and other reasons both types are practiced by some people.

9. Social mobility.

Individuals are recognized in society through the statuses they occupy and the roles they enact. The society as well as individuals is dynamic. Men are normally engaged in endless endeavor to enhance their statuses in society, move from lower position to higher position, secure superior job from an inferior one. For various reasons people of the higher status and position may be forced to come down to a lower status and position. Thus, people in society continue to move up and down the status scale. This movement is called social mobility. The study of social mobility is an important aspect of social stratification. In fact, it is an inseparable aspect of social stratification system because the nature, form, range and degree of social mobility depends on the very nature of stratification system. Stratification system refers to the process of placing individuals in different layers or strata.

Types of Social Mobility

A distinction is made between horizontal and vertical social mobility. The former refers to change of occupational position or role of an individual or a group without involving any change in its position in the social hierarchy, the latter refers essentially to changes in the position of an individual or a group along the social hierarchy. When a rural laborer comes to the city and becomes an industrial worker or a manager takes a position in another company there are no significant changes in their position in the hierarchy. Those are the examples of horizontal mobility. Horizontal mobility is a change in position without the change in statue. It indicates a change in position within the range of the same status. It is a movement from one status to its equivalent. But if an industrial worker becomes a businessman or lawyer he has radically changed his position in the stratification system. This is an example of vertical mobility. Vertical mobility refers to a movement of an individual or people or groups from one status to another. It involves change within the lifetime of an individual to a higher or lower status than the person had to begin with.

Forms of Vertical Social Mobility

The vertical mobility can take place in two ways—individuals and groups may improve their position in the hierarchy by moving upwards or their position might worsen and they may fall down the hierarchy. When individuals get into seats of political position; acquire money and exert influence over others because of their new status they are said to have achieved individual mobility. Like individuals even groups also attain high social mobility. When a dalit from a village becomes an important official it is a case of upward mobility. On the other hand, an aristocrat or a member of an upper class may be dispossessed of his wealth and he is forced to enter a manual occupation. This is an example of downward mobility.

Intergenerational Social Mobility

Time factor is an important element in social mobility. On the basis of the time factor involved in social mobility, there is another type of intergenerational mobility. It is a change in status from that which a child began within the parents, household to that of the child upon reaching adulthood. It refers to a change in the status of family members from one generation to the next. For example, a farmer's son becoming an officer. It is important because the amount of this mobility in a society tells us to what extent inequalities are passed on from one generation to the next. If there is very little intergenerational mobility, inequality is clearly deeply built into the society for people' life chances are being determined at the moment of birth. When there is a mobility people are clearly able to achieve new statuses through their own efforts, regardless of the circumstances of their birth.

Intragenerational Mobility

Mobility taking place in personal terms within the lifespan of the same person is called intragenerational mobility. It refers to the advancement in one's social level during the course of one's lifetime. It may also be understood as a change in social status which occurs within a person's adult career. For example, a person working as a supervisor in a factory becoming its assistant manager after getting promotion.

Structural Mobility

Structural mobility is a kind of vertical mobility. Structural mobility refers to mobility which is brought about by changes in stratification hierarchy itself. It is a vertical movement of a specific group, class or occupation relative to others in the stratification system. It is a type of forced mobility for it takes place because of the structural changes and not because of individual attempts. For example, historical circumstances or labor market changes may lead to the rise of decline of an occupational group within the social hierarchy. An influx of immigrants may also alter class alignments—especially if the new arrivals are disproportionately highly skilled or unskilled.

10. Characteristics of indian village.

1. **Family:** In village community, family is still the basic and most important unit. The whole of the village community structure is dependent on the family. Joint family structure in Indian villages, family as the center of production and consumption in village community, the family is an independent unit, so far as the production and consumption is concerned.
2. **Social stratification:** An order of ranking the individuals based upon relative position in society. Caste and class system are the two major types of social stratification in society. Caste status is and ascribed one while class status is achieved. Certain characteristics or attributes influence the position of individual in stratification system.
3. **Social process:** Social process is the social interactions of groups and individuals with one another. They are mainly competition, conflict, cooperation and accommodation.
4. **Caste system:** Membership of caste, caste restrictions social distance, disabilities and even untouchability are still found in Indian villages. Mostly Indian villages are multicaste villages, even though we have hundreds of different castes in India, the caste composition of villages differ from region-to-region.
5. **Education:** The inadequate physical facilities of the village school, poorly trained and disinterested teacher and inefficient and corrupt administration of the schools contribute much for the problems of village education. Introduction of new educational schemes without proper equipment, facilities, guidance and supervision affect the secondary education in village areas.
6. **Agriculture:** In Indian rural society, there joint family structure, because of agriculture economy. Agriculture is such a job in which a large number of people have to involve.

11. Problems of modern family.

Top 9 issues facing today's family. More than 2,000 people from around the country:
1. Divorce
2. Busyness
3. Absent father figure
4. Lack of discipline
5. Financial pressures
6. Lack of communication
7. Negative media influences
8. Balance of work and family
9. Materialism.

12. Write a note on juvenile delinquencies.

Juvenile delinquency can be defined as a violation of law or ordinance by an individual below the legal adult age of the community. Juvenile delinquency is essentially a legal concept. It does not include all acts of misbehavior or even serious misbehavior by children or youth but only those acts that violate a law.

Adults are considered more responsible for their actions and when they perform juvenile delinquent behavior it is termed as criminal behavior. The legal age dividing juvenile delinquency from adult crime is most often 18 years but can vary country-to-country. The punishment of delinquent behavior is influenced by the attitudes of the local community and the degree of general tolerance of youthful misbehavior.

Causes of Juvenile Delinquency

According to Pauline Young, the most important causes of juvenile delinquency are poverty slums and infected areas, immigrant communities, lack of meaningful and satisfying relationship, family disorganization, war, comic books, bad companionship and social change. According to W Healy and A Bronner, the main causes of juvenile delinquency are bad company, adolescent instability and impulses, early sex experiences, mental conflicts, extreme social instability, love for adventure, motion pictures, school dissatisfaction, sudden impulses and physical conditions of all sorts.

1. **Personal cause:** This may include the biological and psychological conditions of a child.
2. **Environmental cause:** This may include the geographical or ecological causes.
3. **Psychological cause:** These may include feeble-mindedness, emotional strain, and love for adventure, stubborn nature and nonfulfillment of basic wishes, such as recognition, response and security.
4. **Sociocultural factors:** These may be considered to be more important than biological or physical ones as sociologists hold the view that man is not born criminal but made so.
5. **Family:** The home is the first school of the child. His socialization and personality development takes place in the family. Most sociologists have laid much stress on the condition of the family for the causation of juvenile delinquency; broken homes, too much discipline or too less discipline, irresponsible parents, mother working outside the home, too many children, and lonely child are some of the causes.
6. **Economic conditions:** Poverty at home, unemployment of parents, and the instability of the parents to provide the children with adequate facilities create delinquency.
7. **Education:** The absence of education or the lack of proper education may result in juvenile delinquency. Overcrowded schools, uncommitted teachers, and teaching being uninteresting to the young boys and girls may lead to truancy.
8. **Religion and morals:** Religion and morals help the children in their socialization and social control. In the absence of these, the children turn delinquent.
9. **Unhealthy recreations:** Unhealthy recreation like cinema, television and radio also causes delinquency. The young mind is much influenced by the modern media.
10. **Political conditions:** A healthy political situation provides control and welfare of the society. But political instability, corruption, and confusing leadership mislead the young. Political conflicts like war and revolutions also affect their behavior.

SHORT ANSWERS

13. Branches of sociology.

Sorokin has referred to the main currents of recent sociological thoughts in the following four branches of sociology: (1) Cosmosociology, (2) biosociology, (3) general sociology and (4) special sociologies.

Sociology of religion studies, the church as a social institution inquiring into its origin, development and forms as well as into changes in its structure and function.

Sociology of education studies the objectives of the school as a social institution, its curriculum and extracurricular activities and its relationship to the community and its other institutions.

Political sociology studies the social implications of various types of political movements and ideologies and the origin, development and functions of the government and the state.

Sociology of law concerns itself with formalized social control or with the processes whereby members of a group achieve uniformity in their behavior through the rules and regulations imposed upon them by society. It inquires into the factors that bring about the formation of regulatory systems as well as into the reasons for their adequacies and inadequacies as a means of control.

Social psychology seeks to understand human motivation and behavior as they are determined by society and its values. It studies the socialization process of the individual how he becomes a member of society—it also studies the public, crowd, the MOB and various other social groupings and movements. Analysis of mass persuasion or propaganda and of public opinion has been one of its major interests.

Social psychiatry deals with the relationships between social and personal disorganization, its general hypothesis being that society through its excessive and conflicting demands upon the individual is to a large extent responsible for personal maladjustments, such as various types of mental disorder and antisocial behavior. In its applied aspects it is concerned with remedying this situation.

Social disorganization deals with the problems of maladjustment and malfunctioning including problems of crime and delinquency, poverty and dependency, population movements, physical and mental disease. Of these subdivisions crime and delinquency have received perhaps the greatest attention and have developed into the distinct fields of criminology.

Group relations are concerned with studying the problems arising out of the coexistence in a community of diverse racial and ethics groups. New areas and subareas of sociology are continuously evolving over the period of time.

14. AIDS. (See Q. 21, 2016).

15. Race.

A race is a socially constructed category composed of people who share biologically transmitted triads that members of a society consider important. People may classify each other racially based on physical characteristics, such as skin color, facial features, hair textures and body shape. Race is a group which shares in common a certain set of innate physical characters and a geographical origin within certain area. In this way, a race lives in a definite geographical area and has some definite innate characteristics. The biological concept of race arises as result of failure to realize that race is not a sociological term but is distinctly a biological and anthropological concept.

Definitions
1. A race is a large, biological, human grouping with a number of distinctive inherited characteristics which vary within a certain range.
   —AW Green.
2. A race is a large group of people distinguish by inherited physical differences.
   —J Biesanz and M Biesanz.
3. A race is a biologically inherited group possessing a distinctive combination of physical traits that tends to breed true from generation to generation.
   —Hoebel.

Race as a biological concept: Racial group are no doubt refer to biological categories that represent a common observable hereditary traits. Race is a group which share in common a certain set of intimate physical characteristics and geographical origin within a certain area. Historically, three diagnostics traits have been used to divide the human species into races: Skin color, hair, form and various combination of nose, face and lip shapes. The discoveries of fossil man in different parts of the world reveal that man is biologically related to prehistoric men like java man, Neanderthal man and Cro-Magnon man.

16. Crowd.

Human being always belong to groups, group life is organized by social norms.

Definitions
1. Crowd is a gathering of a considerable number of persons around a center or a point of common activities.
   —Kimball Young.
2. Crowd is transitory group spontaneously formed as a result of some common interests. The crowd is a collection of individuals gathered temporarily whose object may be different. Crowd is quickly created and quickly dissolved.
   —RH Thouless.
3. Crowd is a temporary collection of people reacting together to stimuli
   —Horton and Hunt.
4. Crowd is transitory contiguous group organized with completely permeable boundaries, spontaneous formed as a result of some common interest.
   —Thouless.

Characteristics of Crowd
1. **Crowd is a gathering:** Individuals are physically present in a definite place responding to a particular object of attention.
2. **Temporary group:** Crowd is a short lived social group. It is transitory. It is quickly dissolved.
3. **Unorganized group:** A crowd is an unorganized group. It has no definite goals, no aims, social norms and crowd has no leaders and has no social contacts.
4. **Anonymity:** Crowd is an anonymous group. The members of a crowd do not know each other. Among the members of a crowd, there is a lack of personal contacts and individual identity.
5. **Narrow attention:** Crowd directs its attention only to a particular thing or object.
6. **Highly irrational:** Members of a crowd are highly emotional. They do not see any reason in the agreement of others.

7. **Crowd behavior is a part of culture:** Crowd behavior may appear to be spontaneous and unpredicted, but actually, it is not entirely may appear to be spontaneous and unpredictable but actually, it is not entirely so.

17. Exogamy.

Forms of exogamy:
1. **Marriage outside gotra:** Among the Brahmins the prevailing practice is to marry outside the gotra. People who marry within the gotra have repent and treat the woman like a sister or mother.
2. **Marriage outside pravar:** Parvar is a kind of religious and spiritual relation. Besides forbidding marriage within the gotra the Brahmins also forbid marriage between persons belonging to the same pravar. People who utter the name of a common saint at religious functions are believed to belong to the same pravar.
3. **Marriage outside gotras among the Kshatriyas and Vaishyas:** Among Kshatriyas and Vaishyas, it is the gotra of the purohit which is taken into consideration. In these, the ancestry is carried on not through the saint but some follower.
4. **Marriage outside the totem:** In most tribes of India, it is customary to marry outside the totem. Totem is the name given to any specific vegetation or animals with which a tribe believes it has some specific relation.
5. **Village exogamy:** Among many Indian tribes, there is the practice to marry outside the village. This restriction is prevalent in the munda and other tribes of chota Nagpur of Madhya Pradesh..
6. **Panda exogamy:** In Hindu society marriage within the panda is prohibited. Panda means common parentage. According to Brihaspati, offspring from five maternal generations and seven paternal generations are sapinda and they cannot intermarry.

18. Child marriage.

Many people marry their daughters in childhood to escape from dowry, and prepuberty marriage is an evil in itself. On maturity, the boys may or may not be able to adjust with their wives. This crisis situation is by no means left behind after the child marriage is consummated on attaining maturity. If by chance a husband becomes educated or professionally trained and his wife remains uneducated, both partners face crises.

Child marriage in India has been practiced for centuries, with children married off before their physical and mental maturity. The problem of child marriage in India remains rooted in a complex matrix of religious traditions, social practices, economic factors and deeply rooted prejudices. Regardless of its roots, child marriage constitutes a gross violation of human rights, leaving physical, psychological and emotional scars for life. Sexual activity starts soon after marriage, and pregnancy and childbirth at an early age can lead to maternal as well as infant mortality. Moreover, women who marry younger are more likely to experience domestic violence within the home.

19. Closed system.

An isolated system that has no interaction with its external environment. Closed systems with outputs are knowable only thorough their outputs which are not dependent on the system being a closed or open system. Closed systems without any output are knowable only from within.

20. Assimilation.

Assimilation is the process by which when persons and groups come into contact with other cultural groups, in a long run acquire its ways of life. Assimilation is one of the social adjustment. In its process, the individual or group begins to absorb slowly and gradually, somewhat unconsciously, the new circumstances in which it finds itself. It results in the modification of social attitudes. For example in many parts of India, the Hindus and Muslims have become so intimate and well acquainted with each other that they have assimilated many points of each other's cultures into their own and made them integral part of their own social conduct.

Definitions:
1. **Assimilation** denotes conformity and uniformity in respect of culture.
   —Dawson and Getty's.
2. Assimilation is a process of interpenetration and fusion in which persons and group acquire the memories, sentiments and attitudes of other persons or groups and by shaping their experience and history, are incorporated into a common cultural life.
   —Park and Burgess.
3. Assimilation is the process whereby individual or groups once dissimilar become similar, that is become identified in their interests and outlook.
   —Ogburn and Nimkoff.
4. Assimilation is a process whereby attitudes of many persons are united and they thus develop into a unified group.
   —Bogardus.
5. Assimilation is the social process whereby individual and groups come to share the same sentiments and goals.
   —Bissanz and Biesanz.

21. Crime.

A crime is defined as any act that is contrary to legal code or laws. There are many different types of crimes, from crimes against persons to victimless crimes and violent crimes to white collar crimes. With each type of crime also come different sociological phenomena and demographic profiles. In our society, sociologists have identified three general categories of crime:

1. **Crimes against the person:** These are crimes in which an act of violence is either threatened or perpetrated against a person. A mugging is an example of a crime against the person.
2. **Crimes against property:** These are crimes that involve the theft of property or certain forms of damage against the property of another. Arson is an example of a property crime.
3. **Victimless crimes:** These are crimes in which laws are violated, but there is no identifiable victim. Prostitution is often classified as a victimless crime.

22. Nuclear family.

Nuclear family is a universal social phenomenon. In simple words a nuclear family's one, which consists of the husband wife and their children. Soon after their marriage, the children leave their parental home and establish their separate household. Hence, the nuclear family is a small unit free from the control of the elders. Since, there is physical distance between the parent and their children; there is minimum interdependence between them. Thus, a nuclear family is mostly independent.

Function of modern nuclear family:
1. Stable satisfaction of sex need
2. Procreation and upbringing of children
3. Socialization of children
4. Provision of home
5. Self-development of individuals.

2014

Sociology

LONG ESSAYS
1. Define sociology; explain its importance and application in nursing profession.
2. Explain urban community; describe its salient features; list various social problems of urban community.
3. Define social change; explain the factors of social change.

SHORT ESSAYS
4. Nature of society.
5. Difference between primary and secondary groups.
6. Culture and civilization.
7. Man is a social animal, explain.
8. Types of conflict.
9. Causes of juvenile delinquencies.
10. Legislation on Indian marriage and family.
11. Effects of social isolation.
12. Future of caste system in India today.

SHORT ANSWERS
13. Rural community.
14. Matriarchal family.
15. Social dynamics.
16. Cyclic theory of social change.
17. Industrial society.
18. Socialization.
19. Population.
20. Community sentiment.
21. Social group.
22. Social mobility.

LONG ESSAYS

1. Define sociology; explain its importance and application in nursing profession.

The word sociology is derived from Latin word "Societus" meaning society and the Greek word "Logos" meaning the study of science. Thus sociology means science of society. Sociology essentially and fundamentally deals with the network of social relationship we call "Society". Sociology is one of the youngest of social sciences disciplines. The term sociology was coined by Auguste Comte, a French philosopher often referred to as the Father of Sociology. He introduced the word sociology for the first time in his famous work "Cours de Philosophie Positive" at about 1839.

Definitions
1. Sociology is the science of society of social phenomena.
 — LF Ward
2. Sociology is the study of human inter-action and inter-relations, their conditions and consequences.
 — M Ginsberg
3. Sociology is a special social science concentrating on inter-human behaviors on processes of association, on association and dissociation as such.
 — Von Wiese
4. Sociology may be defined as a body of scientific knowledge about human relationships.
 — JF Cuber

Importance of Sociology in Nursing
1. **Sociology makes a scientific study of society:** Scientific knowledge about society is pre-requisites to any marked improvements in the state of human affairs.
2. **Sociology studies roles of the institutions in the development of the individual:** Sociology studies about social institutions and the relation of the individual to each is being made. The home and family, the school and education, the church and religion, the state and government, industry and work, the community and associations these are the great institutions through which society functions.
3. **The study of sociology is indispensable for understanding and planning of society:** Society is a complex phenomenon with a multiple of intricacies. It is well-nigh impossible to understand it and to solve its various problems without study of sociology. A certain amount of knowledge about the society is necessary before any social policies can be carried out. For example, that a policy of decreasing this goal cannot be determined in exclusively economic terms because matters of family organization, customs and traditional values must be taken into account and these requires values must be taken into account and these requires a sociological type of analysis.
4. **Sociology is of great importance in the solution of social problems:** The present world is suffering from many problems which can be solved only through scientific study of the society. It is obvious that social evils do not just happen and everything has its due cause. It is a task of sociology to study the social problems through the methods of scientific research and to find out solution for them.
5. **Sociology has drawn our attention to the intrinsic worth and dignity of man:** Sociology has been instrument in changing our attitude towards human beings. In a huge specialized

society, we are all limited as to the amount of the whole organization and culture that we can experience directly.
6. **Sociology has changed our outlook with regards to the problems of crime, etc.:** Again, it is through the study of sociology that our whole outlook on various aspects of crime has changed. The sciences of criminology and penology and social work and social therapy which are rendering commendable service in understanding social situations and solving individual problems are but handmaids of sociology.
7. **Sociology has made great contribution to enrich human culture:** Human culture has been made richer by the contribution of sociology. It has removed so many cobwebs from our minds and knowledge and enquiry. Sociology also impresses egoistic ambitious and class hatred. In short, its finding stimulates every person to render a full measure of service to every other person and to the common good.
8. **Sociology is of great importance in the solution of international problems:** The progress made by physical sciences has brought the nations of the world has been left behind by the revolutionary progress of the science. We live in twentieth century world that is politically divided in terms of eighteenth century conditions. The consequences are that stresses within and between political units lead time-to-time to war and conflict. Given the workshop of the nation-state, men have failed to bring in peace. The study of sociology of war will help in understanding the underlying causes of war and remove all such causes which promote tensions between nations and ultimately lead to war.
9. **Sociology is useful as a teaching subject:** In the view of its importance. Sociology is becoming popular as a teaching subject also. It is being accorded an important place in the curriculum of colleges and universities.
10. **Sociology as profession:** The value of sociology lies in the fact that it keeps us up-to-date on modern situations; it contribute to making good citizens; it contributes to the solution of community problems; it adds to the knowledge of the society; it identifies good government with community and it helps one to understand causes of things and so on.

2. Explain urban community, describe its salient features, list various social problems of urban community.

The term Urban is derived from the Latin word Urbanus. Urbanus means a city or a town. Towns and cities of India make up the urban communities with about 20% of the population. Compared with other countries, India has a much higher rural population, but the urban population increasing rapidly. Town and cities are overcrowding and always expanding. In urban areas most of the people have to work in connection with industry, the manufacture, trade, transport of goods and materials. In urban, social life relations are for short-time and impersonal. There is no feeling of oneness, and it is a case of each person for himself. There is keen competition. The basis of urban social life is class rather than caste, and social class depends on economic status, some people by working hard, or by other means, may get rich quickly, and move from lower to middle or even upper class.

Urbanism means a way of behavior and thinking. Urbanization refers to certain features like transiency, superficiality, anonymity, impersonal relations, highly mobile and dynamic. This kind of life pattern is extended to rural areas because of vast network of communications. Urbanization is a process of development. It refers to the movement of population from rural to urban areas. It is not merely shifting of people from village to city but also change of work pattern from agriculture to urban type of work like industry, trade, service, etc. According to Anderson, urbanization is a two way process. It involves not only the movement of people from villages to cities change of occupations but involves basic changes in thinking and behavior of people.

Factors Influences Urban Community

Social effects of urbanization: Urbanization and industrialization brought many changes in the society. The family structure, the status of man, caste and class, values of society, social relationships, etc.

1. **Urbanization and family:** Urbanization has affected the family structure, functions and relations. In India, the traditional joint family has be replaced by nuclear family. The trend today is towards a break in joint family. Urban family is based on equalitarian principles. Both husband and wife share their view in decision making. In cities, most of the families both the partners are employed.
2. **Urbanization and castes:** Urbanization caused enormous change in caste and family. The three basic features of caste that are affected by urbanization and education are heredity, hierarchy and endogamy. The urbanites are educated and their relationships are not governed strictly by caste norms. We find change in commensality, material relations, social relations and occupational relations. Another important tendency, one can find is formation of caste associations and struggle for getting more and more governmental concessions in an organized manner.
3. **Urbanization and status of women:** The status of women in ancient India was high. But her position was declined during later periods, women were considered inferior, denied any right. She was suppressed and secluded, subjected to harassment. But after 19th century because of the efforts of reformist's new legislative measures, national movement, establishment of educational institutions, industrialization and urbanization led to the great emancipation of the Indian women.

Common Problems in India

1. **Death and diseases:** In earlier days, the cities suffered from different kinds of epidemics. Medical knowledge was meager and healthcare services were not developed. Hygienic measures were primitive and poor. Consequently, the death rates and incidence of diseases were higher in cities. In modern city nowadays more and more hospitals have been established. Highly qualified and super speciality doctors and well-trained paramedical health team involved in superspecialized medical, surgical and rehabilitative care. Still occurrence of death and diseases are present due new existing social and manmade troubles.
2. **Pollution:** Pollution occurs because of big factories, traffic congestion, smoke, excessive dirt, dust and other types of air contamination, many diseases like respiratory problems, asthma, TB, etc. will spread at a higher rate and there is higher mortality rate. Day-by-day pollutions are increasing at the same time controlling measures also carried out by the exports.
3. **Mental diseases:** City life is very busy, excessive noise, glaring, lights of automobiles, economic pressures create stress and strain. All these create mental tensions and serious problems and leads to mental illness. Isolation is another cause of emotional disturbance such a situation in extreme cases of individuals, leads to suicide.
4. **Slums and housing problems:** Since the dawn of industrial revolution man has gravitated to cities in search of economic opportunities. In cities, he can seek remunerative jobs. Cities made the greatest progress in education, trade, commerce. The new migrants may occupy an area near the place of their work and may construct temporary huts or sheds and began to live in such residential areas. The overcrowding of such areas without any basic amenities become slum.

5. **Transportation congestion:** Transport facility in big cities is a major problem. School children find it difficult to go to their schools because of rush. The increasing the use of automobiles, make the traffic congestion. They pollute the environment with heavy smoke.
6. **Sanitation:** Cities and towns in India have failed to provide good sanitation facility. Municipalities or cooperation have failed to remove the garbage and clean the drains. The sweepers are not sincerely performing their duties. The spread of slum adds to the filth and uncleanliness. Because unhealthy sanitation, the diseases like diarrhea, diphtheria, malaria, etc. spread among citizens.
7. **Corruption:** Corruption is rampant in government offices and city corporations.
8. **Inadequate water supply and drainage system:** Water management is a serious problem in cities. Most of the cities, face the problem of water supply. No city has the facility of supplying water for 24 hours. Many small towns are depending upon tubewells or tanks through the government's aim are to provide clean water supply to all the city dwellers, it has failed to formulate a national policy. Drainage system in cities is equally bad. Stagnant water can be seen in every city to lack of proper drainage and the overcrowding of houses. Consequently, the cities become the breeding places of mosquitoes and cause diseases like malaria, dengue fever, chikungunya, etc.
9. **Poverty:** Poverty is a major social problem in most of the underdeveloped and developing countries. Poverty is less purchasing capacity or poor economy. Poverty is the most important social as well as health problem. Some of the causes of poverty are personal, while others are geographical, economic and social. In capacity of the individual to earn due to faulty heredity, environment, unfavorable physical conditions such as poor natural resources and misdistribution of the available resources.
10. **Unemployment:** Unemployment in youth both educated and uneducated is a major social problem in India. Most of the unemployment is educated youth. The present system of education is responsible for unemployment.
11. **Crime:** Crime is an act forbidden by law and every crime has a penalty presented by law. Crime is always an antisocial act and thus a social problem. Some people commit crime out of frustration due to poverty, unemployment and coercion by superiors and powerful man but others do it because of a craving for the riches, fame and power like business men, professionals and politicians.

Measures to Solve the Urban Problems

In order to solve the problems of the city, effective measures must be taken. The following measures are suggested:
1. Prevention of migration.
2. To arrest the individual growth in a particular place. Decentralization of industries.
3. Systematic urban planning and development.
4. Effective and corrupt free local self-governance.
5. To improve the infrastructure and to provide better healthy civic amenities.
6. Decentralized administration in which the local people must participate.
7. Organization of free health check-up camps and supply of free medicines to poor people.
8. Establishment of health centers in all thickly populated mohallas. Health education must be given about the use of drinking water, nutrition, community health services must be provided by trained health personnel's.

3. Define social change; explain the factors of social change.

The word change indicates a difference in anything seen over some period of time. The difference may be great or it may be negligible. Social change is the change in society. Society is a web of social relationships. Hence, social change is a change in social relationships. MacIver and Page, writing in this context, have observed correctly, it is the change in these which alone we shall regard as social change. Society is not a static phenomenon, but it is a dynamic entity. Social change has occurred in all societies and at all times. Society passes through various stages. It is an ever changing phenomenon growing, decaying, renewing and accommodating itself to changing conditions.

Definitions

1. Social change is a term used to describe variation or modification of any aspects of social processes, social patterns, social interactions or social organizations.
—Jones.
2. Social change as, any alterations as occur in social organization that is the structure and functions of society.
—Kingsley Davis.
3. Social change is change in the social relationships.
—MacIver.
4. Social change may be defined as modification in ways of doing and thinking of people.
—Jenson.
5. Social change may be defined as a new fashion or mode, either modifying or replacing the old in the life of a people or in the operation of society.
–Mazumdar.

Factors of Social Change

Social change is brought about by a number of factors, such as technological, industrial, economic, ideological and religious. Geographical and biological changes too result in sociocultural changes.

The rate of social change varies from place-to-place and time-to-time.

Geographical Factors

Changes in the geographical environment create changes in social life. The geographical factors comprise all those inorganic phenomena which extort an influence on human life. They include climate of the earth and those factors in the outer crust of the earth's surface which condition man's livelihood. The climate influences include temperature, sunshine, rainfall, relative humidity, prevailing winds, the possibility of tornadoes and cyclones, and the electromagnetic atmospherics of the atmosphere. Geographical changes also affect food supply, leading to new dietary habits. The new diet forces physiological adjustments which in turn modify temperament and behavior.

Biological Factors

The biological environment affects the human cultural pattern in much the same way as does the geographical environment. Man utilizes the available plant and animal life in ways determined by his culture, and he wards off enemies (bacteria, poisonous plants, insects, pests, dangerous animals, etc.). With the best means, he has been able to invent. Furthermore, the biological environment is constantly changing as one animal species gains ground at the expense of some other, while the struggle for existence goes on.

Demographic Factors

The relationship between human population, density, environment and culture is a fundamental one in relation to social changes and we must subject it to further analysis. Population increase or decrease determines social institutions and social relations very much. Population explosion creates problems of low standards of life, unemployment, higher density, etc. Modern techniques of family planning, family welfare and population control have brought about changes in the size of the family, sex, and education, attitude towards sex, morals and social values. The quality of the population is also an important factor in social change. People are endowed with certain hereditary characteristics which are limiting factors in personality development and in the achievements the individual will be able to make.

Technological Factors

Technology refers to the body of knowledge about how to adopt or make use of and act upon physical environment and their material resources in order to satisfy human needs. It includes our knowledge and artifacts. It is the most important factor of social change in modern times. Every new invention brings along with it a number of changes in social life. Scientific discoveries and inventions are very important for social change. The motorcar, telephone, railway, steam engine, radio, etc. have had a great impact on society and its institutions. The radio and television influence entertainment, education, politics, transportation and many other types of activities.

Cultural Factors

Edward B Tylor has defined culture as that complex whole which includes knowledge, belief, art, morals, law, custom and any other capabilities and habits acquired by man as a member of society. Culture is the unique possession of human society and it is transmitted from generation to generation. These beliefs, customs, values and traditions exert great influence on human society and also the extent to which a society can accept new patterns. The possibility of innovations depends to a great extent on the existing culture. Diffusion of culture within a society and also from one society to another is an important factor in cultural and social change. Culture also plays an indirect role in social change. A very good example is how man's economic activities are influenced by his religious principles. Besides, social change is influenced by social inventions, for example, social legislations like untouchability act, marriage act, act against prostitution, antidowry act, child marriage act, restraints act, etc.

Psychological Factors

Social change is much facilitated and promoted by new ambitions, aspirations and attitudes of people. These in turn are helped by several factors including education. Dissatisfaction with the existing conditions and facilities are common in these modern days. The revolt, unrest and indiscipline among the contemporary youth in India are due to such dissatisfaction or frustration.

SHORT ESSAYS

4. Nature of society.

Society consists, not of individuals, but in their mutual interactions and mutual interrelations. It is a complex structure formed by these mutual relations; it is a system, a pattern. Individuals or people do not merit the name society but a society is sometimes used to denote people. Some sociologist have viewed society is a web of social relationships. These social relationships are not of one kind. Some of them are simple and some complex, some are permanent and some temporary—these includes behavior, usages, customs, modes of operations, authority, assistance and other types of relations.

Definitions
1. A society is a collection of individuals united by certain relations or modes of behavior which mark them off from other who do not enter into these relations or who differ from them in behavior
   —Ginsberg.
2. Society is a system of usage and procedures of authority and mutual aid, of many groupings and divisions, of controls of human behavior and liberties.
   —MacIver and Page.
3. Society is the union itself, the organization, the sum of formal relations in which associating individuals are bound together.
   —Giddings.

Characteristics of Human Society
1. **Society is abstract:** Thus while describing the nature of society, society is abstract because it is constituted of the social relations, customs and laws, besides other elements. In the words of Odum, in another aspect society may be visualized as the behavior of human being and the consequent problems of relationship and adjustments that arise.
2. **Society is not a group of people:** Some sociologist have viewed society as a group of people. Hankins writes, we may for our purpose here define society as any permanent or continuing group of men, women and children, able to carry on independently the process of racial perpetuation and maintenance on their own cultural level.
3. **Society is an organization of relationships:** Society is an organization, a system or a pattern of relationships among human being. Parsons has written society may be defined as the total complex of human relationships in so far as they grow out of action in terms of means—end relationships, intrinsic or symbolic.
4. **Psychic element in social relationships:** According to MacIver and Giddings and some other sociologist, social relationships invariably possess a psychic element, which takes the form of awareness of another's presence, common objectives, common interest, etc. There is neither any society nor any social relationship without this realization. Society exists only where social being behaved towards one another in a manner determined by recognition of each other.
5. **Liberty:** Human society is dynamic. In society, the individual given liberty in respect of many kinds of changes. In all civilized societies of the world, people have the freedom to get educated, choose a desired profession, marry and beget children, think independently and to express their thoughts in an appropriate manner.
6. **Many group and divisions:** In this way, there are many groups and divisions in each society. Some of these groups are natural while other are constituted intentionally. Keeping in view some specific objectives. Both primary groups like family and neighborhood, and secondary groups like unions, labor unions, etc. are extremely important for the development of social life.
7. **Mutual assistance:** In society, even inequality is based upon mutual relationships. People possessing diverse characteristics often assume complementary roles. People of opposite sexes are able to achieve more intense and intimate relations than individuals of the same sex because each fulfills the deficiency of the other. In the same way, people who differ from one another in respect of income, status, wealth, education, etc. help and assist each other.

8. **Usage and customs:** Man is a social being. His very existence and development is rendered impossible in the absence of society. He has to establish relations with other members of society to fulfill his own needs. These relations lead to mutual behavior. This behavior becomes progressively complex and takes on the form of usage or custom.
9. **Modes of action or procedure:** MacIver has used the word procedures for institutions. In this way, procedures or institutions like marriage, inheritance, education, religious beliefs, political parties, etc. play an important part in society.
10. **Authority:** Authority is indicative of that relation who regulates or controls the related individuals or classes in such a way that one evinces a sense of respect, faith, and subordination towards the other. The cause of authority is the inevitable inequality in society. There is greater similarity than dissimilarity in society but even then inequality is found in every society in some form or other.
11. **Organization:** Every society has its own individual and unique organization in which there is division of labor of one kind or the other. People who are completely disorganized cannot be said to be consisting a society.
12. **Assistance:** Dukheim has expressly said that, due to division of work, there is greater evidence of dissimilarity. The life of society depends upon mutual assistance.
13. **Independence:** An important element in the organization of society is independence. Man cannot satisfy his needs if he leads a solitary life. So he needs society, and stay in society because it is his nature. The members of society are dependent upon each other for the fulfillment of their needs.

5. Difference between primary and secondary groups.

(See Q. 4, 2016)

6. Culture and civilization.

Civilization has a precise standard of measurement but not culture. The products of civilization can be measured quantitatively on the basis of efficiency. A motor car runs faster than bullock cart. A power loom is superior to the handloom. Tractor is more efficient than the hand plough. Money economy is better than the barter system.

There is not yard stick to assess the superiority or inferiority of cultural product. Every community admires its own customs, religion, beliefs, morals, ideals, etc. as better than those of another community. No one can prove that Kalidasa is superior to another.

Culture is internal and an end, while civilization is external and a means. Culture is concerned with internal life of man, his ways of thinking and living. It is related to inner thoughts, feelings, beliefs, ideals, values, etc.

Civilization is concerned with the external life of man. It is concerned with material instruments, techniques and social organizations devised by man to control the conditions of his life. They serve as means to ends. Man uses them to secure certain satisfactions determined by culture. So civilization is the means while culture is an end. Civilization is transmitted without effort, but not culture.

The products of civilization like bus, train, TV, computer, printing press, etc. can be used by all people even if they do not know their mechanism in detail, so they can be transmitted from place-to-place easily and quickly. Underdeveloped countries are importing many fruits of modern civilization from developed countries. Culture is concerned with internal life of man. It is a way of life. It becomes a part of one's personality. It is very difficult to change one's mode of life. A person clings to his culture family. Culture can be transmitted only to the likeminded.

Civilization is always advancing but not culture. The machines, vehicles and other products of civilization are more efficient than those of previous generation. They improved from time-to-time. We cannot say definitely that the art, literature, thoughts, ideals, etc. of today are superior to those of early period. Both fields of life—culture and civilization are created by man to help him in his struggle for existence. They are interrelated and interdependent. One field influences the other.

The product of civilization becomes a symbol of culture. The plough is a symbol of culture of an Indian village. Civilization is a vehicle of culture. The means product by the civilization is used for the development. Progress and spread of culture.

So civilization and culture are not the same. Civilization grows intensively and extensively. It spreads from one country to another. Civilization is checked when it becomes identical with the culture. This happened in the medieval ages. But Renaissance came which completely changed the outlook of man. MacIver observes that civilization tends to proceed more rapidly, more simply, less selectively, always spreading outward from the technological and economic advance.

7. Man is a social animal. Explain.

(See Q. 10, 2016)

8. Types of conflict.

Conflict is a process of seeking something by eliminating or weakening the competitors. It is a competition in its most hostile and personal form. When a competitive endeavor turns into a violent strife among concerned individuals or groups to achieve the same goal, the competitive situation turns into a conflict situation. It arises primarily from a clash of interests within groups. Conflict may also occur without violence, for example, Satyagraha of Gandhi. Conflict is defined as deliberate attempt to oppose, resist or coerce the will of another or others. It is a process which leads two or more persons or groups to try to frustrate the attempts of their opponents to attain certain objectives.

Definitions

1. Kingsley Davis defines conflict, "as modified forms of struggle."
2. MacIver and Page state that, "social conflict included all activity in which men contest against one another for any objective".
3. According to AW Green, "conflict is the deliberate attempt to oppose, resist or coerce the will of another or others."
5. According to Gillin and Gillin, "conflict is the social process in which individuals or groups seek their ends by directly challenging the antagonist by violence or threat of violence."
6. Majumdar opines that, "conflict is an opposition or struggle involving an emotional attitude of hostility as well as violent interference with autonomous choice."

Features of Conflict

1. A dissociative and disintegrative social process.
2. A universal process.
3. A conscious process.
4. A personal process.
5. An intermittent process.
6. Mainly violent in nature.

7. Conflict disregards social norms.
8. Conflict may lead to new consensus.
9. Conflict may bring solidarity in the group.
10. Conflict may lead to change of status of conflicting parties.

Classification of Conflict

Conflict is found in many forms in all societies. Different sociologists have classified conflicts into different forms. Some of these classifications are:
1. MacIver and Page classify conflict into two types, i.e. direct and indirect conflict.
2. Gillin and Gillin classify conflict into five types, such as personal conflict, racial conflict, political conflict, class conflict and international conflict.
3. George Simmel classifies conflict into four major forms, such as war, feud, litigation and conflict of impersonal ideals.

9. Causes of juvenile delinquencies.

(See Q. 13, 2015)

10. Legislation on Indian marriage and family.

In March 1961, when the bill on unequal marriages was being discussed in the Rajya Sabha, one member quoted epic against its inclusion in the institution of Hindu marriage. Dr Radhakrishnan, the then chairman of the Rajya Sabha, had remarked: The ancient history cannot solve the problems of modern society. This is an answer in one sentence to those critics who want to maintain a gap between social opinion and social legislation.

Legislation must meet the social needs of the people; and because the social needs change, legislation also must change from time-to-time. The function of social legislation is to adjust the legal system continually to a society, which is constantly outgrowing that system. The gulf between the current needs of the society and the old laws must be bridged. The laws have got to give recognition to certain de facto changes in society. One of the changes in modern India is the change in the attitude towards marriage; hence the necessity of laws on different aspects of marriage.

The laws enacted in India relate to: (i) age at marriage (ii) field of mate selection, (iii) number of spouses in marriage, (iv) breaking of marriage, (v) dowry to be given and taken, and (vi) remarriage. The important legislations relating to these six aspects of marriage passed from time-to-time are: (i) The Child Marriage Restraint Act, 1929 (dealing with age at marriage), (ii) The Hindu Marriage Disabilities Removal Act 1946 and Hindu Marriage Validity Act, 1949 (dealing with field of mate selection), (iii) The Special Act. 1954 (dealing with age at marriage, freedom to children in marriage without parental consent, bigamy, and breaking up of marriage), (iv) The Hindu Marriage Act, 1955 (dealing with age at marriage with the consent of parents bigamy, and breaking up of marriage) (v) The Dowry Act 1961, and (vi) The Widow Remarriage Act, 1856.

11. Effects of social isolation.

The absence of communicative interaction or social contact is called social isolation. It is a situation deprived of social contacts; both the individuals and the group can be isolated.

Spatial Isolation

Spatial isolation is external. It is an enforced deprivation of contacts as for criminals, when somebody is banished from the community or put to solitary imprisonment. The individual in such cases is deprived of the production of this group. An individual when subjected to spatial isolation becomes aggressive and shows a greater propensity for antisocial behavior. At one point of time, it was thought that solitary confinement could improve the character of the convicts but it proved futile. It leads to melancholic mental conditions, sexual abnormalities and antisocial attributes.

Organic Isolation

Means isolation caused by certain organic defects of the individual, such as deafness or blindness. It is not imposed by any external authority but it is organic. The deaf and the blind are deprived of experiences common to all healthy men.

12. Future of caste system in India today.

Caste is closely connected with the Hindu philosophy and religion, custom and tradition. It is believed to have had a divine origin and sanction. It is deeply rooted social institution in India. There are more than 2,800 castes and subcastes with all their peculiarities. The term caste is derived from the Spanish word caste meaning breed or lineage. The word caste also signifies race or kind. The Sanskrit word for caste is Varna which means color. The caste stratification of the Indian society had its origin in the chaturvarna system. According to this doctrine, the Hindu society was divided into four main varnas—Brahmins, Kashtriyas, Vaishyas and Shudras. The Varna system prevalent during the Vedic period was mainly based on division of labor and occupation. The caste system owns its origin to the Varna system. Ghurye says any attempt to define caste is bound to fail because of the complexity of the phenomenon.

The Indian caste system has played a significant role in shaping the occupations and roles as well as values of Indian society. Religion has been the constant push towards this stratification system for centuries, beginning with the Aryans and continuing down a long road of unfortunate discrimination, segregation, violence, and inequality. Hinduism was the backbone of the purity pollution complex, and it was the religion that influenced the daily lives and beliefs of the Indian people. Even after 69 years of independence, Indians continue to be in the grip of caste consciousness. Historically, India has been surviving as a nation for millennia with closed groups divided by caste, creed and language (Velassery, xi). Work was divided and each had his allotted task since birth, and heredity of occupation was a rule that played a big role in the economics of urban and rural life. Mobility of occupation or caste was restricted, and an individual leaving the occupation of his ancestors in order to follow his/her own path was rarely witnessed. It can be seen that caste continues to play an important role in the dynamic of social and political interactions within India. However, the relationship between caste and hereditary occupations has become less significant now, and there are fewer restrictions on social interaction among castes, especially in urban areas (Sekhon, 55). The present Indian society is moving from its closed systems towards a state of change and progression marked by the assertion of the human spirit irrespective of castes and creeds (Velassery, xii).

SHORT ANSWERS

13. Rural community.

Rural sociology is the branch which studies the life of rural people. It is considered with rural society, its social structure, social institutions and their relationships. It studies the life of rural people and analysis their attitudes and beliefs. India is a land of villages; the majority of the people are living in villages. So villages are the significant aspect of Indian society. Indian villages are considered unique and distinct from villages of other countries. Generally, a village refers to a small group of people living permanently in a definite geographic area who depend mainly on farming activities.

Definitions
1. The village is unit of rural society. It is the theater where in the quantum of rural life unfolds itself and functions.
—AR Desai.
2. The rural community comprises of the constellation of institutions and persons grouped about a small center and sharing common primary interest.
—Elridge and Merrill
3. A village as a unit of compact settlement varying in size, smaller than a town.
—Anthony Giddens.

14. Matriarchal family.

A matriarchy is a social system organized around the principle of mother-rule in which mothers, or females, are at the top of the power structure. There is no solid evidence that a matriarchal society has ever existed. Even in societies with matrilineal descent, the power structure is either egalitarian or dominated formally by the father or some other male figure. In order for a social system to be considered a matriarchy, it would need the support of a culture that defined women's dominance as desirable and legitimate. So, even though women are the authority figures in single-parent families, they are not considered matriarchies. According to the Oxford English Dictionary matriarchy is a "form of social organization in which the mother or oldest female is the head of the family, and descent and relationship are reckoned through the female line; government or rule by a woman or women."

15. Social dynamics.

Social dynamics can refer to the behavior of groups those results from the interactions of individual group members as well to the study of the relationship between individual interactions and group level behaviors. ... The fundamental assumption of the field is that individuals are influenced by one another's behavior.

Dynamics in sociology consisted of studying and tracing interconnections between these many aspects of society as they actually existed and changed in the many types of society in the cumulative process of history. It was a study that is of the actual varieties of societies existing in the world. Social statics is chiefly analytical. Social dynamics is chiefly empirical. Dynamics applies the analysis of statics to the study of actual societies.

16. Cyclic theory of social change.

Cyclical theories: Cyclical theories of social change focus on the rise and fall of civilizations attempting to discover and account for these patterns of growth and decay. Spengler, Toynbee and Sorokin can be regarded as the champions of this theory. Spengler pointed out that the fate of civilizations was a matter of destiny. Each civilization is like a biological organism and has a similar life-cycle, birth, maturity, old-age and death. After making a study of eight major civilizations including the West, he said that the modern Western society is in the last stage, i.e. old age. He concluded that the Western societies were entering a period of decay as evidenced by wars, conflicts and social breakdown that heralded their doom.

17. Industrial society.

Industrial sociology studies development and impact of modern industry on human societies. After the industrial revolution and the introduction of machine, the work culture of human beings changed tremendously, and new organization called factories came into existence. Industrialization has created various problems. So to study industry, its relation, industrial sociology as a special branch came into existence. A very important factor in the history of society has been the industrial revolution which has brought about far-reaching consequences in the structure of societies.

18. Socialization.

Socialization is nothing but a process through which human society converts the newborn human infant into an active member of the society. Socialization is a process of learning. It is a continuous process from the birth to death. Socialization is a vital process in the sense that without the help of this process, it is impossible to convert the newborn human infant into an active member of the society. The human child comes into this world only with animal needs and impulses, such as hunger, thirst, sex, etc. But soon after the birth of the child, it will be ushered into the process of socialization. In fact, the biological drives of man will be channelized into cultural needs through socialization.

The social order is maintained largely by socialization. If they violate the rules of the social group socialization is not possible. It is said that process of socialization starts long before the child is born. The social circumstances preceding his birth lay down to a great extent the kind of life he is lead. Socialization is a process of learning to perform skills and to perform social roles. The term socialization refers to all the processes by which, how an infant acquires skills roles, norms, values and personality patterns.

Socialization is the process whereby the individual learns the folkways, mores, norms and values of his society. In this process, individual learns various techniques of performing different social roles. Green defined "socialization as a process by which the child acquires a cultural content, along with selfhood and personality." Number of agencies is responsible for the socialization of the individual. The family is the first agency of child's socialization. Gradually, the growing child exposed to many other different agencies of socialization.

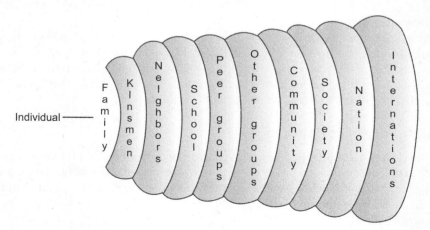

The following figure indicates the fact how the individual gradually expands his relationship with different agencies of socialization.

Definitions

1. Socialization is a process of adaptation by the individual of the conventional patterns of behavior is described as his socialization, because it occurs on account of his integration with others and his exposure to the culture which operates through them.
   —VV Akolar.
2. The development of We-feeling in association and the growth in their capacity and will to act together is called socialization of the individual.
   —EA Ross.
3. Socialization is the process whereby persons learn to behave dependably together on behalf of human welfare and in so doing experience social self-control, social responsibility and balanced personality.
   —Bogardus.
4. Socialization is the process by which the individual learns to conform to the norms of the group.
   —WF Ogburn.
5. Socialization as a process of transmission of culture, the process whereby men learn the rules and practices of social groups.
   —Petter Worsley.
6. Socialization as learning that enables the learner to perform social roles. He further says that it is a process by which individual acquire the already existing culture of groups they come into.
   —Harry M Johnson.
7. Socialization consists of the complex processes of interaction through which the individual learns the habits, beliefs, skills and standards of judgment that are necessary for his effective participation in social groups and communities.
   —Lundberg.

19. Population.

Population studies are broadly defined as the scientific study of human populations. Major areas studied include broad population dynamics; fertility and family dynamics; health, aging, and mortality; and human capital and labor markets. Researchers in population studies also focus on methodology. Population studies are an interdisciplinary area of study; scholars from demography, epidemiology, sociology, economics, anthropology, and various other disciplines study populations. Various associations and centers exist throughout the United States and elsewhere. The Population Association of America, established in 1930, is a scientific, professional organization established to promote the improvement, advancement, and progress through research of problems related to human populations.

20. Community sentiment.

According to Sutherland, Woodward and Maxwell, a community is a local area over which people are using the same language, conforming the some mores, feeling more or less the same sentiments and acting upon the same attitudes. In this way, this community sentiment is extremely essential in the people belonging to a community.

21. Social group.

Social group is a collection of human being. In its elementary sense, a group is a number of units of anything is close proximity to another. Thus, we may speak of a group of houses on a street, of trees in a forest or of buses in a bus stand. In the human field, by group we mean any collection of human beings who are brought into social relationships with one another. A group of social unit which consists of a number of individuals who stand in (more or less) definite status and role relationships to another and which possesses a set of values or norms of its own regulating the behavior of individual members at least in matters of consequences to the group.

Definitions

1. Social groups as masses of people in regular contact or communication as possessing a recognizable structure.
   —Moris Ginsberg.
2. Groups as any collection of human being who is brought into social relationships with one another.
   —MacIver.
3. A group is any number of human being is reciprocal communication.
   —Cuber.
4. A social group grows out of and requires a situation which permits meaningful inter-stimulation and meaningful response between the individuals involved, common focusing of attention, common stimuli and or interest and the development of certain common drives, motivations or emotions.
   —Gillin and Gillin.

22. Social mobility.

Social mobility is an act of moving from one social status to another. People in society continue to move up and down the status scale. This is called social mobility. Mobility may be for groups as well as individuals. In an open class, every individual's struggles to get into higher rank. But it depends on the back-ground of his ascribed status and the available opportunities in the social set up. Individuals are normally recognized in society through the statuses they occupy and the roles they enact. Not only the society is dynamic, but also the individuals are dynamic.

Definitions

1. Social mobility is the movement of a person or persons from one social status to another.
   —Wallace and Wallace.
2. Social mobility refers to the movement of an individual or group from one social class or social stratum to another.
   —Dictionary of Sociology.
3. Social mobility refers to the movement of individuals between different levels of social hierarchy, usually defined occupationally.
   —N Abercrombie.
4. Mobility refers to any transition of an individual or social object or value; anything that has been created or modified by human activity—from one social position to another.
   —Sorokin.
5. The term social mobility refers to the processes by which individuals move from one position to another in society positions which by general consent have been given specific hierarchical values.
   —Lipset and Bendix (1960).

Community Health Nursing

2019

Community Health Nursing-I

LONG ESSAYS
1. a. Define community health nursing. b. Describe the various determinants of health.
2. a. Define demography. b. Describe the methods of data collection, analysis and its interpretation.
3. a. What are the methods of family planning? b. Briefly explain on laparoscopic sterilization.

SHORT ESSAYS
4. General measures to promote health.
5. List the waterborne diseases and its prevention.
6. Food adulteration Act.
7. Uses of epidemiology.
8. Women empowerment.
9. Intrauterine contraceptive devices.
10. Housing standards.
11. Epidemiology of H1N1.
12. Control of rodents.

SHORT ANSWERS
13. Define zoonosis.
14. List common arthropod infections.
15. Define immunity.
16. Define epidemic.
17. List four health problems of children.
18. Define communication.
19. Prevention of anemia.
20. List four health problems of elderly.
21. Importance of rainwater harvesting.
22. Modified risk factors of hypertension.

LONG ESSAYS

1. a. Define community health nursing. b. Describe the various determinants of health.

Community health Nursing is the synthesis of nursing and public health practice applied to promote and protect the health of population. It combines all the basic elements of professional, clinical nursing with public health and community practice.

Community health nursing also called public health nursing or community nursing, combines primary healthcare and nursing practice in a community setting. Community health (CH) nurses provide health services, preventive care, intervention and health education to communities or populations.

Determinants of Health

The range of personal, social, economic, and environmental factors that influence health status are known as determinants of health.

Determinants of health fall under several broad categories:
- Social factors
- Health services
- Individual behavior
- Biology and genetics

It is the interrelationships among these factors that determine individual and population health. Because of this, interventions that target multiple determinants of health are most likely to be effective. Determinants of health reach beyond the boundaries of traditional health care and public health sectors, such as education, housing, transportation, agriculture, and environment can be important allies in improving population health.

Social: Social determinants of health reflect social factors and the physical conditions in the environment in which people are born, live, learn, play, work and age. Also known as social and physical determinants of health, they impact a wide range of health, functioning and quality of life outcomes.

Examples of social determinants include:
1. Availability of resources to meet daily needs, such as educational and job opportunities, living wages, or healthful foods
2. Exposure to crime, violence, and social disorder, such as the presence of trash
3. Social support and social interactions
4. Exposure to mass media and emerging technologies, such as the internet or cell phones
5. Socioeconomic conditions, such as concentrated poverty
6. Quality schools
7. Transportation options
8. Public safety
9. Residential segregation.

Examples of physical determinants include:
1. Natural environment, such as plants, weather, or climate change
2. Built environment, such as buildings or transportation
3. Worksites, schools, and recreational settings
4. Housing, homes, and neighborhoods

5. Exposure to toxic substances and other physical hazards
6. Physical barriers, especially for people with disabilities
7. Aesthetic elements, such as good lighting, trees, or benches.

Individual behavior: Individual behavior also plays a role in health outcomes. For example, if an individual quits smoking, his or her risk of developing heart disease is greatly reduced.

Many public health and healthcare interventions focus on changing individual behaviors, such as substance abuse, diet, and physical activity. Positive changes in individual behavior can reduce the rates of chronic disease in this country.

Examples of individual behavior determinants of health include:
1. Diet
2. Physical activity
3. Alcohol, cigarette, and other drug use
4. Hand washing.

Biology and genetics: Some biological and genetic factors affect specific populations more than others. For example, older adults are biologically prone to being in poorer health than adolescents due to the physical and cognitive effects of aging.

Sickle cell disease is a common example of a genetic determinant of health. Sickle cell is a condition that people inherit when both parents carry the gene for sickle cell. The gene is most common in people with ancestors from West African countries, Mediterranean countries, South or Central American countries, Caribbean islands, India, and Saudi Arabia.

Examples of biological and genetic social determinants of health include:
1. Age
2. Sex
3. HIV status
4. Inherited conditions, such as sickle cell anemia, hemophilia, and cystic fibrosis
5. Carrying the *BRCA1* or *BRCA2* gene which increases risk for breast and ovarian cancer
6. Family history of heart disease.

Social determinants of health: Social determinants of health are economic and social conditions that influence the health of people and communities. These conditions are shaped by the amount of money, power, and resources that people have, all of which are influenced by policy choices. Social determinants of health affect factors that are related to health outcomes.

2. a. Define demography. b. Describe the methods of data collection, analysis and its interpretation. *(See Q. 2, 2015)*

3. a. What are the methods of family planning? b. Briefly explain on laparoscopic sterilization.

Barrier methods of birth control:
1. A condom is a thin latex or polyurethane sheath. The male condom is placed around the erect penis. The female condom is placed inside the vagina before intercourse.
2. A condom must be worn at all times during intercourse to prevent pregnancy.
3. Condoms can be bought in most drug and grocery stores. Some family planning clinics offer free condoms. You do not need a prescription to get condoms.

Diaphragm and cervical cap:
1. A diaphragm is a flexible rubber cup that is filled with spermicidal cream or jelly.
2. It is placed into the vagina over the cervix before intercourse, to prevent sperm from reaching the uterus.
3. It should be left in place for 6 to 8 hours after intercourse.
4. Diaphragms must be prescribed by a woman's provider. The provider will determine the correct type and size of diaphragm for the woman.
5. About 5-20 pregnancies occur over 1 year in 100 women using this method depending on proper use.
6. A similar, smaller device is called a cervical cap.
7. Risks include irritation and allergic reactions to the diaphragm or spermicide, and increased frequency of urinary tract infection and vaginal yeast infection. In rare cases, toxic shock syndrome may develop in women who leave the diaphragm in too long. A cervical cap may cause an abnormal Pap test.

Vaginal sponge:
1. Vaginal contraceptive sponges are soft, and contain a chemical that kills or "disables" sperm.
2. The sponge is moistened and inserted into the vagina, to cover over the cervix before intercourse.
3. The vaginal sponge can be bought at pharmacy without a prescription.

Hormonal methods of birth control: Some birth control methods use hormones. They will have either both an estrogen and a progestin, or a progestin alone. You need a prescription for most hormonal birth control methods.
1. Both hormones prevent a woman's ovary from releasing an egg during her cycle. They do this by affecting the levels of other hormones the body makes.
2. Progestins help prevent sperm from making their way to the egg by making mucus around a woman's cervix thick and sticky.

Types of hormonal birth control methods include:
1. Birth control pills: These may contain both estrogen and progestin, or only progestin.
2. Implants: These are small rods implanted beneath the skin. They release a continuous dose of hormone to prevent ovulation.
3. Progestin injection, such as Depo-Provera, that are given into the muscles of the upper arm or buttocks once every 3 months.
4. The skin patch, such as Ortho Evra, is placed on your shoulder, buttocks, or other place on the body. It releases a continuous dose of hormones.
5. The vaginal ring, such as NuvaRing, is a flexible ring about 2 inches (5 centimeters) wide. It is placed into the vagina. It releases the hormones progestin and estrogen.
6. Emergency (or morning after pill) contraception: This medicine can be bought without a prescription at your drugstore.

Intrauterine device (IUD):
1. The IUD is a small plastic or copper device placed inside the woman's uterus by her provider. Some IUDs release small amounts of progestin. IUDs may be left in place for 5 to 10 years depending on the device used.
2. IUDs can be placed at almost any time.
3. IUDs are safe and work well. Fewer than 1 out of 100 women per year will get pregnant using an IUD.

4. IUDs that release progestin may be for treating heavy menstrual bleeding and reducing cramps. They may also cause periods to stop completely.

Permanent Methods of Birth Control

These methods are best for men, women, and couples who feel certain they do not want to have children in the future. They include vasectomy and tubal ligation. These procedures can sometimes be reversed if a pregnancy is desired at a later time. However, the success rate for reversal is not high.

Birth control methods that do not work very well:
1. Withdrawal of the penis from the vagina before ejaculation can still result in pregnancy. Some semen often escapes before full withdrawal. It can be enough to cause a pregnancy.
2. Douching shortly after sex is not likely to work. The sperm can make their way past the cervix within 90 seconds. Douching is never recommended because it can cause infections in the uterus and tubes.
3. Breastfeeding: Despite the myths, women who are breastfeeding can become pregnant.

Laparoscopic sterilization.

Laparoscopic tubal ligation is a surgical sterilization procedure in which a woman's fallopian tubes are either clamped and blocked or severed and sealed. About 20% of women choose tubal ligation as their contraceptive method, making it the second most common form of female contraception in the United States.

Tubal ligation is surgery to block a woman's fallopian tubes. A tubal ligation is a permanent form of birth control. After this procedure has been performed, an egg cannot move from the ovary through the tubes (a woman has two fallopian tubes), and eventually to the uterus.

Female sterilization (also referred to as tubal ligation) includes a number of different procedures and techniques that provide permanent contraception for women. The most common techniques prevent pregnancy by disrupting the patency of the fallopian tubes. This prevents conception by blocking transport of sperm from the lower genital tract to an ovulated oocyte.

Female sterilization may be performed immediately after childbirth (postpartum sterilization) or at a time unrelated to a pregnancy (interval sterilization). Most postpartum sterilization procedures are performed at time of cesarean delivery or after a vaginal delivery via mini-laparotomy. Most interval sterilization procedures are performed via laparoscopy.

Indications and contraindications: The only indication for sterilization is the patient's desire for permanent contraception. Ultimately, the choice is made by the patient, but the decision requires thorough counseling about permanent sterility and the risk of regret.

There are no medical conditions that are strictly incompatible with laparoscopic sterilization; however, there may be factors that make women more suitable for a particular route of sterilization or other contraceptive options.

SHORT ESSAYS

4. General measures to promote health.

Health promotion is, as stated in the 1986. World health organization (WHO), "the process of enabling people to increase control over, and to improve, their health. To reach a state of complete physical, mental and social well-being, an individual or group must be able to identify and to realize aspirations, to satisfy needs, and to change or cope with the environment. Health is, therefore, seen as a resource for everyday life, not the objective of living. Health is a positive concept emphasizing social and personal resources, as well as physical capacities. Therefore, health promotion is not just the responsibility of the health sector, but goes beyond healthy lifestyles to well-being".

Health Promotion Measures
1. Purpose: Provide basic matters regarding comprehensive promotion of people's health and make the effort to improve public health through implementation of measures for promoting people's health.
2. Cooperation between the government, local governments, health promotion service providers, and other related entities.

Elements of Health Promotion: There are 3 key elements of health promotion:

1. **Good governance for health:** Health promotion requires policy makers across all government departments to make health a central line of government policy. This means they must factor health implications into all the decisions they take, and prioritize policies that prevent people from becoming ill and protect them from injuries.

These policies must be supported by regulations that match private sector incentives with public health goals. For example, by aligning tax policies on unhealthy or harmful products, such as alcohol, tobacco, and food products which are high in salt, sugars and fat with measures to boost trade in other areas. And through legislation that supports healthy urbanization by creating walkable cities, reducing air and water pollution, enforcing the wearing of seat belts and helmets.

2. **Health literacy:** People need to acquire the knowledge, skills and information to make healthy choices, for example, about the food they eat and healthcare services that they need. They need to have opportunities to make those choices. And they need to be assured of an environment in which people can demand further policy actions to further improve their health.

3. **Healthy cities:** Cities have a key role to play in promoting good health. Strong leadership and commitment at the municipal level is essential to healthy urban planning and to build up preventive measures in communities and primary healthcare facilities. From healthy cities evolve healthy countries and ultimately, a healthier world.

5. List the waterborne diseases and its prevention.

Waterborne diseases are caused by pathogenic microorganisms that most commonly are transmitted in contaminated fresh water. Infection commonly results during bathing, washing, drinking, in the preparation of food, or the consumption of food thus infected. Various forms of waterborne diarrheal disease probably are the most prominent examples, and affect mainly children in developing countries; according to the World.

Waterborne diseases include the following:
1. Polio
2. Malaria
3. Cholera
4. Dengue
5. Typhoid
6. Anemia
7. Botulism
8. Fluorosis

9. Trachoma
10. Hepatitis
11. Diarrhea
12. Giardiasis
13. Ascariasis
14. Trichuriasis
15. Arsenicosis
16. Malnutrition.

Waterborne disease is easily transmitted when contaminated water is used for any of the following purposes: Drinking, making ice cubes, washing uncooked fruits and vegetables, making baby formula, brushing teeth and washing dentures or contact lenses. Take the following precautions as applicable when faced with any water that may be unsafe:

1. Do not trust bottled water. Reports of locals filling bottles with tap water, sealing and then selling as purified water have come out of several countries. Since Aquatabs have no unpleasant taste or color, play it safe any time you are faced with suspect water.
2. If you are visiting or living in an area with poor sanitation, be especially wary of the water.
3. If your local Medical Officer of Health has issued a Boil Water Advisory for your community, take the advice seriously.
4. Do not drink untreated water from a spring, stream, river, lake, pond or shallow well. Assume it is contaminated with animal, bird and/or human feces. Disinfect with Aquatabs or boil for 1 to 5 minutes depending on elevation.
5. Prevention is easier than seeking medical treatment once infected. Aquatabs produce no unpleasant taste or color and are safe and simple to use. If you run out of Aquatabs, boil all suspect water for 1 to 5 minutes depending on elevation.
6. Note: Unlike water treated with Aquatabs, boiled water contains no residual chlorine protection from recontamination.
7. Note: Not all filters are capable of removing many bacteria and viruses. Check manufacturers claims carefully and be wary of filters that are not capable of removing viruses. When in doubt, treat with Aquatabs after filtration.
8. Ask for drinks without ice unless the ice is made from bottled or boiled water. Avoid popsicles and flavored ices that may have been made with contaminated water.
9. In many places, the food can be as risky as the water. You should be especially suspicious of salads, uncooked fruits and vegetables, unpasteurized milk, raw meat, shellfish, and any foods sold by street vendors. Avoid eating raw fruits and vegetables unless peeled in your presence. Avoid raw milk and products made from raw milk. Drink only pasteurized or boiled milk.
10. Practice good hygiene, such as frequent hand washing and disinfection of cutlery, cutting boards, etc. Wash hands thoroughly and frequently using soap, in particular after contact with pets or farm animals, or after having been to the toilet.

6. Prevention of food adulteration Act.

Prevention of food adulteration: Prevention of Food Adulteration (PFA) Act was amended in 1964, 1976 and lately in 1986 to make the act more stringent. A minimum imprisonment of 6 months with minimum fine of ₹ 1,000 is envisaged under the act for cases to proven adulteration, whereas for the cases of adulteration which may render the food injurious to cause death or such harm which may amount to grievous hurt (within the meaning of section 320 of IPC) the punishment may go up to life imprisonment and fine which shall not less than ₹ 5,000.

7. Uses of epidemiology.

Epidemiology process is bound to continue in future adding new challenges to the practice of public health. In these circumstances, epidemiology is designed to play an increasingly important role in defining the magnitude of the problems, forecasting their long-term consequences and deriving appropriate strategies for their promotion and control. Presently, the use of epidemiology is mainly confined to following areas:

1. **Disease antecedents:** Epidemiology has always stressed the importance of exploring the natural history of disease in their entirely, with special stress on the identification of disease antecedents rather than disease consequents.
2. **Disease correlates:** Epidemiology has revolutionized the concept of etiology and etiogenesis. Epidemiological studies identified a variety of disease correlates not all of which are casually associated diseases, and some of which behave as risk factors, the risk factors the increase the probability of contracting a particular disease.
3. **Disease behavior:** Epidemiological surveillance is applied to disease of international significance. Disease behavior is studied by a process of epidemiological surveillance whereby diseases are kept under constant observation firstly to identify their normal distribution patterns and normal temporal fluctuations, and secondly to detect any deviation in their expected behavior patterns.
4. **Disease and causation:** Epidemiological studies not only establish cause effect association of many noncommunicable diseases, but also estimate the strength of associations in terms of relative and absolute risks. The most notable example are the cause effect associations established by epidemiological studies between smoking and lung cancer and smoking and coronary heart diseases.
5. **Strategy formulation**: Epidemiology plays an important role in strategy formulation for disease control programs and improves program efficiency and effectiveness. Control and eradication of disease is much more complex than their prevention or treatment. A sound control strategy is one that epidemiologically relevant and operationally feasible.
6. **Program evaluation:** Program performance is evaluated by measuring achievements in various operational areas of the program. Evaluation of public health program is both managerial and epidemiological process.

8. Women empowerment.

Empowerment of women, also called gender empowerment, has become a significant topic of discussion in regards to development and economics. Entire nations, businesses, communities, and groups can benefit from the implementation of programs and policies that adopt the notion of women empowerment.

Process of empowerment: The process which enables individuals/groups to fully access personal/collective power, authority and influence, and to employ that strength when engaging with other people, institutions or society. In other words, "Empowerment is not giving people power; people already have plenty of power, in the wealth of their knowledge and motivation, to do their jobs magnificently. We define empowerment as letting this power out (Blanchard, K)." It encourages people to gain the skills and knowledge that will allow them to overcome obstacles in life or work environment and ultimately, help them develop within themselves or in the society.

Empowerment includes the following, or similar, capabilities:
1. The ability to make decisions about personal/collective circumstances.

2. The ability to access information and resources for decision-making.
3. Ability to consider a range of options from which to choose (not just yes/no, either/or).
4. Ability to exercise assertiveness in collective decision making.
5. Having positive-thinking about the ability to make change.
6. Ability to learn and access skills for improving personal/collective circumstance.
7. Ability to inform others' perceptions though exchange, education and engagement.
8. Involving in the growth process and changes that is never ending and self-initiated.
9. Increasing one's positive self-image and overcoming stigma.
10. Increasing one's ability in discreet thinking to sort out right and wrong.

Ways to empowerment:
1. One way to deploy the empowerment of women is through land rights. Land rights offer a key way to economically empower women, giving them the confidence they need to tackle gender inequalities.
2. Women in developing nations are legally restricted from their land on the sole basis of gender. Having a right to their land gives women a sort of bargaining power that they would not normally have, in turn; they gain the ability to assert themselves in various aspects of their life, both in and outside of the home.
3. Another way to provide women empowerment is to allocate responsibilities to them that normally belong to men. When women have economic empowerment, it is a way for others to see them as equal members of society. Through this, they achieve more self-respect and confidence by their contributions to their communities.
4. Simply including women as a part of a community can have sweeping positive effects. Not only did this drive up the efficiency of the group, but the women gained incredible self-esteem, while others including men, viewed them with more respect.
5. Participation which can be seen and gained in a variety of ways has been argued to be the most beneficial form of gender empowerment. Political participation, be it the ability to vote and voice opinions, or the ability to run for office with a fair chance of being elected, plays a huge role in the empowerment of peoples. It can include participation in the household, in schools, and the ability to make choices for one. It can be said that these latter participations need to be achieved before one can move onto broader political participation. When women have the agency to do what she wants, a higher equality between men and women is established.
6. Governments, organizations, and individuals have caught hold of the lure of microfinance. They hope that lending money and credit allows women to function in business and society, which in turn empowers them to do more in their communities.
7. One of the primary goals in the foundation of microfinance was women empowerment. Loans with low interest rates are given to women in developing communities in hopes that they can start a small business and provide for her family. It should be said, however, that the success and efficiency of microcredit and microloans is controversial and constantly debated.

9. Intrauterine contraceptive devices. (*See* Q. 8, 2014)

10. Housing standards. (*See* Q. 3, 2016)

11. Epidemiology of H1N1.

H1N1 Swine flu is a subtype of influenza A virus (a communicable viral disease), which causes upper, and potentially lower respiratory tract infections in the host it infects, resulting in symptoms, such as nasal secretions, chills, fever, decreased appetite, and possibly lower respiratory tract disease. H1N1 swine influenza is a common infection in pigs worldwide, and that is why it is also known as swine flu. H1N1 swine flu leads to respiratory disease that can potentially infect the respiratory tract of pigs. Sometimes, people who are closely associated with pigs or in the proximity of pigs have developed swine flu (zoonotic swine flu). Swine influenza viruses can potentially cause infections in humans if antigenic characteristics of the virus change through reassortment.

Mode of transmission: Swine influenza (novel H1N1 and H3N2v) spreads from person to person, either by inhaling the virus or by touching surfaces contaminated with the virus, then touching the mouth or nose. Infected droplets are expelled into the air through coughing or sneezing.

Symptoms: The signs and symptoms of swine flu are similar to those of infections caused by other flu strains and can include:
1. Fever (but not always)
2. Chills
3. Cough
4. Sore throat
5. Runny or stuffy nose
6. Watery, red eyes
7. Body aches
8. Headache
9. Fatigue
10. Diarrhea
11. Nausea and vomiting.

Swine influenza is considered one of the most important primary pathogens of swine respiratory disease and infection is primarily with H1N1, H1N2 and H3N2 influenza A viruses. The antigenetic characteristics of these viruses distinguish them from others circulating at a global level in pigs. These viruses have remained endemic in European pig populations but significant differences in the circulation of these strains occur at a regional level across Europe. The dynamic of co-circulation of viruses, impact of prior immunity, husbandry practices and other local factors all contribute to the complex epidemiology.

12. Control of rodents.

Steps to rodent control: Roof rat survival depends upon the existence of 3 basic environmental factors: (1) Food, (2) Water, and (3) Harborage.

Step 1: Eliminate food and water
1. Remove all potential sources of food from the premises, such as bird seed left out for birds. Routinely harvest ripe fruit and pick up all fruit that has fallen to the ground.
2. Store pet food in metal containers with tight sealing lids and do not leave uneaten pet food outdoors.
3. Avoid storing food in garages and storage sheds unless it is in rat-proof covered metal containers.
4. Control snails and clean up pet feces because they are favored food items.
5. Keep trash cans closed at all time with tightly fitted lids.
6. Repair leaking eliminates any other faucets, sprinklers, or other piping. Keep drain covers tightly fastened and unnecessary standing water.

Step 2: Destroy rats
1. Rats should be snap trapped if they are inside a residence or building. Place traps near nesting areas or where rats are likely to hide. Do not place traps where children or pets will disturb or be harmed by them. Remember, snap traps are very DANGEROUS!

2. Poisoning with baits indoors is NOT recommended because a rat may die inside the structure and create an odor and fly problem. Poison baits may be used when following recommended guidelines.
3. Remove dead rats by placing animals in tightly sealed containers for proper disposal. Clean and disinfect the affected areas.

Step 3: Eliminate shelter and harborage

1. Close all openings larger than ¼ inch to exclude rats and mice.
2. Repair or replace damaged vent screens.
3. Remove all trash and debris.
4. Stack woodpiles, lumber and household items at least 18 inches above the ground, and 12 inches away from fences and walls.
5. Trim trees, bushes and vines at least 4 feet away from the roof.
6. Remove heavy vegetation away from buildings and fences.
7. Thin vegetation to allow daylight in and remove rat hiding places.

Step 4: Maintain a rat free property

After rats have been reduced, prevent reinfestation by keeping harborage and food sources to a minimum.

SHORT ANSWERS

13. Define zoonosis. *(See Q. 17, 2014)*

14. List common arthropod infections.

Arthropod-borne diseases are transmitted by arthropods, members of the invertebrate phylum Arthropoda which includes insects, spiders, and crustaceans. Mosquitoes, fleas, ticks, lice, and flies are the arthropods that usually act as vectors for various pathogens (disease-causing microorganisms) including bacteria, viruses, helminths (parasitic worms), and protozoa. Transmission of these pathogens to humans by the arthropod vector can cause a variety of human diseases including malaria, yellow fever, chagas disease, and dengue fever. These and other arthropod-borne diseases can result in a wide range of effects, from mild flulike symptoms to death. Some survivors of arthropod-borne diseases can suffer chronic, crippling after-effects.

15. Define immunity.

The condition of being immune. Immunity can be innate'for example, humans are innately immune to canine distemper'or conferred by a previous infection or immunization. Immunity means being protected from something and being unaffected or not bothered by it.

16. Define epidemic. *(See Q. 20, 2014)*

17. List four health problems of children.

Common Child Health Issues

1. Colds: **Children** get lots of colds—it can be as often as once a month.
2. Gastroenteritis: Lots of **children** get gastroenteritis ('gastro')
3. Conjunctivitis: Conjunctivitis is an infection of **the** lining of **the** eyeball and eyelids.

4. Impetigo
5. Hand, foot and mouth disease
6. Lice
7. Worms
8. Warts.

18. Define communication.

Communication defined as two-way process of reaching mutual understanding in which participants not only exchange (encode-decode) information, news, ideas and feelings but also create and share meaning. In general, communication is a means of connecting people or places. In business, it is a key function of management—an organization cannot operate without communication between levels, departments and employees.

19. Prevention of anemia.

In most cases, anemia is preventable during pregnancy. Here are three ways to make sure you are getting the necessary vitamins and minerals to keep your red blood cell levels in the right range.

1. **Prenatal vitamins:** Prenatal vitamins usually contain iron and folic acid. Taking a prenatal vitamin once a day is an easy way to get essential vitamins and minerals for sufficient red blood cell production.

2. **Iron supplements:** Pregnant women need around 27 mg of iron daily. But depending on the type of iron or iron supplement consumed, the dose will vary.

3. **Proper nutrition:** Most women can get sufficient amounts of iron and folic acid during pregnancy by eating the right foods.

20. List four health problems of elderly.

Getting older can bring senior health challenges. By being aware of these common chronic conditions:
1. Arthritis
2. Heart disease
3. Cancer
4. Respiratory disease
5. Alzheimer's disease
6. Osteoporosis
7. Diabetes
8. Influenza and pneumonia.

21. Importance of rainwater harvesting.

Rainwater harvesting is a sustainable process that helps in preserving rain water for different purposes and for the future needs as well. Rainwater harvesting is a method of collecting and storing rain water to be used for various purposes while it can be used in future as well.

Benefits of Rainwater Harvesting

1. Storing rainwater helps in recharging the aquifers.
2. It helps in preventing urban flooding due to excess rain.
3. The stored water can be used for irrigation practices in farming region.
4. The water can be used for daily use and help in reducing water bills in the towns and cities.
5. Is a helpful way to tackle the scarcity of water in arid and dry regions.
6. It helps in restoring the groundwater level.

22. Modified risk factors of hypertension.

Hypertension is a disease entity of its own. It remains silent being asymptomatic during its clinical course. Because of its asymptomatic appearance, it does immense harm to the body in the form of target organ damage, hence the WHO has named it the "silent killer."

Hypertension is a major cause of cardiovascular morbidity and mortality. Excess dietary salt, low dietary potassium, overweight and obesity, physical inactivity, excess alcohol, smoking, socioeconomic status, psychosocial stressors, and diabetes are considered as modifiable risk factors for hypertension.

2018

Community Health Nursing-I

LONG ESSAYS
1. Define epidemiology and explain the role of community health nurse in each level of prevention.
2. Describe the methods of data collection, analysis and interpretation of demographical data.
3. Define family planning and describe the methods of population control.

SHORT ESSAYS
4. Concept and dimensions of health.
5. Epidemiological triad.
6. Mentall illness.
7. Morbidity and mortality.
8. Food poisoning.
9. Trachoma.
10. Tuberculosis.
11. Epilepsy.
12. Women empowerment.

SHORT ANSWERS
13. Sexual life.
14. Hygiene.
15. Accidents.
16. Family size.
17. Blindness.
18. Demongraphy.
19. Occupational health.
20. Diphtheria.
21. Healthy lifestyle.
22. Health education.

LONG ESSAYS

1. Define epidemiology and explain the role of community health nurse in each level of prevention. *(See Q. 2, 2016)*

2. Describe the methods of data collection, analysis and interpretation of demographical data. *(See Q. 5, 2016)*

3. Define family planning and describe the methods of population control.

"Family planning is a way of thinking and living that it is adopted voluntarily, upon the basis of knowledge, attitude and responsible decisions by individuals and couples in order to promote the health and welfare of the family group and thus contribute effectively to the social development of a country"—WHO, 1971.

Objectives of the family planning

Family planning refers to practices that help individuals or couples to attain certain objectives (WHO, 1971) given below:
1. To avoid unwanted births.
2. To bring about wanted births.
3. To regulate the intervals between pregnancies.
4. To control the time at which birth occurs in relation to the age of the parents.
5. To determine the number of children in the family.

Services that make these practices possible include:
1. Education and counseling on family planning.
2. The provisions of contraceptives.
3. The management of infertility.
4. Education about sex and parenthood.
5. Organizationally related activities, such as genetic and marriage counseling, screening for malignancy, and adoption services.

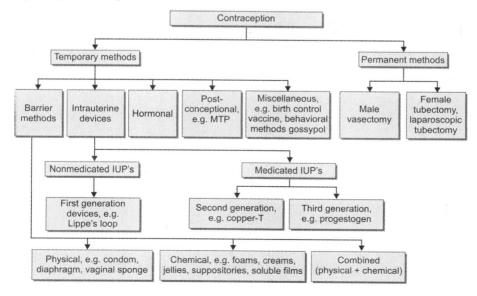

Female Sterilization

Sterilization is a permanent method of contraception whereby the person is rendered infertile. In case of female sterilization there are commonly two methods: These are tubectomy or minilaparotomy and laparoscopy sterilization.

To undergo these procedures certain criteria's should be followed:
1. The client must be married and the spouse must be living together.
2. The female client preferably is below 45 years and above 22 years.
3. The couple should have at least one child with age above 1 year.
4. The client or spouse must not have undergone previous sterilization except in case of failures.
5. The client should give consent for the surgery and its full implications.
6. In case of mentally ill client, a psychiatrist must certify and the legal guardian/spouse should give consent in such cases.

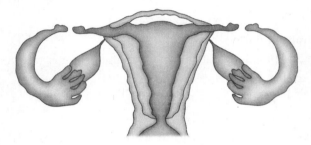

Fig. 1: Tubectomy.

Specific Criteria in Case of Tubectomy (Fig. 1)
1. Within 7 days after the menstrual period.
2. Postpartum sterilization preferably be performed within 7 days of delivery. Since, there should not be any infection or contraindication.
3. PostMTP/along with MTP: Sterilization with medical termination of pregnancy can be performed concurrently in the absence of anemia and infection.
4. Sterilization following spontaneous abortion can be performed with antibiotic coverage in the absence of anemia and other infections.

Counseling for Sterilization
1. As a community health nurse one should explain the client with all methods of family planning in their own language.
2. The nurse must ensure that the client makes informed decision for sterilization voluntarily.
3. The nurse must provide a clear description of the specific procedure prior to the surgery, during surgery, after surgery (in case of tubectomy). Example investigations, clinical examinations, side effects, potential complications, etc.

Advantages
1. It is a safe and simple procedure.
2. It is a permanent procedure for preventing future pregnancies.
3. It does not affect sexual pleasure, ability or performance.
4. It will not affect the client's ability to carry out normal day-to-day work.
5. It has a very less chance of failure even if performed under optimum circumstances.
6. Sterilization does not provide protection against RTI/STD or HIV/AIDS.

Procedures

1.	Make comfortable position of the client on operation theater (OT) table	To get the cooperation
2.	Sterilize the site with betadine solution	To prevent infection
3.	Spread to OT towel and make it sure that the operation site is visible	To cover the area except operation site to prevent infection
4.	Provide injection xylocaine 2% with injection adrenaline (it prevent bleeding) 3–5 mL	For local anesthesia
5.	Surgeons will decide the incision below the umbilicus. 2–2.5 cm with scalpel blade	Depends on physical/skin condition
6.	Then to rectus muscles, peritoneum, the finger will reach fallopian tube (confirm the tube with uterus)	Procedure
7.	Catch the middle of the tube with babcock and tie the tube with white thread—2 times and cut the middle part of the fallopian tube and leave it the place	Procedure
8.	Continue the same procedure to the another side of the fallopian tube	Procedure
9.	Watch for bleeding/vital signs	Nurses responsibility
10.	Stitch the incision with catgut No. 1/No. 2	Since, it is a permenent method
11.	Suture the skin peritoneal	Procedure
12.	Apply sterile dressings	Present infection
13.	Care of the client/article	Responsibilities

Laparoscopic Sterilization (Fig. 2)

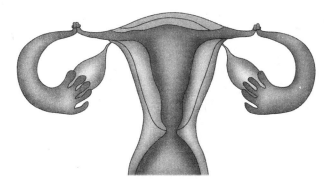

Fig. 2: Laparoscopic sterilization.

1. Here the procedure will be done with the help of laparoscopic instruments.
2. There will be no cutting of fallopian tube takes place.
3. The surgeon tie the tubes with special bands.
4. After this procedure immediately the clients can move to their respective places.
5. There will not be any incision/suture over the abdomen.
6. Dressing seal can be removed after 7 days.
7. She can be continue with her regular functions and duties.

Male Sterilization

Vasectomy: Male sterilization is a permanent method of contraception where by blocking the duct that carries sperm. There are two methods, they are (Fig. 3):
1. Conventional vasectomy.
2. Nonscalpel vasectomy.

Healthy clients with no contraindications should be offered surgery as soon as convenient for them.

Vasectomy sterilization procedure is very simple, easy to perform with least morbidity when compared to female sterilization.

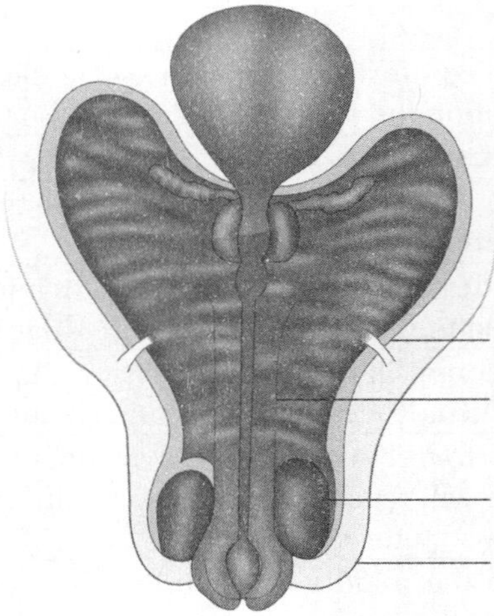

Fig. 3: Vasectomy.

Eligibility Criteria
1. The client must be married and the spouse must be living together.
2. The male client preferably be below 60 years and his wife must be below 45 years of age.
3. The number of children must not be criteria for determining the eligibility for sterilization. However, it is preferable that the couple should have at least one child with age above 1 year.
4. The client or spouse must not have undergone previous sterilization, unless in case of failure.
5. The client must be in the proper state of mind to understand the full implications of the sterilization.

Counseling for Sterilization
1. Explain all the family planning methods in front of the couple/spouse.
2. Make sure that the clients' decisions is voluntarily.
3. Counsel the client in their understandable language.
4. Educate the client regarding the selected method and procedure.

In Case of Male Sterilization
1. It is a safe and simple procedure.
2. It is a permanent procedure for preventing future pregnancies.
3. It does not affect sexual pleasure, ability, or performance.
4. It will not affect the clients to carry out normal day-to-day work.
5. After male sterilization, it is necessary to use a backup contraceptive method either for 20 ejaculations or for a period of 3 months.
6. Sterilization does not provide protection against RTI/STI or HIV/AIDS.
7. It has 1% chance of failure, even if performed under optimum circumstances.
8. In case of any doubts/clarification consult medical officials.

Responsibilities of Nurse
1. Informed consent is must for all clients.
2. Check with the client's case sheet whether they underwent required investigations like hemoglobin %, clotting time/bleeding time, urine analysis, etc.
3. Check the client underwent all required physical assessment and screening.

Preoperative Instruction
1. The client must bathe and wear clean and loose cotton clothing.
2. Should not have heavy food prior to male sterilization.

3. Should shave the part thoroughly.
4. Empty the bladder just before operation.
5. Make sure that injection tetanus toxoid 0.5 mL IM has given/taken.
6. Make sure that test dose of injection xylocaine and ensure that will not be any reactions/allergic to xylocaine/lignocaine.
7. Ensure that premedication has given.

Procedures

1.	Makes comfortable position (Fowler's position)	To get the cooperation
2.	Sterilize/clean the operation site with betadine and spirite	To prevent infection
3.	Spread the operation theater towel and make sure that the operation site/part in visible	To prevent infection, and visualize the operation site
4.	Clips the operation theater towel	To make sure the towel should not move
5.	Inform the client that giving a small injection	To get the cooperation
6.	Injection the local anesthesia to the operational site	Unaware of pain
7.	Make a small incision with scalpel (1 inch)	Procedure
8.	Make sure with vas deferens	To achieve the procedural objectives
9.	Clamp the vas deferens and tie it with thread and with catgut in both sides	Procedure
10.	Close the incision with one stitch	Procedure
11.	Apply sterile dressing and T bandage	To support operated part and the sterile dressing. T bandage is necessary
12.	Allow the person to get up and walk	No hospital stay
13.	Care of the person and articles	Responsibilities
14.	Follow-up visits	Health maintenance

Nonscalpel Vasectomy

1. Procedure is same without incision and stitch.
2. There were no need of scalpel blade and handle.
3. The procedure will perform by the special device which causes the entry and lifting the vas deferens and banding the vas deferens with the special equipment like pliable probe.

Instructions to the Clients

1. Take the antibiotics up to 7 days.
2. Normal food.
3. Normal duties and functions.
4. Any problems inform the junior health assistants at his door step.
5. Visit the surgeon after 1 week. Remove the stitch in case of vasectomy.
6. In case of NSV visit the surgeon, just for examination of operated part and suggestions.

7. Use condoms/nirodh up to 90 days after vasectomy operation to prevent (3 months) pregnancy.
8. Advice the clients to check semen analysis after 3 months.
9. Provide enough health care when it is required.

SHORT ESSAYS

4. Concept and dimensions of health.

There are five dimensions of health: Physical, mental, emotional, spiritual, and social. This inter-relationship between the dimensions of health is one of the key aspects that you need to understand for preliminary physical development, health and physical education (PDHPE).

Physical: The physical dimension of health refers to the bodily aspect of health. It refers to the more traditional definitions of health as the absence of disease and injury. Physical health ranges in quality along a continuum where a combination of diseases, such as cancer, diabetes, cardiovascular disease or hypertension is at one end and a person who is at optimum physical condition is at the other.

Mental: Mental health is more the functioning of the brain, while emotional health refers to the person's mood often connected to their hormones. Mental health then includes many mental health issues, such as Alzheimer's and dementia. It refers to the person's ability to use their brain and think. This may be to solve problems or to recall information, but the focus is on the cognitive aspect of the person.

Emotional: Emotional health is about the persons mood or general emotional state. It is our ability to recognize and express feelings adequately. It relates to self-esteem as well as the ability to control emotions to maintain a realistic perspective on situations. The relationship between emotional and mental health is clear and as such some illnesses relate to both, such as: Depression and anxiety.

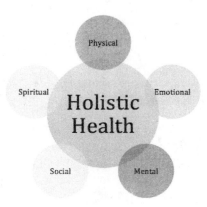

Spiritual: Spiritual health will very easily affect emotional and mental health as having a purpose in life can help you to apply yourself to achieving goals. Having a purpose to life can also help people to maintain a proper perspective on life and overcome adversity. Often people who are spiritual meet together regularly around their spiritual purpose which helps to improve their social health.

Social: The social dimension of health refers to our ability to make and maintain meaningful relationships with others. Good social health includes not only having relationships but behaving appropriately within them and maintaining socially acceptable standards. The basic social unit of relationship is the family, and these relationships impact a person's life the most. Other key relationships are close friends, social networks, teachers, and youth leaders.

5. Epidemiological triad.

A traditional model of infectious disease causation, known as the epidemiologic triad is depicted in Figure 4. The triad consists of an external agent, a host and an environment in which host and agent are brought together causing the disease to occur in the host.

In this model, disease results from the interaction between the agent and the susceptible host, in an environment that supports transmission of the agent from a source to that host. The epidemiologic triad model is helpful when considering association and causation. The triad consists of three factors—1. agent, 2. host and 3. environment. They interact in a variety of ways that result in various states of health in an individual or a community.

Agent: In infectious disease models, the term "agent" originally referred to the entity or microorganism (e.g. virus, bacterium) capable of causing the disease. As a general rule, the agent must be present for the disease to occur. However, the mere presence of the agent is not always sufficient for the disease to occur.

As the scope of epidemiology has expanded, the concept of "agent" has also grown to include chemical and physical components. This model works well with infectious diseases and accidents/injuries and most noninfectious diseases.

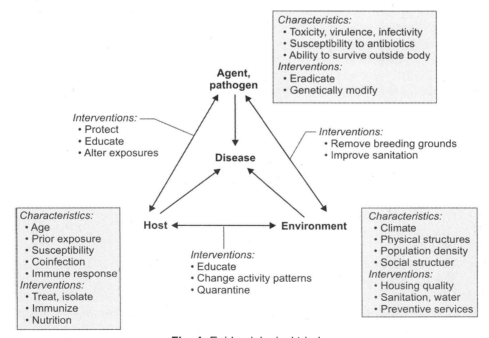

Fig. 4: Epidemiological triad.

Host: "Host" refers to the intrinsic factors that influence an individual's exposure, susceptibility or response to a causative agent. These factors also called risk factors include socioeconomic status, lifestyle, behaviors, and psychological characteristics.

Environment: Environmental factors are extrinsic factors that affect the agent and the opportunity for exposure. They can be physical factors (e.g. climate), biological factors (e.g. insects) or socioeconomic factors (e.g. sanitation, access to health services).

6. Mentall illness.

Mental illness, also called mental health disorders, refers to a wide range of mental health conditions—disorders that affect the mood, thinking and behavior. Examples of mental illness include depression, anxiety disorders, schizophrenia, eating disorders and addictive behaviors.

Causes

Mental illnesses, in general, are thought to be caused by a variety of genetic and environmental factors:

Inherited traits: Mental illness is more common in people whose blood relatives also have a mental illness. Certain genes may increase your risk of developing a mental illness, and your life situation may trigger it.

Environmental exposures: Before birth. Exposure to environmental stressors, inflammatory conditions, toxins, alcohol or drugs while in the womb can sometimes be linked to mental illness.

Brain chemistry: Neurotransmitters are naturally occurring brain chemicals that carry signals to other parts of your brain and body. When the neural networks involving these chemicals are impaired, the function of nerve receptors and nerve systems change, leading to depression and other emotional disorders.

Symptoms: Signs and symptoms of mental illness can vary depending on the disorder, circumstances and other factors. Mental illness symptoms can affect emotions, thoughts and behaviors. Examples of signs and symptoms include:
1. Feeling sad or down
2. Confused thinking or reduced ability to concentrate
3. Excessive fears or worries, or extreme feelings of guilt
4. Extreme mood changes of highs and lows
5. Withdrawal from friends and activities
6. Significant tiredness, low energy or problems sleeping
7. Detachment from reality (delusions), paranoia or hallucinations
8. Inability to cope with daily problems or stress
9. Trouble understanding and relating to situations and to people
10. Problems with alcohol or drug use
11. Major changes in eating habits
12. Sex drive changes
13. Excessive anger, hostility or violence
14. Suicidal thinking.

7. Morbidity and mortality.

Morbidity refers to the unhealthy state of an individual, while mortality refers to the state of being mortal. Both concepts can be applied at the individual level or across a population. For example, a morbidity rate looks at the incidence of a disease across a population and/or geographic location during a single year. Mortality rate is the rate of death in a population. The two are often used together to calculate the prevalence of a disease, e.g. measles and how likely that disease is to be deadly, particularly for certain demographics.

Comparison Chart

	Morbidity	**Mortality**
Definition	Morbidity refers to the state of being diseased or unhealthy within a population	Mortality is the term used for the number of people who died within a population
Demographic reference	Morbidity refers to an incidence of ill health in a population	Mortality refers to the incidence of death or the number of deaths in a population
Database/reports	World Health Statistics (compiled by WHO), MMWR (Morbidity and Mortality Weekly Report, by Center for Disease Control and Prevention, USA), EMDB (European hospital Morbidity Database, Europe), NHMD (National hospital morbidity Database, Australia)	The Human mortality database developed by the Department of Demography at the University of California, Berkeley and the Max Planck Institute for Demographic Research in Rostock Germany.
Units of measurement	Morbidity scores or predicted morbidity are assigned to ill patients with the help of systems, such as the APACHE II, SAPS II and III, Glasgow Coma scale, PIM2, and SOFA	Mortality rates are generally expressed as the number of deaths per 1,000 individuals per year.
Types of data	Data is collected according to the disease type, gender age, area	The mortality rate can be distinguished into crude death rate; perinatal mortality rate; the maternal mortality rate; infant mortality rate; child mortality rate; standardized mortality rate; and age-specific mortality rate.

8. Food poisoning. *(See Q. 11, 2016)*

9. Trachoma. *(See Q. 18, 2015)*

10. Tuberculosis.

Tuberculosis (TB) is caused by bacteria *(Mycobacterium tuberculosis)* that most often affect the lungs. Tuberculosis is curable and preventable. TB is spread from person to person through the air. When people with lung TB cough, sneeze or spit, they propel the TB germs into the air. A person needs to inhale only a few of these germs to become infected.

About one-third of the world's population has latent TB, which means people have been infected by TB bacteria but are not (yet) ill with disease and cannot transmit the disease.

People infected with TB bacteria have a lifetime risk of falling ill with TB of 10%. However persons with compromised immune systems, such as people living with HIV, malnutrition or diabetes, or people who use tobacco, have a much higher risk of falling ill.

When a person develops active TB (disease), the symptoms (cough, fever, night sweats, weight loss, etc.) may be mild for many months. This can lead to delays in seeking care, and results in transmission of the bacteria to others. People ill with TB can infect up to 10-15 other people through close contact over the course of a year. Without proper treatment up to two third of people ill with TB will die.

Symptoms: Although your body may harbor the bacteria that cause TB, your immune system usually can prevent you from becoming sick. For this reason, doctors make a distinction between:

1. Latent TB: In this condition, you have a TB infection, but the bacteria remain in your body in an inactive state and cause no symptoms. Latent TB, also called inactive TB or TB infection, is not contagious. It can turn into active TB, so treatment is important for the person with latent TB and help to control the spread of TB. An estimated 2 billion people have latent TB.

2. Active TB: This condition makes you sick and in most cases can spread to others. It can occur in the first few weeks after infection with the TB bacteria, or it might occur years later.

Signs and symptoms of active TB include:
1. Coughing that lasts 3 or more weeks
2. Coughing up blood
3. Chest pain, or pain with breathing or coughing
4. Unintentional weight loss
5. Fatigue
6. Fever
7. Night sweats
8. Chills
9. Loss of appetite.

Classification of drugs used in antituberculosis treatment	
First-line drugs	**Second-line drugs**
• Isoniazide • Rifammpin • Pyrazinamide • Ethambutol • Streptomycin	• Amikacin • Amino salicyclic acid • Capreomycin • Ciprofloxacin • Clofazimine • Cycloserine • Ethionamide • Levofloxacin • Rifabutin • Rifapentine

Prevention: If the test is positive for latent TB infection, your doctor may advise you to take medications to reduce your risk of developing active tuberculosis. The only type of tuberculosis that is contagious is the active variety, when it affects the lungs.

Protect your Family and Friends
1. **Stay home:** Do not go to work or school or sleep in a room with other people during the first few weeks of treatment for active tuberculosis.
2. **Ventilate the room:** Tuberculosis germs spread more easily in small closed spaces where air does not move. If it is not too cold outdoors, open the windows and use a fan to blow indoor air outside.
3. **Cover the mouth:** Use a tissue to cover your mouth anytime you laugh, sneeze or cough. Put the dirty tissue in a bag, seal it and throw it away.

4. **Wear a mask:** Wearing a surgical mask when you are around other people during the first 3 weeks of treatment may help lessen the risk of transmission.

Vaccinations: In countries where tuberculosis is more common, infants often are vaccinated with bacillus Calmette-Guerin (BCG) vaccine because it can prevent severe tuberculosis in children. The BCG vaccine is not recommended for general use in the United States because it is not very effective in adults. Dozens of new TB vaccines are in various stages of development and testing.

11. Epilepsy. (*See* Q. 17, 2015)

12. Women empowerment. (*See* Q. 10, 2015)

SHORT ANSWERS

13. Sexual life.

According to the current working definition, sexual health is: "…a state of physical, emotional, mental and social well-being in relation to sexuality; it is not merely the absence of disease, dysfunction or infirmity. Sexual health requires a positive and respectful approach to sexuality and sexual relationships, as well as the possibility of having pleasurable and safe sexual experiences, free of coercion, discrimination and violence. For sexual health to be attained and maintained, the sexual rights of all persons must be respected, protected and fulfilled." (WHO, 2006a)

14. Hygiene.

The science of preventive medicine and the preservation of health. Also commonly used as a euphemism for cleanliness and proper sanitation.

Health benefits of hygiene are:
1. It reduces the risk of infection
2. It helps you to stay healthy
3. Avoid Illness
4. Fight against disease-causing germs and bacterial to enter into the body
5. It prevents the transmission of germs
6. It also helps our body from the skin infection
7. Hand washing can avoid the transition of bacteria from food to your body
8. Keeping your house clean and hygiene helps you to stay healthy.

15. Accidents.

Accident defined as an unplanned, unexpected, and undesigned (not purposefully caused) event which occurs suddenly and causes (1) injury or loss, (2) a decrease in value of the resources, or (3) an increase in liabilities. As a technical term 'accident' does not have a clearly defined legal meaning. In insurance terminology, an accident is the events which are not deliberately caused, and which is not inevitable. For example, if a driver (who is covered under personal automobile insurance for injury and losses due to negligence) willfully drives the vehicle into a tree, the resulting injury or loss is not insured.

16. Family size.

Family size may be considered from two perspectives. At the individual (micro) level, it defines one aspect of an individual's family background or environment. As such, it represents a potential influence on the development and accomplishments of family members. At the societal (macro) level, family size is an indicator of societal structure that may vary over time, with concomitant implications for individual development and social relations in different cohorts.

17. Blindness.

Loss of useful sight. Blindness can be temporary or permanent. Damage to any portion of the eye, the optic nerve, or the area of the brain responsible for vision can lead to blindness. There are numerous (actually, innumerable) causes of blindness. The current politically correct terms for blindness include visually handicapped and visually challenged.

18. Demongraphy. (*See* Q. 20, 2016)

19. Occupational health.

Occupational health refers to the identification and control of the risks arising from physical, chemical, and other workplace hazards in order to establish and maintain a safe and healthy working environment. These hazards may include chemical agents and solvents, heavy metals, such as lead and mercury, physical agents, such as loud noise or vibration, and physical hazards, such as electricity or dangerous machinery.

Definition: Occupational health is the promotion and maintenance of the highest degree of physical, mental and social well-being of workers in all occupations by preventing departures from health, controlling risks and the adaptation of work to people, and people to their jobs. (ILO/WHO 1950)

20. Diphtheria.

Diphtheria defined as an acute and highly contagious bacterial disease causing inflammation of the mucous membranes, formation of a false membrane in the throat which hinders breathing and swallowing, and potentially fatal heart and nerve damage by a bacterial toxin in the blood. It is now rare in developed countries owing to immunization.

Diphtheria: An acute infectious upper respiratory tract disease that affects the throat. It is caused by the bacteria *Corynebacterium diphtheriae*. Symptoms include sore throat and mild fever at first. As the disease progresses, a membranous substance forms in the throat that makes it difficult to breathe and swallow. Diphtheria can be deadly. It is one of the diseases that the diphtheria-tetanus (DT), diphtheria-tetanus-pertussis (DTP), and diphtheria-tetanus-acellular-pertussis (DTaP) vaccines are designed to prevent.

21. Healthy lifestyle.

A healthy lifestyle is a way of living that lowers the risk of being seriously ill or dying early. Not all diseases are preventable, but a large proportion of deaths particularly those from coronary heart disease and lung cancer can be avoided. Scientific studies have identified certain types of behavior that contribute to the development of noncommunicable diseases and early death. Health is not only just about avoiding disease. It is also about physical, mental and social well-being. When a healthy lifestyle is adopted, a more positive role model is provided to other people in the family particularly children. This booklet aims to help readers change their behavior and improve their health in order to live healthier, longer lives.

22. Health education.

Health education is any combination of learning experiences designed to help individuals and communities to improve their health, by increasing their knowledge or influencing their attitudes. Health education is the profession of educating people about health. Areas within this profession encompass environmental health, physical health, social health, emotional health, intellectual health, and spiritual health. It can be defined as the principle by which individuals and groups of people learn to behave in a manner conducive to the promotion, maintenance, or restoration of health. However, as there are multiple definitions of health, there are also multiple definitions of health education.

The Joint Committee on Health Education and Promotion Terminology of 2001 defined Health Education as "any combination of planned learning experiences based on sound theories that provide individuals, groups, and communities the opportunity to acquire information and the skills needed to make quality health decisions."

The World Health Organization defined Health Education as "compris[ing] [of] consciously constructed opportunities for learning involving some form of communication designed to improve health literacy, including improving knowledge, and developing life skills which are conducive to individual and community health.

2017

Community Health Nursing-I

LONG ESSAYS
1. a. Define health. b. Enlist the dimensions of health. c. Explain the levels of prevention to promote health.
2. a. Enlist the methods of collection of demographical data. b. Explain any two methods.
3. a. Enlist the intestinal infections, b. Describe the epidemiology and management of hookworm infection.

SHORT ESSAYS
4. Explain about water purification on small scale.
5. Explain different methods of disposal of waste in community.
6. Write about types of ventilation.
7. Measurement of mortality.
8. Explain the steps of epidemiological investigation.
9. Signs and symptoms and management of cholera.
10. Write about DOTS.
11. Explain modes of transmission of HIV.
12. Explain barrier methods of contraception.

SHORT ANSWERS
13. Define eugenics.
14. Mention the types of cohort.
15. Mention the effect of poor lighting.
16. Define sex ratio.
17. Safe period method of fertility control.
18. Define eligible couple.
19. Montoux test.
20. Define food hygiene.
21. Mention the causes of obesity.
22. List for zoonotic diseases.

LONG ESSAYS

1. a. Define health. (*See* Q. 1, 2016) b. Enlist the dimensions of health. (*See* Q. 6, 2014) c. Explain the levels of prevention to promote health.

Levels of Prevention

Three broad categories of determinants of human behavior will be discussed in this study session and you will have an opportunity to learn about the influence of these factors in determining human behavior.

Prevention, as it relates to health, is really about avoiding disease before it starts. It has been defined as the plans for, and the measures taken, to prevent the onset of a disease or other health problem before the occurrence of the undesirable health event. There are three distinct levels of prevention:

1. **Primary prevention**—those preventive measures that prevent the onset of illness or injury before the disease process begins, e.g. include immunization and taking regular exercise.
2. **Secondary prevention**—those preventive measures that lead to early diagnosis and prompt treatment of a disease, illness or injury to prevent more severe problems developing. Here health educators, such as health extension practitioners can help individuals acquire the skills of detecting diseases in their early stages, e.g. include screening for high blood pressure and breast self-examination.
3. **Tertiary prevention**—those preventive measures aimed at rehabilitation following significant illness. At this level health services workers can work to retrain, re-educate and rehabilitate people who have already developed an impairment or disability.

2. a. Enlist the methods of collection of demographical data. b. Explain any two methods. (*See* Q. 5, 2016)

3. a. Enlist the intestinal infections. b. Describe the epidemiology and management of hookworm infection.

Gastrointestinal infections are viral, bacterial or parasitic infections that cause gastroenteritis, an inflammation of the gastrointestinal tract involving both the stomach and the small intestine. Symptoms include diarrhea, vomiting, and abdominal pain. Dehydration is the main danger of gastrointestinal infections, so rehydration is important, but most gastrointestinal infections are self-limited and resolve within a few days. However, in a healthcare setting and in specific populations (newborns/infants, immunocompromized patients or elderly populations), they are potentially serious. Rapid diagnosis, appropriate treatment and infection control measures are therefore particularly important in these contexts.

Gastrointestinal infections can be caused by a large number of microorganisms including:

- *Adenovirus* can cause diarrhea, fever, conjunctivitis, bladder infections and rashes, but the most common symptom is respiratory illness. After rotavirus, it is the most common cause of pediatric diarrhea.
- *Campylobacter* is one of the most common bacterial cause of gastroenteritis worldwide and is frequent in children under two. It can cause diarrhea (sometimes bloody), abdominal cramps, vomiting and fever. It is usually foodborne through raw or undercooked meat (especially poultry) or through contaminated milk.

- *Clostridium difficile* infection is responsible for up to 25% of cases of antibiotic-associated diarrhea most often contracted in hospitals or healthcare institutions. Elderly and immunocompromized patients are most at risk. The recent emergence of highly toxigenic and resistant *C. difficile* strains has led to more frequent and severe outbreaks, increased morbidity and mortality.
- *Escherichia coli*, often called *E. coli*, is the leading cause of travelers' diarrhea and a major cause of diarrheal disease in the developing world, especially among children. People usually contract *E. coli* through ingestion of water contaminated with human or animal feces.
- *Helicobacter pylori*, called *H. pylori*, is a cause of gastritis and is associated with the development of gastric and duodenal ulcers. It can cause stomach pain or nausea, but in many cases there are no symptoms. Infected people have a 10-20% lifetime risk of developing peptic ulcers and 1–2% risk of stomach cancer.
- *Rotavirus* is the most frequent cause of diarrhea in young children and infants and it is responsible for the most severe cases. There is a vaccine for rotavirus, but globally it causes more than ½ million deaths per year in children less than 5 years old. Most of these are in emerging countries.
- *Salmonella and Shigella* are foodborne GI illnesses. *Salmonella* is common and is found in raw meats, poultry, seafood and eggs, as well as milk and dairy products. Acute symptoms include nausea, vomiting, abdominal cramps, diarrhea, fever, and headache. *Shigella* is frequently found in water polluted with human feces. Symptoms of shigellosis (bacillary dysentery) include abdominal pain, cramps, diarrhea, fever, vomiting, and blood, pus, or mucus in stool.
- *Staphylococcus aureus* is the most common cause of food intoxication, characterized by abrupt/violent onset, severe nausea, cramps, vomiting, and diarrhea using lasting 1-2 days. This opportunistic pathogen can be found on humans (skin, infected cuts, noses and throats) and has been associated with a wide range of foods including meat and meat products, poultry and egg products, salads, bakery products, and dairy products.
- *Yersinia enterocolitica*, called *Y. enterocolitica*, is a relatively infrequent cause of diarrhea and abdominal pain. Infection is most often acquired by eating contaminated food, especially raw or undercooked pork products, as well as ice-cream and milk. Common symptoms are fever, abdominal pain, and diarrhea which is often bloody.

Hookworm Infection

Hookworm is a soil transmitted helminth (STH) and is one of the most common roundworm of humans. Infection is caused by the nematode parasites *Necator americanus* and *Ancylostoma duodenale*. Hookworm infections often occur in areas where human feces are used as fertilizer or where defecation onto soil happens.

Geographic distribution: The geographic distributions of the hookworm species that are intestinal parasites in human, *Ancylostoma duodenale* and *Necator americanus* are worldwide in areas with warm, moist climates and are widely overlapping.

Diagnosis: The standard method for diagnosing the presence of hookworm is by identifying hookworm eggs in a stool sample using a microscope. Because eggs may be difficult to find in light infections, a concentration procedure is recommended.

Management

Anthelminthic medications (drugs that rid the body of parasitic worms), such as albendazole and mebendazole are the drugs of choice for treatment of hookworm infections. Infections are generally treated for 1-3 days. The recommended medications are effective and appear to have few side effects. Iron supplements may also be prescribed if the infected person has anemia.

SHORT ESSAYS

4. Explain about water purification on small scale.

1. **Boiling:** Boiling is the oldest and satisfactory method of purification of water on small scale. Boiling for 5 to 10 minutes kills bacteria, spores, cysts and ova of intestinal parasites. It also removes hardness of water and soft water is produced. Boiling is an excellent method of purification of water provided boiling is done in a neat and clean vessel and after boiling it is stored in clean covered container. Preferably water should be boiled in the same container in which it is to be stored. Only that much amount of water should be boiled which can be used within a few hours.

2. **Distillation:** Distillation is also a good method of purification of water. During this method all kinds of dissolved impurities can be removed even the volatile one as well. For this purpose first and last portion of the distillate must be rejected because these portions may contain the volatile ingredients which may again contaminate the distilled water. Distillation is not possible for the purification of water to be used for routine household purposes.

3. **Filtration through muslin cloth:** Muslin cloth acts as a coarse filter which can remove the suspended materials. So water filtered through muslin is not fit for drinking purposes though it can be used for other household purposes like bathing, washing the clothes, etc.

4. **Three pitcher system:** This is very old system of purification of water. In this system three pitchers are used which are kept one above the other on a wooden stand. The top pitcher contains sand, second charcoal and sand; and the lowest collects the purified water. The raw water is filled in the first pitcher from where it percolates through a hole into the 2nd pitcher. From here the water further percolates through the hole to the third pitcher.

5. **Chemicals:** Various types of chemical agents used for disinfection of water are as follows:
   a. **Bleaching powder (Chlorinated lime):** Chemically it is $CaOCl_2$. A fresh sample of bleaching powder contains 33% of available chlorine but on storage it loses chlorine content. Therefore bleaching powder is stored in dry, air-tight containers and at cool and dark places.
   Roughly speaking 2.5 g of a good quality of bleaching powder could be required to disinfect 1,000 liters of water. Bleaching powder will not directly purify the turbid and polluted water. Therefore such water should first be treated with preliminary filtration and then subjected to chlorination.
   b. **Chlorine tablets:** These tablets are good for disinfecting small quantities of water. They are available in different strengths for disinfecting various quantities of water. One tablet of 500

mg is sufficient for disinfecting 20 liters of water. These are available in the market under various trade names, e.g. halozone tablets manufactured by the Boots company.

c. **Quick Lime (calcium oxide):** Some people prefer to use dry slaked lime than ordinary lime. About 360 mg of slaked lime will disinfect 4.5 liters of water. It is cheap, easily available and quite effective. Therefore it is recommended for disinfecting wells and tanks in cholera outbreak. Disadvantage of quick lime is that large doses of it are required for disinfection of water, i.e. 20 times than that of bleaching powder.

d. **High test hypochlorite (HTH):** It is a calcium compound and contains about 65–75 % of available chlorine. This is much stable compound and I g of HTH is needed for one cubic meter of water.

e. **Alum:** Alum is not a germicidal. It is used to purify muddy water and to remove turbidity. 60–240 mg of alum cans purity 4-5 liters of water. Calcium carbonate which is present in all kinds of water also gets precipitated as calcium sulfate and aluminum hydrate. The suspended impurities as well as bacteria also get precipitated which are removed after filtration and clear purified water is obtained.

f. **Potassium permanganate:** It is a strong oxidizing agent and can kill cholera vibrios but it does not destroy other disease producing organisms. It is used for disinfecting wells. Its dose is 0.5 parts per million (0.5 ppm). It is not suitable for disinfecting large volume of water.

Its disadvantages are that it alters the taste, smell and colour of water thus treated. Moreover this method is not considered dependable therefore no longer used for disinfecting the water.

6. **Domestic filters:** Water for drinking purposes can be purified by means of domestic filters which are discussed below:

   a. **Berkefeld filters:** These are cylindrical filters known as 'filter candles' or 'ceramic candles'. They are made up of unglazed porcelain or Kieselguhr and are available in various porosity grades. When water is purified through these candles the pores get clogged which need cleaning from time to time at least once a week by scrubbing with a hard brush and passing the water under pressure from inside to outside direction which will remove the entangled particles from the interstices.

   b. **Pasteur's chamber land filter:** It is made up of unglazed porcelain tubes which can be screwed on to a water tap. They work only under pressure and muddy water cannot be filtered through it because the pores will be immediately blocked.

   Therefore such water must be cleaned to remove mud. For cleaning the filters they are scrubbed from outside with a hard brush and water is made to pass under pressure from inside to outside. They are quick and reliable as they make the water free from all kinds of impurities including bacteria.

5. Explain different methods of disposal of waste in community.

There are eight major groups of waste management methods, each of them divided into numerous categories. Those groups include source reduction and reuse, animal feeding, recycling, composting, fermentation, landfills, incineration and land application. You can start using many techniques right at home like reduction and reuse which works to reduce the amount of disposable material used.

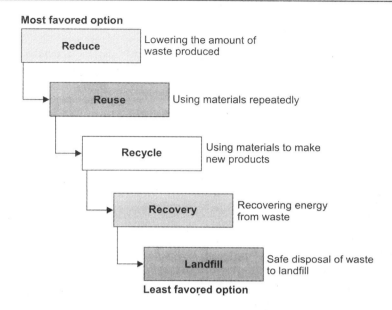

Methods of Waste Disposal

Landfill: The landfill is the most popularly used method of waste disposal used today. This process of waste disposal focuses attention on burying the waste in the land.

Incineration/combustion: Incineration or combustion is a type disposal method in which municipal solid wastes are burned at high temperatures so as to convert them into residue and gaseous products.

Recovery and recycling: Resource recovery is the process of taking useful discarded items for a specific next use. These discarded items are then processed to extract or recover materials and resources or convert them to energy in the form of useable heat, electricity or fuel. Recycling is the process of converting waste products into new products to prevent energy usage and consumption of fresh raw materials. Recycling is the third component of reduce, reuse and recycle waste hierarchy. The idea behind recycling is to reduce energy usage, reduce volume of landfills, reduce air and water pollution, reduce greenhouse gas emissions and preserve natural resources for future use.

Plasma gasification: Plasma gasification is another form of waste management. Plasma is a primarily an electrically charged or a highly ionized gas. Lighting is one type of plasma which produces temperatures that exceed 12,600 °F. With this method of waste disposal, a vessel uses characteristic plasma torches operating at +10,000 °F which is creating a gasification zone till 3,000 °F for the conversion of solid or liquid wastes into a syngas.

6. Write about types of ventilation.

Ventilation is the intentional introduction of outdoor air into a space and is mainly used to control indoor air quality by diluting and displacing indoor pollutants; it can also be used for purposes of thermal comfort or dehumidification.

Natural ventilation: Natural ventilation is the use of wind and temperature differences to create airflows in and through buildings. There are two basic types of natural ventilation effects: buoyancy and wind. Buoyancy ventilation is more commonly referred to as temperature-induced or stack ventilation. Wind ventilation supplies air from a positive pressure through openings on the windward side of a building and exhausts air to a negative pressure on the leeward side. Airflow rate depends on the wind speed and direction as well as the size of openings.

Task ventilation: Traditional ventilation systems supply a mixture of outside and recirculated air in high velocity jets so that the indoor air in rooms is often well mixed. This can be an inefficient method of delivering outside air to an occupant. Task-ambient conditioning (TAC) systems are a ventilation technology with the potential for improved ventilation to the occupant.

Mechanical ventilation: This system supplies the required airflow at a constant rate. Ventilation is supplied by forcing air through the ducting with the use of a fan. The use of the fan however uses a lot of energy and consequently greater CO_2 emissions.

Hybrid ventilation: Hybrid ventilation is the mix of natural and mechanical ventilation. In this project there is only one aspect of mechanical ventilation which contributes to the hybrid one: The fan which enhances the natural stack effect if the conditions are poor.

7. Measurement of mortality.

A mortality rate is a measure of the frequency of occurrence of death in a defined population during a specified interval.

The formula for calculating the mortality rate is as follows:

$$\text{Rate} = \frac{\text{Mortality Number of deaths in a given time period}}{\text{Population from which the deaths occurred in the same time period}} \times 10^n$$

When the mortality rate is based on vital statistics (e.g. counts of birth or death certificates), the denominator is usually the population at the midpoint of the given time period. In the English and Dutch-speaking Caribbean, a factor of 10^3 (1,000) or 10^4 (10,000) is used for most types of mortality rates. Here are some of the measures of mortality used most frequently:

1. Crude mortality rate
2. Cause-specific mortality rate
3. Proportionate mortality rate
4. Case-fatality rate
5. Age-specific rate
6. Neonatal mortality rate
7. Postneonatal mortality rate
8. Infant mortality rate
9. Fetal mortality rate
10. Perinatal mortality rate
11. Maternal mortality rate.

The following table summarizes the values of x, y and 10^n for each of these measures.

Measure	Numerator	Denominator	Expressed per number at risk (10^n)
Crude mortality rate	Total number of deaths reported during a given year	Estimated mid-year population	1,000 or 100,000
Cause-specific mortality rate	Deaths assigned to a specific cuase during a given year time interval	Estimated mid-year population	100,000
Proportionate mortality rate	Deaths assigned to a specific cause during a given year	Total number of deaths from all causes during the same year	100 or 1,000
Case-fatality rate	Deaths assigned to a specific disease during a given year	New cases of that disease reported during the same year	100
Age-specific mortality rate	Deaths in an age group in a year	Estimated mid-year population in that age group	1,000 or 100,000
Neonatgal mortality rate	Deaths under 28 days of age during a year	Live births during the same year	1,000
Postneonatal mortality rate	Deaths under 28 days to but not including 1 year of age during a year	Live births during the same year	1,000
Infant mortality rate	Deaths under 1 year of age during a year	Live births reported during the same year	1,000
Fetal mortality rate	Fetal deaths (28 weeks + gestation) in a year	Live births + fetal deaths during the same year	1,000
Perinatal mortality rate	Fetal deaths (28 weeks + gestation) + infant deaths <7 days of age in a year	Fetal deaths + live births during the same year	1,000
Maternal mortality rate	Deaths assigned to pregnancy related causes during a year	Live births during the same year	100,000

The figure below maps the time periods for some of the rates that apply to early life. You can see that some measures are subsets of others. For example, the infant mortality rate includes both the neonatal mortality rate and the postneonatal mortality rate.

8. Explain the steps of epidemiological investigation.

The primary reason for conducting outbreak investigations is to identify the source in order to establish control and to institute measures that will prevent future episodes of disease. They are also sometimes undertaken to train new personnel or to learn more about the disease and its mechanisms for transmission. Whether an outbreak investigation will be conducted may also be influenced by the severity of the disease, the potential for spread, the availability of resources, and sometimes by political considerations or the level of concern among the general public.

Steps of epidemiological investigation

Step 1: Prepare for field work
Step 2: Establish the existence of an outbreak
Step 3: Verify the diagnosis
Step 4: Define and identify cases
Step 5: Perform descriptive epidemiology
Step 6: Develop hypotheses
Step 7: Evaluate hypotheses
Step 8: Execute additional studies
Step 9: Implement control and prevention measures
Step 10: Communicate findings
Step 11: Follow-up recommendations

9. Signs and symptoms and management of cholera.

Signs and symptoms of cholera:

1. Watery diarrhea (sometimes in large volumes)
2. Rice-water stools
3. Fishy odor to stools.
4. Vomiting.
5. Rapid heart rate.
6. Loss of skin elasticity (washer woman hands sign.
7. Dry mucous membranes (dry mouth)
8. Low blood pressure.

Management of cholera:

Cholera requires immediate treatment because the disease can cause death within hours.

1. **Rehydration:** The goal is to replace lost fluids and electrolytes using a simple rehydration solution, oral rehydration salts (ORS). The ORS solution is available as a powder that can be reconstituted in boiled or bottled water. Without rehydration, approximately half the people with cholera die. With treatment, the number of fatalities drops to less than 1%.
2. **Intravenous fluids:** During a cholera epidemic, most people can be helped by oral rehydration alone, but severely dehydrated people may also need intravenous fluids.
3. **Antibiotics:** Antibiotics are not a necessary part of cholera treatment, some of these drugs may reduce both the amount and duration of cholera-related diarrhea for people who are severely ill.
4. **Zinc supplements:** Zinc may decrease and shorten the duration of diarrhea in children with cholera.

10. Write about DOTS.

Direct observed treatment short course (DOTS) is the WHO recommended strategy for tuberculosis control based on modern management technique. Tuberculosis control failed because of the reluctance of patients to continue treatment once the clinical features have subsided. DOTS involves the observation of the patient swallowing antituberculosis drugs by the doctor, health worker, or a volunteer.

The WHO endorsed strategy DOTS stands for Directly Observed Treatment Short course. DOTS is a very effective method of treatment of tuberculosis. It has a cure rate of 85%. It ensures patient compliance. It safeguards against the development of drug resistance. It was first introduced in 15 project areas, of which 10 in metropolitan cities and 5 in one district each of 5 states. Gradual DOTS is being extended to the entire country.

Following are the five tenets of DOTS:
1. Political commitment for sustained tuberculosis control.
2. Detection of tuberculosis cases by sputum smear microscopy of those who attend a healthcare facility and complain of cough for the past more than 3 weeks.
3. Standard treatment regimens for 6–8 months with direct observation for at least the first month.
4. Regular and uninterrupted supply of antitubercular drugs.
5. Systematic monitoring and accountability for each patient of tuberculosis.

Features
Following are the important features of DOTS:
1. Focus for early detection of tuberculosis is on sputum examination rather than on X-ray of chest.
2. Priority is accorded to the treatment of sputum positive cases.
3. Health workers or community volunteers visit the home of the patient and watch him or her swallow the drugs. This direct observation is continued till the patient is certified cured.
4. The system of patient registration, monitoring and follow-up is made rigorous.
5. Drugs are procured in time and in sufficient quantity, and their delivery is decentralized.

11. Explain modes of transmission of HIV.

HIV is transmitted in human body fluids by three major routes: (1) sexual intercourse through vaginal, rectal, or penile tissues; (2) direct injection with HIV-contaminated drugs, needles, syringes, blood or blood products; and (3) from HIV-infected mother to fetus in utero, through intrapartum inoculation from mother to infant or during breastfeeding (Stine 155). According to the CDC, HIV is not spread by tears, sweat, coughing or sneezing. Nor it is transmitted via a an infected person's clothes, phone, drinking glasses, eating utensils or other objects that HIV-infected people have used that are free of blood.

Sexual transmission: Sexual transmission of HIV happens when infected semen, blood , or vaginal secretions enter the bloodstream of a partner. Although HIV can be transmitted during vaginal or oral penetration, unprotected anal sex by a male or female seems to be the most dangerous. The risk to acquire HIV depends mainly on three factors: (1) the number of sexual partners; (2) the prevalence of HIV infection in these partners; (3) the probability of virus transmission during sexual contact.

Heterosexual HIV transmission: In 1985, less than 2% of AIDS cases were from the heterosexual population. However, by 1993 the number increased to a 8% of the total number of reported cases in the United States. Data demonstrate that heterosexually transmitted HIV infection is growing at a faster rate than homosexual or IDUs (Stine 180).

Injection drug users and HIV transmission: For 1996, from the total cases reported to the CDC, 36% were directly or indirectly associated with injecting-drug use. (Stine 188). Injecting-drug-user associated with AIDS cases include persons who are IDUs, their heterosexual sex partners and children whose mothers were IDUs or sex partners of IDUs.

Is HIV transmitted by insects: Epidemological data from Africa and the Unites States suggests that AIDS was not transmitted by insect bites. If this would be the case, many more cases would be reported among children and elderly people.

Other means of transmission: Rare cases have been reported to the CDC of HIV transmission via acupuncture, artificial insemination, tattoo, and human bite. Most of the incidents have occurred due to the use of a used needle and the transfusion of body fluids such as blood.

12. Explain barrier methods of contraception.

Barrier methods of birth control block sperm from entering the uterus. Using a spermicide with a barrier method gives you the best possible barrier method protection.
1. The spermicide kills most of the sperm that enter the vagina.
2. The barrier method then blocks any remaining sperm from passing through the cervix to fertilize an egg.

Barrier methods include the diaphragm, cervical cap, male condom, and female condom and spermicidal foam, sponges, and film. Unlike other methods of birth control, barrier methods are used only when you have sexual intercourse. Be sure to read the instructions before using a barrier method. It is very important that you use a barrier method correctly every time you have sex.

Barrier methods of birth control act as barriers to keep the man's sperm from reaching the woman's egg. Some barrier methods also protect against sexually transmitted infections (STIs). A few barrier methods (spermicide, condom, and sponge) can be bought in most drugstores. Others (diaphragm and cervical cap) must be prescribed by a healthcare professional.

Advantages of all Barrier Methods
Barrier methods of birth control:
1. Do not affect a woman's or man's future fertility.
2. Are only used at the time of sexual intercourse.
3. Are safe for a woman to use while she is breastfeeding.
4. Do not affect other health conditions, such as highblood pressure or diabetes.
5. Are less expensive than hormonal methods of birth control, and some are available without a prescription.

Condoms and diaphragms may reduce the risk of cervical cancer which is caused by a sexually transmitted human papillomavirus. Condoms also are the best method for reducing the risk of sexually transmitted infections including HIV.

Disadvantages of all barrier methods: Failure rates for barrier methods are higher than for most other methods of birth control. If you are considering using a barrier method for birth control, think through what the emotional and financial costs of an unintended pregnancy would be if the method fails.

To prevent pregnancy with a barrier method, you and your partner must be comfortable with using it and be prepared to use it every time you have sex. For some couples, barrier methods are not a good choice because one or both partners:
1. Find it embarrassing to use.
2. Do not want a barrier method to interrupt foreplay or intercourse.

SHORT ANSWERS

13. Define eugenics.

Eugenics is a movement that is aimed at improving the genetic composition of the human race. Historically, eugenicists advocated selective breeding to achieve these goals. Today we have technologies that make it possible to more directly alter the genetic composition of an individual. However, people differ in their views on how to best (and ethically) use this technology.

14. Mention the types of cohort.

A cohort is a defined group of people who have something in common. The characteristics, which the members of the group have in common, may take many different forms including age, presence of a particular disease, geographical area of residence and dietary habits.

Elements of cohort study
1. Selection of study subjects.
2. Obtaining data on exposure.
3. Comparison of groups.
4. Follow-up.
5. Analysis.

In a cohort study, subjects without the outcome of interest are assembled, classified according to characteristics which might be related to outcome, and then observed through time to determine which of them experience the outcome of interest. Such studies may be prospective, the cohort is assembled in the present and followed into the future (a concurrent cohort study), or retrospective, the cohort is assembled from past records and followed forward from that time (an historical cohort study). What characterizes cohort studies is that subjects are categorized on the basis of the independent variable (the causative variable is usually termed the independent variable and the outcome is termed the dependent variable)?

Types of cohort study:
1. **Prospective cohort study:** This is the most common and most scientific of cohort studies. It begins in the present and proceeds and terminates in the future.

Past	Present	Future	Type
	F →	D	Prospective
F →	D		Retrospective
F →	D + F →	D	Retrospective prospective

2. **Retrospective cohort study:** This is based on the data recorded in the past. The data pertains to persons with as well as persons without F. The data is concerned with both their demographic characteristics and their health status at repeated annual medical examinations. These data are scrutinized to determine how many persons with F and how many without it had developed D.
3. **Retrospective prospective cohort study:** In this first a retrospective cohort study is done. Afterwards the subjects are contacted and initiated into a prospective study.

15. Mention the effect of poor lighting.

1. **Accidents:** One of the most serious problems of bad lighting is accidents. Poor lighting can become a danger in the workplace because it is hard to see things like the proximity, speed, depth, and exact shape of the things around you. This can lead to employees tripping and falling, causing serious injuries in some cases.
2. **Squinting:** When an employee cannot see what they are working on clearly, they start to squint and strain their eyes. This constant straining will make them uncomfortable, and they could end up with irritated eyes including burning, tearing, or dryness.
3. **Headaches:** Whether the light is too dim or too bright, your employees could suffer from extreme headaches. If they are working in the same location frequently, these headaches can start to repeat. Employees who are in pain or discomfort will find it difficult to focus on their work which will also affect what they can get done.
4. **Lack of productivity:** Bad lighting can actually make your employees less productive. And if your employees are less productive than they should be, you are entire business will suffer. Dim lights can cause employees to become drowsy and work slower than normal.
5. **Bad posture/discomfort:** A side effect of feeling drowsy and having to squint and lean forward to see your work is slouching.

16. Define sex ratio.

The sex ratio is the ratio of males to females in a population. In most sexually reproducing species, the ratio tends to be 1:1. This tendency is explained by Fisher's principle. For various reasons, however, many species deviate from anything like an even sex ratio, either periodically or permanently.

17. Safe period method of fertility control.

The fertility awareness method (FAM) is a natural family planning strategy that women can use to help prevent pregnancy. ... In the rhythm method and in FAM, you abstain from sex (periodic abstinence) during your most fertile days. Alternately, you can use backup contraception on your fertile days.

These are some common methods incorporated into fertility awareness:

Calendar rhythm method: Use past menstrual cycles to estimate the time of your ovulation. When used on its own, this is the least reliable method of birth control. It should be avoided if your menstrual cycles are shorter than 26 days or longer than 32 days.

Temperature method: Basal body temperature for several cycles by using a very sensitive basal thermometer to take the temperature before you get out of bed each morning. Due to hormonal surges, your BBT goes up right after ovulation.

Cervical mucus method: Track the color, thickness, and texture of the cervical mucus to monitor your fertility. The cervical mucus becomes thinner, slippery, and stretchy when you ovulate.

18. Define eligible couple.

- Definition: A currently married couple wherein the wife is in the reproductive age (i.e. 15–49 years of age)
- Approximately 150–180 eligible couples per 1,000 population in India
- These couples are in need of family planning services
- The "eligible couple register" is maintained and updated by the ANM/MPHW/ASHA.

19. Mantoux test.

The Mantoux test or Mendel–Mantoux test (also known as the Mantoux screening test, tuberculin sensitivity test, Pirquet test, or PPD test for purified protein derivative) is a tool for screening for tuberculosis (TB) and for tuberculosis diagnosis.

20. Define food hygiene.

Food hygiene is the conditions and measures necessary to ensure the safety of food from production to consumption. Food can become contaminated at any point during slaughtering or harvesting, processing, storage, distribution, transportation and preparation. Lack of adequate food hygiene can lead to foodborne diseases and death of the consumer.

21. Mention the causes of obesity.

Obesity generally is on account of overnutrition and is called "regulatory obesity." Genetic, endocrinal, metabolic, and other non-nutritional causes account for a small fraction of obesity; these are the cases of "metabolic obesity."

Regulatory obesity is because of an imbalance between the needs and the intake of energy.

The obese person is consuming more food than necessary for the body and is indulging in less activity than that required for burning the food.

Obesity results from eating excessive amounts of sweets, chocolates, toffees, ghee, egg, butter, fried foods, and the like. Often the foundation of adulthood obesity is laid when the infant is overfed. Such overfeeding increases the number of infant's adipose cells. In later life, these abundant cells help store excessive amounts of fat and produce obesity.

Psychological factors can lead to overeating: For instance, the individual, who is under constant emotional strain, finds satisfaction in food; in other words eating provides him an outlet for his pent-up unpleasant feelings. Another motive for overeating is the yearning for companionship. This forces the individual to spend much time in the company of friends and foods.

22. List for zoonotic diseases. (See Q. 17, 2014)

2016

Community Health Nursing-I

LONG ESSAYS

1. a. Define health. b. Explain the factors which influence the health of an individual.
2. a. Define epidemiology. b. List the uses of epidemiology. c. As a community health nurse what are the steps you will follow to investigate an epidemic.
3. a. What are the general accepted goals of housing. b. Explain the minimum standards for housing.

SHORT ESSAYS

4. Scope of family planning as stated by WHO expert committee 1970.
5. Methods of data collection.
6. Three widely used methods of pasteurization.
7. Prevention and control of air pollution.
8. Approaches to control noise.
9. Controlled tipping as a method of refuse disposal.
10. Clinical features of chickenpox.
11. Prevention and control of food poisoning.
12. Causes of obesity.

SHORT ANSWERS

13. Define prevalence.
14. Enlist role of VCT in HIV prevention and care.
15. Define wholesome water.
16. Define infant mortality rate.
17. Mention two uses of epidemiology.
18. Iceberg phenomena of disease.
19. Active immunity.
20. Define demography.
21. Four causes of iron deficiency anemia.
22. Define food fortification.

LONG ESSAYS

1. a. Define health. b. Explain the factors which influence the health of an individual.

Definition

Health is defined as a "state characterized by anatomic, physiologic, and psychological integrity; ability to perform personally valued family, work, and community roles; ability to deal with physical, biologic, psychological, and social stress". Then, in 1948, in a radical departure from previous definitions, the WHO proposed a definition that aimed higher, linking health to well-being, in terms of "physical, mental, and social well-being, and not merely the absence of disease and infirmity". Although this definition was welcomed by some as being innovative and exciting, it was also criticized as being vague, excessively broad, and unmeasurable. For a long time, it was set aside as an impractical ideal and most discussions of health returned to the practicality of the biomedical model.

Factors which influence the health of an individual.

Many factors combine together to affect the health of individuals and communities. Whether people are healthy or not, is determined by their circumstances and environment. To a large extent, factors, such as where we live, the state of our environment, genetics, our income and education level, and our relationships with friends and family all have considerable impacts on health, whereas the more commonly considered factors, such as access and use of healthcare services often have less of an impact.

The determinants of health include:
1. The social and economic environment,
2. The physical environment, and
3. The person's individual characteristics and behaviors.

The context of people's lives determines their health, and so blaming individuals for having poor health or crediting them for good health is inappropriate. Individuals are unlikely to be able to directly control many of the determinants of health. These determinants or things that make people healthy or not include the above factors, and many others:

1. **Income and social status:** Higher income and social status are linked to better health. The greater the gap between the richest and poorest people, the greater the differences in health.
2. **Education:** Low education levels are linked with poor health, more stress and lower self-confidence.
3. **Physical environment:** Safe water and clean air, healthy workplaces, safe houses, communities and roads all contribute to good health. Employment and working conditions—people in employment are healthier particularly those who have more control over their working conditions.
4. **Social support networks:** Greater support from families, friends and communities are linked to better health. Culture—customs and traditions, and the beliefs of the family and community all affect health.
5. **Genetics:** Inheritance plays a part in determining lifespan, healthiness and the likelihood of developing certain illnesses. Personal behavior and coping skills-balanced eating, keeping active, smoking, drinking, and how we deal with life's stresses and challenges all affect health.
6. **Health services:** Access and use of services that prevent and treat disease influences health
7. **Gender:** Men and women suffer from different types of diseases at different ages.

2. a. Define epidemiology. b. List the uses of epidemiology. c. As a community health nurse, what are the steps you will follow to investigate an epidemic.

Epidemiology is the study of frequency, distribution and determinants of health-related states in human populations. The study is followed by establishing programs to prevent or control health problems. The objective of epidemiology is to determine the effective strategies for the control of diseases. These are based on the elimination, modification and manipulation of the determinants and risk factors of diseases. Epidemiology is a body of knowledge culled through field studies. The aim of these studies is to find out the differences between (a) those persons who have the disease and those who do not, (b) those places where the disease is common and those places where it is rare, and (c) those times when the disease is common and those when it is uncommon.

Definitions

1. Epidemiology is the study of various factors and conditions that determine the occurrence and distribution of health, disease defect, disability and death among groups of individuals (Clark 1965).
2. Epidemiology is the study of the distribution of a disease or a physiological condition in human population and of the factors that influence this distribution (Lilienfeld 1980).
3. Epidemiology is the study of distribution and determinants of disease frequency in man (Mohom 1960).

Uses of Epidemiology

1. **Epidemiology completes the natural history of disease** by providing information about the behavior of the disease in its early stages (before it has become serious or advanced enough to require hospitalization). This information complements the conventional knowledge about it based on the study of its advanced cases found in hospitals.
2. **Epidemiology helps identify the precursors of disease:** Leukoplakia as the precursor of for oral cancer, and *Helicobacter pylori* infection as that of duodenal ulcer were identified by epidemiological studies.
3. **Epidemiology helps identify syndromes:** For instance, it has enabled the epidemiologist to learn that the following clinical features do not indicate separate disease entities, but constitute the single syndrome of AIDS: Chronic cough. Loss of weight in spite of normal eating habits.
4. **Epidemiology helps identify the spectrum of diseases** occurring as the sequelae of a single condition. Diseases of heart, kidney and brain can all follow hypertension.
5. **Epidemiology helps elucidate the risk factors of diseases** where they are not known. Examples are the administration of oxygen to infants as the risk factor for retrolental fibroplasias, the use of thalidomide by pregnant women as that for phocomelia in their babies, and raised serum cholesterol as that for coronary artery disease.
6. **Epidemiology helps determine the effective methods of control** of diseases where they are not known. The historical example of this is the epidemiological study of the cholera epidemic in Broad street of London by Dr John Snow and his recommendation that the handle of the contaminated borewell be removed (so that people would not be able to drink its contaminated water).
7. **Epidemiology helps in community diagnosis:** Community diagnosis is the assessment of the health needs of the community. Data about population, births, deaths, diseases, health resources and people's lifestyles are obtained through epidemiological studies. The data are

analyzed to determine what the priority health problems of the community are. A plan of action to address these is then prepared.
8. **Epidemiology helps predict the future** behavior of the disease. Based on the epidemiologically noted fact that AIDS predisposes to tuberculosis, it can be predicted that the incidence of tuberculosis will show a rise in the years to come.
9. **The other uses of epidemiology are the following:** a. It helps identify factors that block the ongoing control programs, b. It provides guidelines for revising medical education syllabus in the country, c. It helps identify the priority areas for medical research, d. It facilitates the standardization of biostatistician techniques.

Nurses Role

Epidemiology process is bound to continue in future adding new challenges to the practice of public health. In these circumstances, epidemiology is designed to play an increasingly important role in defining the magnitude of the problems, forecasting their long-term consequences and deriving appropriate strategies for their promotion and control. Presently, the use of epidemiology is mainly confined to following areas:
1. **Disease antecedents:** Epidemiology has always stressed the importance of exploring the natural history of disease in their entirely, with special stress on the identification of disease antecedents rather than disease consequents.
2. **Disease correlates:** Epidemiology has revolutionized the concept of etiology and etiogenesis. Epidemiological studies identified a variety of disease correlates not all of which are casually associated diseases, and some of which behave as risk factors the risk factors the increase the probability of contracting a particular disease.
3. **Disease behavior:** Epidemiological surveillance is applied to disease of international significance. Disease behavior is studied by a process of epidemiological surveillance whereby diseases are kept under constant observation firstly to identify their normal distribution patterns and normal temporal fluctuations, and secondly to detect any deviation in their expected behavior patterns.
4. **Disease and causation:** Epidemiological studies not only establish cause effect association of many noncommunicable diseases, but also estimate the strength of associations in terms of relative and absolute risks. The most notable example are the cause effect associations established by epidemiological studies between smoking and lung cancer and smoking and coronary heart diseases.
5. **Strategy formulation**: Epidemiology plays an important role in strategy formulation for disease control programs and improves program efficiency and effectiveness. Control and eradication of disease is much more complex than their prevention or treatment. A sound control strategy is one that epidemiologically relevant and operationally feasible.
6. **Program evaluation:** Program performance is evaluated by measuring achievements in various operational areas of the program. Evaluation of public health program is both managerial and epidemiological process.

3. a. What are the general accepted goals of housing? b. Explain the minimum standards for housing.

Maslow's classic model places human needs on a hierarchy. This means that new needs emerge when those lower on the hierarchy are relatively well gratified. So necessities in man's life demands for shelter in which he makes his abode (a home) for healthy living. The natural tendency of man's behavior for shelter is wide, that has resulted in creating modern dwelling to live.

Meaning of Housing

Housing" means homes to live in. House refers to a physical structure where unit of society, the family lives but the concept is slowly changing to "Human settlement" which allow the extended out look of a house, where people live, interact and pursue their goals. A WHO Expert Group (1961) has coined the word residential environment which is used by man for his activity and desired devices for his family well-being.

Importance of Housing

Healthy housing plays a vital role in the total welfare of the individuals, families and community. If the houses are poor in construction and sanitation, and are overcrowded, they will lead to diseases, accidents, etc. where by the welfare of whole community as a whole is effected eventually. Therefore good housing is essential for every individual.

Need of Housing

Every person or family lives in different types of houses based on their need and economical status. The following needs of a man have to be fulfilled through good housing:
1. **Physical needs:** A house should be well ventilated with fresh air, adequate lighting to provide comfort.
2. **Physiological needs:** Like privacy and family life. This will provide man's satisfaction.
3. **Psychological needs:** A man will have feeling of having dignity, status in community life, respect of family and satisfaction.
4. **Health needs:** Health needs like adequate water, sanitary latrine, balanced diet, protection from insects and animals through good housing.
5. **Protective needs:** Like safety from accidents. Protection from fire hazards, defaults in electricity, poor flooring can be prevented through strong safe dwellings.

Goals of Housing

Goals are statements about desirable conditions. The goals of housing are:
1. **Shelter:** It is a basic need. The house should provide a sanitary shelter.
2. **Family life:** House should provide adequate space for family life and related activities viz., preparation and storage of food, meeting, sleeping, etc.
3. **Access to community facilities:** One of the important elements of housing is accessibility to community services like health services, schools, shopping areas, places of worships, etc.
4. **Economic stability:** Housing is a form of investment. It provides economic stability and well-being of the family.
5. **Family participation:** In community life, family is a part of community. It is an important source of friends. Community focuses on to improve their living conditions.

The implementation of goals of housing by government should be:
a. Introduce housing schemes.
b. Establish housing standards.
c. Create financial support to improve the housing.

Healthful Housing

American Public Health Association has given basic principles of healthful housing on similar lines. WHO has given following healthful housing criteria:
1. It gives physical protection and shelter.
2. Adequate provision for cooking, eating, washing and excretory functions.
3. It prevents spread of infections and communicable diseases.
4. Protects from noise.

5. Protects from atmosphere pollutions.
6. Housing material is free from toxic and harmful chemicals.
7. Encourage personality development.
8. Promote mental health.
9. To attain social goals like:
    a. Family life.
    b. Access to community facility.
    c. Social participation.
    d. Economic stability.

Basic Factors in Housing or Housing Standards

Housing is the modern concept is broadening of houses. Various factors are taken into consideration in determining housing standards. These standards vary from one region to another region.

Aim

Improvement of housing and environmental conditions for the majority of families within the limits set by available resources and objectives. Environmental Hygiene Committee of Government of India has given some minimum housing standards that are to be maintained by building regulations through municipality, corporation, town planning and urban development authorities.

Site

The site should be elevated from its surroundings:
- Adequate width
- Away from breedy places of flies.
- Away from nuisance, such as noise, smoke, dust.
- Should have clean surroundings.
- Structure should be well drained.

1. Site of house: In an elevated place in a residential area of town and subsoil water must be below 10 feet.
2. Set back: The built up area is restricted to 2/3rd of site. Wind direction and ventilation are considered.
3. Cubic space: It should be 500 cubic feet per person.
4. Floor: Pucca floor, no crack and damp floor.
5. Floor Area: 100 square feet per person.
6. Roof: It should be more than 10 feet.
7. Walls: Strong and weather resistant.
8. Rooms: According to family size and need of privacy, number of rooms is suggested.
9. Windows: Window area should be 1/5th of floor area.
10. Lightening: It is expected to have a day light factor (DF) of 1.0 or above 1.0.
11. Water supply: Safe and whole some water supply is guaranteed.
12. Washing: Should have provision for washing facility
13. Bathing facility: House should have adequate bathing facility.
14. Kitchen: Adequate provision of separate sanitary area for food preparation.
15. Privy: Sanitary RCA latrine and water carriage system is a must under criteria of healthful housing.
16. Refusal disposal: Daily disposal and transport for sanitary disposal is advocated.

SHORT ESSAYS

4. Scope of family planning as stated by WHO expert committee 1970.

Family planning basically means planning the number of children in the family. It is "limiting the size of the family by conscious efforts." The motto of family planning is "child by choice and not by chance". Family planning can be defined as an instrument of social transformation which aims at creating better parents, healthier children and happier homes. It seeks to inject social responsibility into married life. Family planning is described by an Expert Committee of the WHO in the following manner. "Family planning refers to practices that help individuals or couples to attain certain objectives".
1. To avoid unwanted births
2. To bring about wanted births
3. To regulate the intervals between pregnancies
4. To control the time at which births occur in relation to the ages of the parent; and
5. To determine the number of children in the family. "Family planning as a basic human right".

The United Nations Conference on Human Rights at Tehran in 1968 recognized family planning as a basic human right. The World Conference of the Women's Year in 1975 also declared – "the right of women to decide freely and responsibly on the number and spacing of their children and to have access to the information and means to enable them to exercise that right."

Scope of Family Planning Services

It is unfair to think that family planning is just equal to birth control. In fact, it is something more than mere birth control. WHO Expert Committee (1970) has stated that family planning includes in its purview the following aspects: 1. The proper spacing and limitation of births, 2. Advice on sterility, 3. Education for parenthood, 4. Sex education, 5. Genetic counseling, 6. Premarital consultation and examination, 7. Carrying out pregnancy tests, 8. Marriage counseling, 9. Preparation of couples for the arrival of their first child, 10. Providing services for unmarried mothers, 11. Teaching home economics and nutrition. 12. Providing adoption services. These activities vary from country-to-country according to national objectives and policies with regard to family planning.

Renaming of "Family Planning Program" as "Family Welfare Program"

The Government of India evinced greater interest in controlling population growth in 1976. During the emergency (1976–78) compulsory sterilization was carried on at great speed through coercive measures in various places in North India. For example, in 1976, more than 76 lakh sterilizations were carried out against a target of 43 lakh. Coercive methods adopted for the implementation of the program during this period resulted in people's discontentment. Hence the Janata Government, which came to power soon after emergency, wanted to follow a soft policy. It announced a comprehensive population policy in that year. Family planning program was renamed as "Family Welfare Program". This welfare program has experienced several ups and downs in its performance over time.

Government's efforts at controlling population through family planning/welfare program have not yielded consistent results. The program has experienced several ups and downs in its performance over time. For example, the number of sterilizations increased from around 7,000 in 1956 to 1.84 million in 1970–71. This figure increased to 2.19 million during 1971–72 but it came down to 0.94 million during 1973–74. This decline was particularly due to abandonment of camp approach. During the emergency period (1975–77) sterilization performance of sterilizations was really good (about 8.26 million sterilization cases in 1976–77 alone).

The performance of sterilization came down particularly after emergency. But the trend nowadays is slowly changing in favor of family welfare program. Particularly, in the nineties the total program seems to have greater acceptance among the public. The central government has been investing more and more money for the implementation of the family welfare programs through its five-year plans. The Government, for example, spent a meagre amount of ₹ 65 lakhs for this purpose in the First Five-Year Plan. The Government, however, started spending more and more money towards the program in the other Plans. For example, it spent ₹ 27 crores in the Third Plan, ₹ 497 crores in the Fifth Plan, ₹ 1,010 crores in the Sixth Plan, ₹ 3,221 crores in the Seventh Plan and ₹ 6,792 crores in the Eighth Plan. The Ninth Plan allocated ₹ 14,194 crores for this program.

5. Methods of data collection.

There are various methods of data collection. A 'Method' is different from a 'Tool.' While a method refers to the way or mode of gathering data, a tool is an instrument used for the method. For example, a schedule is used for interviewing. The important methods are (a) observation, (b) interviewing, (c) mail survey, (d) experimentation, (e) simulation, and (f) projective technique. To collect primary data during the course of doing experiments in an experimental research but in case we do research of the descriptive type and perform surveys, whether sample surveys or census surveys, then we can obtain primary data either through observation or through direct communication with respondents in one form or another or through personal interviews.

This, in other words, means that there are several methods of collecting primary data, particularly in surveys and descriptive researches. Important ones are: (i) observation method, (ii) interview method, (iii) through questionnaires, (iv) through schedules and (v) other methods which include (a) warranty cards; (b) distributor audits; (c) pantry audits; (d) consumer panels; (e) using mechanical devices; (f) through projective techniques; (g) depth interviews, and (h) content analysis. Observations involves gathering of data relating to the selected research by viewing and or listening. Interviewing involves face-to-face conversation between the investigator and the respondent. Mailing is used for collecting data by getting questionnaires completed by respondents. Experimentation involves a study of independent variables under controlled conditions. Experiments may be conducted in a laboratory or in field in a natural setting. Simulation involves creation of an artificial situation similar to the actual life situation. Projective methods aim at drawing inferences on the characteristics of respondents by presenting to them stimuli. Even method has its advantages and disadvantages.

1. **Registration:** The registers and licensees are particularly valuable for complete enumeration, but are limited to variables that change slowly, such as numbers of fishing vessels and their characteristics
2. **Questionnaires:** The forms which are completed and returned by respondents. An inexpensive method that is useful where literacy rates are high and respondents are cooperative.
3. **Interviews:** The forms which are completed through an interview with the respondent. More expensive than questionnaires, but they are better for more complex questions, low literacy or less cooperation.
4. **Direct observations:** The making direct measurements is the most accurate method for many variables, such as catch, but is often expensive. Many methods, such as observer programs, are limited to industrial fisheries.
5. **Reporting:** The main alternative to making direct measurements is to require fishers and others to report their activities. Reporting requires literacy and cooperation, but can be backed up by a legal requirement and direct measurements.

6. **Census:** It is a population estimate and is a process of complete enumeration of all individuals in a country on a fixed day. It contains aspects like general, economic, social, cultural, migration, establishments, fertility and special information. First recorded census in the world was done in 1749 at Sweden. In India, it started in 1872 and every ten years since then. Recent census, the fourteenth decennial census of India took place in 2001. Depending on requirement and utility, improvements are made in each census. The legal basis is provided by the Central Act of 1948. Based on census data, various indicators are developed and used in national health planning.
7. **Ad-hoc survey:** The surveys for evaluating the health status of a population that is community diagnosis of problems of health and disease. It is information about the distribution of these problems over time and space that provides the functional basis for planning and developing needed services.

6. Three widely used methods of pasteurization.

Pasteurization is a heat treatment that destroys pathogenic organisms (bacteria, viruses, protozoa, molds and yeasts) in foodstuffs to reduce the total bacterial count. The process, introduced in 1862 by the French scientist, Louis Pasteur, is vitally important to the food, beverage and dairy industries, ensuring the safe consumption of such foods as milk, cream, cheese, fruit juices, honey and eggs, as well as extending their shelf lives. Pasteur established that by heating milk to 145° F for 30 minutes, 99.9% of the bacteria present were destroyed. Since then series of time-temperature curves have been developed for all known microorganisms to consistently provide "a 5-log kill," the industry's terminology for the destruction of 99.999% of the microorganisms present in a product. Unlike sterilization, pasteurization is not intended to kill all the microorganisms in the food or dairy product and is designed to cause little, if any, degradation of the foodstuff in terms of color, aroma or flavor.

1. **High-temperature short-time (HTST) pasteurization,** or flash pasteurization, is the most common method these days, especially for higher volume processing. This method is faster and more energy efficient than batch pasteurization. Though the higher temperature may give the milk a slightly cooked flavor, HTST pasteurization has been used for so long that people are used to the flavor. HTST milk is forced between metal plates or through pipes heated on the outside by hot water, and the milk is heated to 72°C (161°F) for 15 seconds.
2. **UHT,** also known as ultra-heat-treating, processing holds the milk at a temperature of 140°C (284 °F) for 4 seconds.
3. **Batch (or "vat") pasteurization** is the simplest and oldest method for pasteurizing milk. Milk is heated to 154.4°F (63°C) in a large container and held at that temperature for 30 minutes. This process can be carried out at home on the stovetop using a large pot or, for small-scale dairies, with steam-heated kettles and fancy temperature control equipment. In batch processing, the milk has to be stirred constantly to make sure that each particle of milk is heated.

7. Prevention and control of air pollution.

Air Pollution
It is an undesirable change in the physical, chemical or biological characteristics of air.

Air Pollutants
They are the substances which pollute the air. Some of the common pollutants are dust, soot, ash, carbon monoxide, excess of carbon dioxide, sulfur dioxide, oxides of nitrogen, hydrocarbons,

chlorofluorocarbons (CFC), lead compounds, asbestos dust, cement dust, pollens and radioactive rays.

Sources of Air Pollution

The pollution of air can be caused by natural processes or by human activities.

The sources of air pollution are classified into two groups:
1. Natural sources
2. Manmade sources.

Natural sources of air pollution: They are dust storms, forest fires, ash from smoking volcanoes, decay of organic matters and pollen grains floating in air.

Manmade sources of air pollution: They are population explosion, deforestation, urbanization and industrialization, whose effects can be explained as follows:
1. Burning of fuels like wood, cow dung cakes, coal and kerosene in homes pollute the air.
2. Exhaust gases emitted by motor vehicles which pollute the air are the major source of air pollution in big cities.
3. Industries pollute air by releasing various types of pollutants, such as sulfur dioxide, oxides of carbon, nitrogen oxide, chlorine, asbestos dust and cement dust.
4. Thermal power plants pollute air by emitting sulfur dioxide and fly-ash.
5. Nuclear power plants pollute air by releasing radioactive rays.
6. Use of fertilizers and pesticides in agriculture pollute the air.
7. Mining activities releases particulate matter into the air and pollutes it.
8. Indiscriminate cutting of trees and clearing of forests increases the amount of carbon dioxide in the atmosphere and thereby pollutes it.
9. Use of chlorofluorocarbons in refrigeration, fire extinguishers and aerosol sprayers pollutes air by depleting the ozone layer.
10. Smoking pollutes air by emitting carbon monoxide and nicotine.

Harmful Effects of Air Pollution
1. Air pollution affects respiratory system causing breathing difficulties and diseases, such as bronchitis, asthma, lung cancer, tuberculosis and pneumonia.
2. Air pollution affects the central nervous system causing carbon monoxide poisoning. CO has more affinity for hemoglobin than oxygen and thus forms a stable compound carboxyhemoglobin (COHb), which is poisonous and causes suffocation and death.
5. Air pollution causes depletion of ozone layer due to which ultraviolet radiations can reach the earth and cause skin cancer, damage to eyes and immune system.
6. It causes acid rain which damages crop plants, trees, buildings, monuments, statues and metal structures and also makes the soil acidic.
7. It causes greenhouse effect or global warming which leads to excessive heating of earth's atmosphere, further leading to weather variability and rise in sea level. The increased temperature may cause melting of ice caps and glaciers, resulting in floods.
8. Air pollution from certain metals, pesticides and fungicides causes serious ailments.
    a. Lead pollution causes anemia, brain damage, convulsions and death.
    b. Certain metals cause problem in kidney, liver, circulatory system and nervous system.
    c. Fungicides cause nerve damage and death.
    d. Pesticides like dichloro diphenyl trichloroethane (DDT) which are toxic enter into our food chain and gets accumulated in the body causing kidney disorders and problems of brain and circulatory system.

Prevention and Control of Air Pollution

Different techniques are used for controlling air pollution caused by 'gaseous pollutants' and that caused by 'particulate pollutants'.

1. **Methods of controlling gaseous pollutants:** The air pollution caused by gaseous pollutants like hydrocarbons, sulfur dioxide, ammonia, carbon monoxide, etc. can be controlled by using three different methods—combustion, absorption and adsorption.
2. **Combustion:** This technique is applied when the pollutants are organic gases or vapors. The organic air pollutants are subjected to 'flame combustion or catalytic combustion' when they are converted to less harmful product carbon dioxide and a harmless product water.
3. **Absorption:** In this method, the polluted air containing gaseous pollutants is passed through a scrubber containing a suitable liquid absorbent. The liquid absorbs the harmful gaseous pollutants present in air.
4. **Adsorption:** In this method, the polluted air is passed through porous solid adsorbents kept in suitable containers. The gaseous pollutants are adsorbed at the surface of the porous solid and clean air passes through.
5. **Methods of controlling particulate emissions:** The air pollution caused by particulate matter like dust, soot, ash, etc. can be controlled by using fabric filters, wet scrubbers, electrostatic precipitators and certain mechanical devices.
    I. **Mechanical devices:** It works on the basis of following:
       Gravity: In this process, the particulate settle down by the action of gravitational force and get removed.
       Sudden change in the direction of air flow: It brings about separation of particles due to greater momentum.
    II. **Fabric filters:** The particulate matter is passed through a porous medium made of woven or filled fabrics.
        a. The particulate present in the polluted air are filtered and gets collected in the fabric filters, while the gases are discharged.
        b. The process of controlling air pollution by using fabric filters is called 'bag filtration'.
    III. **Wet scrubbers:** They are used to trap SO_2, NH_3 and metal fumes by passing the fumes through water.
    IV. **Electrostatic precipitators:** When the polluted air containing particulate pollutants is passed through an electrostatic precipitator, it induces electric charge on the particles and then the aerosol particles get precipitated on the electrodes.

Some other methods of controlling air pollution

1. Tall chimneys should be installed in factories.
2. Better designed equipment and smokeless fuels should be used in homes and industries.
3. Renewable and nonpolluting sources of energy like solar energy, wind energy, etc. should be used.
4. Automobiles should be properly maintained and adhere to emission control standards.
5. More trees should be planted along roadsides and houses.

8. Approaches to control noise.

A noise problem starts with a noise source, such as a stream of traffic on a highway. The noise is transmitted through a path and then arrives at the receiver. The noise will be perceived as a problem when the noise is so high as to be a nuisance to the receiver.

Impacts of Noise
Some of the adverse effects are summarized below:
- **Annoyance:** It creates annoyance to the receptors due to sound level fluctuations. The aperiodic sound due to its irregular occurrences causes displeasure to hearing and causes annoyance.
- **Physiological effects:** The physiological features like breathing amplitude, blood pressure, heart-beat rate, pulse rate, blood cholesterol are effected.
- **Loss of hearing:** Long exposure to high sound levels cause loss of hearing. This is mostly unnoticed, but has an adverse impact on hearing function.
- **Human performance:** The working performance of workers/human will be affected as they will be losing their concentration.
- **Nervous system:** It causes pain, ringing in the ears, feeling of tiredness, thereby effecting the functioning of human system.
- **Sleeplessness:** It affects the sleeping there by inducing the people to become restless and lose concentration and presence of mind during their activities.
- **Damage to material:** The buildings and materials may get damaged by exposure to infrasonic/ultrasonic waves and even get collapsed.

Noise Control at Source
The noise pollution can be controlled at the source of generation itself by employing techniques like:
- Reducing the noise levels from domestic sectors: The domestic noise coming from radio, tape recorders, television sets, mixers, washing machines, cooking operations can be minimized by their selective and judicious operation. By usage of carpets or any absorbing material, the noise generated from felling of items in house can be minimized.
- Maintenance of automobiles: Regular servicing and tuning of vehicles will reduce the noise levels. Fixing of silencers to automobiles, two wheelers, etc. will reduce the noise levels.
- Control over vibrations: The vibrations of materials may be controlled using proper foundations, rubber padding, etc. to reduce the noise levels caused by vibrations.
- Low voice speaking: Speaking at low voices enough for communication reduces the excess noise levels.
- Prohibition on usage of loud speakers: By not permitting the usage of loudspeakers in the habitant zones except for important meetings/functions. Nowadays, the urban administration of the metro cities in India, is becoming stringent on usage of loudspeakers.
- Selection of machinery: Optimum selection of machinery tools or equipment reduces excess noise levels. For example selection of chairs, or selection of certain machinery/equipment which generate less noise (sound) due to its superior technology, etc. is also an important factor in noise minimization strategy.
- Maintenance of machines: Proper lubrication and maintenance of machines, vehicles, etc. will reduce noise levels. For example, it is a common experience that, many parts of a vehicle will become loose while on a rugged path of journey. If these loose parts are not properly fitted, they will generate noise and cause annoyance to the driver/passenger. Similarly is the case of machines. Proper handling and regular maintenance is essential not only for noise control but also to improve the life of machine.

The severity of the problem depends on the strength of the noise source (such as heavy or light traffic) or the length of the path, that is, how large is the separation between the noise

source and the receiver. An effective approach to noise control approach will usually consist of the following three steps (in order):
1. **Eliminate:** It is the noise necessary in the first place? Is there an alternative way to achieve the same outcome? For example, through different processes, using different machinery or adapting existing machinery (including using different parts).
2. **Isolate:** If the noise cannot be eliminated, can the machinery be enclosed to reduce the noise? Can it be placed in another area away from people?
3. **Minimize:** If it is not possible to eliminate or isolate the noise, how can it be minimized? For example, can people be moved around the plant to reduce their exposure? Are the correct classes of hearing protection devices (HPDs) being worn? To help you identify the best solution for your workplace, you should first undertake some analysis of the problem.

9. Controlled tipping as a method of refuse disposal.

Sanitary landfill, method of controlled disposal of municipal solid waste (refuse) on land. The method was introduced in England in 1912 (where it is called controlled tipping). Waste is deposited in thin layers (up to 1 meter, or 3 feet) and promptly compacted by heavy machinery (e.g. bulldozers); several layers are placed and compacted on top of each other to form a refuse cell (up to 3 meters, or 10 feet, thick). At the end of each day the compacted refuse cell is covered with a layer of compacted soil to prevent odors and windblown debris. All modern landfill sites are carefully selected and prepared (e.g. sealed with impermeable synthetic bottom liners) to prevent pollution of ground water or other environmental problems. When the landfill is completed, it is capped with a layer of clay or a synthetic liner in order to prevent water from entering. A final topsoil cover is placed, compacted, and graded, and various forms of vegetation may be planted in order to reclaim otherwise useless land e.g. to fill declivities to levels convenient for building parks, golf courses, or other suitable public projects.

Controlled tipping or controlled burial is similar in principle to sanitary landfill but at a smaller scale that is appropriate in rural areas. In controlled tipping/burial, solid waste is disposed of into a dug pit and is regularly covered with soil to avoid attracting disease vectors, such as flies and rodents. Covering the waste also stops it from being blown by the wind and avoids bad smells—hence 'controlled'. Note that various similar terms may be used to describe different types of waste disposal pit. A refuse pit is a simple pit used to dispose of household refuse, which may or may not be used for controlled tipping (with soil). Some wastes will need to be buried under soil as soon as they are disposed of, in which case the pit may be referred to as a burial pit.

When there is a need for preparing a refuse pit for households, you should advise them that sites for controlled tipping should be 10 m away from the house (preferably at the back of the house), at least 15 m and preferably 30–50 m away from water wells and at a lower ground level. At community level, a communal refuse pit should be 100 m away from houses and they will also need to consider the direction of wind. The site should be easily accessible, with adequate space, and should be fenced, so that it is not accessible to children and domestic animals.

Care must be taken to avoid creating places that could harbor rats or encourage the breeding of flies and other insects. Waste from individual households should be taken to the site in suitable containers such as sacks, plastic bags or buckets. For a community waste disposal pit, it should be a collective responsibility to keep communal areas clean. Animal carcasses need to be disposed of carefully because they can encourage the breeding of flies and rodents, and attract scavenger animals. They can be disposed of in a common burial pit for the community. Burning of waste is another possible, though less desirable, method of final disposal. A burning site should be sited downwind and well away from houses. Noncombustible materials, such as broken bottles, bones, etc. should be separated and buried at a safe location, not used by farming. Ashes that remain after burning can be used as fertilizer or, if mixed with mud, can be used for plastering of earth walls or floors.

10. Clinical features of chickenpox.

Chickenpox infection appears 10–21 days after exposure to the virus and usually lasts about 5–10 days. The rash is the telltale indication of chickenpox. Chickenpox appears as a very itchy rash that spreads from the torso to the neck, face and limbs. Lasting 7–10 days, the rash progresses from red bumps to fluid-filled blisters (vesicles) that drain and scab over. Vesicles may also appear in the mouth, on the scalp, around the eyes or on the genitals and can be very painful. This cycle repeats itself in new areas of the body until finally, after about 2 weeks; all of the sores have healed. The disease is contagious until all the spots have dried up. Unfortunately, the virus is also contagious for at least 1 day before the rash breaks out. Other signs and symptoms which may appear 1–2 days before the rash include:
1. Fever
2. Loss of appetite
3. Headache
4. Tiredness and a general feeling of being unwell (malaise).

Once the chickenpox rash appears, it goes through three phases:
1. Raised pink or red bumps (papules) which break out over several days.
2. Small fluid-filled blisters (vesicles) forming from the raised bumps over about 1 day before breaking and leaking.
3. Crusts and scabs which cover the broken blisters and take several more days to heal.

New bumps continue to appear for several days. As a result, you may have all three stages of the rash—bumps, blisters and scabbed lesions—at the same time on the second day of the rash. Once infected, you can spread the virus for up to 48 hours before the rash appears, and you remain contagious until all spots crust over.

The disease is generally mild in healthy children. In severe cases, the rash can spread to cover the entire body, and lesions may form in the throat, eyes and mucous membranes of the urethra, anus and vagina. New spots continue to appear for several days.

11. Prevention and control of food poisoning.

Food poisoning is illness resulting from consumption of contaminated food or water. Food can be contaminated by bacteria, viruses, parasites or fungi, or by toxins produced by them. Food poisoning is one of the most common illnesses in Australia, with an estimated 4–7 million cases of foodborne illness each year.

General Guidelines to Prevent Food Poisoning

1. Make sure that food from animal sources (meat, dairy, eggs) is cooked thoroughly or pasteurized. Use a thermometer to check the temperature of the food.
2. Avoid eating raw or spoiled meats and eggs. Check expiration dates on meats and eggs before purchasing and again before preparing.
3. Carefully select and prepare fish and shellfish to ensure quality and freshness.
4. If you are served an undercooked meat or egg product in a restaurant, send it back for further cooking. You should also ask for a new plate.
4. Be careful that you do not let juices or drippings from raw meat, poultry, shellfish, or eggs contaminate other foods.

6. Do not leave eggs, meats, poultry, seafood, or milk for extended periods of time at room temperature. Promptly refrigerate leftovers and food prepared in advance.
7. Wash hands, cutting boards, and knives with antibacterial soap and warm to hot water after handling raw meat, poultry, seafood, or eggs. Wooden cutting boards are not recommended, because they can be harder to clean.
8. Avoid unpasteurized milk or foods made from unpasteurized milk.
9. Do not thaw foods at room temperature. Thaw foods in the refrigerator and use them promptly. Do not refreeze foods once they have been completely thawed.
10. Keep the refrigerator at 40°F or lower, and the freezer at 0°F or lower.
11. Wash raw vegetables and fruits thoroughly before eating, especially those that will not be cooked. Avoid eating alfalfa sprouts until their safety can be assured. Methods to decontaminate alfalfa seeds and sprouts are being investigated.
12. Drink only pasteurized juice or cider. Commercial juice with an extended shelf life that is sold at room temperature (juice in cardboard boxes, vacuum sealed juice in glass containers) has been pasteurized, although this is generally not indicated on the label. Juice concentrates are also heated sufficiently to kill bacteria.
13. Be aware of proper home-canning procedures. Instructions on safe home-canning can be obtained from county extension services or from the US Department of Agriculture.
14. If you are ill with diarrhea or vomiting, do not prepare food for others, especially infants, the elderly, and those with weakened immune systems, because they are more vulnerable to infection.
15. Wash hands with soap after handling reptiles, turtles, birds, or after contact with human or pet feces.
16. Breastfeed your baby if possible. Mother's milk is the safest food for young infants. Breastfeeding may prevent many food-borne illnesses and other health problems.
17. Those at high-risk, such as pregnant women, people with weakened immune systems, infants.
18. Avoid soft cheeses, such as feta, Brie, Camembert, blue-veined, and Mexican-style cheese. (hard cheeses, processed cheeses, cream cheese, and cottage cheese are safe.)
19. Cook foods until they are steaming hot, especially leftover foods or ready-to-eat foods, such as hot dogs.
20. Although the risk of foodborne disease associated with foods from deli counters is relatively low, pregnant women and people with weakened immune systems may choose to avoid these foods or thoroughly reheat cold cuts before eating.

12. Causes of obesity.

Lack of Energy Balance

A lack of energy balance most often causes overweight and obesity. Energy balance means that your energy IN equals your energy OUT. Energy IN is the amount of energy or calories you get from food and drinks. Energy OUT is the amount of energy your body uses for things like breathing, digesting, and being physically active.

Other Causes

An inactive lifestyle: Many Americans are not very physically active. One reason for this is that many people spend hours in front of TVs and computers doing work, schoolwork, and leisure activities. In fact, more than 2 hours a day of regular TV viewing time has been linked to overweight and obesity. Other reasons for not being active include: Relying on cars instead of walking, fewer physical demands at work or at home because of modern technology and conveniences, and lack of physical education classes in schools.

Environment: Our environment does not support healthy lifestyle habits; in fact, it encourages obesity. Some reasons include:
1. Lack of neighborhood sidewalks and safe places for recreation. Not having area parks, trails, sidewalks, and affordable gyms makes it hard for people to be physically active.
2. Work schedules. People often say that they do not have time to be physically active because of long work hours and time spent commuting.
3. Oversized food portions. Americans are exposed to huge food portions in restaurants, fast food places, gas stations, movie theaters, supermarkets, and even at home. Some of these meals and snacks can feed two or more people. Eating large portions means too much energy IN. Over time, this will cause weight gain if it is not balanced with physical activity.
4. Lack of access to healthy foods. Some people do not live in neighborhoods that have supermarkets that sell healthy foods, such as fresh fruits and vegetables, or for some people, these healthy foods are too costly.
5. Food advertising. Americans are surrounded by ads from food companies. Often children are the targets of advertising for high-calorie, high-fat snacks and sugary drinks. The goal of these ads is to sway people to buy these high-calorie foods, and often they do.

Genes and Family History

Studies of identical twins who have been raised apart show that genes have a strong influence on a person's weight. Overweight and obesity tend to run in families. Your chances of being overweight are greater if one or both of your parents are overweight or obese.

Your genes also may affect the amount of fat you store in your body and where on your body you carry the extra fat. Because families also share food and physical activity habits, a link exists between genes and the environment.

Children adopt the habits of their parents. A child who has overweight parents who eat high-calorie foods and are inactive will likely become overweight too. However, if the family adopts healthy food and physical activity habits, the child's chance of being overweight or obese is reduced.

Health Conditions

Some hormone problems may cause overweight and obesity, such as underactive thyroid (hypothyroidism), Cushing's syndrome, and polycystic ovarian syndrome (PCOS). Underactive thyroid is a condition in which the thyroid gland does not make enough thyroid hormone. Lack of thyroid hormone will slow down your metabolism and cause weight gain. You will also feel tired and weak.

Cushing's syndrome is a condition in which the body's adrenal glands make too much of the hormone cortisol. Cushing's syndrome also can develop if a person takes high doses of certain medicines, such as prednisone for long periods.

People who have Cushing's syndrome gain weight, have upper-body obesity, a rounded face, fat around the neck, and thin arms and legs.

PCOS is a condition that affects about 5–10% of women of childbearing age. Women who have PCOS often are obese, have excess hair growth, and have reproductive problems and other health issues. These problems are caused by high levels of hormones called androgens.

Medicines: Certain medicines may cause you to gain weight. These medicines include some corticosteroids, antidepressants, and seizure medicines. These medicines can slow the rate at which your body burns calories, increase your appetite, or cause your body to hold on to extra water. All of these factors can lead to weight gain.

Emotional factors: Some people eat more than usual when they are bored, angry, or stressed. Over time, overeating will lead to weight gain and may cause overweight or obesity.

Smoking: Some people gain weight when they stop smoking. One reason is that food often tastes and smells better after quitting smoking. Another reason is because nicotine raises the rate at which your body burns calories, so you burn fewer calories when you stop smoking. However, smoking is a serious health risk, and quitting is more important than possible weight gain.

Age: As you get older, you tend to lose muscle, especially if you are less active. Muscle loss can slow down the rate at which your body burns calories. If you do not reduce your calorie intake as you get older, you may gain weight. Midlife weight gain in women is mainly due to aging and lifestyle, but menopause also plays a role. Many women gain about 5 pounds during menopause and have more fat around the waist than they did before.

Pregnancy: During pregnancy, women gain weight to support their babies' growth and development. After giving birth, some women find it hard to lose the weight. This may lead to overweight or obesity, especially after a few pregnancies.

Lack of sleep: Research shows that lack of sleep increases the risk of obesity. For example, one study of teenagers showed that with each hour of sleep lost, the odds of becoming obese went up. Lack of sleep increases the risk of obesity in other age groups as well. People who sleep fewer hours also seem to prefer eating foods that are higher in calories and carbohydrates, which can lead to overeating, weight gain, and obesity.

Sleep helps maintain a healthy balance of the hormones that make you feel hungry (ghrelin) or full (leptin). When you do not get enough sleep, your level of ghrelin goes up and your level of leptin goes down. This makes you feel hungrier than when you are well-rested. Sleep also affects how your body reacts to insulin, the hormone that controls your blood glucose (sugar) level. Lack of sleep results in a higher than normal blood sugar level, which may increase your risk for diabetes.

SHORT ANSWERS

13. Define prevalence.

Prevalence is a statistical concept referring to the number of cases of a disease that are present in a particular population at a given time, whereas incidence refers to the number of new cases that develop in a given period of time. The proportion of individuals in a population having a disease or characteristic. Prevalence is a statistical concept referring to the number of cases of a disease that are present in a particular population at a given time, whereas incidence refers to the number of new cases that develop in a given period of time.

Prevalence is a measure of disease that allows us to determine a person's likelihood of having a disease. Therefore, the number of prevalent cases is the total number of cases of disease existing in a population. A prevalence rate is the total number of cases of a disease existing in a population divided by the total population. So, if a measurement of cancer is taken in a population of 40,000 people and 1,200 were recently diagnosed with cancer and 3,500 are living with cancer, then the prevalence of cancer is 0.118. (Or 11,750 per 100,000 persons).

14. Enlist role of VCT in HIV prevention and care.

1. Educed HIV transmission among specific high-risk populations.
2. Strengthened the capacity of the Government of Nepal and Nepali civil society in policy formulation.

3. Provided technical leadership to improve the planning, collection, analysis and use of strategic information.
4. Worked with the Government of Nepal and partner organizations to improve access to HIV services for people living with HIV and those at high-risk for HIV transmission.
5. Collaborated with the government and all stakeholders in planning, implementing and monitoring HIV programs.

15. Define wholesome water.

Wholesome water is fit to use for drinking, cooking, food preparation or washing without any potential danger to human health by meeting the requirements of regulations made under Section 67 (Standards of Wholesomeness) of the Water Act 1991. These stipulate the criteria that the water must meet in order to protect the lifelong health of the population. These parameters include limits on:
1. Biological quality (including levels of bacteria and oocysts).
2. Chemical quality (including levels of metals, solvents, pesticides and hydrocarbons).
3. Physical qualities (including color, taste and odor).

The quality of water that is supplied through public water mains is strictly controlled by legislation to ensure that it is wholesome, and is also subject to regular testing at the consumer's tap to prevent any loss of quality during transmission and storage.

16. Define infant mortality rate.

Infant mortality rate (IMR) is defined as "the ratio of infant deaths registered in a given year to the total number of live births registered in the same year; usually expressed as a rate per 1,000 live births" (87). It is given by the formula:

$$\text{IMR} = \frac{\text{Number of deaths of children less than 1 year of age in a year}}{\text{Number of live births in the same year}} \times 10$$

IMR is universally regarded not only as a most important indicator of the health status of a community but also of the level of living of people in general, and effectiveness of MCH services in particular. Infant mortality is given a separate treatment by demographers because: (a) infant mortality is the largest single age—category of mortality; (b) deaths at this age are due to a peculiar set of diseases and conditions to which the adult population is less exposed or less vulnerable; (c) infant mortality is affected rather quickly and directly by specific health programs and hence may change more rapidly than the general death rate.

17. Mention two uses of epidemiology.

1. To study the history of the health of populations.
2. To diagnose the health of the community—"population medicine"; incidence, prevalence, disability and mortality.
3. To study the working of health services and how to improve them.
4. To estimate individual risks, on average, from population estimates.
5. To identify syndromes by describing the distribution of clinical phenomena.
6. To complete the clinical picture of chronic diseases and describe their natural history: Across ethnicities, gender, age groups, etc. by exposure level(s)
7. To search for causes of health and disease.

18. Iceberg phenomena of disease.

Iceberg phenomenon of disease gives a picture of the spectrum of diseases in a community. The visible part of the iceberg denotes the clinically apparent cases of disease in the community. The part of the iceberg below the water level denoted the latent, subclinical, undiagnosed and carrier states in the community, which forms the major part. The hidden part is especially important in disease like hypertension, diabetes and malnutrition.

Some diseases exhibiting iceberg phenomenon:
1. Diabetes
2. Hypertension
3. Malnutrition
4. Polio
5. Leprosy.

The **iceberg phenomenon** describes a situation in which a large percentage of a problem is subclinical, unreported, or otherwise hidden from view. Thus, only the "tip of the iceberg" is apparent to the epidemiologist. Uncovering disease that might otherwise be below "sea-level" by screening and early detection often allows for better disease control (Fig. 1).

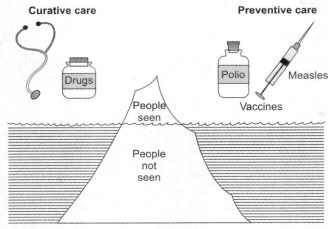

Fig. 1: The iceberg.

Consider:
1. For every successful suicide attempt, there are many more unsuccessful attempts and a still larger number of people with depressive illness that might be severe enough to have them wish to end their lives. With appropriate treatment, depressives with suicidal tendencies would be less likely to have suicidal ideation and be less likely to attempt suicide.
2. Reported cases of AIDS represents only the tip of HIV infections. With proper antiretroviral therapy, clinical illness may delayed and transmission averted.
3. Serious dog bite injuries often go undetected. For each fatal dog bite, there are about 670 dog bite hospitalizations, 16,000 emergency department visits, 21,000 medical visits to other clinics, and 187,000 nontreated bites. With effective recognition, animal control programs can be put into place to prevent dog bite injuries.

19. Active immunity.

Active immunity is immunity that develops from creating antibodies to a disease or illness. Immunity refers to having a resistance to a disease or illness. Taking this into consideration, you could further break down active immunity by defining it as gaining resistance to a particular disease or illness by creating antibodies to the disease or illness.

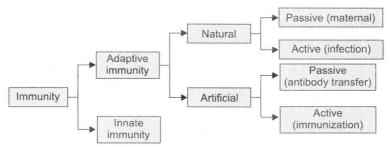

The first type of active immunity comes from being exposed to the pathogen that causes the disease. The term for this is **natural active immunity.** When an infectious organism, like a bacteria or virus, enters your body, it will begin to mount an immune response to try to attack the pathogen. The **T-cells** in your bloodstream will attach to the pathogen and then present the pathogen to the B-cells in the bloodstream. The **B-cells** are the ones that create the antibody that can attack and kill the pathogen. **Antibodies** are proteins that are specifically made to deactivate and kill pathogens.

20. Define demography.

Demography is derived from two Greek words "demos" meaning the people and "graphein" meaning the record. Demography deals with the study of the size, the composition and the distribution of human population at a point of time. Community health nursing and population plays a significant relationship. People are the basic unity of community health care.

Definitions of Demography

Demography is as branch of science which studies the human population and their elements. The elements are change in the size of population, structure of population and geographical distribution of population.

Demography is the scientific study of human population, such as changes in population size, the composition of the population and distribution of population in space. It also deals with five "demographic process" namely fertility, mortality, marriage, migration and social mobility.

21. Four causes of iron deficiency anemia.

According to the American society of hematology, iron deficiency is the most common cause of anemia. There are many reasons why a person might become deficient in iron. These include:

Inadequate Iron Intake

Eating too little iron over an extended amount of time can cause a shortage in your body. Foods, such as meat, eggs, and some green leafy vegetables are high in iron. Because iron is essential during times of rapid growth and development, pregnant women and young children may need even more iron-rich foods in their diet.

Pregnancy or blood loss due to menstruation: In women of childbearing age, the most common causes of irondeficiency anemia are heavy menstrual bleeding and blood loss during childbirth.

Internal bleeding: Certain medical conditions can cause internal bleeding which can lead to irondeficiency anemia. Examples include an ulcer in your stomach, polyps (tissue growths) in the colon or intestines, or colon cancer. Regular use of pain relievers, such as aspirin can also cause bleeding in the stomach.

Inability to absorb iron: Certain disorders or surgeries that affect the intestines can also interfere with how your body absorbs iron. Even if you get enough iron in your diet, celiac disease or intestinal surgery, such as gastric bypass, may limit the amount of iron your body can absorb.

22. Define food fortification.

Food fortification is the practice of adding essential vitamins and minerals (e.g. iron, vitamin A, folic acid, iodine) to staple foods to improve their nutritional content. Fortification is a safe, effective way to improve public health that has been used around the world since the 1920s.

Many diets, especially those of the poor, contain insufficient amounts of vitamins and minerals due to lack of variation and/or consumption of predominantly processed foods. Adequate amounts of vitamins and minerals in the diet, also called micronutrients since they are only needed in small amounts are critical to an individual's health and development. Since most populations in resource-poor settings do not have access to adequate quantities of fruits, vegetables, and meats where micronutrients are abundant, and because providing vitamin tablets poses logistical and economic constraints, food fortification is a practical and inexpensive alternative.

2015

Community Health Nursing-I

LONG ESSAYS
1. Explain in detail the epidemiology and management of malaria.
2. Define demography, which are the methods of collecting demographic data, describe the demographic cycle.
3. Explain the different methods of waste disposal in India.

SHORT ESSAYS
4. Air pollution.
5. Housing standards.
6. Levels of prevention.
7. Mumps.
8. Oral contraceptive pills.
9. Obesity.
10. Women empowerment.
11. Malnutrition.
12. Mode of disease transmission.

SHORT ANSWERS
13. Safe and wholesome water.
14. Immunoglobulins.
15. Tubectomy.
16. Types of diabetes.
17. Epilepsy.
18. Trachoma.
19. Purchasing power.
20. Incubation period.
21. Spectrum of health.
22. Ascariasis.

LONG ESSAYS

1. Explain in detail the epidemiology and management of malaria.

Till 1950, malaria was considered to be a major health problem of India. An estimate of the disease in 1953 showed an annual incidence of 75 million cases, and 8 lakhs deaths. The National Malaria Control and Eradication Programs launched in 1953 and 1958 respectively gave a deathblow to malaria; by 1971, the incidence of malaria declined to just over 1 million cases and no deaths. The disease which was on its way to eradication reappeared. In 1976, the incidence of malaria score to a peak of 6.47 million cases (of which 7,42,247 were falciparum cases) with 59 deaths.

Pathogenesis
1. **Agent factors:** Malaria caused by *plasmodium vivax, P. malariae, P. Falciparum* and *P. ovale*. As parasites *P. vivax, P. ovale* and *P. malariae* may persist for years in the liver and are responsible for the chronic carrier state. Because blood transfusions and street-drug paraphernalia also can spread malaria, drug-addicts have a higher incidence of the disease.
2. **Host factors:** Malaria affects all ages. Newborn infants have considerable resistance to infection with *P. falciparum*. Males are more frequently exposed to the risk of acquiring malaria than females in India. Malaria is predominantly a rural disease and is closely related to agriculture practices.
3. **Environmental factors:** Malaria is a seasonal disease, in most parts of India, the maximum prevalence is from July to November. Rain in general provides opportunities for the breeding of mosquitoes and may give rise to epidemics of malaria. Burrow pits, garden pools, irrigation channels and engineering projects have led to the breeding of mosquitoes and an increase in malaria. Malaria consequent on human undertaking is called "Manmade malaria".
4. **Mode of transmission:** Malaria is transmitted by the bite of female anopheles mosquitoes. Direct transmissions occur may be induced accidentally by hypodermic intramuscular and intrainjections of blood or plasma. Congenital infection of the newborn from an infected mother may also occur but it is comparatively rare.
5. **Incubation period:** This is the length of time between the infective mosquito bite and the first appearance of clinical signs of which fever is most common. This period is usually not less than 10 days.

Clinical Features
After an incubation period of 12–30 days, the patient may report malaria's prodromal signs and symptoms, such as chills fever, headache, fatigue and myalgia interspersed with periods of well-being. Acute attacks occur when erythrocytes rupture. These attacks have three stages:
1. **Cold stage:** These attacks have three stages from chills to extreme shaking.
2. **Hot stage:** Lasting for 3–4 hours, characterized by a high fever (up to 107°F) accompanied by cough, headache backache, abdominal pain, nausea, vomiting and delirium.
3. **Wet stage:** Lasting for 2–4 hours characterized by profuse sweating.

The Government of India introduced a modified plan of operation from 1977 to tackle the situation effectively. Efforts are now being made to contain the disease. By 1984, the incidence of malaria was brought down to 2.1 million cases, since then the epidemiological situation has not shown any great improvement. It seems to have reached a plateau, which is causing concern. By the end of 2001, about 2.05 million cases of malaria (with about 1 million cases of falciparum malaria) and 1015 deaths were reported from different states. The 1994 resurgence of malaria compelled the Government of India to appoint an Expert Committee on Malaria to identify the problem areas and to suggest specific measures against the different paradigms of malaria. Thus, the Malaria Action Program (MAP) was evolved and is being implemented.

The objectives of this new Malaria Action Program are:
1. Management of serious and complicated malaria cases.
2. Prevention of mortality with particular reference to high-risk groups.
3. Reduction of morbidity.
4. Control of outbreaks and epidemics.
5. Reduction of falciparum.
6. Incidence and containment resistance malaria.
7. Maintenance of low incidence status.
8. The recent resurgence of malaria in many parts of the country necessitated the need to strengthen the health promotion component of the program.
9. It has been decided to observe antimalaria month before the onset of monsoon, i.e. month of June every year.

2. Define demography, which are the methods of collecting demographic data, describe the demographic cycle.

Demography is derived from two Greek words "demos" meaning the people and "graphein" meaning the record. Demography deals with the study of the size, the composition and the distribution of human population at a point of time. Community health nursing and population plays a significant relationship. People are the basic unity of community health care.

Definitions of Demography

Demography is as branch of science which studies the human population and their elements. The elements are change in the size of population, structure of population and geographical distribution of population.

Demography is the scientific study of human population, such as changes in population size, the composition of the population and distribution of population in space. It also deals with five "demographic process" namely—fertility, mortality, marriage, migration and social mobility.

History of Demographic Studies

The historical roots of demography are spread over centuries. The earliest records of census operations have been traced as far back as 4000 BC in Babylonia, 3000 BC in China and 2500 BC in Egypt.

Canada was the first country to operate census on Modern lines in 1666, followed by United States in 1790 and England in 1801. Countrywide census operation was introduced in India in 1881.

During 17th century, the growing importance of vital registration and laws enforcing compulsory registration of vital events, the process also spread in other regions of the world. The first act of this spread was introduced in India in 1886. The voluntary registration of births, deaths and civil marriages act for compulsory vital registration was passed in 1969.

Sources of Demography

Census

The word census originated from the Latin word 'censere' which means to:
1. **Assess or to rate:** The first census of India was conducted in 1872, hence the census of 1881 is considered as the first systematic census of India. Census 2001 is the 14th census the 6th census of independent India and the first of 21st century.

2. **Vital registration:** It is a process of recording vital events that occur in a population from-time-to-time, the events registered related to births, deaths and marriage. Vital registration helps in planning, implementation and evaluation of community health services/programs.
3. **Institutional records:** The records are routinely maintained by various categories of hospitals and healthcare institutions, operating at various levels, have limited public health relevance.

Demographic Cycle

1. **High stationary stage:** This characterized by high crude birth rate and crude death rate with a negligible demographic gap between two.
2. **Early expanding stage:** This is characterized by a crude birth rate that continues to remain high and a crude death rate that starts declining.
3. **Late expanding stage:** This is characterized by a crude birth rate that continues to fall and crude birth rate that starts declining.
4. **Low stationary stage:** This is characterized by a low crude birth rate and a low crude death rate with a negligible demographic gap.
5. **Declining stage:** This is characterized by a low crude birth rate and a low crude death rate with a negligible demographic gap.

Demographic Trends

Global Level

The population of the world is not uniformly distributed over the globe. It is mainly concentrated in the developing countries.

Demographic profile of these countries and their health status is greatly influenced by their levels of socioeconomic development. UNICEF has grouped the countries of the world into three categories—industrialized, developing and least developed. The world population stood at 6 billion by year 2000 and the population growth was 6 billion in 2000. The statistical indices used to assess the health profile of the countries of the world are both crude and specific. The difference between crude birth rate and crude death rate for comparing the health status of countries are infant mortality rate (IMR), under-five mortality rate (UFMR) and maternal mortality rate (MMR).

Indian Level

India is the second populous country in the world. The population size is about 1,027 million in 2001. The population size is about 1,000 million between 1991 and 2001. According to 2001 census, the child population, the total number of children of 0–6 years 15.78 crores out of which male children are 8.19 crores and female children are 7.59 crores. The sex ratio in India has been generally adverse to women, i.e. 1 number of women per 1,000 men has generally been less than.

Urbanization: It is a recent phenomenon in the developing countries. The proportion of the urban population in India has increased from 10.84% in 1901 to 25.72% in 1991 and was 27.8 in the year 2001. The another factor expectancy at birth has continued to increase globally over the living longer and they have a right to a long life in good health rather than one of pain and disability.

Demographic Trends in India

Some important facts related to population derived from Census of India-2001 are the following:
1. At 00-00 hours 1st March 2001, the interim population of India was declared 1,02,70,15,247 persons. In this, number of males was 53,12,77,078 and that of females was 49,57,38,169.
2. The annual increase rate of population has decreased from 2.14 to 1.93%.

3. In the last 10 years, population of India has increased from 84 crores 63 lacs to 102 crores and 70 lacs.
4. Sex ratio has improved. In the earlier decade of 1981-1991, the number of women per thousand men was 927, which has increased to 933 at present.
   The ratio of literates in the population has increased from 52.2 to 65.4%.
   Population figures show that due to increase in literacy, the population growth is decreasing.
5. In decade 1991-2001, population has increased by 21.34%. The total increase of the population in this decade is more than the total population of the fifth largest country of the world, Brazil.
6. Kerala is the most literate state where 90.92% population is educated whereas in Bihar, less than half of the population, 47.53% people is literate. Bihar has proved to be the most backward state of the country.
7. Compared to the previous decade, the ratio of children in the population has reduced which shows that fertility rate has come down.
8. The highest density of population is in Delhi, 9,294 person per square kilometer and it is lowest in Arunachal Pradesh with 13 persons per square kilometer.
9. According to Census-2001, the population growth has come down in most of the states. The highest decline is in Andhra Pradesh. In the decade of 1981-1991, the growth rate of population in Andhra Pradesh was 24.2%, whereas in 1991-2001, the growth rate is 13.86%.

3. Explain the different methods of waste disposal in India.

Waste management is the process of treating solid wastes and offers variety of solutions for recycling items that do not belong to trash. It is about how garbage can be used as a valuable resource. Waste management is something that each and every household and business owner in the world needs. Waste management disposes of the products and substances that you have use in a safe and efficient manner.

Landfill

The landfill is the most popularly used method of waste disposal used today. This process of waste disposal focuses attention on burying the waste in the land. Landfills are found in all areas. There is a process used that eliminates the odors and dangers of waste before it is placed into the ground. While it is true, this is the most popular form of waste disposal, it is certainly far from the only procedure and one that may also bring with it an assortment of space. This method is becoming less these days although, thanks to the lack of space available and the strong presence of methane and other landfill gases, both of which can cause numerous contamination problems. Many areas are reconsidering the use of landfills.

Incineration/Combustion

Incineration or combustion is a type of disposal method in which municipal solid wastes are burned at high temperatures so as to convert them into residue and gaseous products. The biggest advantage of this type of method is that it can reduce the volume of solid waste to 20–30% of the original volume, decreases the space they take up and reduce the stress on landfills. This process is also known as thermal treatment where solid waste materials are converted by incinerators into heat, gas, steam and ash. Incineration is something that is very in countries where landfill space is no longer available which includes Japan.

Recovery and Recycling

Resource recovery is the process of taking useful discarded items for a specific next use. These discarded items are then processed to extract or recover materials and resources or convert them to energy in the form of useable heat, electricity or fuel. Recycling is the process of converting waste products into new products to prevent energy usage and consumption of fresh raw materials. recycling is the third component of reduce, reuse and recycle waste hierarchy. The idea behind recycling is to reduce energy usage, reduce volume of landfills, reduce air and water pollution, reduce greenhouse gas emissions and preserve natural resources for future use.

Plasma Gasification

Plasma gasification is another form of waste management. Plasma is a primarily an electrically charged or a highly ionized gas. Lighting is one type of plasma which produces temperatures that exceed 12,600°F. With this method of waste disposal, a vessel uses characteristic plasma torches operating at +10,000°F which is creating a gasification zone till 3,000°F for the conversion of solid or liquid wastes into a syngas. During the treatment solid waste by plasma gasification, the waste's molecular bonds are broken down as result of the intense heat in the vessels and the elemental components. Thanks to this process, destruction of waste and dangerous materials is found. This form of waste disposal provides renewable energy and an assortment of other fantastic benefits.

Composting

Composting is a easy and natural biodegradation process that takes organic wastes, i.e. remains of plants and garden and kitchen waste and turns into nutrient rich food for your plants. Composting, normally used for organic farming, occurs by allowing organic materials to sit in one place for months until microbes decompose it. Composting is one of the best methods of waste disposal as it can turn unsafe organic products into safe compost. On the other side, it is slow process and takes lot of space.

Waste-to-Energy (Recover Energy)

Waste-to-Energy (WtE) process involves converting of nonrecyclable waste items into useable heat, electricity, or fuel through a variety of processes. This type of source of energy is a renewable energy source as nonrecyclable waste can be used over and over again to create energy. It can also help to reduce carbon emissions by offsetting the need for energy from fossil sources. Waste-to-Energy, also widely recognized by its acronym WtE is the generation of energy in the form of heat or electricity from waste.

Avoidance/Waste Minimization

The easier method of waste management is to reduce creation of waste materials thereby reducing the amount of waste going to landfills. Waste reduction can be done through recycling old materials like jar, bags, repairing broken items instead of buying new one, avoiding use of disposable products like plastic bags, reusing second hand items, and buying items that uses less designing. Recycling and composting is a couple of the best methods of waste management. Composting is so far only possible on a small scale, either by private individuals or in areas where waste can be mixed with farming soil or used for landscaping purposes. Recycling is widely used around the world, with plastic, paper and metal leading the list of the most recyclable items. Most material recycled is reused for its original purpose.

SHORT ESSAYS

4. Air pollution.

It is a fact, that pure air is impossible, because foreign substances have been present in the air at all times at all places. The term "air pollution" is, therefore applied when there is an excessive concentration of foreign matter in the outdoor atmosphere which is harmful to man or his environment. In broadest sense, air pollution results from the presence of foreign materials in the air and is either natural or manmade.

Air pollution is a growing menace to health throughout the universe. Recent surveys show that air pollution is on the increase in India due to increased industrialization, urbanization and increased density of population.

Sources of Air Pollution
1. Industrial process—chemical, metallurgical, fertilizer, oil refineries, etc.
2. Combustion industrial and domestic combustion of coal, oil and other fuel which emit smoke and soot.
3. Vehicles—motor vehicles, trucks, trains, aircrafts, buses, and diesel engines, etc.
4. Incinerators and sewers burning refuse.
5. Agricultural activities spraying insecticides, grain dust, etc.
6. Radioactive substances.

Actually, all human activities bring people into contact with some form of air pollution. The main classes of human generated air pollution are:
1. Carbon monoxide, a major part of automobile exhaust.
2. Sulfur oxides, produced mostly by combustion of coal, fuel oils and natural gas.
3. Hydrocarbons, a family of compounds containing carbon and hydrogen.
4. Nitrogen oxides, mainly emitted by power plants and in transportation vehicle exhausts.
5. Particulate matter, such as dust, soot or ash, e.g. particulates in cosmetics, aerosols, in spray cans, fibrous particles from rugs, blankets, draperies and clothes and radon.

5. Housing standards.

Housing means homes to live in. House refers to a physical structure where unit of society, the family lives but the concept is slowly changing to "Human settlement" which allow the extended outlook of a house, where people live, interact and pursue their goals. A WHO Expert Group (1961) has coined the word residential environment which is used by man for his activity and desired devices for his family well-being.

Basic Factors in Housing or Housing Standards

Housing is the modern concept is broadening of houses. Various factors are taken into consideration in determining housing standards. These standards vary from one region to another region.

Aim

Improvement of housing and environmental conditions for the majority of families within the limits set by available resources and objectives. Environmental hygiene Committee of Government of India has given some minimum housing standards that are to be maintained by building regulations through municipality, corporation, town planning and urban development authorities.

Site

The site should be elevated from its surroundings:
- Adequate width
- Away from breedy places of flies.
- Away from nuisance, such as noise, smoke, dust.

- Should have clean surroundings.
- Structure should be well drained.
    1. Site of house: In an elevated place in a residential area of town and subsoil water must be below 10 feet.
    2. Set back: The built up area is restricted to 2/3rd of site. Wind direction and ventilation are considered.
    3. Cubic space: It should be 500 cubic feet per person.
    4. Floor: Pucca floor, no crack and damp floor.
    5. Floor area: 100 square feet per person.
    6. Roof: It should be more than 10 feet.
    7. Walls: Strong and weather resistant.
    8. Rooms: According to family size and need of privacy, number of rooms is suggested.
    9. Windows: Window area should be 1/5th of floor area.
    10. Lightening: It is expected to have a day light factor (DF) of 1.0 or above 1.0.
    11. Water supply: Safe and whole some water supply is guaranteed.
    12. Washing: Should have provision for washing facility.
    13. Bathing facility: House should have adequate bathing facility.
    14. Kitchen: Adequate provision of separate sanitary area for food preparation.
    15. Privy: Sanitary RCA latrine and water carriage system is a must under criteria of healthful housing.
    16. Refusal disposal: Daily disposal and transport for sanitary disposal is advocated.

6. Levels of prevention.

Primary prevention seeks to prevent the onset of specific diseases via risk reduction: By altering behaviors or exposures that can lead to disease, or by enhancing resistance to the effects of exposure to a disease agent. Examples include smoking cessation and vaccination. Primary prevention reduces the incidence of disease by addressing disease risk factors or by enhancing resistance. Some approaches involve active participation, as with regular tooth brushing and flossing to prevent dental caries. Other approaches are passive: Adding fluoride to the municipal drinking water to harden tooth enamel and prevent caries. Primary prevention generally targets specific causes and risk factors for specific diseases, but may also aim to promote healthy behaviors, improve host resistance, and foster safe environments that reduce the risk of disease, for instance, thorough cleaning of operating rooms to prevent postoperative infection.

Secondary prevention includes procedures that detect and treat preclinical pathological changes and thereby control disease progression. Screening procedures (such as mammography to detect early stage breast cancer) are often the first step leading to early interventions that are more cost effective than intervening once symptoms appear. Routine blood sugar testing for people over 40 would be an example relevant to detecting Catherine's diabetes early. Screening is usually undertaken by health professionals, either at the level of individual doctor-patient encounters (e.g. routine blood pressure checks) or via public health screening programs (e.g. mammography screening). The criteria for implementing a screening program are described.

Tertiary prevention can include modifying risk factors, such as assisting a cardiac patient to lose weight, or making environmental modifications to reduce an asthmatic patient's exposure to allergens. In the example of Catherine Richards, it might include ensuring regular check-ups to monitor her condition including eye test to check for possible adverse outcomes of her diabetes. Where the condition is not reversible, tertiary prevention focuses on rehabilitation, assisting the patient to accommodate to his disability. For reversible conditions, such as many types of heart disease, tertiary prevention will reduce the population prevalence, whereas for incurable conditions it may increase prevalence if it prolongs survival. The key goal for tertiary prevention is to enhance quality of life.

7. Mumps.

Mumps is a contagious disease caused by a virus that passes from one person to another through saliva, nasal secretions, and close personal contact. The condition primarily affects the parotid glands. Parotid glands also called salivary glands are the organs responsible for producing saliva. There are three sets of salivary glands on each side of your face, located behind and below your ears. The hallmark symptom of mumps is swelling of the salivary glands.

Symptoms of mumps usually appear within 2 weeks of exposure to the virus. Flu-like symptoms may be the first to appear including:
1. Fatigue
2. Body aches
3. Headache
4. Loss of appetite
5. Low-grade fever.

Treatment

Because mumps is a virus, it does not respond to antibiotics or other medications. However, you can treat the symptoms to make yourself more comfortable while you are sick:
1. Rest when you feel weak or tired.
2. Take over-the-counter pain relievers, such as acetaminophen and ibuprofen, to bring down your fever.
3. Soothe swollen glands by applying ice packs.
4. Drink plenty of fluids to avoid dehydration due to fever.
5. Eat a soft diet of soup, yogurt, and other foods that are not hard to chew (chewing may be painful when your glands are swollen).
6. Avoid acidic foods and beverages that may cause more pain in your salivary glands.

8. Oral contraceptive pills.

Oral contraceptives (birth-control pills) are used to prevent pregnancy. Estrogen and progestin are two female sex hormones. Combinations of estrogen and progestin work by preventing ovulation (the release of eggs from the ovaries). They also change the lining of the uterus (womb) to prevent pregnancy from developing and change the mucus at the cervix (opening of the uterus) to prevent sperm (male reproductive cells) from entering. Oral contraceptives are a very effective method of birth control, but they do not prevent the spread of human immunodeficiency virus [HIV, the virus that causes acquired immunodeficiency syndrome (AIDS)] and other sexually transmitted diseases. Some brands of oral contraceptives are also used to treat acne in certain patients. Oral contraceptives treat acne by decreasing the amounts of certain natural substances that can cause acne.

Some oral contraceptives (Beyaz, Yaz) are also used to relieve the symptoms of premenstrual dysphoric disorder (physical and emotional symptoms that occur before the menstrual period each month) in women who have chosen to use an oral contraceptive to prevent pregnancy.

1. Oral contraceptives (the pill) are hormonally active pills which are usually taken by women on a daily basis. They contain either two hormones combined (progestogen and estrogen) or a single hormone (progestogen).
2. Combined oral contraceptives suppress ovulation. Progestogen-only contraceptives also suppress ovulation in about half of women (they are slightly less effective). Both types cause a thickening of the cervical mucus, blocking sperm penetration.
3. Oral contraceptives are 92–99% effective. A woman can decide to start taking the pill if she is sexually active or planning to become sexually active and is certain she is not pregnant. Some pills are taken daily for 21 days and stopped for 7 days before starting a new package.
4. Other kinds are taken continuously for 28 day cycles. Oral contraceptives should be taken in order, at a convenient and consistent time each day. They are appropriate for women who are willing to use a method that requires action daily and who will be able to obtain supplies on a continuous basis.
5. The pill offers continuous protection against pregnancy, it produces regular and shorter periods (and frequently a decrease in menstrual cramps), and it protects against ovarian and endometrial cancer, ectopic pregnancies and infections of the fallopian tubes.
6. Possible side effects include nausea, breast tenderness, mild headaches, weight gain or loss. Very rarely, it can lead to serious health risks (e.g. blood clots, heart attack, and stroke). Risks are higher for women over 35 years who smoke.
7. The pill does not protect against sexually transmitted infections (STIs, including HIV). To protect against STIs, a male or female condom must be used.

9. Obesity.

Obesity increases the risk of many diseases. Fat is deposited on our bodies when the energy (kilojoules) we consume from food and drink is greater than the energy used in activities and at rest. Small imbalances over long periods of time can cause you to become overweight or obese.

Obesity and other noncommunicable diseases (NCDs), such as cardiovascular diseases, cancers and diabetes are now the world's biggest killers causing an estimated 35 million deaths each year, 60% of all deaths globally, with 80% in low- and middle-income countries.

Body Mass Index

Overweight and obesity are defined by the World Health Organization using the body mass index (BMI). BMI is a measure of body size and is used to indicate level of risk for morbidity (disease risk) and mortality (death rates) at the population level. It is calculated by dividing your weight in kilograms by your height in meters squared. For example, a person who is 165 cm tall and weighs 64 kg would have a BMI of 24.

People with a BMI of 25 or more are classified as overweight. People with a BMI of 30 or greater are classified as obese. BMI calculations used for adults are not a suitable measure of weight for children or adolescents. A dietitian or your doctor can assess your child's weight using a special BMI chart, together with weight and height growth charts.

The distribution of fat is important when assessing overweight and obesity, and the associated disease risk. Increased abdominal obesity is related to a higher risk of cardiovascular disease, type 2 diabetes and cancer. Abdominal obesity is measured using waist circumference.

When identifying health risk in adults, it is recommended that you combine BMI with waist circumference as a measurement of disease risk. A waist circumference above 94 cm in men and above 80 cm in women is regarded as overweight and an indicator of serious chronic disease risk. A waist circumference above 102 cm in men and 88 cm in women is regarded as obesity.

Causes of Obesity

A range of factors can cause obesity. Factors in childhood and adolescence are particularly influential, since a high proportion of obese children and adolescents grow up to be obese adults. Factors known to increase the risk of obesity include:

1. **Eating more kilojoules than you use**—whatever your genetic background, you will deposit fat on your body if you eat more energy (kilojoules) than you use.
2. **Modern living**—most modern conveniences, such as cars, computers, televisions and home appliances reduce the need to be physically active.
3. **Socioeconomic factors**—people with lower levels of education and lower incomes are more likely to be overweight or obese. This may be because they have less opportunity to eat healthy foods and take part in physical activities.
4. **Changes in the food supply**—availability and marketing of energy-dense, nutrient poor foods and drinks have increased and the relative cost of them has decreased.
5. **Inactivity**—for most of us, physical activity is no longer a natural part of our daily schedule. Obese people tend to live sedentary lifestyles.
6. **Genes**—researchers have found that genetics play a part in regulating body weight. However, these genes explain only a small part of the variation in body weight. Parental overweight or obesity is associated with increased risk of child overweight or obesity.
7. **Birth factors**—some studies suggest that a person is more likely to become obese later in life if they experienced poor nutrition in utero, maternal smoking, or had a low birth weight. However, other studies show that high birth weight (especially above 4 kg) is a stronger risk for becoming overweight. There is convincing evidence showing that breastfeeding infants compared with formula feeding is associated with a reduced risk of becoming obese.

10. Women empowerment.

Women empowerment refers to the creation of an environment for women where they can make decisions of their own for their personal benefits as well as for the society.

Women empowerment refers to increasing and improving the social, economic, political and legal strength of the women, to ensure equal right to women, and to make them confident enough to claim their rights, such as:

1. Freely live their life with a sense of self-worth, respect and dignity
2. Have complete control of their life, both within and outside of their home and workplace
3. To make their own choices and decisions
4. Have equal rights to participate in social, religious and public activities
5. Have equal social status in the society
6. Have equal rights for social and economic justice
7. Determine financial and economic choices
8. Get equal opportunity for education
9. Get equal employment opportunity without any gender bias
10. Get safe and comfortable working environment.

Importance of Women Empowerment is Important

1. **Underemployed and unemployed:** Women population constitutes around 50% of the world population. A large number of women around the world are unemployed. The world economy suffers a lot because of the unequal opportunity for women at workplaces.
2. **Equally competent and intelligent:** Women are equally competent. Nowadays, women are even ahead of men in many socioeconomic activities.

3. **Talented:** Women are as talented as men. Previously, women were not allowed higher education like men and hence their talents were wasted. But nowadays, they are also allowed to go for higher studies and it encourages women to show their talents which will not only benefit her individually but to the whole world at large.
4. **Overall development of society:** The main advantage of women empowerment is that there will be an overall development of the society. The money that women earn does not only help them and or their family, but it also help develop the society.
5. **Economic benefits:** Women empowerment also leads to more economic benefits not to the individuals but to the society as well. Unlike earlier days when they stayed at home only and do only kitchen stuffs, nowadays, they roam outside and also earns money like the male members of the society. Women empowerment helps women to stand on their own legs, become independent and also to earn for their family which grows country's economy.
6. **Reduction in domestic violence:** Women empowerment leads to decrease in domestic violence. Uneducated women are at higher risk for domestic violence than educated women.
7. **Reduction in corruption:** Women empowerment is also advantageous in case of corruption. Women empowerment helps women to get educated and know their rights and duties and hence can stop corruption.
8. **Reduce poverty:** Women empowerment also reduces poverty. Sometimes, the money earned by the male member of the family is not sufficient to meet the demands of the family. The added earnings of women helps the family to come out of poverty trap.
9. **National development:** Women are increasingly participating in the national development process. They are making the nation proud by their outstanding performances almost every spheres including medical science, social service, engineering, etc.
10. **Irreplaceable in some sectors:** Women are considered irreplaceable for certain jobs.

11. Malnutrition.

Malnutrition occurs when a person does not receive adequate nutrients from diet. This causes damage to the vital organs and functions of the body. Lack of food is the most cause of malnutrition in the poorer and developing countries.

The causes of malnutrition include:
1. Lack of food: This is common among the low income group as well as those who are homeless.
2. Those having difficulty eating due to painful teeth or other painful lesions of the mouth. Those with dysphagia or difficulty swallowing are also at risk of malnutrition. This could be due to a blockage in the throat or mouth or due to sores in the mouth.
3. Loss of appetite: Common causes of loss of appetite include cancers, tumors, depressive illness and other mental illnesses, liver or kidney disease, chronic infections, etc.
4. Those with a limited knowledge about nutrition tend to follow an unhealthy diet with not enough nutrients, vitamins and minerals and are at risk of malnutrition.
5. Elderly living alone, disabled persons living alone or young students living on their own often have difficulty cooking healthy balanced meals for themselves and may be at risk of malnutrition.
6. The elderly (over 65 years of age are), especially those living in care facilities are at a higher risk of malnutrition. These individuals have long-term illnesses that affect their appetite and ability to absorb nutrients from food and they may also have difficulty feeding themselves.

In addition, there may be concomitant mental ailments like depression that affect appetite and food intake.
7. Those who abuse drugs or are chronic alcoholics.
8. Those with eating disorders like anorexia nervosa have difficulty maintaining adequate nutrition.
9. Those with digestive illnesses like ulcerative colitis or Crohn's disease or malabsorption syndrome have difficulty in assimilating the nutrients from diet and may suffer from malnutrition.
10. Those with diarrhea or persistent nausea or vomiting.
11. Some medications tend to alter the body's ability to absorb and break down nutrients and taking these may lead to malnutrition.
12. The demand for energy from food exceeds the amount of food taken. This includes those who have suffered a serious injury, burn or after major surgical procedures. This also includes pregnant women and children whose growth and needs for the unborn baby causes increased demand for nutrients and calories that may be deficient in a normal diet.
13. Among children lack of knowledge of adequate feeding among parents is the leading cause of malnutrition worldwide.
14. Premature babies are at a higher risk of malnutrition as are infants at the time of weaning.
15. Childhood cancers, heart defects from birth (congenital heart disease), cystic fibrosis and other major long-term diseases in children are the leading cause of malnutrition.
16. Neglected children, orphans and those living in care homes are at risk of malnutrition.

Symptoms of Malnutrition in Adults

The most common symptom is a notable weight loss. For example, those who have lost more than 10% of their body weight in the course of three months and are not dieting could be malnourished. This is usually measured using the body mass index or the BMI. This is calculated by the weight in kilograms divided by the height in meters squared. A healthy BMI for adults usually lies between 18.5 and 24.9. Those with a BMI between 17 and 18.5 could be mildly malnourished, those with BMIs between 16 and 18 could be moderately malnourished and those with a BMI less than 16 could be severely malnourished.

Other Symptoms Include

1. Weakness of muscles and fatigue. The muscles of the body appear to waste away and may be left without adequate strength to carry out daily activities.
2. Many people complain of tiredness all day and lack of energy. This may also be due to anemia caused by malnutrition.
3. Increased susceptibility to infections.
4. Delayed and prolonged healing of even small wounds and cuts.
5. Irritability and dizziness
6. Skin and hair becomes dry. Skin may appear dry, and flaky and hair may turn dry, lifeless, dull and appear like straw. Nails may appear brittle and break easily.
7. Some patients suffer from persistent diarrhea or long-term constipation.
8. Menstruation may be irregular or stop completely in malnourished women.
9. Depression is common in malnutrition. This could be both a cause as well as an effect of malnutrition.

Symptoms of Malnutrition in Children

Symptoms of malnutrition in children include:
1. Growth failure: This may be manifested as failure to grow at a normal expected rate in terms of weight, height or both.

2. Irritability, sluggishness and excessive crying along with behavioral changes like anxiety, attention deficit are common in children with malnutrition.
3. The skin becomes dry and flaky and hair may turn dry, dull and straw like in appearance. In addition, there may be hair loss as well.
4. Muscle wasting and lack of strength in the muscles. Limbs may appear stick like.
5. Swelling of the abdomen and legs. The abdomen is swollen because of lack of strength of the muscles of the abdomen. This causes the contents of the abdomen to bulge out making the abdomen swollen. Legs are swollen due to edema. This is caused due to lack of vital nutrients. These two symptoms are seen in children with severe malnutrition.
6. There are classically two types of protein-energy malnutrition (PEM) in children. These are: Marasmus and Kwashiorkor.
7. In Marasmus, there may be obvious weight loss with muscle wasting. There is little or no fat beneath the skin. The skin folds are thin and the face appears pinched like an old man or monkey. Hair is sparse or brittle.
8. In Kwashiorkor the child is between 1 and 2 with hair changing color to a listless red, gray or blonde. Face appears round with swollen abdomen and legs. Skin is dry and dark with splits or stretch marks like streaks where stretched.
9. In nutritional dwarfism the patient appears stunted in growth.

Treatment of Malnutrition at Home

This is suitable for patients who are able to eat and digest food normally. Treatment at home involves:
1. The diet planner and advisor discuss the diet with the patient and makes recommendations and diet plans to improve nutrient intake.
2. In most patients with malnutrition the intake of protein, carbohydrates, water, minerals and vitamins need to be gradually increased.
3. Supplements of vitamins and minerals are often advised.
4. Those with protein energy malnutrition may need to take protein bars or supplements for correction of the deficiency.
5. The body mass index is regularly monitored to check for improvement or responsiveness to dietary interventions.
6. Occupational therapists and a team of physicians of different specialties may be necessary for people with disability who cannot cook or shop for themselves or those who have mental disorders, dementia or long-term illnesses.
7. Those who have difficulty in swallowing, chewing or eating may need to be given very soft or pureed food for easy eating.

Treatment of malnutrition at the hospital: The team of physicians and healthcare providers who manage malnutrition patients includes a gastroenterologist who specializes in treating digestive conditions, a dietician, a nutrition nurse, a psychologist and a social worker. Nasogastric tube feeding, PEG feeding and intravenous infusion or parenteral nutrition may be done in the hospital for moderate to severely malnourished patients who are unable to take food via the mouth.

12. Mode of disease transmission.

There are six common modes of transmission of infection. If the mode of transmission is known, precautions can be put in place to prevent outbreaks. Precautions will vary according to the microorganism involved and the context of the case. For instance, a case of influenza in a normal household setting does not require strict precautions, where as one in a long-term care home might. In hospitals, the infection control team can be a source of advice on which precautions to use. Outside hospitals, the local public health authority can be consulted.

I. Contact
Direct: Direct physical contact (body surface to body surface) between infected individual and susceptible host. For example, influenza virus; infectious mononucleosis; chlamydia. Precautions: Hand hygiene; masks; condoms.

Indirect: Infectious agent deposited onto an object or surface (fomite) and survives long enough to transfer to another person who subsequently touches the object. For example, RSV; Norwalk; rhinovirus, perhaps influenza. Precautions: Sterilizing instruments; disinfecting surfaces and toys in school.

Droplet: Via coughing or sneezing, or (in health care) during suctioning. Droplets are relatively large (>5 μm) and can be projected up to about one meter. For example, *Meningococcus*; influenza (though there is some debate); respiratory viruses. Precautions: Masks; cover mouth; stand clear.

II. Noncontact
Airborne: Transmission via aerosols (airborne particles <5 μm) that contain organisms in droplet nuclei or in dusts. Can be spread via ventilation systems. For example, TB; measles; chickenpox; smallpox (and may be influenza: controversial, as more likely via droplets). Precautions: Masks; negative pressure rooms in hospitals.

Vehicle: A single contaminated source spreads the infection (or poison). This can be a common source or a point source. For example, (a) Point source: Foodborne outbreak from infected batch of food; cases typically cluster around the site (such as a restaurant), (b) Common source: The Listeriosis outbreak in Canada in 2008 was linked to a meat production facility in Ontario. It caused 20 cases across five provinces. Cases may be widely dispersed due to transport and distribution of the vehicle. Precautions: Normal safety and disinfection standards. Deliberate contamination of Tylenol in 1982 led to the use of tamper-proof containers for medicines.

Vector-borne: Transmission by insect or animal vectors. For example, mosquitoes, malaria vector, ticks, Lyme disease vector. Precautions: Protective barriers (window screens, bed nets); insect sprays; culling animals.

SHORT ANSWERS

13. Safe and wholesome water.
Safe and wholesome water is defined as that which is:
1. Free from pathogenic agents
2. Free from harmful chemical substances
3. Pleasant to taste, colorless and odorless
4. Usable for domestic purposes.

If water does not fulfill the above criteria, it is said to be polluted or contaminated. Water pollution is a growing hazard in many developing countries owing to human activity. It is not possible to provide positive health to the community without ample and safe drinking water.

14. Immunoglobulins.

Immunoglobulins (Igs) are glycoprotein molecules also called antibodies (Abs) that are produced in response to foreign substances entering the living body—antigens or immunogens (viruses, bacteria, or toxins, etc.) binding to them and forming antigen-antibody complexes resulting in Ag elimination and protection of the body of the host). Igs are produced by the lymphocytes and are found in fraction of blood called gamma globulin. Gerald M Edelman and Rodney Robert Porter are the notable researchers who worked extensively on purification and structural analysis of Igs, particularly the IgG type. Igs are synthesized with a molecular arrangement that fits the shape of molecules on the antigens or immunogens, in order to allow effective binding of the Abs. Igs binding to Ags basically help to inactivate, weaken or enhance phagocytosis of Ags.

15. Tubectomy.

A tubectomy refers to the blocking or cutting a small portion of the fallopian tubes. These tubes are roughly 10 cm long structures, present within a woman's abdomen and are attached to either side of the uterus. They open into the uterus at one end and on to the ovaries at the other end. The main function of this tube is to carry the ovum (egg)—after it is released from the ovary—into the uterus to help it fertilize. During a tubectomy, the surgeon reaches the fallopian tubes by either cutting open the abdomen (open surgery) or using laparoscopic techniques (minimally invasive surgery). The tubes are then cut and ligated (tied) or a clip is placed at one particular point, thereby stopping the passage of eggs into the uterus. This prevents the possibility of any further pregnancies.

16. Types of diabetes.

Diabetes is a chronic, often debilitating and sometimes fatal disease, in which the body either cannot produce insulin or cannot properly use the insulin it produces. Insulin is a hormone that controls the amount of glucose (sugar) in the blood. Diabetes leads to high blood sugar levels which can damage organs, blood vessels and nerves. The body needs insulin to use sugar as an energy source.

Type 1 diabetes occurs when the immune system mistakenly attacks and kills the beta cells of the pancreas. No, or very little, insulin is released into the body. As a result, sugar builds up in the blood instead of being used as energy. About 5–10% of people with diabetes have type 1 diabetes. Type 1 diabetes generally develops in childhood or adolescence, but can develop in adulthood.

Type 1 diabetes is always treated with insulin. Meal planning also helps with keeping blood sugar at the right levels.

Type 1 diabetes also includes latent autoimmune diabetes in adults (LADA), the term used to describe the small number of people with apparent type 2 diabetes who appear to have immune-mediated loss of pancreatic beta cells.

Type 2 diabetes occurs when the body cannot properly use the insulin that is released (called insulin insensitivity) or does not make enough insulin. As a result, sugar builds up in the blood instead of being used as energy. About 90% of people with diabetes have type 2 diabetes. Type 2 diabetes more often develops in adults, but children can be affected. Depending on the severity of type 2 diabetes, it may be managed through physical activity and meal planning, or may also require medications and/or insulin to control blood sugar more effectively.

A third type of diabetes, gestational diabetes, is a temporary condition that occurs during pregnancy. It affects approximately 2–4% of all pregnancies (in the nonaboriginal population) and involves an increased risk of developing diabetes for both mother and child.

17. Epilepsy.

Epilepsy is a chronic disorder, the hallmark of which is recurrent, unprovoked seizures. Many people with epilepsy have more than one type of seizure and may have other symptoms of neurological problems as well. Sometimes EEG testing, clinical history, family history and outlook are similar among a group of people with epilepsy. In these situations, their condition can be defined as a specific epilepsy syndrome. The human brain is the source of human epilepsy. Although the symptoms of a seizure may affect any part of the body, the electrical events that produce the symptoms occur in the brain. The location of that event, how it spreads and how much of the brain is affected, and how long it lasts all have profound effects. These factors determine the character of a seizure and its impact on the individual. Having seizures and epilepsy can also affect one's safety, relationships, work, driving and so much more. How epilepsy is perceived or how people are treated often is a bigger problem than the seizures.

Causes of epilepsy vary by age of the person. Some people with no clear cause of epilepsy may have a genetic cause. But what is true for every age is that the cause is unknown for about half of everyone with epilepsy.

1. Some people with no known cause of epilepsy may have a genetic form of epilepsy. One or more genes may cause the epilepsy or epilepsy may be caused by the way some genes work in the brain. The relationship between genes and seizures can be very complex and genetic testing is not available yet for many forms of epilepsy.
2. About 3 out of 10 people have a change in the structure of their brains that causes the electrical storms of seizures.
3. Some young children may be born with a structural change in an area of the brain that gives rise to seizures.
4. About 3 out of 10 children with autism spectrum disorder may also have seizures. The exact cause and relationship is still not clear.
5. Infections of the brain are also common causes of epilepsy. The initial infections are treated with medication, but the infection can leave scarring on the brain that causes seizures at a later time.
6. People of all ages can have head injuries, though severe head injuries happen most often in young adults.
7. In middle age, strokes, tumors and injuries are more frequent.
8. In people over 65, stroke is the most common cause of new onset seizures. Other conditions, such as Alzheimer's disease or other conditions that affect brain function can also cause seizures.

18. Trachoma.

Trachoma is a bacterial infection that affects your eyes. It is contagious, spreading through contact with the eyes, eyelids, and nose or throat secretions of infected people. It can also be passed on by handling infected items, such as handkerchiefs. At first, trachoma may cause mild itching and irritation of your eyes and eyelids. Then you may notice swollen eyelids and pus draining from the eyes. Untreated trachoma can lead to blindness. Trachoma is the leading preventable cause of blindness worldwide. The World Health Organization (WHO) estimates that 6 million people have been blinded by trachoma. Most blinding trachoma occurs in poor areas of Africa. Among children under 5, prevalence of active trachoma infections can be 60% or more.

19. Purchasing power.

The alternative to using market exchange rates is to use purchasing power parities (PPPs). The purchasing power of a currency refers to the quantity of the currency needed to purchase a given unit of a good, or common basket of goods and services. Purchasing power is clearly determined by the relative cost of living and inflation rates in different countries. Purchasing power parity means equalizing the purchasing power of two currencies by taking into account these cost of living and inflation differences.

20. Incubation period.

The incubation period is the time between being exposed to a disease and when the symptoms start. If your child was around someone who is sick and the incubation time has gone by, then your child was probably not infected and would not get sick. It is also possible that your child's body had already developed antibodies to fight the infection.

21. Spectrum of health.

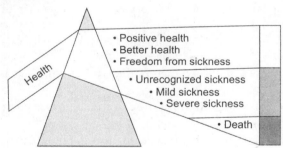

22. Ascariasis.

Ascariasis is an infection of the small intestine caused by *Ascaris lumbricoides* (*A. lumbricoides*), which is a species of roundworm. man can become infected with ascariasis after accidentally ingesting the eggs of the *A. lumbricoides* roundworm. The eggs can be found in soil contaminated by human feces or uncooked food contaminated by soil that contains roundworm eggs. Children often become infected when they put their hands in their mouths after playing in contaminated soil, according to WHO. Ascariasis can also be passed directly from person-to-person. After ingestion, the *A. lumbricoides* roundworm reproduces inside your intestine. The worm goes through several stages:
1. Swallowed eggs first hatch in the intestine.
2. The larvae then move through your bloodstream to your lungs.
3. After maturing, the roundworms leave your lungs and travel to your throat.
4. You will either cough up or swallow the roundworms in your throat. The worms that are swallowed will travel back to your intestine.
5. Once they are back in your intestine, the worms will mate and lay more eggs.
6. The cycle continues. Some eggs are excreted through your feces. Other eggs hatch and return to the lungs.

2014

Community Health Nursing-I

LONG ESSAYS
1. Explain the epidemiologic features and nursing management of typhoid fever.
2. What are the causes of population explosion? and explain the impact on social, economic development of individual, society and community.
3. What are the criteria for healthful housing? Explain the housing standards.

SHORT ESSAYS
4. Effects of noise.
5. Types of ventilation.
6. Dimensions of health.
7. Composting.
8. Intrauterine device.
9. Poliomyelitis.
10. Mode of direct transmission of disease.
11. Women empowerment.
12. Target free approach.

SHORT ANSWERS
13. Carrier.
14. Passive immunity.
15. Crude death rate.
16. No scalpel vasectomy.
17. Zoonosis.
18. Flurosis.
19. Demographic cycle.
20. Epidemic.
21. Chickenpox.
22. Reservoir of infection.

LONG ESSAYS

1. Explain the epidemiologic features and nursing management of typhoid fever.

Typhoid fever is an acute illness associated with fever caused by the *Salmonella typhi* bacteria. It can also be caused by *Salmonella paratyphi*, a related bacterium that usually causes a less severe illness. The bacteria are deposited in water or food by a human carrier and are then spread to other people in the area.

Typhoid fever is characterized by severe systemic illness with fever and abdominal pain. The organism classically responsible for the enteric fever syndrome is *S. enterica* serotype typhi (formerly S. typhi). Other Salmonella serotypes, particularly *S enterica* serotype paratyphi A, B, or C, can cause a similar syndrome; however, it is usually not clinically useful or possible to reliably predict the causative organism based on clinical findings. The term "enteric fever" is a collective term that refers to both typhoid and paratyphoid fever.

Fecal-oral transmission route: The bacteria that cause typhoid fever spread through contaminated food or water and occasionally through direct contact with someone who is infected. In developing nations, where typhoid fever is endemic, most cases result from contaminated drinking water and poor sanitation. The majority of people in industrialized countries pick up typhoid bacteria while traveling and spread it to others through the fecal-oral route. This means that *S. typhi* is passed in the feces and sometimes in the urine of infected people. You can contract the infection if you eat food handled by someone with typhoid fever who has not washed carefully after using the toilet. You can also become infected by drinking water contaminated with the bacteria.

Typhoid carriers: Even after treatment with antibiotics, a small number of people who recover from typhoid fever continue to harbor the bacteria in their intestinal tracts or gallbladders, often for years. These people, called chronic carriers, shed the bacteria in their feces and are capable of infecting others, although they no longer have signs or symptoms of the disease themselves.

Signs and symptoms are likely to develop gradually—often appearing 1–3 weeks after exposure to the disease.

Early illness: Once signs and symptoms do appear, you are likely to experience:
1. Fever that starts low and increases daily, possibly reaching as high as 104.9°F (40.5°C)
2. Headache
3. Weakness and fatigue
4. Muscle aches
5. Sweating
6. Dry cough
7. Loss of appetite and weight loss
8. Abdominal pain
9. Diarrhea or constipation
10. Rash
11. Extremely swollen abdomen
12. Later illness.

If you do not receive treatment, you may:
1. Become delirious
2. Lie motionless and exhausted with your eyes half-closed in what is known as the typhoid state.

Complications

Intestinal bleeding or holes: The most serious complications of typhoid fever—intestinal bleeding or holes (perforations) in the intestine—may develop in the third week of illness. A perforated intestine occurs when your small intestine or large bowel develops a hole, causing intestinal contents to leak into your abdominal cavity and triggering signs and symptoms, such as severe abdominal pain, nausea, vomiting and bloodstream infection (sepsis). This life-threatening complication requires immediate medical care.

Other, less common complications:
- Inflammation of the heart muscle (myocarditis)
- Inflammation of the lining of the heart and valves (endocarditis)
- Pneumonia
- Inflammation of the pancreas (pancreatitis)
- Kidney or bladder infections
- Infection and inflammation of the membranes and fluid surrounding your brain and spinal cord (meningitis)
- Psychiatric problems, such as delirium, hallucinations and paranoid psychosis.

Management: Commonly prescribed antibiotics.

Ciprofloxacin (Cipro): In the United States, doctors often prescribe this for nonpregnant adults.

Ceftriaxone (Rocephin): This injectable antibiotic is an alternative for people who may not be candidates for ciprofloxacin, such as children.

These drugs can cause side effects, and long-term use can lead to the development of antibiotic-resistant strains of bacteria.

Problems with antibiotic resistance: In the past, the drug of choice was chloramphenicol. Doctors no longer commonly use it, however, because of side effects, a high rate of health deterioration after a period of improvement (relapse) and widespread bacterial resistance.

In fact, the existence of antibiotic-resistant bacteria is a growing problem in the treatment of typhoid fever, especially in the developing world. In recent years, S. typhi also has proved resistant to trimethoprim-sulfamethoxazole and ampicillin.

2. What are the causes of population explosion? and explain the impact on social, economic development of individual, society and community.

Population explosion is a self-created catastrophe which the mankind has brought upon itself. Population is one of the primary factor have brought in their wake widespread pollution of air, water and land as well as deforestation, desertification, accidents involving chemicals and the danger of extinction of some plant and animal species.

Causes of population Explosion

Reasons related to high birth rate: Hot climate lack of recreation, child marriage, poverty, polygamy, lack of education, family planning, religious superstitions, housing problems and lack of social security.

Reasons for reduced death rate: Improvement in medical and health services control of epidemics, improvement in economic conditions and increase for increase in the population—lack of political determination and will power regarding family planning.

Effects of population explosion:
1. Low standard of living

2. Shortage of food
3. Old persons have to work beyond the age of retirement
4. Young person work at the cost of education
5. Unemployment, housing and law and order problems

Conflicts and wars: Overpopulation in developing countries puts a major strain on the resources it should be utilizing for development. Conflicts over water are becoming a source of tension between countries, which could result in wars. It causes more diseases to spread and makes them harder to control. Starvation is a huge issue facing the world and the mortality rate for children is being fuelled by it. Poverty is the biggest hallmark we see when talking about overpopulation. All of this will only become worse if solutions are not sought out for the factors affecting our population. We can no longer prevent it, but there are ways to control it.

Rise in unemployment: When a country becomes overpopulated, it gives rise to unemployment as there fewer jobs to support large number of people. Rise in unemployment gives rise to crime as people will steal various items to feed their family and provide them basic amenities of life.

High cost of living: As difference between demand and supply continues to expand due to overpopulation, it raises the prices of various commodities including food, shelter and healthcare. This means that people have to pay more to survive and feed their families.

Solutions to Overpopulation

Better education: One of the first measures is to implement policies reflecting social change. Educating the masses helps them understand the need to have one or two children at the most. Families that are facing a hard life and choose to have four or five children should be discouraged. Family planning and efficient birth control can help in women making their own reproductive choices. Open dialogue on abortion and voluntary sterilization should be seen when talking about overpopulation.

Making people aware of family planning: As population of this world is growing at a rapid pace, raising awareness among people regarding family planning and letting them know about serious after effects of overpopulation can help curb population growth. One of the best way is to let them know about various safe sex techniques and contraceptives methods available to avoid any unwanted pregnancy.

Tax benefits or concessions: Government of various countries might have to come with various policies related to tax exemptions to curb overpopulation. One of them might be to waive of certain part of income tax or lowering rates of income tax for those married couples who have single or two children. As we humans are more inclined towards money, this may produce some positive results.

3. What are the criteria for healthful housing? Explain the housing standards.

Maslow's classic model places human needs on a hierarchy. This means that new needs emerge when those lower on the hierarchy are relatively well-gratified. So, necessities in man's life demands for shelter in which he makes his abode (a home) for healthy living. The natural tendency of man's behavior for shelter is wide, that has resulted in creating modern dwelling to live.

Housing means homes to live in. House refers to a physical structure where unit of society, the family lives but the concept is slowly changing to "Human settlement" which allow the extended outlook of a house, where people live, interact and pursue their goals. A WHO Expert Group (1961) has coined the word residential environment which is used by man for his activity and desired devices for his family well-being.

Importance: Healthy housing plays a vital role in the total welfare of the individuals, families and community. If the houses are poor in construction and sanitation, and are overcrowded, they will lead to diseases, accidents, etc. where by the welfare of whole community as a whole is effected eventually. Therefore, good housing is essential for every individual.

Need of housing: Every person or family lives in different types of houses based on their need and economical status. The following needs of a man have to be fulfilled through good housing:
1. **Physical needs:** A house should be well-ventilated with fresh air, adequate lighting to provide comfort.
2. **Physiological needs:** Like privacy and family life. This will provide satisfaction to mankind.
3. **Psychological needs:** A man will have feeling of having dignity, status in community life, respect of family and satisfaction.
4. **Health needs:** Health needs like adequate water, sanitary latrine, balanced diet, protection from insects and animals through good housing.
5. **Protective needs:** Like safety from accidents. Protection from fire hazards, defaults in electricity, poor flooring can be prevented through strong safe dwellings.

Goals of housing: Goals are statements about desirable conditions. The goals of housing are:
1. **Shelter:** It is a basic need. The house should provide a sanitary shelter.
2. **Family life:** House should provide adequate space for family life and related activities viz. preparation and storage of food, meeting, sleeping, etc.
3. **Access to community facilities:** One of the important elements of housing is accessibility to community services like health services, schools, shopping areas, places of worships, etc.
4. **Economic stability:** Housing is a form of investment. It provides economic stability and well-being of the family.
5. **Family participation:** In community life, family is a part of community. It is an important source of friends. Community focuses on to improve their living conditions.

The implementation of goals of housing by Government should be:
a. Introduce housing schemes.
b. Establish housing standards.
c. Create financial support to improve the housing.

Healthful housing: American Public Health Association has given basic principles of healthful housing on similar lines. WHO has given following healthful housing criteria:
1. It gives physical protection and shelter.
2. Adequate provision for cooking, eating, washing and excretory functions.
3. It prevents spread of infections and communicable diseases.
4. Protects from noise.
5. Protects from atmosphere pollutions.
6. Housing material is free from toxic and harmful chemicals.
7. Encourage personality development.
8. Promote mental health.
9. To attain social goals like:
    a. Family life.
    b. Access to community facility.
    c. Social participation.
    d. Economic stability.

SHORT ESSAYS

4. Effects of noise.

1. **Hearing problems:** Any unwanted sound that our ears have not been built to filter can cause problems within the body. Our ears can take in a certain range of sounds without getting damaged. Man-made noises, such as jackhammers, horns, machinery, airplanes and even vehicles can be too loud for our hearing range. Constant exposure to loud levels of noise can easily result in the damage of our ear drums and loss of hearing. It also reduces our sensitivity to sounds that our ears pick up unconsciously to regulate our body's rhythm.
2. **Health issues:** Excessive noise pollution in working areas, such as offices, construction sites, bars and even in our homes can influence psychological health. Studies show that the occurrence of aggressive behavior, disturbance of sleep, constant stress, fatigue and hypertension can be linked to excessive noise levels. These in turn can cause more severe and chronic health issues later in life.
3. **Sleeping disorders:** Loud noise can certainly hamper your sleeping pattern and may lead to irritation and uncomfortable situations. Without a good night sleep, it may lead to problems related to fatigue and your performance may go down in office as well as at home. It is therefore recommended to take a sound sleep to give your body proper rest.
4. **Cardiovascular issues:** Blood pressure levels, cardiovascular disease and stress related heart problems are on the rise. Studies suggest that high intensity noise causes high blood pressure and increases heart beat rate as it disrupts the normal blood flow. Bringing them to a manageable level depends on our understanding noise pollution and how we tackle it.
5. **Trouble communicating:** High decibel noise can put trouble and may not allow two people to communicate freely. This may lead to misunderstanding and you may get difficult understanding the other person. Constant sharp noise can give you severe headache and disturb your emotional balance.
6. **Effect on wildlife:** Wildlife faces far more problems than humans because noise pollution since they are more dependent on sound. Animals develop a better sense of hearing than us since their survival depends on it. The ill-effects of excessive noise begin at home. Pets react more aggressively in households where there is constant noise. They become disoriented more easily and face many behavioral problems. In nature, animals may suffer from hearing loss, which makes them easy prey and leads to dwindling populations. Others become inefficient at hunting, disturbing the balance of the ecosystem.

Species that depend on mating calls to reproduce are often unable to hear these calls due to excessive man-made noise. As a result, they are unable to reproduce and cause declining populations. Others require sound waves to echo-locate and find their way when migrating. Disturbing their sound signals means they get lost easily and do not migrate when they should. To cope up with the increasing sound around them, animals are becoming louder which may further add to the pollution levels. This is why understanding noise pollution can help us lower the impact it has on the environment.

5. Types of ventilation.

Natural ventilation is the use of wind and temperature differences to create airflows in and through buildings. There are two basic types of natural ventilation effects: Buoyancy and wind. Buoyancy ventilation is more commonly referred to as temperature-induced or stack ventilation. Wind ventilation supplies air from a positive pressure through openings on the windward side of a building and exhausts air to a negative pressure on the leeward side. Air flow rate depends on the wind speed and direction as well as the size of openings. In summer, the indoor-outdoor temperature difference is not high enough to drive buoyancy ventilation, and wind is used to supply as much fresh air as possible. In winter, however, the indoor is much warmer than outdoors, providing an opportunity for buoyancy ventilation.

6. Dimensions of health.

The term wellness can refer to a variety of conditions within the body. While many people associate their wellness to their physical health. It can also be used to describe your environmental, mental, intellectual, occupational, emotional or spiritual well-being. These different dimensions of health will interact together to help determine your full quality of life.

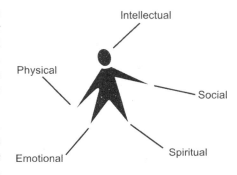

Wellness: It is much more than merely physical health, exercise or nutrition. It is the full integration of states of physical, mental, and spiritual well-being. The model used by our campus includes social, emotional, spiritual, environmental, occupational, intellectual and physical wellness. Each of these seven dimensions act and interact in a way that contributes to our own quality of life.

Social wellness: It is the ability to relate to and connect with other people in our world. Our ability to establish and maintain positive relationships with family, friends and coworkers contributes to our social wellness.

Emotional wellness: It is the ability to understand ourselves and cope with the challenges life can bring. The ability to acknowledge and share feelings of anger, fear, sadness or stress; hope, love, joy and happiness in a productive manner contributes to our emotional wellness.

Spiritual wellness: It is the ability to establish peace and harmony in our lives. The ability to develop congruency between values and actions and to realize a common purpose that binds creation together contributes to our spiritual wellness.

Environmental wellness: It is the ability to recognize our own responsibility for the quality of the air, the water and the land that surrounds us. The ability to make a positive impact on the quality of our environment be it our homes, our communities or our planet contributes to our environmental wellness.

Occupational wellness: It is the ability to get personal fulfillment from our jobs or our chosen career fields while still maintaining balance in our lives. Our desire to contribute in our careers to make a positive impact on the organizations we work in and to society as a whole leads to occupational wellness.

Intellectual wellness: It is the ability to open our minds to new ideas and experiences that can be applied to personal decisions, group interaction and community betterment. The desire to learn new concepts, improve skills and seek challenges in pursuit of lifelong learning contributes to our intellectual wellness.

Physical wellness: It is the ability to maintain a healthy quality of life that allows us to get through our daily activities without undue fatigue or physical stress. The ability to recognize that our behaviors have a significant impact on our wellness and adopting healthful habits (routine check-ups, a balanced diet, exercise, etc.) while avoiding destructive habits (tobacco, drugs, alcohol, etc.) will lead to optimal physical wellness.

7. Composting.

The process of natural decomposition is very important to one type of waste disposal. **Composting** is a form of waste disposal where organic waste decomposes naturally under oxygen-rich conditions. Although, all waste will eventually decompose, only certain waste items are considered compostable and should be added to compost containers, food waste, such as banana peels, coffee grinds and eggshells, are great items to compost. Adding meat products to compost should be avoided because as it decomposes, it will attract large animals and will smell very badly! In addition to food waste, yard waste, such as grass clippings and leaves, can also be added to compost containers. These items will help increase decomposition and help reduce odor as materials break down. As with household food waste, there are also some types of yard waste that should be avoided. Perennial weeds which are plants that come back year after year, should not be added to compost because they will grow back and spread.

Once these waste items are placed in a pile, the composting process can start. The organic materials are broken down naturally by earthworms, bacteria and other organisms that live in soil. Although, the composting process can occur without any further human involvement, most composting involves the addition of water and oxygen—which occurs by turning the compost—to speed up the overall process. After several months, when all the organic material is broken down, the final product is created and is often referred to as humus.

Benefits of composting: As of 2013, over 27% of all municipal solid waste in the United States was comprised of yard and food waste. By composting these items, it makes it possible to reduce the overall amount of waste being sent to landfills and mass-burn incinerators. In addition to reducing waste, the process of composting also creates a usable product. The final compost, humus, is nutrient-rich and can be used to amend poor soils and fertilize gardens instead of using chemical fertilizers. The added compost also helps soil retain water and therefore can improve growing conditions.

Examples of composting: Although, decomposition can occur anywhere naturally, composting is more controlled and occurs in two different types of locations. Composting can occur on a large scale through a city or town's municipality. As of 2012, there were over 3,000 municipal composting programs in the United States. Combined, these facilities recycle around 37% of yard waste in the country.

8. Intrauterine device.

Intrauterine device is inserted into the cavity to prevent conception. The device which are placed in the womb. The device may be inert or medicated. The inert device is made up of plastic material only and the medicated devices are fortified with copper, silver or a progestation preparation. The device which are placed in the womb. The device may be inert or medicated.

1. Lippes loop: It is a double S-shaped serpentine device made of polythene impregnated with barium sulfate for radio-opacity.

Two pieces of nylon (transcervical threads) are attached to the lower end of the loop forming tail, the nylon tail projects into the vagina. Periodic feeling for the tail reassures the user that the loop is in place. The tail also helps in easy removal of the device.

Advantages
1. No moral objection.
2. Easy, cheap to acquired.

3. Once inserted, no further attention is needed, through follow-up to be done in between.
4. Free of systematic side effects.
5. Reversible.
6. Once inserted can be left as long as the individual requires.
7. Insertion is simple and takes only few minutes.

9. Poliomyelitis.

Poliomyelitis also called polio and infantile paralysis. In poliomyelitis, there will be inflammation of the gray matter of the spinal cord.
1. Poliomyelitis is an acute communicable disease caused by the poliovirus. Most patients present with minor illness (fever, malaise, headache, sore throat and vomiting), but a few develop aseptic meningitis and paralytic illness.
2. Poliomyelitis is an acute systemic disease caused by an RNA virus which replicates mainly in the gastrointestinal tract. In some cases, the virus may reach the CNS and damage anterior horn cells of the spinal cord and occasionally the medulla and motor cortex.

Pathogenesis

1. **Agent:** The virus is resistant and stable, remaining viable for months outside the body.
2. **Reservoir of infection:** Man is the only known reservoir of infection. Most infections are subclinical. It is the mild and subclinical infection that play a dominant role in the spread of infection.
3. **Source of infection:** The virus is found in the feces and oropharyngeal secretions of an infected person.
4. **Host factor:** In India, about 50% of cases are reported in infancy. The most vulnerable age is between 6 months and 3 years.
5. **Environmental factors:** Approximately 60% of cases recorded in India were during June to September. The environmental sources of infection are contaminated water, food and flies.
6. **Mode of transmission:** Fecal-oral route is the main route of spread in developing countries. The infection may spread directly through contaminated fingers where hygiene is poor or indirectly through contaminated water, milk, foods, flies and articles of daily use. Droplet infection—this may occur in the acute phase of disease when the virus occurs in the throat.
7. **Incubation period:** Usually 7–14 days.

Prevention of Polio

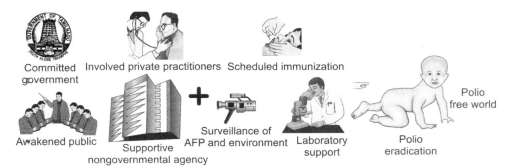

Preventive Measures of Poliomyelitis
1. **Active immunization:** Two types of polio vaccine are used (a) Salk inactivated polio vaccine (IPV) administered by injection, (b) Sabin oral live attenuated vaccine (OPV). It is the recommended vaccine in most countries.
2. **Passive immunization:** With 5–15 mL according to age of child of gamma globulin. Some measures of protection are afforded for 6 weeks. Indications—newborn in hospital are exposed to infection, unimmunized children in hospital ward in which a case of poliomyelitis develops.

Polio vaccines (Sabin): Oral polio vaccine (OPV) has been recommended by the WHO as the vaccine of choice for the eradication of poliomyelitis as it is the only vaccine suitable for carrying out supplementary activities, including PPIs and outbreak control measures. The OPV has several advantages including ease of administration, lower costs and the familiarity of the health staff, other health care providers and the community with the use of OPV.

The advantages of OPV include:
1. Only vaccine suitable for polio eradication strategies and recommended by the WHO for the elimination of wild polioviruses from the environmen.t
2. Case of administration.
3. Familiarity of health personnel with this vaccine.
4. Low cost.
5. Suitability for use in outbreaks.
6. Equally effective as injectable polio vaccine (IPV) under field conditions.
7. Provides immunity to the community vaccine vial monitor (VVM).

10. Provide mode of direct transmission of disease.

Infectious diseases are often spread through direct contact. Types of direct contact include:
1. Person-to-person contact: Infectious diseases are commonly transmitted through direct person-to-person contact. Transmission occurs when an infected person touches or exchanges body fluids with someone else. This can happen before an infected person is aware of the illness. Sexually transmitted diseases (STDs) can be transmitted this way. Pregnant women can also transmit infectious diseases to their unborn children via the placenta. Some STDs including gonorrhea can be passed from mother to baby during childbirth.
2. Droplet spread: The spray of droplets during coughing and sneezing can spread an infectious disease. You can even infect another person through droplets created when you speak. Since droplets fall to the ground within a few feet, this type of transmission requires close proximity.

2. Copper-T: The copper-T is made of plastic but is wrapped with fine copper which enhances its contraceptive effect. Its acceptance is higher than that of the loop. It is T-shaped bioactive contraceptive device made of polyethylene or any other polymer and reinforced with copper metal. The devices are impregnated with barium sulfate for radio-opacity and are fitted with two transcervical threads at the tail end. Metallic copper possess a strong antifertility action.

11. Women empowerment.

(*See* Q. 10, 2015)

12. Target free approach.

Family Welfare Program is to be implemented from the 1st April 1996 on the bases of target free approach. Now the family welfare service is a integrated approach under reproductive and child health services (RCH). The RCH includes family planning + CSSM + precaution of RTI and STD and AIDS + a client approach to provide family welfare and healthcare services. The National Family Welfare Program moves from the target based activity to client centered driven quality services program.

The objective of the family planning programmers to reduce the birth rate. Contraception is only an instrument for bringing about reduction in birth rate. The success of program with reference to the objective can judged only on the basis of the reduction in the birth rate. Grass root level worker like ANM, multipurpose health worker both male and female are to give an estimate of the various family welfare activities required in the areas/population covered by them. It is expected that at the PHC level plan, the local NGO activities primary school teachers, pradhans and panchayat members, private practioners of indigenous systems of medicines would be involved in the formulation of the PHC based family welfare health care. Aggregation of all such estimates of grass root workers of various subcenters and at the primary health center shall be prepared at each PHC in the distinct.

Although, the input requirement for family welfare activities shall be based on the requirement given by grass root level worker like ANM, the monitoring in the performance of ANM shall not be merely on the basis of achievements in this regard alone, but would be done with the help of indicators to improvements and quality service.

SHORT ANSWERS

13. Carrier.

The term "carrier" is used for any person who is symptom-free (or has only very mild symptoms) despite having a medical condition. The two main types are—carriers of genetic diseases and carriers of infectious diseases. Genetic carriers can occur in any recessive but not in a dominant genetic disease. For example, X-linked recessive diseases affect only males, with women being symptom-free carriers of a genetic defect, passed onto their male children. Both males and females can be carriers of autosomal recessive genetic diseases. Genetic carriers are not contagious; they can only pass the disease onto their own children through genetics. Infectious disease carriers are those who have a low-level infection with a disease but without symptoms. Carriers of infectious diseases can be contagious even if they do not have symptoms. Whether an infectious carrier is contagious depends on the type of condition.

14. Passive immunity.

Passive immunity means that you gained resistance to the disease without having to actively do anything to gain resistance. In other words, you have received the antibodies that you needed to fight off an infection without your own immune system having to create the antibodies. This is in contrast to active immunity, in which your immune system has to be exposed to the disease in order to actually create the antibodies that are needed to fight the disease.

There are two main ways that passive immunity is acquired. One way is experienced by babies worldwide everyday during fetal development. The baby acquires the antibodies in the mother's body, which she has created over her lifetime. This is called natural passive immunity.

We all experienced a little passive immunity at least once in life. There is another added benefit for babies that are breastfed. The first milk to come out is also packed with antibodies from the mother's body. This is a lot of the reason why pediatricians recommend breastfeeding, and why studies have shown that breastfed babies are healthier overall. The antibodies circulate for about 6 weeks and then they are no longer in the blood.

15. Crude death rate.

The total number of deaths per year per 1,000 people. As of 2014, the crude death rate for the whole world is 7.89 per 1,000 (down from 8.37 per 1,000 in 2009) according to the current CIA World Fact book. Note that the crude death rate can be misleading.

16. No scapel vasectomy.

The no scalpel vasectomy is a technique used to do the vasectomy through one single puncture. The puncture is made in the scrotum and requires no suturing or stitches. The primary difference compared to the conventional vasectomy is that the vas deferens is controlled and grasped by the surgeon in a less traumatic manner. This results in less pain and fewer postoperative complications. This procedure is done with the aid of a local anesthetic called 'Xylocaine' (similar to 'Novocain'). The actual interruption of the vas which is done with the no scalpel technique is identical to the interruption used with conventional techniques. The no scalpel technique is simply a more elegant and less traumatic way for the surgeon to control the vas and proceed with its interruption.

17. Zoonosis.

Zoonosis or a **zoonotic disease** is one that can be passed between humans and animals. Humans often consider themselves separate from the 'wild world' of animals, but we are actually just another species and part of the big biological picture. Zoonotic diseases are so common, in fact, that the Centers for Disease Control and Prevention has estimated that roughly six of every ten infectious diseases qualify as zoonotic. Many can be fatal if left untreated.

Usually, some type of physical contact is required. This can be via contact with the animal itself, through contact with bodily fluids (such as blood, saliva, urine, or feces) or through contact with something that has been contaminated by the animal or its bodily fluids. So, a bite from an insect or tick can transmit disease to a human. Interacting with animals at a state fair, a petting zoo, a farm, or a pet store can transmit disease. Even eating or drinking contaminated food or water can transmit disease.

18. Flurosis.

Ingestion of excess fluoride, most commonly in drinking-water, can cause fluorosis which affects the teeth and bones. Moderate amounts lead to dental effects, but long-term ingestion of large amounts can lead to potentially severe skeletal problems. Paradoxically, low levels of fluoride intake help to prevent dental caries. The control of drinking-water quality is therefore critical in preventing fluorosis. Fluorosis is caused by excessive intake of fluoride. The dental effects of fluorosis develop much earlier than the skeletal effects in people exposed to large amounts of fluoride. Clinical dental fluorosis is characterized by staining and pitting of the teeth. In more severe cases all the enamel may be damaged. However, fluoride may not be the only cause of dental enamel defects. Enamel opacities similar to dental fluorosis are associated with other conditions, such as malnutrition with deficiency of vitamins D and A or a low protein-energy diet. Ingestion of fluoride after six years of age will not cause dental fluorosis.

Chronic high-level exposure to fluoride can lead to skeletal fluorosis. In skeletal fluorosis, fluoride accumulates in the bone progressively over many years. The early symptoms of skeletal fluorosis include stiffness and pain in the joints. In severe cases, the bone structure may change and ligaments may calcify, with resulting impairment of muscles and pain. Acute high-level exposure to fluoride causes immediate effects of abdominal pain, excessive saliva, nausea and vomiting. Seizures and muscle spasms may also occur.

19. Demographic cycle.

Demography is the scientific study of human population. It focuses its attention on the following three observable human phenomenon:
1. Change in population size (growth or decline).
2. Composition of population.
3. Distribution of population in space.

The demographic processes which determine these phenomena are:
1. Fertility
2. Mortality
3. Marriage
4. Migration
5. Social mobility.

Demographic cycle: A look back into the history shows that every nation passes through five stages of demographic cycle:
1. First stage (high stationary): It is characterized by high birth rate and high death rate which cancel each other. So, the population remains stationary. India was in this stage till 1920.
2. Second stage (early expanding): There is a decline in death rate while the birth rate remains unchanged. So, the population expands. Many developing countries of Asia and Africa are in this stage.
3. Third stage (late expanding): Death rate declines further and birth rate begins to fall. Yet there is an increase in population since birth exceeds deaths. India appears to have entered this stage.
4. Fourth stage (low stationary): Low birth rate and low death rate. So, the population becomes stationary. Sweden, Belgium, Denmark and Switzerland are in this stage.
5. Fifth stage (declining): Population begins to decline as birth rate is lower than death rate. East European countries like Germany and Hungary are now in this stage.

20. Epidemic.

An epidemic is the rapid spread of infectious disease to a large number of people in a given population within a short period of time, usually two weeks or less. Epidemics **occur when an agent and susceptible hosts are present in adequate** numbers, and the agent can be effectively conveyed from a source to the susceptible hosts. More specifically, an epidemic may result from:
1. A recent increase in amount or virulence of the agent.
2. The recent introduction of the agent into a setting where it has not been before.
3. An enhanced mode of transmission so that more susceptible persons are exposed.
4. A change in the susceptibility of the host response to the agent.
5. Factors that increase host exposure or involve introduction through new portals of entry.

21. Chickenpox.

Also known as varicella, chickenpox is a virus that often affects children. It is characterized by itchy, red blisters that appear all over the body. Chickenpox was once so common it was considered a childhood rite of passage. It is very rare to have the chickenpox infection more than once.

Symptoms: A rash is the most common symptom of the chickenpox. However, you will be contagious several days before the rash develops and will experience other symptoms first, such as:
1. Fever.
2. Headache.
3. Loss of appetite.

About 2 days after you experience the symptoms mentioned above, the rash will begin to develop. The rash goes through three different phases before you recover from the virus. These phases include:
1. Developing red or pink bumps all over your body.
2. Bumps filled with fluid that leak.
3. Bumps that scab over and begin to heal.

The bumps on your body will not all be in the same phase at the same time. New bumps will appear throughout your infection. You are still contagious until all the bumps on your body have scabbed over.

Causes: The varicella-zoster virus causes the chickenpox infection. Most cases occur through contact with an infected person. The virus may be contagious several days before blisters appear, and it remains contagious until all blisters have crusted over. It is spread through:
1. Saliva.
2. Coughing.
3. Sneezing.
4. Contact with blisters.

22. Reservoir of infection.

Reservoir includes places in the environment where the pathogen lives (this includes people, animals and insects, medical equipment, and soil and water).

Medical-Surgical Nursing

2019

Medical-Surgical Nursing-I

LONG ESSAYS

1. a. Define and classify anemia. b. Explain the etiological factors, clinical manifestations and management of iron deficiency anemia. c. Describe the role of nurse in prevention of iron deficiency anemia.
2. a. Describe the etiopathophysiology and clinical manifestations of pulmonary tuberculosis. b. Describe the diagnostic measures and medical management of pulmonary tuberculosis. c. Describe the role of nurse in prevention of pulmonary tuberculosis.
3. Mr Suresh is diagnosed with colorectal cancer and is posted for colostomy: a. Define the term ostomy, b. List the types of ostomies, c. Explain the postoperative management of Mr Suresh with colostomy.

SHORT ESSAYS

4. Explain the pathophysiology of acute inflammatory process.
5. Describe the management of client with acute renal failure.
6. Explain the different treatment modalities for fracture.
7. Define myocardial infection and discuss the nursing management of a patient with acute-myocardial infraction.
8. Explain pathophysiology and management of nephritic syndrome.
9. Describe the management of client after amputation.
10. Describe the acute and chronic complications of diabetes mellitus.
11. Explain the causes and management of psoriasis.
12. Explain the drug therapy for HIV infection.

SHORT ANSWERS

13. List the methods of prevention of hepatitis B.
14. Differentiate between disinfection and sterilization.
15. List the complications of valve replacement surgery.
16. What is paget's disease?
17. Name the specific blood investigation to rule out typhoid fever.
18. List the clinical features of myxedema.
19. What is acne vulgaris?
20. What is cardiopulmonary resuscitation?

21. Define hemorrhoids.
22. List the clinical manifestations of Cushings syndrome.

LONG ESSAYS

1. a. Define and classify anemia. b. Explain the etiological factors, clinical manifestations and management of iron deficiency anemia, c. Describe the role of nurse in prevention of iron deficiency anemia

Refers to a deficit of RBC or Hb is blood resulting in decreased oxygen carrying capacity.

Classification: Acquired anemia: Anemia due to deficiency of factors for the production of anemia.
1. Iron deficiency anemia.
2. Megaloblastic anemia.
3. Pernicious anemia.
4. Aplastic anemia.
5. Hemolytic anemia: Anemia resulting from excessive RBC destruction.
6. Hemorrhagic anemia: Anemia due to excessive blood loss.
7. Sickle cell anemia, thalassemia.

Etiology

1. **Blood loss due to:** Trauma and ulceration, decreased production of platelets, increased destruction of platelets, and decreased of clotting factors.
2. **Impaired RBC production:** Nutritional deficiencies, iron deficiency most common, folic acid, vitamin B_{12} or B_6 deficiency.
3. **Deceased erythrocyte production:** Secondary hemolytic anemia associated with chronic infections, renal disease, drugs, diarrhea, bone marrow depression, leukemia, aplastic anemia, transient erythrocytopenia of childhood.
4. **Increased RBC destruction:** Drugs, chemicals, parvovirus infections.
   Antibody reactions—RH, ABO incompatibility, lack of absorption, inadequate intake of nutrients, excessive blood loss.

Clinical Manifestations

Early symptoms: Listlessness, fatigability, anorexia, nausea, constipation, hemorrhoids, weight loss, diarrhea, headache, dizziness, numbness, twinkling of extremities, irritabilities and paralysis. Late symptoms pallor, palpitations tachycardia, weakness, tachypnea, shortness of breath on exertion.

Repeated Infections

Diagnostic Evaluations

1. Complete blood count
2. Physical examination
3. Serum iron, total iron binding capacity
4. Serum ferritin
5. Vitamin B_{12}, B_6 and folate levels
6. Hb level
7. Stool examination for worms.

Management

1. Oral iron at a dose of 6 mg/kg/day.
2. Dietetic management—reduce top milk, and increase iron fortified cereals, bread products, green leafy vegetables, egg, etc.
3. Inferon injections—intramuscular injections are given in Z tract to avoid staining of muscles oxygen therapy.
4. Blood transfusion.

Nursing Management

1. Collect detail history related to the life pattern, diet and hygiene.
2. Assess pallor and fatigability.
3. Observe for exertional dyspnea.
4. Stool examination for worm infestation.
5. Monitor weight of the patient.
6. Monitor HB level.

2. a. Describe the etiopathophysiology and clinical manifestations of pulmonary tuberculosis. b. Describe the diagnostic measures and medical management of pulmonary tuberculosis. c. Describe the role of nurse in prevention of pulmonary tuberculosis.

Pulmonary tuberculosis is an infectious disease of lung parenchyma caused by *Mycobacterium tuberculi*. It is also transmitted to bone, meninges, kidney and lymph nodes.

Risk Factors

1. Close contact
2. Immunosuppressed patients
3. Overcrowding, substance abuse.

Etiology

Mycobacterium tuberculosis, a gram-positive, acid-fast bacilli, is usually spread via air-borne droplets which are produced when the infected individual coughs, sneezes or speaks. Once released into a room, the organisms are dispersed and can be inhaled. Brief exposure to a tubercle bacilli rarely causes an infection. Rather it is more commonly spread to the individual who has had repeated close contact with an infected person. It is not highly infective and transmitted. It usually requires close, frequent or prolonged exposure. The disease cannot be spread by hands, books, glasses, dishes or other fomites.

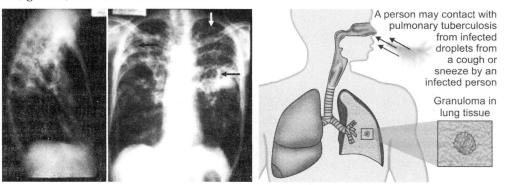

Pathophysiology

When an individual with no previous exposure to TB (negative tuberculin reactor) inhales a sufficient number of tubercle bacilli into the alveoli, tuberculosis infection occurs. The body's reaction to the TB bacilli depends on the susceptibility of the individual, the size of the dose and the virulence of the organisms. Inflammation occurs within the alveoli (parenchyma) of the lungs, and natural body defenses attempt to counteract the infection.

When the bacilli are inhaled, they pass down the bronchial system and implant themselves on the respiratory bronchioles or alveoli. The lower part of the lungs is usually the site of initial bacterial implantation. After implantation, the bacilli multiply with no initial resistance from the host. The organisms are engulfed by phagocytosis (initially neutrophils and later macrophages) and may continue to multiply within the phagocytes.

Macrophages ingest the organism and present the microbacterial antigens to the T cells. CD4 cells secrete lymphokine that enhance the capacity of the macrophages to ingest and kill bacteria. Lymph nodes in the hilar region of the lung become enlarged on their filter drainage from the infected site. The inflammatory process and the cellular reaction produce a small, firm, white nodules called the 'primary tubercle'. The center of the nodules contains tubercle bacilli. Cells gather around the center and usually the outer portion becomes fibrosed. Thus, blood vessels are compressed, nutrition of tubercle is impaired, and necrosis occurs at the center. The area becomes walled off by fibrotic tissue, and the center gradually becomes soft and cheesy in consistency. This later process is known as "Caseation necrosis". This material may become calcified (calcium deposits) or it may liquify (liquification necrosis). The liquified material maybe coughed up, leaving a cavity or hole in the parenchyma of the lung. This cavity or cavities are visible on chest X-ray films and results in the diagnosis of cavitary disease. The only X-ray evidence of TB infection is a calcified nodule known as "Ghon's tubercle". Ghon's tubercle is referred to as the "primary complex". When a tuberculosis lesion regresses and heals, the infection enters a latent period in which it may persist without producing a clinical illness. The infection may develop into clinical disease if the persisting organism begins to multiply rapidly, or it may remain dormant. If the initial immune response is not adequate, control of the organisms is not maintained and clinical disease results. Certain individuals are at a higher risk for clinical disease including those who are immunosuppressed, e.g. HIV, cancer, person who received chemotherapy or corticosteroid therapy or have diabetes mellitus. Dormant but viable organism persists for years. Reactivation of TB can occur if the host defense mechanisms become impaired.

Clinical Manifestation

In the early stages of TB, the person is usually free of symptoms. Many cases are found incidentally when routine chest X-rays are taken especially in older adults. Systemic manifestation may initially consist of fatigue, malaise, anorexia, weight loss, low-grade fever (especially in late afternoons) and night sweats. The weight loss may not be excessive until late in the disease and is often attributed to overwork or other factors. Irregular menses may also be present in premenopausal women.

A characteristic pulmonary manifestation is cough that becomes frequent and produces mucoid or macopurulents sputum. Chest pain characterized as dull or tight may also be present. Hemoptysis is not a common finding and is usually associated with more advanced cases Sometimes TB has more acute, sudden manifestation. The patient has high fever, chills, generalized Flu-like symptoms, pleuritic pain and a production of cough.

The complication of TB is miliary tuberculosis, pleural effusion, TB pneumonia, involvement of other organs, e.g. bone, kidney, brain, etc.

Diagnostic Investigations

History, chest X-ray, sputum for AFP and culture, Mantoux test.

Mantoux test: By using a tuberculin syringe, 0.1 mL of PPD is introduced in the forearm, and the indurations is measured after 48-72 hours. The reading of 10 mm or above shows highly significant infection, 5-9 is exposed to infection, 0-4 no sensitivity.

Medical Management

Treatment regimen		Regimen
Category of treatment	Type of patient	
Category I	New sputum smear-positive Seriously ill sputum smear-negative Seriously ill extrapulmonay	2(HRZE)3 4(HR)3
Category II	Sputum smear-positive relapse Sputum smear-positive failure Sputum semar-positive treatment after default	2(HRZES)3 1(HRZES)3 5(HRE)3
Category III	Sputum smear-negative Not seriously ill, extrapulmonary	2(JRX)3 4(HR)3

Pharmacological: Isoniazid (INH), refampicin (RIF), ethambutal (EMB), pyrizinamide (PZA), streptomycin (SM)

Directly observed treatment short (DOTS) course therapy

The number before the letters refers to the number of months of treatment. The subscript after the letters refers to the number of doses per week. H: Isoniazid (600 mg), R: Rifampicin (450 mg), Z: Pyrazinamide (1500 mg), E: Ethambutol (1200 mg), S: Streptomycin (750 mg). Patients who weigh more than 60 kg receive additional rifampicin 150 mg. Patients more than 50-year-old receive streptomycin 500 mg. Patients in categories I and II who have positive sputum smear at the end of the initial intensive phase receive an additional month of intensive phase treatment.

Nursing Management

1. Treat the patient with antituberculoid drugs.
2. Advice to cover the nose and mouth while sneezing and coughing.
3. Advice the patient to take the medicine continuously.
4. Dispose the waste properly.
5. Tracheobronchial suctioning.
6. Postural drainage.
7. Coughing exercise.
8. Explain the treatment regimen and side effects.
9. Instruct the personal hygiene.
10. Small and frequent feeds.
11. Increased fluid intake.

3. **Mr Suresh is diagnosed with colorectal cancer and is posted for colostomy: a. Define the term ostomy. b. List the types of ostomies. c. Explain the postoperative management of Mr Suresh with colostomy.**

(See Q. 8, 2015 for a and b)

Postprocedure Care
1. When return flow is complete, remove the Mackintosh clean the skin around the colostomy opening of and dry use skin thoroughly.
2. Apply a clean dressing or a clear colostomy bad over the stoma.
3. Change the dressing of incision aspects technique.
4. Take all the articles in utility room. Clean the equipments immediately.
5. Patients are instructed for the care and deamy of colostomy bags to prolong its life and keep it fete from odor.
6. Chart the procedure in the patient's record.

SHORT ESSAYS

4. **Explain the pathophysiology of acute inflammatory process.**

(See Q. 5, 2015)

5. **Describe the management of client with acute renal failure.**

Acute renal failure is an acute loss of kidney function that occurs over days to weeks and results in an inability to appropriately excrete nitrogenous wastes and creatinine. Electrolyte disturbances and loss of fluid homeostasis may occur. In spite of this rapid decline in kidney function, patients with acute renal failure often have few symptoms.

Pathophysiology: Creatinine is a metabolic waste product excreted by the kidneys. When the GFR is normal, creatinine is filtered through the glomerulus into the tubules and then excreted. Creatinine is also secreted by tubular cells. Medications, such as trimethoprim [Proloprim; with sulfamethoxazole (Bactrim, Septra)] and cimetidine (Tagamet) can inhibit tubular secretion and falsely elevate the serum creatinine level. Formulas to estimate the glomerular filtration rate (GFR) in patients with acute renal failure should not be used to adjust medication dosages because the serum creatinine level is not in a steady state and continues to fluctuate.

Management
Treatment for acute kidney failure involves identifying the illness or injury that originally damaged your kidneys. the treatment options depend on what's causing your kidney failure. The doctor will also work to prevent complications and allow your kidneys time to heal. Treatments that help prevent complications include:
1. **Treatments to balance the amount of fluids in your blood:** If your acute kidney failure is caused by a lack of fluids in the blood, your doctor may recommend intravenous (IV) fluids. In other cases, acute kidney failure may cause you to have too much fluid leading to swelling in your arms and legs. In these cases, your doctor may recommend medications (diuretics) to cause your body to expel extra fluids.
2. **Medications to control blood potassium:** If the kidneys are not properly filtering potassium from the blood, the doctor may prescribe calcium, glucose or sodium polystyrene sulfonate (Kionex) to prevent the accumulation of high levels of potassium in your blood. Too much

potassium in the blood can cause dangerous irregular heartbeats (arrhythmias) and muscle weakness.
3. **Medications to restore blood calcium levels:** If the levels of calcium in your blood drop too low, your doctor may recommend an infusion of calcium.
4. **Dialysis to remove toxins from your blood:** If toxins build up in the blood, you may need temporary hemodialysis- often referred to simply as dialysis—to help remove toxins and excess fluids from the body while your kidneys heal. Dialysis may also help remove excess potassium from the body. During dialysis, a machine pumps blood out of your body through an artificial kidney (dialyzer) that filters out waste. The blood is then returned to your body.

6. Explain the different treatment modalities for fracture.

A broken bone or bone fracture occurs when a force exerted against a bone is stronger than the bone can bear. This disturbs the structure and strength of the bone, and leads to pain, loss of function and sometimes bleeding and injury around the site. Our skeleton is made up of bones. Bones are a type of connective tissue, reinforced with calcium and bone cells. Bones have a softer center called marrow where blood cells are made. The main functions of our skeleton are supporting our body enabling movement and protecting our internal organs.

Broken bones heal by themselves—the aim of medical treatment is to make sure the pieces of bone are lined up correctly. The bone needs to recover fully in strength, movement and sensitivity. Some complicated fractures may need surgery or surgical traction (or both).

Depending on where the fracture is and how severe, treatment may include:
1. Splints: To stop movement of the broken limb
2. Braces: To support the bone
3. Plaster cast: To provide support and immobilise the bone
4. Traction: A less common option
5. Surgically inserted metal rods or plates: To hold the bone pieces together
6. Pain relief.

Immobilization: The most common type of fracture management is with immobilization. There are different types of immobilization including splint, braces, casts, slings, and others.

Cast immobilization is the most common method where a material (typically plaster or fiberglass) is wrapped around an injured extremity and allowed to harden. Casts come in an endless number of shapes and sizes and require proper cast care.

Fractures treated with immobilization must be adequately aligned to allow for healing with good results. If the alignment of the fracture is not sufficient, further treatment will be needed.

Reducing (resetting) the broken bone: A procedure called a fracture reduction, or reducing a fracture, is an intervention to better align the broken bones. A fracture reduction can either be done as a closed reduction (nonsurgical) or an open reduction (surgery). A typical closed reduction is performed either by providing local anesthetic to the broken bone or a general anesthesia, followed by a specific maneuver to attempt to realign the broken bone. After a closed reduction, a splint or cast would be applied to hold the bones in the improved alignment.

Traction: Traction is an older form of fracture management that is used much less commonly today. However, there are certain situations where traction can be a very useful treatment option. Traction involves gentle pulling of the extremity to align the bones. Often a metal pin is placed in the bone on the far side of the fracture, this is called skeletal traction. Ropes and weights are attached to the pin to gently pull the bone fragments into alignment.

Pins: Pins are often used to stabilize smaller bones (For example, hands and wrist) when a closed reduction can be used to improve alignment, but a cast is insufficient to hold the bones in place. Pins are typically placed through the skin in a procedure called a closed reduction with percutaneous pinning (CRPP). The pins are placed in an operating room, but can typically be removed in your doctor's office and there is little discomfort in most pin removal procedures. If there is discomfort, the removal can be performed in the operating room.

External fixation: External fixation also uses pins that enter the skin but are held together outside the body with a frame to maintain alignment. External fixation is an excellent option with severe trauma as they can be applied quickly, they can be adjusted as needed, and they allow access to the skin and soft-tissue wounds. External fixation is often used with open fractures vs. closed fracture. External fixation can also be helpful when there is significant swelling that could make surgery too risky. By temporarily immobilizing the fracture, the swelling can improve, and internal fixation can be considered at a later time.

Open reduction with internal fixation: Open reduction means to surgically open the site of the fracture, align the bone fragments, and then hold them in place. The most common type of internal fixation are metal plates and screws, although there are many devices that can be used to stabilize different types of fractures.

Intrameduallary rodding: Intramedullary IM rodding is a surgical procedure to stabilize a broken bone by inserting a metal rod in the hollow medullary canal of the bone. This part of the bone (where the bone marrow is) can be used to hold the rod and allow for early movement and weight bearing. IM rodding is often the preferred treatment for fractures of the lower extremity long bones that are not close to the joints (bone ends). In these cases, patients can resume walking much sooner than with other types of fracture treatment.

Operation Procedure for Bone Fractures

A cast made from plaster of Paris is one of the most common ways of immobilizing a limb. This cast is made from a preparation of gypsum that sets hard when water is added. Depending on the location and severity of the fracture, the operation procedures can include:

1. **Closed or simple fractures:** The two ends of the broken bone are lined up and held in place. The limb is thoroughly bandaged, then the wet plaster is applied. Sometimes, once the plaster is dry, the cast is split into two and the two halves are rebandaged on the outside. This allows for any swelling that may occur
2. **Open or compound fractures:** These are thoroughly cleaned in the operating room to remove debris before being set because a broken bone exposed to the open air may become infected.
3. **Long bones:** Long bones, such as the bone of the thigh (femur) are difficult to keep aligned. In adults these are often treated by internal nailing. A child may need traction for a couple of days before setting the bone in a cast. Once the two ends of bone start to show signs of healing, the leg and hip joint are immobilized in plaster of Paris. In other cases, pins are inserted above and below the fracture and secured to an external frame or 'fixator'. This is done under a general anesthetic.

Immediately after an operation on a bone fracture: After surgery, your doctor will check that you have full feeling in the area. For example, if you have a broken arm in plaster, they may ask you to wiggle your fingers. They will also check your limb for tingling, pallor (pale color) or coolness. These tests check whether the splint is affecting your limb's nerve and blood supply. The injured part is kept as still as possible in the first few days. Nurses will offer you pain-relieving medication. They will determine the difference between the pain of the fracture and any pain that could be caused by the splint, traction, plaster cast, poor alignment of the limb or swelling of the limb.

7. Define myocardial infection and discuss the nursing management of a patient with acute myocardial infraction.

The term "myocardial infarction" focuses on the myocardium (the heart muscle) and the changes that occur in it due to the sudden deprivation of circulating blood. The main change is necrosis (death) of myocardial tissue. The word "infarction" comes from the Latin "infarcire" meaning "to plug up or cram." It refers to the clogging of the artery.

Myocardial infarction (MI) is used synonymously with coronary occlusion and heart attack, yet MI is the most preferred term as myocardial ischemia causes acute coronary syndrome (ACS) that can result in myocardial death.
1. In an MI, an area of the myocardium is permanently destroyed because plaque rupture and subsequent thrombus formation result in complete occlusion of the artery.
2. The spectrum of ACS includes unstable angina, non-ST-segment elevation MI, and ST-segment elevation MI.

Nursing Management
The nursing management involved in MI is critical and systematic, and efficiency is needed to implement the care for a patient with MI.

Nursing Assessment
One of the most important aspects of care of the patient with MI is the assessment.
1. Assess for chest pain not relieved by rest or medications.
2. Monitor vital signs, especially the blood pressure and pulse rate.
3. Assess for presence of shortness of breath, dyspnea, tachypnea, and crackles.
4. Assess for nausea and vomiting.
5. Assess for decreased urinary output.
6. Assess for the history of illnesses.
7. Perform a precise and complete physical assessment to detect complications and changes in the patient's status.
8. Assess IV sites frequently.

Diagnosis: Based on the clinical manifestations, history, and diagnostic assessment data, major nursing diagnosis may include.

Ineffective cardiac tissue perfusion related to reduced coronary blood flow.

Risk for ineffective peripheral tissue perfusion: Related to decreased cardiac output from left ventricular dysfunction.
Deficient knowledge related to post-MI self-care.

Planning and Goals
To establish a plan of care, the focus should be on the following:
1. Relief of pain or ischemic signs and symptoms.
2. Prevention of myocardial damage.
3. Absence of respiratory dysfunction.
4. Maintenance or attainment of adequate tissue perfusion.
5. Reduced anxiety.
6. Absence or early detection of complications.
7. Chest pain absent/controlled.
8. Heart rate/rhythm sufficient to sustain adequate cardiac output/tissue perfusion.
9. Achievement of activity level sufficient for basic self-care.

10. Anxiety reduced/managed.
11. Disease process, treatment plan, and prognosis understood.
12. Plan in place to meet needs after discharge.

Nursing Priorities
1. Relieve pain, anxiety.
2. Reduce myocardial workload.
3. Prevent/detect and assist in treatment of life-threatening dysrhythmias or complications.
4. Promote cardiac health, self-care.

Nursing Interventions
Nursing interventions should be anchored on the goals in the nursing care plan.
1. Administer oxygen along with medication therapy to assist with relief of symptoms.
2. Encourage bed rest with the back rest elevated to help decrease chest discomfort and dyspnea.
3. Encourage changing of positions frequently to help keep fluid from pooling in the bases of the lungs.
4. Check skin temperature and peripheral pulses frequently to monitor tissue perfusion.
5. Provide information in an honest and supportive manner.
6. Monitor the patient closely for changes in cardiac rate and rhythm, heart sounds, blood pressure, chest pain, respiratory status, urinary output, changes in skin color, and laboratory values.

Evaluation
After the implementation of the interventions within the time specified, the nurse should check if:
1. There is an absence of pain or ischemic signs and symptoms.
2. Myocardial damage is prevented.
3. Absence of respiratory dysfunction.
4. Adequate tissue perfusion maintained.
5. Anxiety is reduced.

Discharge and Home Care Guidelines
The most effective way to increase the probability that the patient will implement a self-care regimen after discharge is to identify the patient's priorities.

Education: This is one of the priorities that the nurse must teach the patient about heart-healthy living.

Home care: The home care nurse assists the patient with scheduling and keeping up with the follow-up appointments and with adhering to the prescribed cardiac rehabilitation management.

Follow-up monitoring: The patient may need reminders about follow-up monitoring including periodic laboratory testing and ECGs, as well as general health screening.

Adherence: The nurse should also monitor the patient's adherence to dietary restrictions and prescribed medications.

Documentation Guidelines
To ensure that every action documented is an action done, documentation must be secured. The following should be documented:
1. Individual findings.
2. Vital signs, cardiac rhythm, presence of dysrhythmias.

3. Plan of care and those involved in planning.
4. Teaching plan.
5. Response to interventions, teaching, and actions performed.
6. Attainment or progress towards desired outcomes.
7. Modifications to plan of care.

8. Explain pathophysiology and management of nephritic syndrome.
(See Q. 11, 2015)

9. Describe the management of client after amputation.

Lower extremity amputations are most commonly performed because of advanced chronic peripheral arterial disease. Amputation can relieve signs and symptoms, improve function, and maintain or improve the patient's quality of life. Most postoperative nursing care priorities are the same as for any surgical patient: assessing and maintaining the patient's airway, breathing, and circulation; monitoring vital signs; managing pain; taking steps to prevent respiratory complications and venous thromboembolism; and watching for signs and symptoms of hemorrhage.

1. After surgery, the patient will have a soft dressing or a rigid dressing made of fiberglass or plaster.
2. Assess the surgical dressing for integrity and drainage. Elevate the stump for the first 24 to 48 hours.
3. Move and turn the patient gently and slowly to prevent severe muscle spasms.
4. Reposition the patient every 2 hours, turning the patient from side to side and prone, if possible.
5. Lying prone helps reduce hip flexion contractures. Avoid placing pillows between the patient's legs or under the back.
6. Unwrap the stump dressing every 4–6 hours for the first 2 days postoperatively as prescribed and then at least once daily.
7. Assess the stump for signs and symptoms of infection and skin irritation or breakdown.
8. Assess the color, temperature, and most proximal pulse on the stump before rewrapping it, comparing findings to the contralateral extremity.
9. Before rewrapping the stump, provide periwound skin care as ordered, but avoid lotion.
10. Wrap the stump when it is elevated to prevent edema and vascular stasis. Follow your facility's policy for replacing the bandage, such as every 2–4 days or sooner if it becomes soiled.
11. Help the patient perform range-of-motion and muscle-strengthening exercises. Encourage the patient to push the residual limb into a soft pillow, then into a firmer pillow, and finally against a hard surface to prepare for prosthesis fitting and to reduce the incidence of phantom limb pain and sensation.
12. Encourage the patient to eat a well-balanced diet.
13. Provide emotional support and patient teaching to help your patient deal with altered body image and lifestyle changes.

10. Describe the acute and chronic complications of diabetes mellitus.

High blood sugar levels can seriously damage parts of your body including your feet and your eyes. These are called the complications of diabetes.

Chronic Complications

Neuropathy

Nerve damage from diabetes is called diabetic neuropathy (new-ROP-uh-thee). About half of all people with diabetes have some form of nerve damage.

Cataracts: A cataract is a thickening and clouding of the lens of the eye. The lens is the part of the eye that helps you focus on. Cataracts can make a person's vision blurry or make it hard to see at night.

Retinopathy: Another eye problem, called diabetic retinopathy (pronounced: reh-tih-NAH-puh-thee) involves changes in the retina, the light-sensitive layer at the back of the eye. These changes happen because of damage or growth problems in the small blood vessels of the retina.

Glaucoma: People with diabetes also have a greater chance of getting glaucoma. In this disease, pressure builds up inside the eye which can decrease blood flow to the retina and optic nerve and damage them. At first, a person may not have trouble seeing. But if it is not treated, glaucoma can cause a person to lose vision. The risk increases as a person gets older and has had diabetes longer. People with glaucoma take medications to lower the pressure inside the eye and sometimes need surgery.

Foot complications: Neuropathy (which can cause numbness in the feet) as well as other complications.

Kidney disease (nephropathy): Keep your diabetes and blood pressure under control to lower the chance of getting kidney disease.

Stroke: Maintain target levels for blood glucose, blood pressure, and cholesterol to reduce your risk of stroke.

Acute Complications

Hypoglycemia: Hypoglycemia is low blood glucose (blood sugar). It is possible for your blood glucose to drop, especially if you are taking insulin or a sulfonylurea drug (those make your body produce insulin throughout the day). With these medications, if you eat less than usual or were more active, your blood glucose may dip too much.

Skin complications: Stay alert for symptoms of skin infections and other skin disorders common in people with diabetes.

DKA (ketoacidosis) and ketones: Warning signs of DKA and check urine for ketones, especially when you're sick.

High blood pressure: Also called hypertension—raises your risk for heart attack, stroke, eye problems, and kidney disease.

11. Explain the causes and management of psoriasis. (*See* Q. 9, 2016)

Psoriasis is a common skin condition that speeds up the life cycle of skin cells. It causes cells to build up rapidly on the surface of the skin. The extra skin cells form scales and red patches that are itchy and sometimes painful. Psoriasis is a chronic disease that often comes and goes. The main goal of treatment is to stop the skin cells from growing so quickly.

Causes

The cause of psoriasis is not fully understood, but it is thought to be related to an immune system problem with T cells and other white blood cells, called neutrophils, in your body.

T cells normally travel through the body to defend against foreign substances, such as viruses or bacteria.

But if you have psoriasis, the T cells attack healthy skin cells by mistake, as if to heal a wound or to fight an infection.

Overactive T cells also trigger increased production of healthy skin cells, more T cells and other white blood cells, especially neutrophils. These travel into the skin causing redness and sometimes pus in pustular lesions. Dilated blood vessels in psoriasis-affected areas create warmth and redness in the skin lesions.

The process becomes an ongoing cycle in which new skin cells move to the outermost layer of skin too quickly in days rather than weeks. Skin cells build up in thick, scaly patches on the skin's surface, continuing until treatment stops the cycle.

Just what causes T cells to malfunction in people with psoriasis is not entirely clear. Researchers believe both genetics and environmental factors play a role.

Topical corticosteroids: These drugs are the most frequently prescribed medications for treating mild to moderate psoriasis. They reduce inflammation and relieve itching and may be used with other treatments.

Mild corticosteroid ointments are usually recommended for sensitive areas, such as your face or skin folds, and for treating widespread patches of damaged skin.

Your doctor may prescribe stronger corticosteroid ointment for smaller, less sensitive or tougher-to-treat areas.

Long-term use or overuse of strong corticosteroids can cause thinning of the skin. Topical corticosteroids may stop working over time. It is usually best to use topical corticosteroids as a short-term treatment during flares.

Vitamin D analogues: These synthetic forms of vitamin D slow skin cell growth. Calcipotriene (Dovonex) is a prescription cream or solution containing a vitamin D analogue that treats mild to moderate psoriasis along with other treatments. Calcipotriene might irritate your skin. Calcitriol (Vectical) is expensive but may be equally effective and possibly less irritating than calcipotriene.

Anthralin: This medication helps slow skin cell growth. Anthralin (Dritho-Scalp) can also remove scales and make skin smoother. But anthralin can irritate skin, and it stains almost anything it touches. It is usually applied for a short time and then washed off.

Topical retinoids: These are vitamin A derivatives that may decrease inflammation. The most common side effect is skin irritation. These medications may also increase sensitivity to sunlight, so while using the medication apply sunscreen before going outdoors.

The risk of birth defects is far lower for topical retinoids than for oral retinoids. But tazarotene (Tazorac, Avage) is not recommended when you are pregnant or breastfeeding or if you intend to become pregnant.

Calcineurin inhibitors: Calcineurin inhibitors-tacrolimus (Prograf) and pimecrolimus (Elidel)-reduce inflammation and plaque buildup. Calcineurin inhibitors are not recommended for long-term or continuous use because of a potential increased risk of skin cancer and lymphoma. They may be especially helpful in areas of thin skin, such as around the eyes, where steroid creams or retinoids are too irritating or may cause harmful effects.

Salicylic acid: Available over-the-counter (nonprescription) and by prescription, salicylic acid promotes sloughing of dead skin cells and reduces scaling. Sometimes it is combined with other medications, such as topical corticosteroids or coal tar to increase its effectiveness. Salicylic acid is available in medicated shampoos and scalp solutions to treat scalp psoriasis.

Coal tar: Derived from coal, coal tar reduces scaling, itching and inflammation. Coal tar can irritate the skin. It is also messy, stains clothing and bedding, and has a strong odor.

Coal tar is available in over-the-counter shampoos, creams and oils. It is also available in higher concentrations by prescription. This treatment is not recommended for women who are pregnant or breastfeeding.

Moisturizers: Moisturizing creams alone would not heal psoriasis, but they can reduce itching, scaling and dryness. Moisturizers is an ointment base are usually more effective than are lighter creams and lotions. Apply immediately after a bath or shower to lock in moisture.

Light Therapy (Phototherapy)

This treatment uses natural or artificial ultraviolet light. The simplest and easiest form of phototherapy involves exposing your skin to controlled amounts of natural sunlight.

Other forms of light therapy include the use of artificial ultraviolet A (UVA) or ultraviolet B (UVB) light either alone or in combination with medications.

Sunlight: Exposure to ultraviolet (UV) rays in sunlight or artificial light slows skin cell turnover and reduces scaling and inflammation. Brief, daily exposures to small amounts of sunlight may improve psoriasis, but intense sun exposure can worsen symptoms and cause skin damage. Before beginning a sunlight regimen, ask your doctor about the safest way to use natural sunlight for psoriasis treatment.

UVB phototherapy: Controlled doses of UVB light from an artificial light source may improve mild to moderate psoriasis symptoms. UVB phototherapy, also called broadband UVB, can be used to treat single patches, widespread psoriasis and psoriasis that resists topical treatments. Short-term side effects may include redness, itching and dry skin. Using a moisturizer may help decrease these side effects.

Narrow band UVB phototherapy: A newer type of psoriasis treatment, narrow band UVB phototherapy may be more effective than broadband UVB treatment. It is usually administered two or three times a week until the skin improves, and then maintenance may require only weekly sessions. Narrow band UVB phototherapy may cause more-severe and longer lasting burns, however.

Goeckerman therapy: Some doctors combine UVB treatment and coal tar treatment which is known as Goeckerman treatment. The two therapies together are more effective than either alone because coal tar makes skin more receptive to UVB light.

Psoralen plus ultraviolet A (PUVA): This form of photochemotherapy involves taking a light-sensitizing medication (psoralen) before exposure to UVA light. UVA light penetrates deeper into the skin than does UVB light, and psoralen makes the skin more responsive to UVA exposure. This more aggressive treatment consistently improves skin and is often used for more-severe cases of psoriasis. Short-term side effects include nausea, headache, burning and itching. Long-term side effects include dry and wrinkled skin, freckles, increased sun sensitivity, and increased risk of skin cancer including melanoma.

Excimer laser: This form of light therapy used for mild to moderate psoriasis treats only the involved skin without harming healthy skin. A controlled beam of UVB light is directed to the psoriasis plaques to control scaling and inflammation. Excimer laser therapy requires fewer sessions than does traditional phototherapy because more powerful UVB light is used. Side effects can include redness and blistering.

12. Explain the drug therapy for HIV infection.

HIV treatment involves taking medicines that slow the progression of the virus in your body. HIV is a type of virus called a retrovirus, and the combination of drugs used to treat it is called antiretroviral therapy (ART). ART is recommended for all people living with HIV, regardless of how long they have had the virus or how healthy they are. ART must be taken every day, exactly as your healthcare provider prescribes.

Antiretroviral therapy: Antiretroviral therapy is the use of HIV medicines to treat HIV infection. People on ART take a combination of HIV medicines (called an HIV treatment regimen) every day. ART is recommended for everyone who has HIV. ART cannot cure HIV, but HIV medicines help people with HIV live longer, healthier lives. ART also reduces the risk of HIV transmission.

Mechanism of Working

HIV attacks and destroys the infection-fighting CD4 cells of the immune system. Loss of CD4 cells makes it hard for the body to fight off infections and certain HIV-related cancers.

HIV medicines prevent HIV from multiplying (making copies of itself) which reduces the amount of HIV in the body (also called the viral load). Having less HIV in the body gives the immune system a chance to recover.

Even though there is still some HIV in the body, the immune system is strong enough to fight off infections and certain HIV-related cancers.

By reducing the amount of HIV in the body, HIV medicines also reduce the risk of HIV transmission. A main goal of ART is to reduce a person's viral load to an undetectable level. An undetectable viral load means that the level of HIV in the blood is too low to be detected by a viral load test. People with HIV who maintain an undetectable viral load have effectively no risk of transmitting HIV to their HIV-negative partner through sex.

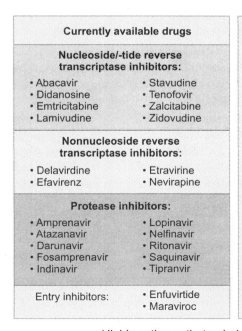
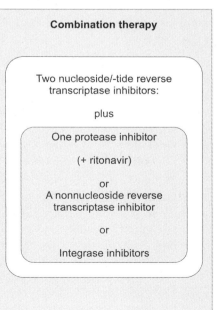

Highly active antiretroviral (HIV) therapy (HAART)

SHORT ANSWERS

13. List the methods of prevention of hepatitis B.

Hepatitis B is a vaccine-preventable disease. More than 1 billion doses of the hepatitis B vaccine have been given worldwide, and it is considered to be a very safe and effective vaccine to protect infants, children and adults from hepatitis B.

All sexual partners, family and close household members living with a chronically infected person should be tested and vaccinated. It is important to remember that hepatitis B is not spread casually! It is not spread by coughing, sneezing, hugging, cooking and sharing food. It is spread through direct contact with infected blood and bodily fluids.

Additional Prevention Measures

In addition to vaccination, there are other simple ways to help stop the spread of hepatitis B:
- Wash your hands thoroughly with soap and water after any potential exposure to blood
- Use condoms with sexual partners
- Avoid direct contact with blood and bodily fluids
- Clean up blood spills with a fresh diluted bleach solution (mix 1 part bleach with 9 parts water)
- Cover all cuts carefully
- Avoid sharing sharp items, such as razors, nail clippers, toothbrushes, and earrings or body rings
- Discard sanitary napkins and tampons into plastic bags
- Avoid illegal street drugs (injecting, inhaling, snorting, or popping pills)
- Make sure new, sterile needles are used for ear or body piercing, tattoos, and acupuncture.

14. Differentiate between disinfection and sterilization.

Disinfection and sterilization are both decontamination processes. While disinfection is the process of eliminating or reducing harmful microorganisms from inanimate objects and surfaces, sterilization is the process of killing all microorganisms. That is the main difference between sterilizing and disinfection.

	Disinfection	**Sterilize**
Definition	To disinfect means to eliminate most harmful microorganisms (not including their spores) from surfaces or objects; inactivate viruses	To sterilize means to kill ALL microbes—whether harmful or not and their spores present on a surface or object
Methods	Phenolic disinfectants, heavy metals, halogens (e.g. chlorine), bleach, alcohols, hydrogen peroxide, detergents, heating and pasteurization	Heat, chemicals, irradiation, high pressure, and filtration
Types	Air disinfectants, alcohols, aldehydes, oxidizing agents, phenolics	Steam, heating, chemical sterilization, radiation sterilization, sterile filtration
Application	Disinfection is used mostly to decontaminate surfaces and air	Sterilization is used for food, medicine and surgical instruments

15. List the complications of valve replacement surgery.

Risks associated with aortic valve repair and aortic valve replacement surgery may include:
- Bleeding
- Blood clots
- Valve dysfunction in replacement valves
- Heart rhythm problems
- Infection
- Stroke
- Death.

16. What is paget's disease.

Paget's disease is a chronic condition which interferes with your body's normal bone remodeling process. Over time, the disease can cause affected bones to become fragile and misshapen. Paget's disease of bone most commonly occurs in the pelvis, skull, spine and legs. Symptoms: Hearing loss; Bone fracture.

17. Name the specific blood investigation to rule out typhoid fever.

According to the World Health Organization (WHO), a definitive diagnosis of typhoid requires isolation of the *S. Typhi* bacterium through blood or bone marrow culture. These methods are considered the gold standard for typhoid diagnosis, though both still have serious practical limitations. Blood culture is expensive and requires specialized personnel and laboratory facilities to perform.

Blood culture facilities are rare in many low-resource countries and are often limited to major hospitals in large cities. When it is possible to perform a blood culture, only 40–60% of typhoid cases are correctly identified due to the low levels of bacteria in the blood during illness. The best time to test is the early days of infection, but the incubation period means that the highest levels of bacteria in the blood are likely present before clinical symptoms develop.

The Widal test is one method that may be used to help make a presumptive diagnosis of enteric fever, also known as typhoid fever. Although the test is no longer commonly performed in the United States or other developed countries, it is still in use in many emerging nations where enteric fever is endemic and limited resources require the use of rapid, affordable testing alternatives. While the method is easy to perform, concerns remain about the reliability of the Widal test.

18. List the clinical features of myxedema.

Along with the signs and symptoms of severe hypothyroidism, symptoms of myxedema crisis can include:
- Decreased breathing (respiratory depression)
- Lower than normal blood sodium levels
- Hypothermia (low body temperature)
- Confusion or mental slowness
- Shock
- Low blood oxygen levels
- High blood carbon dioxide levels
- Coma.

19. What is acne vulgaris? (*See* Q. 15, 2014)

20. What is cardiopulmonary resuscitation? (*See* Q. 10, 2015)

21. Define hemorrhoids.

Dilated (enlarged) veins in the walls of the anus and sometimes around the rectum usually caused by untreated constipation but occasionally associated with chronic diarrhea. Symptoms start with bleeding after defecation. If untreated, hemorrhoids can worsen, protruding from the anus. Treatment involves changing the diet to prevent constipation and avoid further irritation, the use of topical medication, and sometimes surgery. Also known as piles.

22. List the clinical manifestations of Cushing's syndrome.

- Weight gain
- Obesity
- Fatty deposits especially in the midsection, the face (causing a round, moon-shaped face), and between the shoulders and the upper back (causing a buffalo hump)
- Purple stretch marks on the breasts, arms, abdomen, and thighs
- Thinning skin that bruises easily.

2018

Medical-Surgical Nursing-I

LONG ESSAYS
1. a. Define and classify chest injury. b. List the clinical manifestations and diagnostic measures in a client with chest injury. c. Explain the management of a client with chest tube drainage
2. a. Define Benign prostatic hypertrophy. b. Explain the pathophysiological basis of clinical manifestation in a client with Benign prostatic hypertrophy. c. Write the postoperative nursing management following TURP.
3. a. Explain the etiopathophysiology and clinical manifestations of rheumatic heart disease. b. Decribe the preoperative management of a client undergoing valve replacement surgery.

SHORT ESSAYS
4. Pathophysiology of cirrhosis of liver.
5. Complications of acute myocardial infarction.
6. Phases of acute renal failure.
7. Hyperthyroidism.
8. Eczema.
9. Bone healing.
10. Diagnostic studies of HIV infection.
11. Complications of hypertension.
12. Drug therapy in pulmonary tuberculosis.

SHORT ANSWERS
13. Sickle cell anemia.
14. Pleural effusion.
15. Treadmill test.
16. Cor pulomale.
17. Splints.
18. Cellulitis.
19. Prevention of deep vein thrombosis.
20. List four causes of acute abdomen.
21. Prevention of hepatitis B.
22. Male contraceptive methods.

LONG ESSAYS

1. a. Define and classify chest injury. b. List the clinical manifestations and diagnostic measures in a client with chest injur. c. Explain the management of a client with chest tube drainage. *(See* **Q. 4, 2014)**

2. a. Define benign prostatic hypertrophy. b. Explain the pathophysiological basis of clinical manifestation in a client with benign prostatic hypertrophy. c. Write the postoperative nursing management following TURP.

Benign prostatic hyperplasia (BPH) also called prostate gland enlargement—is a common condition as men get older. An enlarged prostate gland can cause uncomfortable urinary symptoms, such as blocking the flow of urine out of the bladder. It can also cause bladder, urinary tract or kidney problems.

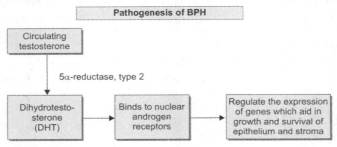

Symptoms: The severity of symptoms in people who have prostate gland enlargement varies, but symptoms tend to gradually worsen over time. Common signs and symptoms of BPH include:
- Frequent or urgent need to urinate
- Increased frequency of urination at night (nocturia)
- Difficulty starting urination
- Weak urine stream or a stream that stops and starts
- Dribbling at the end of urination
- Inability to completely empty the bladder.

Less common signs and symptoms include:
- Urinary tract infection
- Inability to urinate
- Blood in the urine.

Complications

Complications of an enlarged prostate can include:
1. **Sudden inability to urinate (urinary retention):** You might need to have a tube (catheter) inserted into your bladder to drain the urine. Some men with an enlarged prostate need surgery to relieve urinary retention.
2. **Urinary tract infections (UTIs):** Inability to fully empty the bladder can increase the risk of infection in your urinary tract. If UTIs occur frequently, you might need surgery to remove part of the prostate.

3. **Bladder stones:** These are generally caused by an inability to completely empty the bladder. Bladder stones can cause infection, bladder irritation, blood in the urine and obstruction of urine flow.
4. **Bladder damage:** A bladder that has not emptied completely can stretch and weaken over time. As a result, the muscular wall of the bladder no longer contracts properly, making it harder to fully empty your bladder.
5. **Kidney damage:** Pressure in the bladder from urinary retention can directly damage the kidneys or allow bladder infections to reach the kidneys.

Postoperative Nursing Management Following TURP

Transurethral resection of the prostate (TURP) is a surgery used to treat urinary problems due to an enlarged prostate. A combined visual and surgical instrument (resectoscope) is inserted through the tip of the penis and into the tube that carries urine from the bladder (urethra). The prostate surrounds the urethra. Using the resectoscope, your doctor trims away excess prostate tissue that's blocking urine flow.

Postoperative care: After a TURP, the cavity left in the prostate will take between 8 to 12 weeks to heal completely and the full benefits of the procedure appreciated.

Fluid intake: During the first 1-2 weeks after the operation it is important to drink plenty of fluid to flush any new bleeding from the bladder. The amount of fluid drunk usually depends on the amount of blood in your urine. If your urine is quite bloodstained you may need to drink up to 3 L of water per day. If you urine stops being bloodstained and the prostate cavity has healed then a fluid intake of 2 L per day is adequate. Avoid alcohol and coffee for the first few weeks after the procedure as this may make urinary frequency and urgency worse.

Antibiotics: Sometimes after a TURP patients are discharged on antibiotics. This usually occurs in patients who had a catheter in before the operation or who had been having urinary infections before the operation. It is important that if you are discharged on antibiotics that the full course be completed.

Activity: To lower the risk of bleeding after the operation, it is important not to be too active. Avoid lifting, gardening, golf or other demanding activities in the first 2 weeks or so after surgery. Normal daily activities, such as normal walking can occur immediately after the procedure however try to avoid driving a car for at least a week after the procedure. Sexual activity should be avoided for at least 4 weeks.

Bowels: It is important not to become constipated as the need to strain to empty the bowel may cause bleeding. Extra fiber in the diet and a larger fluid intake helps to make sure the bowel actions are soft and regular. If you are prone to constipation let the doctor and the nursing staff know and you may be prescribed a laxative to take whilst in hospital and after discharge.

Bleeding: Within the first few weeks after surgery, the scab where prostate tissue has been removed may sometimes loosen and cause some bleeding. By resting when this happens and drinking plenty of fluid, the bleeding will usually stop.

3. a. Explain the etiopathophysiology and clinical manifestations of rheumatic heart disease. b. Decribe the preoperative management of a client undergoing valve replacement surgery.

Rheumatic heart disease (RHD) is a chronic and progressive form of damage to the heart valves resulting in dysfunction of the heart. It is a complication of an autoimmune disorder called acute rheumatic fever (ARF) which is in turn precipitated by group A streptococcal infections of the throat.

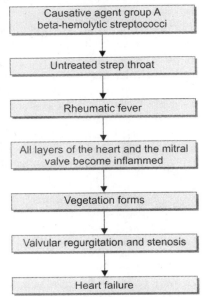

Risk Factors of Rheumatic Heart Disease

Risk factors include poverty, overcrowding and reduced access to medical care. Stopping episodes of recurrent ARF can prevent rheumatic heart disease. Once acute rheumatic fever is diagnosed, stopping further episodes of ARF can halt progression of the disease. Treatment can manage symptoms and reduce the risk of complications.

Symptoms of Rheumatic Heart Disease

Rheumatic heart disease (RHD) does not always cause symptoms. When it does, symptoms may include:
1. Chest pain
2. Heart palpitations
3. Breathlessness on exertion
4. Breathing problems when lying down (orthopnoea)
5. Waking from sleep with the need to sit or stand up (paroxysmal nocturnal dyspnea)
6. Swelling (edema)
7. Fainting (syncope)
8. Stroke
9. Fever associated with infection of damaged heart valves.

Diagnosis of Rheumatic Heart Disease

Diagnosis may include:
1. Physical examination—while a heart murmur may suggest RHD, many patients with RHD do not have a murmur
2. Medical history—including evidence of past ARF or strep infection
3. Chest X-ray—to check for enlargement of the heart or fluid on the lungs
4. Electrocardiogram (ECG)—to check if the chambers of the heart have enlarged or if there is an abnormal heart rhythm (arrhythmia)

5. Echocardiogram—to check the heart valves for any damage or infection and assessing if there is heart failure. This is the most useful test for finding out if RHD is present.

Treatment of Rheumatic Heart Disease

Treatment depends on the severity of rheumatic heart disease, but may include:
1. Hospital admission to treat heart failure
2. Antibiotics for infection (especially of the heart valves)
3. Blood-thinning medicine to prevent stroke or thin blood for replacement valves
4. Balloons inserted through a vein to open up stuck valves
5. Heart valve surgery to repair or replace damaged heart valves.

Complications of Rheumatic Heart Disease

Medical treatment of rheumatic heart disease includes reducing the risk of complications. Options may include:
1. Regular check-ups with a cardiologist (heart specialist) to monitor the heart
2. Up-to-date flu (influenza and pneumococcal) vaccinations
3. Regular (preventative) antibiotic to prevent Group A *Streptococcus* throat infections and recurring ARF
4. Early presentation, diagnosis and, where appropriate, antibiotic treatment of sore throats
   - Good dental hygiene (tooth brushing and flossing, dental check-ups, fluoridated water supply), as oral bacteria entering the bloodstream can increase the risk of complications, such as inflammation of the inner lining of the heart
   - Antibiotics—may be given to some people before some dental or surgical procedures to prevent bacterial infection of the damaged areas of the heart
   - Good prenatal care, as pregnancy can make rheumatic heart disease worse.

Preoperative Management of a Client Undergoing Valve Replacement Surgery.

The principles of nursing care for this group of patients are similar to those undergoing other forms of cardiac surgery. There are special considerations for patients who may already have chronic arrhythmias, altered left ventricular function and pulmonary hypertension. Great care is required with fluid management and haemodynamic monitoring.

Nurses can help patients understand the nature of their disease and the risks and benefits of surgery. While medical treatment may provide symptomatic control and surgery can offer improved long-term outcomes, there is an important role for secondary prevention for these patients who may not be perceived as having the same risks as those with coronary artery disease.

Nurses can provide support for patients as they adapt to living with a prosthetic valve. Those with a mechanical prosthesis will start long-term anticoagulation therapy that will demand changes in lifestyle and self-management. The risks of native and prosthetic valve endocarditis should be raised with patients who are waiting for or who have had valve surgery; education about prophylactic antibiotic therapy for dental and other invasive procedures should be discussed.

Hospital-acquired infection plays a greater role in infective endocarditis than has previously been emphasized. Good infection control practices in hospital can reinforce education messages given to valve patients who are learning to reduce the risk of developing infective endocarditis.

Those undergoing surgical intervention require specialist support throughout their diagnosis and treatment. Surgery can affect the long-term outcomes for these patients, but quality of life and benefit from surgery is likely to be enhanced by effective patient education and by encouraging patients to be involved in decision-making.

SHORT ESSAYS

4. Pathophysiology of cirrhosis of liver. (*See* Q. 2, 2016)

5. Complications of acute myocardial infarction.

Myocardial infarction (MI) is usually the result of thrombosis in a coronary artery, triggered by fissuring or rupture of an atheromatous plaque. Platelets and fibrin are deposited on the damaged plaque resulting in the formation of a clot and the occlusion of the artery. This article is an overview of the most common complications associated with MI.

Sudden death: Fatality from MI remains formidably high, with 50 per cent of patients who die after an acute coronary occlusion doing so within the first hour after the onset of symptoms. Death is commonly due to the dysrhythmia, ventricular fibrillation.

Disturbance of rate, rhythm and conduction: Dysrhythmias are experienced more frequently than any other MI complication, with the incidence of some type of disturbance at virtually 100 per cent. Although these may be life-threatening, many patients experience only self-limiting dysrhythmias of minimal haemodynamic consequence.

Cardiogenic shock: The term cardiogenic shock is used to describe a complex syndrome associated with inadequate perfusion of vital organs - most significantly the brain, kidneys and heart. It occurs in 15 per cent of MI patients and of these, 90 per cent will die in spite of recent advances in therapy. Patients with an anterior MI or who have lost more than 40 per cent of functional myocardium are at greatest risk.

Cardiac rupture: After arrhythmias and cardiogenic shock, the commonest cause of death after acute MI is rupture. Cardiac rupture complicates 10 per cent of acute MIs and occurs in the healing stages at around 5–9 days. **Heart failure:** Heart failure is one of the more severe complications of MI and results from the heart's inability to provide an adequate cardiac output for the body's metabolic requirements

Angina pectoris: Recurrent and persistent anginal symptoms may occur in the early post-infarction period and have been associated with an unfavourable prognosis. Anginal pain is due to the increased oxygen demand on the viable myocardium. Cardiac catheterisation and surgical revascularisation may be indicated in these patients.

Pericarditis: This is often acute and usually occurs 24-72 hours post-MI. It is seen in 20% of patients following a Q-wave MI. It is usually transient, benign and self-limiting but symptoms may be distressing. Pain is typically felt in the region of the heart, is worse on inspiration and relieved by sitting up or leaning forward.

Ventricular septal defect: This structural complication occurs in two per cent of cases as a late complication around days three to five. A hole occurs in the intraventricular septum, resulting in a left to right shunt with subsequent cardiogenic shock, pulmonary circuit overload and severe pulmonary oedema.

Ventricular aneurysm: Aneurysm formation results in 10-15% of cases following extensive destruction of cardiac muscle, and its replacement by scar tissue. During ventricular systole the aneurysm bulges outwards and reduces the ejection fraction by absorbing the force of myocardial contraction

Shoulder hand syndrome: Left shoulder pain and stiffness is felt 2–8 weeks after MI and there may be pain and swelling of the hand. With early mobilization of the patient it has become a rare complication. It is treated with physiotherapy and is usually resolved after 2 years.

6. Phases of acute renal failure.

1. **Onset phase:** Kidney injury occurs.
2. **Oliguric (anuric) phase:** Urine output decreases from renal tubule damage.
3. **Diuretic phase:** The kidneys try to heal and urine output increases, but tubule scarring and damage occur.
4. **Recovery phase:** Tubular edema resolves and renal function improves.

This table describes the features and durations of the four phases of acute kidney injury (AKI).

Phase	Features	Duration
Onset phase	- Common triggering events: Significant blood loss, burns, fluid loss, diabetes insipidus - Renal blood flow—25% of normal - Tissue oxygenation—25% of normal - Urine output below 0.5 mL/kg/hour	Hours to days
Oliguric (anuric)	- Urine output below 400 mL/day, phase possibly as low as 100 mL/day - Increases in blood urea nitrogen (BUN) and creatinine levels - Electrolyte disturbances, acidosis, and fluid overload (from kidney's inability to excrete water)	8–14 days or longer, depending on nature of AKI and dialysis initiation
Diuretic phase	- Occurs when cause of AKI is corrected - Renal tubule scarring and edema - Increased glomerular filtration rate (GFR) - Daily urine output above 400 mL - Possible electrolyte depletion from excretion of more water and osmotic effects of high BUN	7–14 days
Recovery phase	- Decreased edema - Normalization of fluid and electrolyte balance - Return of GFR to 70 or 80% of normal	Several months–1 year

7. Hyperthyroidism.

Hyperthyroidism (overactive thyroid) occurs when your thyroid gland produces too much of the hormone thyroxine. Hyperthyroidism can accelerate the body's metabolism causing unintentional weight loss and a rapid or irregular heartbeat. Several treatments are available for hyperthyroidism. Doctors use antithyroid medications and radioactive iodine to slow the production of thyroid hormones. Sometimes, hyperthyroidism treatment involves surgery to remove all or part of your thyroid gland.

Causes of Hypothyroidism

The causes of hypothyroidism include:
1. **Iodine deficiency disorder**—lack of sufficient iodine in the diet can prevent the thyroid gland from making hormones. The thyroid enlarges as it attempts to comply with the pituitary gland's ceaseless chemical messages to produce more hormones. An enlarged thyroid is known as a goiter. Babies and children can be stunted and severely brain damaged by iodine deficiency because thyroid hormones are needed for normal growth and development.
2. **Hashimoto's disease**—an autoimmune disorder. White blood cells and antibodies of the immune system attack and destroy the cells of the thyroid gland. Without treatment, death can occur within 10 to 15 years.
3. **Treatment for hyperthyroidism**—treatments for hyperthyroidism (including drugs, surgery and radioactive iodine) frequently lead to hypothyroidism.
4. **Surgery**—the primary treatment for thyroid cancer, and also a treatment for hyperthyroidism, surgery will lead to hypothyroidism if the thyroid gland is removed or if insufficient is left in place.
5. **X-rays**—radiation treatments (in the past used for acne, tonsillitis and adenoid problems) can lead to hypothyroidism in later life. These treatments are not used today.
6. **Particular drugs**—including lithium and the heart drug amiodarone can interfere with the normal processing of iodine and the production of thyroid hormone.
7. **Birth defects**—sometimes a baby is born with a congenital defect of the thyroid gland (which affects hormone production) or the thyroid may be completely absent. Without treatment, this can lead to brain damage and stunted growth.
8. **Pituitary gland dysfunction**—the pituitary gland does not make enough thyroid stimulating hormone to prompt the thyroid to produce T3 and T4.
9. **Hypothalamic dysfunction**—the functioning of the pituitary is influenced by another brain structure called the hypothalamus, through the thyrotropin-releasing hormone. Problems with the hypothalamus can affect the pituitary and in turn, the thyroid gland.

Symptoms

The symptoms of hyperthyroidism include:
1. Accelerated heart rate or palpitations
2. Muscle weakness and trembling
3. Unexplained weight loss
4. Sensitivity to heat
5. Diarrhea
6. Sleeping difficulties
7. Sweating
8. Irritability
9. Nervousness, agitation and anxiety
10. Changes in menstruation including scantier flow and increased cycle length.

Treatment for hypothyroidism

Iodine deficiency can be easily relieved by increasing the intake of iodine through iodized salt or iodine rich foods. Hypothyroidism may be caused by the failure of or damage to the thyroid gland, pituitary or hypothalamus. In these cases, treatment focuses on boosting thyroid hormone levels with thyroxine tablets, a form of hormone replacement.

8. Eczema.

It is the superficial inflammation of the skin that is characterized by: Vesicles, redness, edema, oozing crusting, scaling, and itching.

It is classified into as acute, subacute, or chronic: The skin responds to wide variety of noxious stimuli. Inflammatory cells infiltrate the upper dermis and epidermis and breakdown of epidermal cells. Vesicles or bullae form when fluid accumulates between epidermal cells or when there are changes within the cell itself. The result of inflammatory process is a skin surface that is erythematous (from vasodilatation), edematous, exudative or eroded (from vesicle formation) and crusted or scabbed (from infection or an accumulation of serous exudates). Thickening and scaling occur from attempted or exaggerated repair efforts (hyperkeratosis or parakeratosis).

Medications prescribed are antipyretic agents like antihistamines, antianxiety agents, corticosteroids, antiinfective agents to treat secondary agents, topical antifungal, keratolytics.

General management: It is saline and plain water dressings, occlusive dressings, oil-in-water compresses, and hydration.

Nursing diagnosis: Impaired skin intergrity, pruitus, and body image disturbance.

Patient education: 1. Instruct the patient about the application of compresses, soaks, and scrubs using aseptic technique. 2. Instruct the patient in the use and side effects of medications. 3. Inform the patient and the family that successful treatment/therapy requires patience, that therapy may be long-term and the results may not be immediate. 4. Teach the patient the signs and symptoms of secondary infection and to seek medical treatment if they occur.

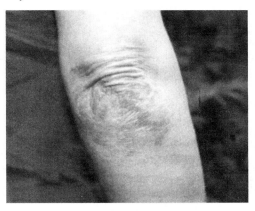

9. Bone healing.

A fracture occurs when the continuity of a bone is broken and local blood supply is interrupted. If the overlying soft tissues are also injured, fracture healing may be delayed or disrupted, particularly in anatomic regions with decreased vascular networks, such as the tibial diaphysis. Bone is unique in its ability to regenerate itself.

Healing occurs via reactivation of embryologic processes resulting in the formation of bone not scar. Fracture healing can be described in three conceptual stages. An understanding of the timing and mechanisms associated with each stage is important in planning fracture treatment. The bone healing process has three overlapping stages: Inflammation, bone production and bone remodeling.

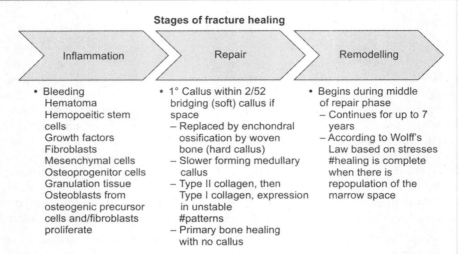

Stages of fracture healing

Inflammation
- Bleeding
  Hematoma
  Hemopoeitic stem cells
  Growth factors
  Fibroblasts
  Mesenchymal cells
  Osteoprogenitor cells
  Granulation tissue
  Osteoblasts from osteogenic precursor cells and/fibroblasts proliferate

Repair
- 1° Callus within 2/52 bridging (soft) callus if space
  – Replaced by enchondral ossification by woven bone (hard callus)
  – Slower forming medullary callus
  – Type II collagen, then Type I collagen, expression in unstable #patterns
  – Primary bone healing with no callus

Remodelling
- Begins during middle of repair phase
  – Continues for up to 7 years
  – According to Wolff's Law based on stresses #healing is complete when there is repopulation of the marrow space

Inflammation starts immediately after the bone is fractured and lasts for several days. When the bone is fractured, there is bleeding into the area leading to inflammation and clotting of blood at the fracture site. This provides the initial structural stability and framework for producing new bone.

Repair

The reparative phase begins a few days after the injury with the arrival of mesenchymal cells able to differentiate into fibroblasts, chondroblasts and osteoblasts. The repair phase persists for several months; it can be divided into two distinct phases: soft and hard callus formation.

1. "Soft callus" formation lasts for approximately 6 weeks from the time of injury. During this preliminary stage of repair, pain and swelling subside and bony fragments become united by fibrous and cartilagenous tissue. Woven bone is formed. While this creates some stability, the fracture may still angulate at this stage if not held with stable external support, such as a cast or external fixator, or internal support provided by plates, screws or intramedullary devices.
2. "Hard callus" formation—during this second stage of repair, woven bone is transformed into lamellar bone. This takes approximately 3 months.

Bone production begins when the clotted blood formed by inflammation is replaced with fibrous tissue and cartilage (known as soft callus). As healing progresses, the soft callus is replaced with hard bone (known as hard callus) which is visible on X-rays several weeks after the fracture.

Bone remodeling, the final phase of bone healing, goes on for several months. In remodeling, bone continues to form and becomes compact returning to its original shape.

Remodeling is the process by which bone is removed in tiny increments and then replaced by new bone. After a fracture, remodeling may continue for months or even years. The adult human skeleton continuously replaces itself at rate of 10-18% per year. The rate of remodeling is accelerated in children and during fracture repair. In addition to being an essential part of fracture healing, remodeling plays an important role in calcium homeostasis. During the remodeling phase the woven bone is converted to lamellar bone and the medullary canal is reconstituted. During this phase, bone responds to loading characteristics according to Wolff's law. Some angular deformity may correct during this stage in children with sufficient growth remaining.

10. Diagnostic studies of HIV infection.

Blood tests are the most common way to diagnose HIV. These tests look for antibodies to the virus that the body creates in an attempt to fight the virus. People exposed to the virus should get tested immediately, although it can take the body anywhere from six weeks to a year to develop antibodies to the virus. Follow-up tests may be needed depending on the initial time of exposure. Most healthcare providers offer HIV testing, often with appropriate counseling. Anonymous and free testing also is available. During testing, your doctor will ask about your symptoms, medical history and risk factors, and perform a physical examination.

Tests for HIV and AIDS

The primary tests for diagnosing HIV and AIDs include:

ELISA test: ELISA which stands for enzyme-linked immunosorbent assay is used to detect HIV infection. If an ELISA test is positive, the Western blot test is usually administered to confirm the diagnosis. If an ELISA test is negative, but you think you may have HIV, you should be tested again in 1–3 months. ELISA is quite sensitive in chronic HIV infection, but because antibodies are not produced immediately upon infection, you may test negative during a window of a few weeks to a few months after being infected. Even though your test result may be negative during this window, you may have a high level of the virus and be at risk of transmitting infection.

Home tests: The only home test approved by the US Food and Drug Administration is called the home access express test which is sold in pharmacies.

Saliva tests: A cotton pad is used to obtain saliva from the inside of your cheek. The pad is placed in a vial and submitted to a laboratory for testing. Results are available in three days. Positive results should be confirmed with a blood test.

Viral load test: This test measures the amount of HIV in your blood. Generally, it is used to monitor treatment progress or detect early HIV infection. Three technologies measure HIV viral load in the blood: 1. Reverse transcription polymerase chain reaction (RT-PCR) 2. Branched DNA (bDNA) and 3. Nucleic acid sequence-based amplification assay (NASBA). The basic principles of these tests are similar. HIV is detected using DNA sequences that bind specifically to those in the virus. It is important to note that results may vary between tests.

Western Blot: This is a very sensitive blood test used to confirm a positive ELISA test result.

11. Complications of hypertension.

The excessive pressure on your artery walls caused by high blood pressure can damage the blood vessels as well as organs in your body. The higher the blood pressure and the longer it goes uncontrolled, the greater the damage.

Uncontrolled high blood pressure can lead to complications including:

1. **Heart attack or stroke:** High blood pressure can cause hardening and thickening of the arteries (atherosclerosis) which can lead to a heart attack, stroke or other complications.
2. **Aneurysm:** Increased blood pressure can cause your blood vessels to weaken and bulge, forming an aneurysm. If an aneurysm ruptures, it can be life-threatening.
3. **Heart failure:** To pump blood against the higher pressure in your vessels, the heart has to work harder. This causes the walls of the heart's pumping chamber to thicken (left ventricular hypertrophy). Eventually, the thickened muscle may have a hard time pumping enough blood to meet your body's needs which can lead to heart failure.

4. **Weakened and narrowed blood vessels in your kidneys:** This can prevent these organs from functioning normally.
5. **Thickened, narrowed or torn blood vessels in the eyes:** This can result in vision loss.
6. **Metabolic syndrome:** This syndrome is a cluster of disorders of your body's metabolism, including increased waist circumference; high triglycerides; low high-density lipoprotein (HDL) cholesterol, the "good" cholesterol; high blood pressure and high insulin levels. These conditions make you more likely to develop diabetes, heart disease and stroke.
7. **Trouble with memory or understanding:** Uncontrolled high blood pressure may also affect your ability to think, remember and learn. Trouble with memory or understanding concepts is more common in people with high blood pressure.
8. **Dementia:** Narrowed or blocked arteries can limit blood flow to the brain leading to a certain type of dementia (vascular dementia). A stroke that interrupts blood flow to the brain also can cause vascular dementia.

12. Drug therapy in pulmonary tuberculosis. (*See* Q. 11, 2016)

SHORT ANSWERS

13. Sickle cell anemia.

Sickle cell anemia is an inherited form of anemia—a condition in which there are not enough healthy red blood cells to carry adequate oxygen throughout the body.

Signs of anemia include:
- Paleness, often seen in the skin, lips, or nail beds
- Tiredness
- Dizziness
- Being short of breath
- Feeling lightheaded
- Being irritable
- Trouble paying attention
- A fast heartbeat.

14. Pleural effusion. (*See* Q. 13, 2015)

15. Treadmill test.

A treadmill exercise stress test is used to determine the effects of exercise on the heart. Exercise allows doctors to detect abnormal heart rhythms (arrhythmias) and diagnose the presence or absence of coronary artey disease. This test involves walking in place on a treadmill while monitoring the electrical activity of your heart. Throughout the test, the speed and incline of the treadmill increase. The results show how well your heart responds to the stress of different levels of exercise.

16. Cor pulomale.

Cor pulmonale is a condition that most commonly arises out of complications from high blood pressure in the pulmonary arteries (pulmonary hypertension). It is also known as right-sided heart failure because it occurs within the right ventricle of your heart. Cor pulmonale causes the right ventricle to enlarge and pump blood less effectively than it should. The ventricle is then pushed to its limit and ultimately fails.

This condition is often prevented when the high pressure of blood going to the lungs is controlled. However, untreated pulmonary hypertension can eventually lead to cor pulmonale along with other related, life-threatening complications.

Symptoms of Cor Pulmonale

The symptoms of cor pulmonale may not be noticeable at first because they are similar to the feelings you get after a hard workout. They include:
1. Shortness of breath
2. Tiredness
3. An increased heart rate
4. Lightheadedness.

17. Splints.

A splint is defined as "a rigid or flexible device that maintains in position a displaced or movable part; also used to keep in place and protect an injured part" or as "a rigid or flexible material used to protect, immobilize, or restrict motion in a part." Splints can also be used to relieve pain in damaged joints.

Types
- Ankle stirrup: Used for the ankles.
- Finger **splints**: Used for the fingers
- Nasal **splint**
- Posterior lower leg
- Posterior full leg
- Posterior elbow
- Sugar tong: Used for the forearm or wrist
- Thumb spica: Used for the thumb.

18. Cellulitis.

Cellulitis is a common, potentially serious bacterial skin infection. The affected skin appears swollen and red and is typically painful and warm to the touch. Cellulitis usually affects the skin on the lower legs, but it can occur in the face, arms and other areas.

Symptoms

Possible signs and symptoms of cellulitis which usually occur on one side of the body include:
- Red area of skin that tends to expand
- Swelling
- Tenderness
- Pain
- Warmth
- Fever
- Red spots
- Blisters
- Skin dimpling.

19. Prevention of deep vein thrombosis.

Deep vein thrombosis is a condition in which blood clots (or thrombi) form in deep veins in the legs or other areas of the body. Veins are the blood vessels that carry blood from the body's tissues to the heart. Deep veins are located deep in the body away from the skin's surface.
- Lose weight, if you are overweight
- Stay active
- Exercise regularly; walking is fine
- Avoid long periods of staying still
- Get up and move around at least every hour whenever you travel on a plane, train, or bus, particularly if the trip is longer than 4 hours
- Do heel toe exercises or circle your feet if you cannot move around
- Stop at least every 2 hours when you drive, and get out and move around
- Drink a lot of water and wear loose fitted clothing when you travel
- Talk to your doctor about your risk of clotting whenever you take hormones whether for birth control or replacement therapy, or during and right after any pregnancy
- Follow any self-care measures to keep heart failure, diabetes, or any other health issues as stable as possible.

20. List four causes of acute abdomen.

- Acute appendicitis
- Acute peptic ulcer and its complications
- Acute cholecystitis
- Acute pancreatitis
- Acute intestinal ischemia
- Acute diverticulitis
- Ectopic pregnancy with tubal rupture
- Ovarian torsion.

21. Prevention of hepatitis B. (*See* Q. 13, 2019)

22. Male contraceptive methods.

Male contraceptives, also known as male birth control are methods of preventing pregnancy that solely involve the male physiology. The most common kinds of male contraception include condoms, withdrawal or pulling out, outer course, and vasectomy.

2017

Medical-Surgical Nursing-I

LONG ESSAYS

1. a. Define diabetes mellitus. b. Explain the treatment modalities of diabetes mellitus. c. Brief the micro- and macrovascular complications of diabetes mellitus.
2. a. Discuss the etiology pathophysiology and diagnostic measures of acute pancreatitis. b. Explain the surgical management of a patient suffering from chronic pancreatitis.
3. Discuss the pathophysiology, assessment, findings and the management of acute glomerulonephritis.

SHORT ESSAYS

4. Risk factors of coronary artery diseases.
5. Urinary tract infection.
6. Respiratory rehabilitation.
7. Nurses responsibility in administration of blood and blood products.
8. Types of fracture.
9. Hepatitis.
10. Prevention of deep vein thrombosis in bed ridden patients.
11. Pneumonia.
12. Arrhythmias.

SHORT ANSWERS

13. Endocarditis.
14. Orthopedic prosthesis.
15. Pneumothorax.
16. Hypospadiasis.
17. Postoperative nursing management of thyroidectomy.
18. Psoriasis.
19. Hypovalumic shock.
20. Pott's spine.
21. Malaria.
22. Defibrillation.

LONG ESSAYS

1. a. Define diabetes mellitus. b. Explain the treatment modalities of diabetes mellitus. c. Brief the micro- and macrovascular complications of diabetes mellitus. *(See Q. 12, 2015)*

2. a. Discuss the etiology, pathophysiology and diagnostic measures of acute pancreatitis. b. Explain the surgical management of a patient suffering from chronic pancreatitis.

Pancreatitis is inflammation of the pancreas which can either be acute (sudden and severe) or chronic (ongoing). The pancreas is a gland that secretes both digestive enzymes and important hormones. Heavy alcohol consumption is one of the most common causes of chronic pancreatitis followed by gallstones. Pancreatitis is one of the least common diseases of the digestive system. Treatment options include abstaining from alcohol, fasting until the inflammation subsides, medication and surgery.

Causes of Pancreatitis

Around half of all people with acute pancreatitis have been heavy drinkers which makes alcohol consumption one of the most common causes. Gallstones cause most of the remaining cases. In rare cases, pancreatitis can be caused by:
1. Trauma or surgery to the pancreas region
2. Inherited abnormalities of the pancreas
3. Inherited disorders of metabolism
4. Viruses (particularly mumps)
5. Medication (including some diuretics) which can also trigger inflammation.

Acute Pancreatitis

Acute pancreatitis is a sudden, debilitating attack of severe upper abdominal pain. Pancreatic enzymes irritate and burn the pancreas and leak out into the abdominal cavity. Complications include respiratory, kidney or heart failure, all of which can be fatal.

The most common cause of severe acute pancreatitis is gallstones blocking the pancreatic duct. This can sometimes occur even if the gallbladder has been previously removed. When triggered by excessive alcohol consumption, acute pancreatitis usually resolves itself with rest and abstinence from drinking.

Common symptoms of an acute attack include:
1. Severe abdominal pain, often spreading through into the back
2. Bloating
3. Fever
4. Sweating
5. Nausea
6. Vomiting
7. Collapse.

The symptoms of acute pancreatitis can sometimes be confused with symptoms of other emergencies, such as heart attack, biliary colic (gallbladder stones) or perforation of a gastric or duodenal ulcer. Acute pancreatitis generally causes severe pain and the sufferer will need emergency treatment in a hospital.

Diagnosis of Pancreatitis
Pancreatitis is generally diagnosed quickly by examination of the abdomen, and confirmed using a series of medical tests including:
1. General tests—such as blood tests, physical examination and X-rays.
2. Ultrasound—sound waves form a picture that detects the presence of gallstones.
3. CT scan—a specialized X-ray takes three-dimensional pictures of the pancreas.
4. MRI scan—this uses a strong magnetic field rather than radiation to take pictures of the abdomen. A special form of MRI called MRCP can also be used to get images of the ducts of the pancreas and help determine the cause of pancreatitis and the extent of damage.

Treatment for Acute Pancreatitis
Treatment may include:
1. Hospital care—in all cases of acute pancreatitis
2. Intensive care in hospital—in cases of severe acute pancreatitis
3. Fasting and intravenous fluids—until the inflammation settles down
4. Pain relief—adequate pain relief is essential and is often given into the vein (intravenously). With appropriate pain relief, a person with pancreatitis is able to draw deep breaths which helps to avoid lung complications, such as pneumonia
5. Endoscopy—a thin tube is inserted through your esophagus to allow the doctor to see your pancreas. This device is used to inject dye into the bile ducts and pancreas. Gallstones can be seen and removed directly
6. Surgery—if gallstones are present, removing the gallbladder will help prevent further attacks. In rare cases, surgery is needed to remove damaged or dead areas of the pancreas
7. Lifestyle change—not drinking alcohol.

Treatment for Chronic Pancreatitis
Treatment may include:
1. Lowering fat intake
2. Supplementing digestion by taking pancreatic enzyme tablets with food
3. Cutting out alcohol
4. Insulin injections, if the endocrine function of the pancreas is compromised
5. Analgesics (pain-relieving medication).

Surgery for Chronic Pancreatitis
Doctors may recommend surgery for people with chronic pancreatitis when the organ cannot drain pancreatic fluids properly due to tissue scarring. Your surgeon can create a new duct, or passageway, to allow the fluid to drain and reduce inflammation. He/she may also remove scarred or diseased tissue.

NYU Langone doctors use different surgical approaches based on the type of damage and where it appears in the pancreas.

A Puestow procedure is used to treat damage to the middle and end portions of the pancreas, also referred to as the body and tail. In this surgery, surgeons open the main pancreatic duct, which runs along the body of the pancreas, from end to end, and attach a portion of the pancreas and the duct directly to the small intestine—a technique called lateral pancreaticojejunostomy.

In a Frey's procedure, damaged tissue is removed from the head of the pancreas, the widest part that sits toward the center of the abdomen. Surgeons may also perform a lateral pancreaticojejunostomy with this procedure to widen the connection between the pancreas and small intestine.

3. Discuss the pathophysiology, assessment, findings and the management of acute glomerulonephritis.

Glomerulonephritis is inflammation of the tiny filters in your kidneys (glomeruli). Glomeruli remove excess fluid, electrolytes and waste from your bloodstream and pass them into your urine. Glomerulonephritis can come on suddenly (acute) or gradually (chronic). Glomerulonephritis occurs on its own or as part of another disease, such as lupus or diabetes. Severe or prolonged inflammation associated with glomerulonephritis can damage the kidneys.

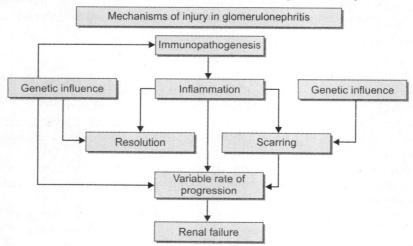

Symptoms

Signs and symptoms of glomerulonephritis depend on whether you have the acute or chronic form and the cause. Glomerulonephritis signs and symptoms include:
1. Pink or cola-colored urine from red blood cells in your urine (hematuria)
2. Foamy urine due to excess protein (proteinuria)
3. High blood pressure (hypertension)
4. Fluid retention (edema) with swelling evident in your face, hands, feet and abdomen.

Complications

Glomerulonephritis can damage your kidneys so that they lose their filtering ability. As a result, dangerous levels of fluid, electrolytes and waste build up in your body.

Possible complications of glomerulonephritis include:
- **Acute kidney failure:** Loss of function in the filtering part of the nephron can result in rapid accumulation of waste products. You might need emergency dialysis an artificial means of removing extra fluids and waste from the blood—typically by an artificial kidney machine.
- **Chronic kidney disease:** Your kidneys gradually lose their filtering ability. Kidney function that deteriorates to less than 10% of normal capacity results in end-stage kidney disease which requires dialysis or a kidney transplant to sustain life.
- **High blood pressure:** Damage to your kidneys and the resulting buildup of wastes in the bloodstream can raise your blood pressure.
- **Nephrotic syndrome:** With this syndrome, too much protein in your urine results in too little protein in your blood. Nephrotic syndrome can be associated with high blood cholesterol and swelling (edema) of the eyelids, feet and abdomen.

Investigation

- **Urine test:** A urinalysis might show red blood cells and red cell casts in your urine, an indicator of possible damage to the glomeruli. Urinalysis results might also show white blood cells, a common indicator of infection or inflammation, and increased protein, which can indicate nephron damage. Other indicators, such as increased blood levels of creatinine or urea, are red flags.
- **Blood tests:** These can provide information about kidney damage and impairment of the glomeruli by measuring levels of waste products, such as creatinine and blood urea nitrogen.
- **Imaging tests:** If your doctor detects evidence of damage, he/she may recommend diagnostic studies that allow visualization of your kidneys, such as a kidney X-ray, an ultrasound examination or a CT scan.
- **Kidney biopsy:** This procedure involves using a special needle to extract small pieces of kidney tissue for microscopic examination to help determine the cause of the inflammation. A kidney biopsy is almost always necessary to confirm a diagnosis of glomerulonephritis.

Treatment: Treatment of glomerulonephritis and your outcome depend on:
- Whether you have an acute or chronic form of the disease
- The underlying cause
- The type and severity of your signs and symptoms.

Some cases of acute glomerulonephritis, especially those that follow a strep infection, might improve on their own and require no treatment. If there is an underlying cause, such as high blood pressure, an infection or an autoimmune disease, treatment will be directed to the underlying cause.

In general, the goal of treatment is to protect your kidneys from further damage.

Therapies for associated kidney failure: For acute glomerulonephritis and acute kidney failure, dialysis can help remove excess fluid and control high blood pressure. The only long-term therapies for end-stage kidney disease are kidney dialysis and kidney transplant. When a transplant is not possible, often because of poor general health, dialysis is the only option.

SHORT ESSAYS

4. Risk factors of coronary artery diseases.

Risk factors for coronary artery disease include:

Age: Simply getting older increases your risk of damaged and narrowed arteries.

Sex: Men are generally at greater risk of coronary artery disease. However, the risk for women increases after menopause.

Family history: A family history of heart disease is associated with a higher risk of coronary artery disease, especially if a close relative developed heart disease at an early age. Your risk is highest if your father or a brother was diagnosed with heart disease before age 55 or if your mother or a sister developed it before age 65.

Smoking: People who smoke have a significantly increased risk of heart disease. Exposing others to your secondhand smoke also increases their risk of coronary artery disease.

High blood pressure: Uncontrolled high blood pressure can result in hardening and thickening of your arteries, narrowing the channel through which blood can flow.

High blood cholesterol levels: High levels of cholesterol in your blood can increase the risk of formation of plaque and atherosclerosis. High cholesterol can be caused by a high level of low-density lipoprotein (LDL) cholesterol, known as the "bad" cholesterol. A low level of high-density lipoprotein (HDL) cholesterol, known as the "good" cholesterol can also contribute to the development of atherosclerosis.

Diabetes: Diabetes is associated with an increased risk of coronary artery disease. Type 2 diabetes and coronary artery disease share similar risk factors, such as obesity and high blood pressure.

Overweight or obesity: Excess weight typically worsens other risk factors.

Physical inactivity: Lack of exercise is also associated with coronary artery disease and some of its risk factors, as well.

High stress: Unrelieved stress in your life may damage your arteries as well as worsen other risk factors for coronary artery disease.

Unhealthy diet: Eating too much food that has high amounts of saturated fat, trans fat, salt and sugar can increase your risk of coronary artery disease.

5. Urinary tract infection.

Urinary tract infections (UTIs) are very common—particularly in women, babies and older people. Around one in two women and one in 20 men will get a UTI in their lifetime.

The kidneys control the amount of water in the blood and filter out waste products to form urine. Each kidney has a tube called a ureter, which joins the kidney to the bladder.

Causes of Urinary Tract Infections

When bacteria enter the urinary tract and multiply, they can cause a UTI. To infect the urinary system, a microorganism usually has to enter through the urethra or, rarely, through the bloodstream. The most common bacterium to cause UTIs is *Escherichia coli* (*E. coli*). It is usually spread to the urethra from the anus.

Other microorganisms, such as mycoplasma and chlamydia, can cause urethritis in both men and women. These microorganisms are sexually transmitted so, when these infections are detected both partners need medical treatment to avoid reinfection.

Symptoms of Urinary Tract Infections

Some of the symptoms of UTIs include:
1. Wanting to urinate more often and urgently, if only a few drops
2. Burning pain or a 'scalding' sensation when urinating
3. A feeling that the bladder is still full after urinating
4. Pain above the pubic bone
5. Cloudy, bloody or very smelly urine.

Risk Factors for Developing Urinary Tract Infections

Some people are at greater risk than others of developing UTIs. These include:
1. Women—sexually active women are vulnerable in part because the urethra is only four centimetres long and bacteria have only this short distance to travel from the outside to the inside of the bladder
2. People with urinary catheters, such as people who are critically ill who cannot empty their own bladder

3. People with diabetes—changes to the immune system make a person with diabetes more vulnerable to infection
4. Men with prostate problems, such as an enlarged prostate gland that can cause the bladder to only partially empty
5. Babies—especially those born with physical problems (congenital abnormalities) of the urinary system.

Prevention of Urinary Tract Infections

Although not always backed up by clinical research, some women have found some suggestions useful in reducing their risk of developing urinary tract infections including:
1. Drink plenty of water and other fluids to flush the urinary system.
2. Treat vaginal infections, such as thrush or trichomonas quickly.
3. Avoid using spermicide-containing products, particularly with a diaphragm contraceptive device.
4. Go to the toilet as soon as you feel the urge to urinate, rather than holding on.
5. Wipe yourself from front to back (urethra to anus) after going to the toilet.
6. Empty your bladder after sex.
7. Avoid constipation.

6. Respiratory rehabilitation.

Pulmonary rehabilitation is a supervised program that includes exercise training, health education, and breathing techniques for people who have certain lung conditions or lung problems due to other condition. Pulmonary rehabilitation can helps to gain strength, reduce symptoms of anxiety or depression, and make it easier to manage routine activities, work, and outings or social activities that you enjoy.

Pulmonary rehabilitation has few risks. Rarely, physical activity during the program can cause problems, such as injuries to the muscles and bones. If serious problems occur during the supervised sessions, your pulmonary rehabilitation team will stop the physical activity right away, give you the appropriate treatment, and contact your doctor.

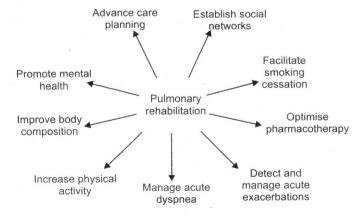

Components: The improvements attributable to individual elements of a program are difficult to assess due to the multidisciplinary nature of pulmonary rehabilitation and to the wide range of therapeutic modalities used.

Exercise Training

1. Physical aerobic training particularly of the lower extremities is mandatory. Any patient capable of undergoing training will benefit from a program that includes leg exercise.
2. Most rehabilitation programs include endurance training.
3. In patients unable to tolerate high-intensity exercise, an alternative is interval training, which consists of 2–3 minutes of high-intensity training alternating with equal periods of rest.
4. The optimal exercise intensity, modality, level of supervision, duration and maintenance program remain to be determined. Although high-intensity training is often prescribed, lower-intensity physical training up to the tolerance level of the individual patient can still produce benefits; in fact, greater emphasis on individual prescription of the appropriate amount of exercise is recommended.
5. Although different exercise training programs have been safely used in various respiratory diseases, they should not be considered in COPD patients until optimal medical control of the disease has been achieved.
6. The varying severity and complexity of different COPD phenotypes suggest that different options should be used for training respiratory and/or peripheral muscles; thus, although it is not possible to generalize, modalities, such as interval training, supported exercise and neuromuscular electrical stimulation have been proposed in order to include the most disabled.

Other Interventions

1. Supportive strategies including nutritional supplementation and advice, and/or pharmacological agents (e.g. testosterone or anabolic drugs), can help improve functional outcome, especially in patients suffering from weight loss and muscle wasting. The contribution of education alone remains unclear.
2. A physiotherapy technique that was previously used as part of rehabilitation encouraged patients to coordinate the breathing process; this technique now receives less emphasis.
3. The term 'breathing retraining' generally refers to such techniques including pursed-lip and diaphragmatic breathing.
4. Pursed-lip breathing is often used subconsciously by COPD patients to enhance exercise tolerance in the face of severe breathlessness and increased ventilatory demand. Pursed-lip breathing results in slower and deeper breaths with a shift in respiratory muscle recruitment from the diaphragm to the accessory muscles of breathing leading to decreased breathlessness and improved oxygenation on exercise.
5. Respiratory muscle training increases the strength and endurance of the respiratory muscles. However, the beneficial effect of respiratory muscle training on the exercise capacity and ADL of COPD patients is still an issue of debate.
6. Neuromuscular electrical stimulation is a possible therapy method for patients with severe chronic respiratory disease who are bed-bound or suffering from extreme skeletal muscle weakness.

7. Nurses responsibility in administration of blood and blood products.

Blood transfusions are a life-sustaining and life-saving treatment but they are not without risk. Conditions that warrant blood transfusions range from acute trauma to intraoperative blood loss to compromised blood cell production secondary to disease or treatment. If you are a nurse on the front line of patient care, you must be adept at administering blood products safely and managing adverse reactions with speed and confidence.

Blood and blood components are selected and given as based on the client's specific needs. The different blood products and their components are described below:
1. **Packed red blood cells**: Packed red blood cells are used when the client is in need of increased oxygen transporting red blood cells as may occur postoperatively and with an acute hemorrhage.
2. **Platelets**: Platelets are administered to clients who are adversely affected with a platelet deficiency or a serious bleeding disorder, such as thrombocytopenia or platelet dysfunction that requires the clotting factors that are in platelets.
3. **Fresh frozen plasma**: Fresh frozen plasma which does not contain any red blood cells is administered to clients who are in need of clotting factors or are in need of increased blood volume as occurs with hypovolemia and hypovolemic shock. Fresh frozen plasma does not have to be typed and cross matched to the client's blood type because plasma does not contain antigen carrying red blood cells.
4. **Albumin**: Albumin is administered to clients who need expanded blood volume and/or plasma proteins.
5. **Clotting factors and cryoprecipitate**: Clotting factors and cryoprecipitate are administered to clients affected with a clotting disorder including the lack of fibrinogen.
6. **Whole blood**: Whole blood is typically reserved for only cases of severe hemorrhage. Whole blood contains clotting factors, red blood cells, white blood cells, plasma, platelets, and plasma proteins.

Before Starting the Transfusion

Safe practice starts with accurate collection of pretransfusion blood samples for typing and crossmatching. Some facilities may require a second authorized staff member to witness and sign the form as the phlebotomist obtains the specimen. Also take these other key actions before you begin the transfusion:
1. Verify that an order for the transfusion exists.
2. Conduct a thorough physical assessment of the patient (including vital signs) to help identify later changes.
3. Document your findings. Confirm that the patient has given informed consent.
4. Teach the patient about the procedures associated risks and benefits, what to expect during the transfusion, signs and symptoms of a reaction, and when and how to call for assistance.
5. Check for an appropriate and patent vascular access.
6. Make sure necessary equipment is at hand for administering the blood product and managing a reaction, such as an additional free IV line for normal saline solution, oxygen, suction, and a hypersensitivity kit.
7. Be sure you are familiar with the specific product to be transfused, the appropriate administration rate, and required patient monitoring. Be aware that the type of blood product and patients condition usually dictates the infusion rate. For example, blood must be infused faster in a trauma victim who's rapidly losing blood than in a 75-year-old patient with heart failure who may not be able to tolerate rapid infusion.
8. Know what personnel will be available in the event of a reaction, and how to contact them. Resources should include the on-call physician and a blood bank representative.
9. Before hanging the blood product, thoroughly double-check the patients identification and verify the actual product. Check the unit to be transfused against patient identifiers, per facility policy.
10. Infuse the blood product with normal saline solution only using filtered tubing.

Administering the Transfusion

Make sure you know the window of time during which the product must be transfused starting from when the product arrives from the blood bank to when the infusion must be completed. Failing to adhere to these time guidelines increases the risk of such complications as bacterial contamination.

Detecting and managing transfusion reactions: During the transfusion, stay alert for signs and symptoms of a reaction, such as fever or chills, flank pain, vital sign changes, nausea, headache, urticaria, dyspnea, and bronchospasm. Optimal management of reactions begins with a standardized protocol for monitoring and documenting vital signs. As dictated by facility policy, obtain the patients vital signs before, during, and after the transfusion.

If you suspect a transfusion reaction, take these immediate actions:
1. Stop the transfusion.
2. Keep the IV line open with normal saline solution.
3. Notify the physician and blood bank.
4. Intervene for signs and symptoms as appropriate.
5. Monitor the patient's vital signs.

8. Types of fracture.

Different types of fracture include:
1. Closed (simple) fracture—the broken bone has not pierced the skin.
2. Open (compound) fracture—the broken bone juts out through the skin, or a wound leads to the fracture site. Infection and external bleeding are more likely.
3. Greenstick fracture—a small, slender crack in the bone. This can occur in children, because their bones are more flexible that an adult's bones.
4. Hairline fracture—the most common form is a stress fracture, often occurring in the foot or lower leg as a result of repeated stress from activities, such as jogging or running.
5. Complicated fracture—structures surrounding the fracture are injured. There may be damage to the veins, arteries or nerves, and there may also be injury to the lining of the bone (the periosteum).
6. Comminuted fracture—the bone is shattered into small pieces. This type of complicated fracture tends to heal more slowly.
7. Avulsion fracture—muscles are anchored to bone with tendons, a type of connective tissue. Powerful muscle contractions can wrench the tendon free and pull out pieces of bone. This type of fracture is more common in the knee and shoulder joints.
8. Compression fracture—occurs when two bones are forced against each other. The bones of the spine, called vertebrae can have this type of fracture. Older people, particularly those with osteoporosis, are at higher risk.

Not all fractures are of a person's arm or leg. Trauma to the head, chest, spine or pelvis can fracture bones, such as the skull and ribs. These fractures are further complicated by the underlying body structure that the bone normally protects. Some of these fractures can be very difficult to manage using first-aid principles only as they may represent life-threatening injuries. Always seek emergency assistance if you suspect this type of fracture.

9. Hepatitis.

Hepatitis means inflammation (swelling and pain) of the liver. The liver is important for a range of functions in the body. These include regulating metabolism, making proteins, storing vitamins and iron, removing toxins and producing bile. If the liver does not work properly, it can cause serious illness or sometimes even death. Hepatitis may be caused by infection, viruses, chemicals, alcohol and other drug use and other factors. Chronic hepatitis means ongoing inflammation of the liver, irrespective of the underlying cause.

The various forms of viral hepatitis are named after different letters of the alphabet. These include hepatitis A, B, C, D and E. They are also sometimes called hep A, hep B, hep C, and so on. While all these viruses affect the liver, they are spread in different ways and have different treatments. The most common types of viral hepatitis in Australia are hepatitis A, B and C.

Symptoms of Hepatitis

Not everyone with hepatitis has symptoms. Generally speaking, when symptoms occur, they may include:
1. Fever
2. Nausea
3. Abdominal discomfort
4. Dark urine
5. Lethargy (tiredness)
6. Painful joints
7. Edema (swelling)
8. Easy bruising
9. Jaundice (yellow skin and eyes).

Hepatitis A: Anyone can be infected if they come in direct contact with the hepatitis A virus through food, drinks or objects contaminated by the feces (poop) of an infected person. Symptoms may last several weeks but the person usually recovers completely. Infection with hepatitis A will give lifelong immunity. However, this does not offer immunity against the other types of hepatitis A vaccine is available to protect against hepatitis A.

Hepatitis B: Spread when blood, semen, vaginal secretions or other body fluids from someone infected with hepatitis B enter the bloodstream of someone who is not infected with hepatitis B. Activities that might enable the spread of hepatitis B include unsafe sex, or the use of unsterile injecting equipment. Hepatitis B can also be passed from mother to child either through the womb (rarely), at the time of birth or shortly after birth.

People who are exposed to the hepatitis B virus may develop long-term hepatitis B (where the virus stays in their body for their entire life). Babies and children who become infected are far more likely than adults to develop long-term hepatitis B

Hepatitis C: Blood-borne virus that is spread when blood from a person with hepatitis C enters another person's bloodstream. In Australia, the most common way it is transmitted is through sharing unsterile injecting drug equipment. Around 20–30% of people who become infected with hepatitis C may clear the virus from their blood with no treatment. These people no longer have hepatitis C and cannot pass it on. Treatment with direct-acting antiviral medicines has greatly improved the outcomes for people with hepatitis C. These treatments can help decrease inflammation in the liver and can clear the virus in up to 90% of people, and there are minimal side effects. There is no vaccine available to prevent hepatitis C infection.

Hepatitis D: Hepatitis D infection is uncommon in Australia, but is prevalent in countries that have a high incidence of hepatitis B. Hepatitis D virus can be acquired either as a coinfection (occurs at the same time) with hepatitis B virus or as a superinfection in people who are hepatitis B positive.

Hepatitis E: Hepatitis E is most common in developing countries. There is no chronic (long-term) infection associated with this virus. Hepatitis E is more severe among pregnant women, especially in the third trimester. The hepatitis E virus is found in the feces of infected people and animals and is spread by eating or drinking contaminated food or water. Transmission from person to person occurs less commonly than with hepatitis A virus.

Pregnant women from Australia are strongly advised not to travel to areas where there is a lot of hepatitis E, especially during the last 3 months of pregnancy.

Diagnosis of Hepatitis

Tests used to diagnose hepatitis may include blood tests and a liver ultrasound or fibroscan (a quick and noninvasive test that uses ultrasound to measure the 'stiffness' of your liver).

Treatment for Hepatitis

Treatment depends on the type of hepatitis. Talk to your doctor about the treatment that is recommended for you. Chronic viral hepatitis whether due to hepatitis B or C can after many years lead to cirrhosis and primary cancer of the liver.

10. Prevention of deep vein thrombosis in bed ridden patients.

Deep vein thrombosis (DVT) is a blood clot or **thrombus** in a deep vein. Most of these clots develop in the leg or thigh. But they may form in a vein in the arm, or other part of the body.

Part of the blood clot may separate from the vein. This is called an **embolus**. It may travel to the lungs and form a pulmonary embolus. This can cut off the flow of blood to a portion of or to the entire lung. A blood clot in the lungs is a medical emergency and may cause death.

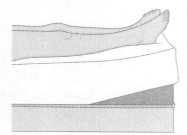
Raise your mattress 5 to 6 inches using a foam wedge.

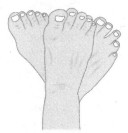
Wiggle your toes and move your ankles in circles.

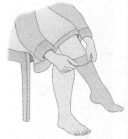
Wear support to elastic stockings as instructed.

Symptoms

Deep vein thrombosis usually occur in the legs. The most common symptoms of DVT include:
- Swelling in the affected leg
- Pain in the leg (may feel like cramping in the calf)
- Warmth in the affected area
- Redness or other changes in skin color, such as the skin turning more pale or more blue than usual.

A DVT can also occur without any noticeable symptoms.

Symptoms of a pulmonary embolism (PE), a blood clot that has traveled to the lungs, include:
- Difficulty breathing
- Sharp chest pain that worsens after taking deep breaths
- Coughing up blood
- Lightheadedness, fainting, and unconsciousness (for very large clots).

Prevention
1. **Preventive treatment with blood-thinning medication.**
2. **Elastic compression stockings:** These stockings, worn on the legs, provide gentle, graduated pressure to keep blood from pooling in the legs. Compression stockings are custom-fit and obtained by prescription. Stockings should be put on after waking and worn throughout the day; they can be removed to bathe and at bedtime.
3. **Movement breaks on long trips:** The overall risk of developing a DVT while traveling is low, although it increases on trips over 4 hours long, especially in long airplane or car trips. You can decrease this risk by moving and flexing your legs and periodically walking around. If you are at high risk of developing a DVT or blood clot, your healthcare provider may recommend that you wear compression stockings while traveling.

Other methods are:
- Lose weight, if you are overweight
- Stay active
- Exercise regularly; walking is fine
- Avoid long periods of staying still
- Get up and move around at least every hour whenever you travel on a plane, train, or bus, particularly if the trip is longer than 4 hours
- Do heel toe exercises or circle your feet if you cannot move around
- Stop at least every two hours when you drive, and get out and move around
- Drink a lot of water and wear loose fitted clothing when you travel
- Talk to your doctor about your risk of clotting whenever you take hormones, whether for birth control or replacement therapy, or during and right after any pregnancy
- Follow any self-care measures to keep heart failure, diabetes, or any other health issues as stable as possible.

11. Pneumonia.

Pneumonia is a type of lung infection caused by a virus or bacteria. The lungs are filled with thousands of tubes called bronchi which end in smaller sacs called alveoli. Each one has a fine mesh of capillaries. This is where oxygen is added to the blood and carbon dioxide is removed.

Causes of Pneumonia

Pneumonia can be triggered by a cold or bout of flu which allows the germs to gain access to the alveoli. In about half of all cases, no cause is ever found. Some of the microorganisms that can cause pneumonia include:
- **Bacteria**—symptoms include rust or green-colored phlegm. Anyone of any age can be affected, but susceptible groups include babies, the elderly, alcoholics, and people recovering from surgery or coping with other illnesses (such as lung disease).
- **Viruses**—symptoms are similar to a severe bout of flu. It is thought that around 50% of pneumonia cases are caused by viral infections.
- **Mycoplasma (a special kind of bacteria)**—symptoms can include white phlegm, nausea and vomiting. Pneumonia caused by mycoplasma organisms is generally mild, but recovery takes longer.

Symptoms of Pneumonia

The symptoms of pneumonia depend on the age of the person, the cause and severity of the infection, and any existing problems with immunity. Some of the symptoms may include:
- Rapid breathing

- Breathing difficulties
- Fever
- General malaise
- Loss of appetite
- Abdominal pain
- Headache
- Chest pain
- Cough
- Blue colouration of the skin around the mouth (cyanosis), caused by lack of oxygen.

If a person has pneumonia, the alveoli in one or both lungs fill with pus and fluids (exudate), which interferes with the gas exchange. This is sometimes known as 'consolidation and collapse of the lung'.

Diagnosis for Pneumonia

If your child seems to be recovering well from a cold or flu, but then relapses, they may have a chest infection. See your doctor immediately, since pneumonia can be life-threatening to babies and young children. Pneumonia is diagnosed using a variety of tests, such as general examination and chest X-rays.

Treatment for Pneumonia

In many cases, the person's own immune system can deal with the infection, but antibiotics may sometimes assist recovery. Treatment depends on the age of the individual and the type of infection, but can include:
- **Hospital admission**—for babies, young children and the elderly. Mild or moderate cases of pneumonia in people who are otherwise well can often be treated at home.
- **Plenty of fluids**—taken orally or intravenously
- **Antibiotics**—to kill the infection, if bacteria are the cause
- **Medications**—to relieve pain and reduce fever
- **Rest**—sitting up is better than lying down.

Immunization for Pneumonia

One of the most common types of bacterial pneumonia is pneumococcal pneumonia, caused by infection with *Streptococcus pneumoniae*. There are vaccines against this strain that reduce the risk of infection.

It is recommended that certain people be immunized including:
- Young children
- Older people over the age of 65 years
- People with chronic illnesses, such as diabetes, asthma or respiratory disorders
- People with reduced immunity
- People who have had an organ transplant
- People who have damaged spleens or have had their spleens surgically removed
- Aboriginal and Torres Strait Islander people over the age of 50 years

12. Arrhythmias.

An irregular heartbeat is an arrhythmia (also called dysrhythmia). Heart rates can also be irregular. A normal heart rate is 50–100 beats per minute. Arrhythmias and abnormal heart rates do not necessarily occur together. Arrhythmias can occur with a normal heart rate, or with heart rates that are slow (called bradyarrhythmias—less than 50 beats per minute). Arrhythmias can also occur with rapid heart rates (called tachyarrhythmias—faster than 100 beats per minute).

Types of Arrhythmia

There are several types of arrhythmia:

Atrial fibrillation: This is irregular beating of the atrial chambers—nearly always too fast. Atrial fibrillation is common and mainly affects older patients. Instead of producing a single, strong contraction, the chamber fibrillates (quivers).

Atrial flutter: While fibrillation consists of many random and different quivers in the atrium, atrial flutter is usually from one area in the atrium that is not conducting properly, so the abnormal heart conduction has a consistent pattern.

Supraventricular tachycardia (SVT): A regular, abnormally rapid heartbeat. The patient experiences a burst of accelerated heartbeats that can last from a few seconds to a few hours. Typically, a patient with SVT will have a heart rate of 160-200 beats per minute. Atrial fibrillation and flutter are classified under SVTs.

Ventricular tachycardia: Abnormal electrical impulses that start in the ventricles and cause an abnormally fast heartbeat. This often happens if the heart has a scar from a previous heart attack. Usually, the ventricle will contract more than 200 times a minute.

Ventricular fibrillation: An irregular heart rhythm consisting of very rapid, uncoordinated fluttering contractions of the ventricles. The ventricles do not pump blood properly, they simply quiver.

Long QT syndrome: A heart rhythm disorder that sometimes causes rapid, uncoordinated heartbeats. This can result in fainting, which may be life-threatening. It can be caused by a genetic susceptibility or certain medications.

Diagnosis of Arrhythmia

The following tests might be ordered:
- Blood and urine tests
- Electrocardiogram (EKG)
- Holtermonitor—a wearable device that records the heart for 1-2 days
- Echocardiogram
- Chest X-ray
- Tilt-table test
- Electrophysiologic testing (or EP studies)
- Heart catheterization.

Complications of Arrhythmia

Stroke—fibrillation (quivering) means that the heart is not pumping properly. This can cause blood to collect in pools and clots can form. If one of the clots dislodges it may travel to a brain artery, blocking it, and causing a stroke. Stroke can cause brain damage and can sometimes be fatal.

Heart failure—prolonged tachycardia or bradycardia can result in the heart not pumping enough blood to the body and its organs—this is heart failure. Treatment can usually help improve this.

SHORT ANSWERS

13. Endocarditis.

Endocarditis occurs when bacteria enter your bloodstream, travel to the heart, and lodge on abnormal heart valves or damaged heart tissue. Abnormal growths (vegetations) that contain collections of bacteria may form in your heart at the site of the infection and damage the heart valves which can cause them to leak.

Common signs and symptoms of endocarditis include:
- Flu-like symptoms, such as fever and chills
- A new or changed heart murmur which is the heart sounds made by blood rushing through your heart
- Fatigue
- Aching joints and muscles
- Night sweats
- Shortness of breath
- Chest pain when you breathe
- Swelling in your feet, legs or abdomen.

14. Orthopedic prosthesis.

An orthopedic implant is a device surgically placed into the body designed to restore function by replacing or reinforcing a damaged structure. For the treatment of back pain, orthopedic implants, such as bone plates and bone screws are used in spinal fusion surgery and fixation of fractured bone segments, as well as implant components used for hip and joint replacement. The material used in orthopedic implants must be biocompatible to avoid rejection by the body. Other risks associated with orthopedic implants include implants coming loose or breaking in the bone causing painful inflammation and infection to surrounding tissue.

Orthopedic prosthesis is medical devices that are utilized to substitute or make an available fixation of bone or replace joint surfaces. In modest words, they are used to replace troubled joints. The prosthesis surgeries are successfully achieved by extremely trained and expert orthopedic surgeons. The surgical process for every prosthesis involves exclusion of damaged joints and an artificial implant replacement.

15. Pneumothorax.

A pneumothorax is a collapsed lung. A pneumothorax occurs when air leaks into the space between your lung and chest wall. This air pushes on the outside of your lung and makes it collapse.

A pneumothorax can be caused by a blunt or penetrating chest injury, certain medical procedures, or damage from underlying lung disease. Or it may occur for no obvious reason. Symptoms usually include sudden chest pain and shortness of breath. On some occasions, a collapsed lung can be a life-threatening event.

Symptoms: The main symptoms of a pneumothorax are sudden chest pain and shortness of breath.

Treatment for a pneumothorax usually involves inserting a needle or chest tube between the ribs to remove the excess air. However, a small pneumothorax may heal on its own.

16. Hypospadiasis.

Hypospadias is a birth defect (congenital condition) in which the opening of the urethra is on the underside of the penis instead of at the tip. The urethra is the tube through which urine drains from your bladder and exits the body. Hypospadias is common and does not cause difficulty in caring for your infant. Surgery usually restores the normal appearance of your child's penis. With successful treatment of hypospadias, most males can have normal urination and reproduction.

Signs and symptoms of hypospadias may include:
- Opening of the urethra at a location other than the tip of the penis
- Downward curve of the penis (chordee)
- Hooded appearance of the penis because only the top half of the penis is covered by foreskin
- Abnormal spraying during urination.

17. Postoperative nursing management of thyroidectomy.

Thyroid surgery can cause potentially fatal complications during the early postoperative phase. It is essential that nurses have the knowledge and skills to detect early signs and symptoms of potential complications and take appropriate action. Early detection and rapid response are key to maintaining patient safety and minimising harm.

1. Wound **care**
2. Placed ice bag on the neck wound. This will reduce swelling and pain
3. Diet
4. The patient may have cold liquid food when fully aware
5. Activity and movement
6. Elevate the head of the bed 25–35°
7. Please be attentive to rest and only have
8. Little exercise for 2-3 weeks after surgery.

18. Psoriasis.

Psoriasis is a chronic skin condition caused by an overactive immune system. Symptoms include flaking, inflammation, and thick, white, silvery, or red patches of skin. Psoriasis treatments include steroid creams, occlusion, light therapy and oral medications, such as biologics psoriasis signs and symptoms are different for everyone. Common signs and symptoms include:
- Red patches of skin covered with thick, silvery scales
- Small scaling spots (commonly seen in children)
- Dry, cracked skin that may bleed
- Itching, burning or soreness
- Thickened, pitted or ridged nails
- Swollen and stiff joints.

19. Hypovalumic shock.

Hypovolemic shock is an emergency condition in which severe blood or fluid loss makes the heart unable to pump enough blood to the body. This type of shock can cause many organs to stop working.

Cause: Losing about one-fifth or more of the normal amount of blood in the body causes hypovolemic shock.

Blood loss can be due to:
- Bleeding from cuts
- Bleeding from other injuries
- Internal bleeding, such as in the gastrointestinal tract.

The amount of circulating blood in your body also may drop when you lose too much body fluid from other causes. This can be due to:
- Burns
- Diarrhea
- Excessive perspiration
- Vomiting.

20. Pott's spine.

Pott's disease, is a form of tuberculosis that occurs outside the lungs whereby disease is seen in the vertebrae. Tuberculosis can affect several tissues outside the lungs including the spine, a kind of tuberculosis arthritis of the intervertebral joints.

Pott's disease is usually located in the thoracic, or upper, spine. Early signs of tuberculosis are fever, night sweats and weight loss. Severe back pain is the most common indication that the TB has spread to the spine. As the disease worsens, patients will have difficulty standing.

21. Malaria.

Malaria is a disease caused by a parasite. The parasite is transmitted to humans through the bites of infected mosquitoes. People who have malaria usually feel very sick, with a high fever and shaking chills. Each year, approximately 210 million people are infected with malaria, and about 440,000 people die from the disease. Most of the people who die from the disease are young children in Africa.

Symptoms

A malaria infection is generally characterized by the following signs and symptoms:
- Fever
- Chills
- Headache
- Nausea and vomiting
- Muscle pain and fatigue.

Other signs and symptoms may include:
- Sweating
- Chest or abdominal pain
- Cough.

22. Defibrillation.

Defibrillators are devices that restore a normal heartbeat by sending an electric pulse or shock to the heart. They are used to prevent or correct an arrhythmia, a heartbeat that is uneven or that is too slow or too fast. Defibrillators can also restore the heart's beating if the heart suddenly stops.

The use of a carefully controlled electric shock, administered either through a device on the exterior of the chest wall or directly to the exposed heart muscle, to normalize the rhythm of the heart or restart it.

Different types of defibrillators work in different ways. Automated external defibrillators (AEDs), which are in many public spaces, were developed to save the lives of people experiencing sudden cardiac arrest. Even untrained bystanders can use these devices in an emergency.

Other defibrillators can prevent sudden death among people who have a high-risk of a life-threatening arrhythmia. They include implantable cardioverter defibrillators (ICDs) which are surgically placed inside your body, and wearable cardioverter defibrillators (WCDs) which rest on the body. It can take time and effort to get used to living with a defibrillator, and it is important to be aware of possible risks and complications.

2016

Medical-Surgical Nursing-I

LONG ESSAYS
1. Mr Raju, 45-years-old diagnosed to have cholelithiasis is suggested for cholecystectomy: a. Define cholelithiasis. b. List down the methods of nonsurgical removal of gallstones. c. Describe the postoperative nursing care of Mr Raju.
2. Mr Kiran, 47-year-old got admitted in medical ward with cirrhosis of liver: a. Define cirrhosis of liver. b. List the etiology and clinical manifestations. c. Prepare a nursing care plan for Mr Kiran using nursing process.
3. Mr Rajiv, 42-year-old man is admitted with severe pain due to renal calculi: a. Mention the types of renal calculi. b. List the clinical manifestations and diagnostic procedures used to diagnose renal calculi. c. Describe the pre- and postoperative nursing care for Mr Rajiv.

SHORT ESSAYS
4. Explain the role of nurse in organ donation.
5. Describe the preoperative preparation of patient undergoing abdominal surgery.
6. Explain the current CPR guidelines.
7. Describe the nursing responsibilities during thrombolytic therapy.
8. Explain pathophysiology of diabetes mellitus.
9. Explain the causes and management of psoriasis.
10. Enumerate on biomedical waste management followed in medical ward.
11. Explain the current schedule of short course chemotherapy for tuberculosis.
12. Explain about prevention of transmission of HIV infection among adults.

SHORT ANSWERS
13. Write about any two specific noninvasive diagnostic procedures done in cardiac diseases.
14. Indicate two reasons to follow rotation of site for insulin administration.
15. Name two opportunistic infections among AIDS patients.
16. Classify hemophilia.
17. List two suture materials and its uses.
18. List four major duties of scrub nurse.
19. Specify the incubation period for poliomyelitis.
20. Write two important clinical manifestations of left ventricular failure.
21. What is DASH diet?
22. List two complications of tracheostomy.

LONG ESSAYS

1. Mr Raju, 45-years-old, diagnosed to have cholelithiasis is suggested for cholecystectomy: (a) Define cholelithiasis. (b) List down the methods of nonsurgical removal of gallstones. (c) Describe the postoperative nursing care of Mr Raju.

Gallstones can occur anywhere in the biliary tree. The cholelithiasis refer to stone formation in the gallbladder. Either acute or chronic inflammation termed as "cholecytitis" can result, precipitated by the presence of stones. When stones form in or migrate to the common bile duct the condition is termed as choledocholelithasis.

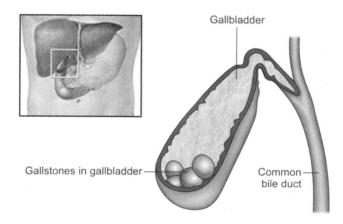

Etiology

Cholecystitis is most commonly associated with stones, when it occurs in the absence of stones it is thought to be caused by bacteria reaching gallbladder via the vascular or lymphatic route or chemical irritant in the bile. *E. coli*, streptococci, and *Salmonellae* are common bacteria. Other causative factors include adhesions, neoplasms, extensive fasting, frequent weight fluctuations, anesthesia and narcotics.

The actual cause of cholelithiasis is unknown. It develops when the valarice that keeps cholestrol, bile salts and calcium in solutions is altered so that precipitation of these substances occurs. Conditions that upset this balance include infection and disturbance in the metabolism of cholestrol. A high percentage of gallstones are precipitated of cholestrol. Other components of bile that precipitates into stone are bile salts, bilirubin, calcium and proteins. Stones sometimes are mixed. The risk factors for cholestrol gallstones are obesity, middle age, pregnancy, multiparity, use of oral contraceptives, rapid weight loss, diseases of the ileum and hypercholesterolemia.

Pathophysiology

Bile is primarily composed of water plus conjugated bilirubin, organic and inorganic ions, small amounts of proteins and three lipids, bile salts, lecithin, and cholesterol. When the balance of these three lipids remains intact, cholesterol is held in solution. If the balance is upset cholesterol can be precipitated. Cholesterol gallstone formation is enhanced by the production of a mucin glycoprotein, which traps cholesterol particles. Supersaturation of the bile with cholesterol also impairs gallbladder mobility and contributes to stasis.

Cholestrol stones are hard, white or yellow-brown in color, radiolucent and can be quite large up to 4 cm. Black-pigmented stones form as the result of an increase of unconjugated billirubin and calcium with a corresponding decrease in bile salts. Gallbladder motility may also be impaired. Brown stones develop in the intra- and extrahepatic ducts and are usually preceded by bacterial invasion.

Clinical Manifestations

Manifestation of cholecystitis varies from indigestion and moderate to severe pain, fever and jaundice. Initial symptoms of acute cholecystitis include indigestion and pain and tenderness in the right upper quadrant (RUQ), which may be referred to the right shoulder and scapula. The pain may be accompanied by anorexia, nausea and possibly vomiting, restlessness and diaphoresis. Manifestation of inflammation include leukocytosis and fever.

Physical findings include RUQ tenderness and abdominal rigidity. Symptoms of chronic cholecystitis include history of fat intolerance, dyspepsia, heartburn and flatulence. Cholelithiasis may produce severe symptom or none at all. The severity of symptoms depend on whether the stones are stationary or mobile and whether obstruction is present.

Clinical manifestations caused by obstructed blood flow are as follows:
1. Obstructive jaundice due to no bile flow into duodenum.
2. Dark amber urine which forms when shaken is due to soluble bilirubin in urine.
3. No urobilirubin in urine due to no bilirubin reaching small intestine to be converted to urobilirubin.
4. Clay-colored stools urobilirubin.
5. Pruritis due to deposition of bile salts in skin tissues.
6. Intolerance for fatty foods—no bile in small intestine for fat digestion.
7. Bleeding tendencies—lack or decreased absorption of vitamin K resulting in decreased production of prothrombins.
8. Steatorrhea—no bile salts in duodenum, preventing fat emulsion and digestion.
9. Billary colic—Murphy sign, i.e. pain colicy and more steady flow. Complications of cholecystitis include subphrenic abscess, pancreatitis, cholangitis (inflammation of bile ducts), biliary cirrhosis, fistulas, and rupture of gallbladder which can produce bile peritonitis.

Diagnostic Study
1. Ultrasound.
2. Cholecystogram or IV cholengiogram.
3. Liver function studies.
4. WBC counts and.
5. Serum bilirubin.

Preoperative

Patient with complete preoperative preparations at home before their arrival on the day of surgery. The nurse will verify that the patient has had NPO and completed any required bowel preparation. Preoperative teaching includes:
1. Teach patient the importance of frequent breathing and use of incentive spirometer because the high incision and RUQ pain predispose the patient to atelectasis and right lower lobe pneumonia.
2. Explain the types of biliary drainage tubes which are anticipated if any.
3. Teach the patient about the pain control plan to be used in the postoperative period.

Postoperative

1. Place the patient in low-Fowler's position, assist to change position frequently.
2. Urge patient to deep breathing at regular intervals (every 1–2 hours) and to cough if secretions are present until ambulating well. Assist patient to effectively splint the incision. Encourage use of incentive spirometer.
3. Give analgesics fairly liberally for the first 2–3 days.
4. Use patient-controlled analgesia if possible. Meperidine has been the drug of choice because it is believed to minimize spasms in the bile ducts, but morphine is being used with increasing frequency.
5. Maintain a dry, intact dressing, usually a drain is inserted near the stump of the cyst duct; some serous fluid drainage is normal initially.
6. Encourage progressive ambulation when permitted.
7. Increase diet gradually to be regular with fat content as tolerated (appetite and fat tolerance may be diminished if there is external biliary drainage).

Biliary Drainage

1. Connect any biliary drainage tubes to be closed gravity drainage.
2. Attach sufficient tubing so the patient can move without restriction.
3. Explain to patient the importance of avoiding kinks, clamping or pulling of the tube.
4. Monitor the amount and color of drainage frequently, measure and record drainage at least every shift.
5. Report any signs of peritonitis (abdominal pain, rigidity or fever) to the concerned doctor.
6. Monitor color of urine and stools; stools will be grayish white if the bile is flowing out a drainage tube, but the normal color should gradually reappear as external drainage diminishes and disappears.

2. Mr Kiran, 47-year old got admitted in medical ward with cirrhosis of liver: a. Define cirrhosis of liver. b. List the etiology and clinical manifestations. c. Prepare a nursing care plan for Mr Kiran using nursing process.

Cirrhosis is a chronic disease characterized by replacement of normal liver tissue with diffuse fibrosis that disrupts the structure and function of the liver. Cirrhosis, or scarring of the liver, is divided into three types: 1. Alcoholic, most frequently due to chronic alcoholism and the most common type of cirrhosis; 2. Postnecrotic, a late result of a previous acute viral hepatitis; and 3. Biliary, a result of chronic biliary obstruction and infection (least common type of cirrhosis).

Clinical Manifestations

1. **Compensated cirrhosis:** Usually found secondary to routine physical examination; vague symptoms.
2. **Decompensated cirrhosis:** Symptoms of decreased proteins, clotting factors, and other substances and of portal hypertension.
3. **Liver enlargement** early in the course (fatty liver); later in course, liver size decreases from scar tissue.
4. **Portal obstruction and ascites:** Chronic dyspepsia, constipation or diarrhea, splenomegaly; spider telangiectases may be observed.
5. **Gastrointestinal varices:** Distended abdominal blood vessels; varices or hemorrhoids; hematemesis; profuse hemorrhage from the stomach; and esophageal varices in about 25% of patients.

6. **Edema**, jaundice, fever.
7. Vitamin deficiency (A, C, and K) and anemia.
8. Mental deterioration with impending hepatic encephalopathy and hepatic coma.

Pathophysiology in cirrhosis of liver: Characterized by diffuse inflammation and fibrosis resulting in drastic structural changes and significant loss of liver function. The basic changes, liver cell death and replacement of normal tissue by scar tissue, results in modules of normal liver parenchyma surrounded by fibrous tissue and fat, because of which obstruction of the splanchnic vein and portal blood flow occurs which leads to fluid retention, increasing edema, ascites, hydrothorax, increased portal hypertension causing increased venous pressure, vascular homeostasis, varicose veins, hemorrhoids and esophageal varices.

Alterations in physiology are usually seen late in the progression of the disease because of the large reserve capacity of the liver. As much as three fourths of the liver can be destroyed before physiologic function is altered.

Assessment and Diagnostic Methods
1. **Liver function tests** [e.g. serum alkaline phosphates AST (SGOTI), ALT (SGPT), GGT, and bilirubin], prothrombin time, ABGs, laparoscopy, in conjunction with biopsy.
2. Ultrasound scanning.
3. Computed tomography (CT) scan.
4. Magnetic resonance imaging (MRI).
5. Radioisotopic liver scans.

Medical Management
Medical management is based on presenting symptoms:
1. Treatment includes antacids, vitamins, balanced diet, and nutritional supplements; Potassium-sparing diuretics (for ascites); avoidance of alcohol.
2. Colchicines may increase the length of survival in patients with mild-to-moderate cirrhosis.

Nursing Management
Assessment
1. Focus on dietary intake, nutritional status, onset of symptoms, history of precipitating factors, including long-term alcohol abuse, exposure to toxic agents, medications.
2. Assess mental status through interview and interaction with patient; note orientation to time, place, and person.
3. Note relationships with family, friends, and coworkers regarding incapacitation secondary to alcohol abuse and cirrhosis.
4. Note abdominal distention and bloating, gastrointestinal bleeding, bruising, and weight changes.
5. Document exposure to toxic agents, such as hepatotoxic medications or illicit drugs.

Nursing Diagnoses
Activity intolerance related to fatigue, general debility, muscle wasting, and discomfort

Imbalanced nutrition: Less than body requirements, related to chronic gastritis, decreased gastrointestinal motility, and anorexia

Impaired skin integrity related to compromised immunologic status, edema, and poor nutrition. Risk for injury and bleeding related to altered clotting mechanisms.

Collaborative Problems/Potential Complications
1. Bleeding and hemorrhage.

2. Hepatic encephalopathy.
3. Fluid volume excess.

Planning and goals: Goals may include independence in activities, improved nutritional status, and improved skin integrity, decreased potential for injury, improved mental status, and absence of complications.

Nursing Interventions

I. Providing Rest
1. Position bed for maximal respiratory efficiency; provide oxygen if needed.
2. Initiate efforts to prevent respiratory, circulatory, and vascular disturbances.
3. Encourage patient to increase activity gradually and plan rest with activity and mild exercise.

II. Improving Nutritional Status
1. Provide a nutritious, high-protein diet supplemented by B-complex vitamins and others including A, C, and K and folic acid if there is no indication of impending coma.
2. Provide small, frequent meals, consider patient preferences, and encourage patient to eat; provide protein supplements, if indicated.
3. Provide nutrients by feeding tube or total parenteral nutrition (PN).
4. Provide patients who have fatty stools (steatorrhea) with water-soluble forms of fat-soluble vitamins A, O, and E, and give folic acid and iron to prevent anemia.
5. Provide a low-protein diet temporarily if patient shows signs of impending or advancing coma; restore protein intake to moderate (1 to 1.5/Kg) when patient's condition permits.

III. Providing Skin Care
1. Change position frequently.
2. Avoid using irritating soaps and adhesive tape.
3. Provide lotion to soothe irritated skin.
4. Take measures to prevent patient from scratching the skin.

IV. Reducing Risk of Injury
1. Use padded side rails if patient becomes agitated or restless.
2. Orient to time, place, and procedures to minimize agitation.
3. Instruct patient to ask for assistance to get out of bed.
4. Provide safety measures to prevent injury or cuts (electric razor, soft toothbrush).
5. Apply pressure to venipuncture sites to minimize bleeding.

V. Monitoring and Managing Complications
Preventing bleeding due to decreased production of prothrombin and monitoring for hepatic encephalopathy are the primary concerns.
1. Observe for melena, and check stools for blood.
2. Take precautionary measures (e.g. use padded side rails, apply pressure to injection site for long period of time, and avoid sharp objects).
3. Use appropnate dietary modification and stool softeners to prevent straining during defecation.
4. Monitor closely for gastrointestinal bleeding. Keep equipment to treat hemorrhage from esophageal varices readily available; intravenous fluids, medications, Sengstaken-Blakemore tube.
5. Monitor closely to identify early evidence of condition.
6. Explain event and treatment if complication noted. Patient may need to be treated in ICU.

VI. Promoting Home and Community-based Care

Prepare for discharge by providing dietary instruction including exclusion of alcohol.
1. Refer to alcoholics anonymous if indicated.
2. Continue sodium restriction; stress avoidance of raw shellfish.
3. Provide written instructions, teaching, support, and reinforcement to patient and family.
4. Encourage rest and probably a change in lifestyle (adequate, well-balanced diet and elimination of alcohol).
5. Instruct family about symptoms of impending encephalopathy and possibility of bleeding tendencies and infection.
6. Refer patient to home care nurse, and assist in transition from hospital to home.

3. Mr Rajiv, 42-year-old man is admitted with severe pain due to renal calculi: a. Mention the types of renal calculi. b. List the clinical manifestations and diagnostic procedures used to diagnose renal calculi. c. Describe the pre- and postoperative nursing care for Mr Rajiv.

Kidney stones, or renal calculi, are solid masses made of crystals. Kidney stones usually originate in your kidneys, but can develop anywhere along your urinary tract. The urinary tract includes the kidneys, ureters, bladder, and urethra. Kidney stones are known to be one of the most painful medical conditions. The causes of kidney stones vary according to the type of stone.

Types of Kidney Stones

Not all kidney stones are made up of the same crystals. The different types of kidney stones include:

Calcium: Calcium stones are the most common. They can be made of calcium oxalate (most common), phosphate, or maleate. Eating fewer oxalate-rich foods can reduce your risk of developing this type of stone. High-oxalate foods include potato chips, peanuts, chocolate, beets, and spinach.

Uric acid: This type of kidney stone is more common in men than in women. They can occur in people with gout or those going through chemotherapy. This type of stone develops when urine is too acidic. A diet rich in purines can increase urine's acidic level. Purine is a colorless substance in animal proteins, such as fish, shellfish, and meats.

Struvite: This type of stone is found mostly in women with urinary tract infections. These stones can be large and cause urinary obstruction. These stones are caused by kidney infection. Treating an underlying infection can prevent the development of struvite stones.

Cystine: Cystine stones are rare. They occur in both men and women who have the genetic disorder cystinuria. With this type of stone, cystine—an acid that occurs naturally in the body, leaks from the kidneys into the urine.

Causes of Kidney Stones

A kidney stone can form when substances, such as calcium, oxalate, cystine or uric acid are at high levels in the urine, although stones can form even if these chemicals are at normal levels.

Medications used for treating some medical conditions, such as kidney disease, cancer or HIV can also increase your risk of developing kidney stones.

A small number of people get kidney stones because of some medical conditions which can lead to high levels of calcium, oxalate, cystine or uric acid in the body.

Symptoms of Kidney Stones

Many people with kidney stones have no symptoms. However, some people do get symptoms, which may include:
1. A gripping pain in the back (also known as 'renal colic')—usually just below the ribs on one side, radiating around to the front and sometimes towards the groin. The pain may be severe enough to cause nausea and vomiting.
2. Blood in the urine.
3. Shivers, sweating and fever—if the urine becomes infected.
4. Small stones like gravel, passing out in the urine, often caused by uric acid stone.
5. An urgent feeling of needing to urinate, due to a stone at the bladder outlet.

Diagnosis of Kidney Stones

Many stones are discovered by chance during examinations for other conditions. Urine and blood tests can help with finding out the cause of the stone. Further tests may include:
1. Ultrasound.
2. CT scans.
3. X-rays, including an intravenous pyelogram (IVP), where dye is injected into the bloodstream before the X-rays are taken.

If you pass a stone, collect it and take it to your doctor for analysis. Analysis of a stone is very useful.

Complications of Kidney Stones

Kidney stones can range in size from a grain of sand to that of a pearl or even larger. They can be smooth or jagged, and are usually yellow or brown. A large stone may get stuck in the urinary system. This can block the flow of urine and may cause strong pain.

Kidney stones can cause permanent kidney damage. Stones also increase the risk of urinary and kidney infection, which can result in germs spreading into the bloodstream.

Treatment for Kidney Stones

Most kidney stones can be treated without surgery. 90% of stones pass by themselves within 3–6 weeks. In this situation, the only treatment required is pain relief. However, pain can be so severe that hospital admission and very strong pain-relieving medication may be needed. Always seek immediate medical attention if you are suffering from strong pain. Small stones in the kidney do not usually cause problems, so there is often no need to remove them. A doctor specializing in the treatment of kidney stones is the best person to advise you on treatment. If a stone does not pass and blocks urine flow or causes bleeding or an infection, then it may need to be removed. New surgical techniques have reduced hospital stay time to as little as 48 hours.

Other treatments include:
1. Extracorporeal shock-wave lithotripsy (ESWL)—ultrasound waves are used to break the kidney stone into smaller pieces, which can pass out with the urine. It is used for stones less than 2 cm in size.
2. Percutaneous nephrolithotomy—a small cut is made in your back, then a special instrument is used to remove the kidney stone.
3. Endoscope removal—an instrument is inserted into the urethra, passed into the bladder and then to where the stone is located. It allows the doctor to remove the stone or break it up so it can pass more easily.

4. Surgery—if none of these methods is suitable, the stone may need to be removed using traditional surgery. This will require a cut in your back to access your kidney and ureter to remove the stone.

Management of Kidney Stones

For most people with recurrent calcium stones, a combination of drinking enough fluids, avoiding urinary infections and specific treatment with medications will significantly reduce or stop new stone formation. Certain drugs, such as thiazide diuretics or indapamide reduce calcium excretion and decrease the chance of another calcium stone. Potassium citrate (Hydralyte, Pedialyte, Urocit-K), or citric juices are used to supplement thiazide treatment and are used by themselves for some conditions where the urine is too acidic. For people who have a high level of uric acid in their urine, or who make uric acid stones, the drug allopurinol will usually stop the formation of new stones.

Preoperative Care

1. Assess knowledge and understanding of the procedure, providing information as needed. Anxiety is reduced, and recovery is enhanced and hastened when the client is fully prepared for surgery.
2. Follow directions from the radiology department, physician, or anesthetist for withholding food and fluids and for bowel preparation prior to surgery. Conscious sedation, general anesthesia, or spinal anesthesia may be required depending on the procedure. Fecal material in the bowel may impede fluoroscopic visualization of the kidney and stone.

Postoperative Nursing Interventions

Relieving Pain

- Administer opioid analgesics (IV or intramuscular) with IV NSAID as prescribed.
- Encourage and assist patient to assume a position of comfort.
- Assist patient to ambulate to obtain some pain relief.
- Monitor pain closely and report promptly increases in severity.

Monitoring and Managing Complications

- Encourage increased fluid intake and ambulation.
- Begin IV fluids if patient cannot take adequate oral fluids.
- Monitor total urine output and patterns of voiding.
- Encourage ambulation as a means of moving the stone through the urinary tract.
- Strain urine through gauze.
- Crush any blood clots passed in urine, and inspect sides of urinal and bedpan for clinging stones.
- Instruct patient to report decreased urine volume, bloody or cloudy urine, fever, and pain.
- Instruct patient to report any increase in pain.
- Monitor vital signs for early indications of infection; infections should be treated with the appropriate antibiotic agent before efforts are made to dissolve the stone.

Health Education

- Explain causes of kidney stones and ways to prevent recurrence.
- Encourage patient to follow a regimen to avoid further stone formation, including maintaining a high fluid intake.
- Encourage patient to drink enough to excrete 3,000 to 4,000 mL of urine every 24 hours.
- Recommend that patient have urine cultures every 1–2 months the first year and periodically thereafter.

- Recommend that recurrent urinary infection be treated vigorously.
- Encourage increased mobility whenever possible; discourage excessive ingestion of vitamins (especially vitamin D) and minerals.
- If patient had surgery, instruct about the signs and symptoms of complications that need to be reported to the physician; emphasize the importance of follow-up to assess kidney function and to ensure the eradication or removal of all kidney stones to the patient and family.
- Provide instructions for any necessary home care and follow-up.

SHORT ESSAYS

4. Explain the role of nurse in organ donation.

The nurse can be very helpful in supporting families through the organ and tissue request process, as the Albany ICU RNs have demonstrated. As the process begins, the first and most important thing the nurse can provide is a private area in which the family can discuss all the issues. There, the staff member designated to make the request, whether a formal transplant coordinator, a social worker, chaplain or nurse can offer the family clarification of what defines brain death since the support system must remain in place even after the client is pronounced dead, for vital organ retrieval (i.e., heart, lungs, kidneys, and liver).

The nurse's job is to reinforce explanations throughout the organ retrieval process. The family must know who legally can give final consent, what options there are for organ or tissue donation, and how donation will affect burial or cremation. Any nurse who could be working in this capacity should review their state's organ retrieval laws and institutional policies and procedures regarding the final consent process.

When a patient is awaiting an organ transplant, he is under intensive medical care. In many transplant centers, each patient has a nurse assigned to him who sees him regularly, follows up on lab work and acts as a liaison between the patient and the transplant physicians. A transplant nurse not only coordinates care and makes sure that the patients is getting all the treatments and testing he needs for the transplant, but also educates her patients about the transplant process and provides emotional support.

Procurement nurses: Procurement nurses work with the transplant team. They initiate contact with the family of the patient whose organs might be suitable for transplant—then coordinate the timing of the organ harvest from the donor with the transplant into the recipient. The procurement nurse also might assist with the surgical removal of organs from the donor and ensure that the organs are properly transported to maintain viability when they reach the recipients.

Surgical RNs: The transplant team consists of doctors and nurses specially trained in transplant, which involves two patients: The donor and the recipient. Separate surgical teams might handle the removal of the organs from the donor and the placement into the recipient, or the same team might perform both surgeries. The donor and the recipient are often not in the same hospital or even in the same state.

5. Describe the preoperative preparation of patient undergoing abdominal surgery.

Before Surgery

The client needs to have a preoperative physical exam by primary or referring physician within 7 days of the scheduled surgery. Patient will be given instructions for cleansing the colon (bowel).

Day of surgery: On the day of surgery, report to the admitting area to register. A nurse will take patient's vital signs (blood pressure, pulse and temperature) and will ask him/her a list of questions to ensure that he/she is ready for surgery. If the doctor or anesthesiologist requires a chest X-ray or EKG and these were not done as a part of patient preoperative examination, patient's may have them done at the hospital. However, this may delay patient surgery. Blood will be drawn and sent back to the laboratory for current test results. Patient may also be asked to give a urine specimen. His/her family will be directed to the surgical waiting room and he/she will go to a preop room. The anesthesiologist will talk with him/her about options for anesthesia and pain control. An intravenous (IV) line will be started to prevent him/her from becoming dehydrated. It will remain in place for several days after his/her surgery until he/she are able to take liquids by mouth. Before surgery, he/she may be given antibiotics through the IV to decrease the risks of infection after surgery. He/she will receive medication to relax.

In the operating room: Once patient's asleep, a catheter may be placed in his/her bladder to collect and record urine output. A nasogastric (NG) tube may be passed through his/her nose, down the throat and into the stomach. This tube removes secretions from the stomach that may cause postoperative nausea and vomiting. In most cases, the tube is removed before patient wake up. The length of surgery varies from patient to patient and is determined by the general health of the patient and how complicated the surgery is.

6. Explain the current CPR guidelines.

1. CPR begins with compressions delivered hard and fast in the middle of the victim's chest. The rescuer should place the heel of one hand on the center of the victim's chest and the other hand right on top of the first with fingers intertwined.
2. Each compression should be at least 2" deep and delivered at a rate of at least 100/minute. After giving 30 compressions a rescuer who is able to breathe for the victim should do so. If a rescuer is unable to breathe for the victim they should provide continuous high quality compressions until professional rescuers arrive.
3. Breaths for the victim start by adjusting their airway. Tilt the victim's head by the forehead back and lifting the chin to open the airway. Pinch shut the victim's nose using the forefinger and thumb.
4. Each breath given to the victim should be a normal breath for the rescuer and delivered over 1 second while looking for the victims chest to rise.
5. A total of two breaths should be given to the patient and then the rescuer should immediately start chest compressions again.
6. The cycle of 30 compressions and 2 breaths should be continued until the rescuer is physically unable to do so or professional rescuers arrive.
7. As soon as an automated external defibrillator (AED) becomes available it should be turned on and its instructions followed to connect it to the patient. An AED will only work on someone who will benefit from it and will not harm someone who will not benefit from it.

7. Describe the nursing responsibilities during thrombolytic therapy.

Preinfusion Care
- Obtain nursing history, and perform a physical assessment. Information obtained from the history and physical exam helps determine whether thrombolytic therapy is appropriate. The goal is to initiate thrombolytic therapy within 30 minutes of arrival

- Evaluate for contraindications to thrombolytic therapy: Recent surgery or trauma (including prolonged CPR), bleeding disorders or active bleeding, cerebral vascular accident, neurosurgery within the last 2 months, gastrointestinal ulcers, diabetic hemorrhagic retinopathy, and uncontrolled hypertension. Thrombolytic agents dissolve clots and therefore, may precipitate intracranial, internal, or peripheral bleeding
- Inform the client of the purpose of the therapy. Discuss the risk of bleeding and the need to keep the extremity immobile during and after the infusion. Minimal movement of the extremity is necessary to prevent bleeding from the infusion site.

During the Infusion

- Assess and record vital signs and the infusion site for hematoma or bleeding every 15 minutes for the first hour, every 30 minutes for the next 2 hours, and then hourly until the intravenous catheter is discontinued. Assess pulses, color, sensation, and temperature of both extremities with each vital sign check. Vital signs and the site are frequently assessed to detect possible complications
- Remind the client to keep the extremity still and straight. Do not elevate head of bed above 15°. Extremity immobilization helps prevent infusion site trauma and bleeding. Hypotension may develop, keeping the bed flat helps maintain cerebral perfusion
- Maintain continuous cardiac monitoring during the infusion. Keep antidysrhythmic drugs and the emergency cart readily available for treatment of significant dysrhythmias. Ventricular dysrhythmias commonly occur with reperfusion of the ischemic myocardium.

Postinfusion Care

- Assess vital signs, distal pulses, and infusion site frequently as needed. The client remains at high-risk for bleeding following thrombolytic therapy
- Evaluate response to therapy: Normalization of ST segment, relief of chest pain, reperfusion dysrhythmias, early peaking of the CK and CK-MB band. These are signs that the clot has been dissolved and the myocardium is being reperfused
- Maintain bed rest for 6 hours. Keep the head of the bed at or below 15°. Reinforce the need to keep the extremity straight and immobile. Avoid any injections for 24 hours after catheter removal. Precautions, such as these are important to prevent bleeding
- Assess puncture sites for bleeding. On catheter removal hold direct pressure over the site for at least 30 minutes. Apply a pressure dressing to any venous or arterial sites as needed. Perform routine care in a gentle manner to avoid bruising or injury. Thrombolytic therapy disrupts normal coagulation. Peripheral bleeding may occur at puncture sites, and there may not be sufficient fibrin to form a clot. Direct or indirect pressure may be needed to control the bleeding
- Assess body fluids including urine, vomitus, and feces, for evidence of bleeding; frequently assess for changes in level of consciousness and manifestations of increased intracranial pressure, which may indicate intracranial bleeding. Assess surgical sites for bleeding. Monitor hemoglobin and hematocrit levels, prothrombin time (PT), and partial thromboplastin time (PTT). These provide additional means of assessing for bleeding
- Administer platelet-modifying drugs (e.g. aspirin, dipyridamole) as ordered. Platelet inhibitors decrease platelet aggregation and adhesion and are used to prevent reocclusion of the artery
- Report manifestations of reocclusion including changes in the ST segment, chest pain, or dysrhythmias.

8. Explain pathophysiology of diabetes mellitus.

Type-2 diabetes is caused by either inadequate production of the hormone insulin or a lack of response to insulin by various cells of the body.

Normal regulation of blood sugar: Glucose is an important source of energy in the body. It is mainly obtained from carbohydrates in the diet which are broken down into glucose for the various cells of the body to utilize. The liver is also able to manufacture glucose from its glycogen stores. In a healthy person, a rise in blood sugar after a meal triggers the pancreatic beta cells to release the hormone insulin. Insulin, in turn, stimulates cells to take up the glucose from the blood. When blood glucose levels fall, during exercise, for example, as well as insulin stimulating the uptake of glucose from the blood by body cells, it also induces the:
1. Stimulates the conversion of glucose to pyruvate (glycolysis) to release free energy.
2. Conversion of excess glucose to glycogen for storage in the liver (glycogenesis).
3. Uptake and synthesis of amino acids, proteins, and fat.

Pathophysiology: In type-2 diabetes, the body either produces inadequate amounts of insulin to meet the demands of the body or insulin resistance has developed. Insulin resistance refers to when cells of the body, such as the muscle, liver and fat cells fail to respond to insulin, even when levels are high. In fat cells, triglycerides are instead broken down to produce free fatty acids for energy; muscle cells are deprived of an energy source and liver cells fail to build up glycogen stores. This also leads to an overall rise in the level of glucose in the blood. Glycogen stores become markedly reduced and there is less glucose available for release when it may be needed. Obesity and lack of physical activity are thought to be major causes of insulin resistance.

9. Explain the causes and management of psoriasis.

Psoriasis is a chronic, noninfectious, inflammatory disease of the skin in which the production of epidermal cells occur faster than normal. Onset may occur at any age but is most common between the ages of 15 and 35 years. Main sites of the body affected are the scalp, areas over the elbows and knees, lower part of the back, and genitalia, as well as the nails. Bilateral symmetry often exists. Psoriasis may be associated with asymmetric rheumatoid factor–negative arthritis of multiple joints. An exfoliative psoriatic state may develop in which the disease progresses to involve the total body surface (erythrodermic psoriatic state).

Pathophysiology: The basal skin cells divide too quickly, and the newly formed cells become evident as profuse scales or plaques of epidermal tissue. As a result of the increased number of basal cells and rapid cell passage, the normal events of cell maturation and growth cannot occur, which prevents the normal protective layers of the skin to form. Current evidence supports an immunologic basis for psoriasis. The primary defect is unknown. Periods of emotional stress and anxiety aggravate the condition, and trauma, infections, and seasonal and hormonal changes also are trigger factors.

Medical management: Goals of management are to slow the rapid turnover of epidermis, to promote resolution of the psoriatic lesions, and to control the natural cycles of the disease. There is no known cure. The therapeutic approach should be understandable, cosmetically acceptable, and not too disruptive of lifestyle. First, any precipitating or aggravating factors are addressed. An assessment is made of lifestyle, because psoriasis is significantly affected by stress. The most important principle of psoriasis treatment is gentle removal of scales (bath oils, coal tar preparations, and a soft brush used to scrub the psoriatic plaques). After bathing, the application of emollient creams containing alpha-hydroxy acids (Lac-Hydrin, Penederm) or salicylic acid will continue to soften thick scales. Three types of therapy are standard: Topical, systemic, and phototherapy.

10. Enumerate on biomedical waste management followed in medical ward.

Biomedical waste management has recently emerged as an issue of major concern not only to hospitals, nursing home authorities but also to the environment. The biomedical wastes generated from healthcare units depend upon a number of factors, such as waste management methods, type of healthcare units, occupancy of healthcare units, specialization of healthcare units, ratio of reusable items in use, availability of infrastructure and resources, etc. The proper management of biomedical waste has become a worldwide humanitarian topic today. Although hazards of poor management of biomedical waste have aroused the concern world over, especially in the light of its far-reaching effects on human, health and the environment.

Definition: According to Biomedical Waste (Management and Handling) Rules, 1998 of India "Any waste which is generated during the diagnosis, treatment or immunization of human beings or animals or in research activities pertaining thereto or in the production or testing of biologicals."

Need of biomedical waste management in hospitals
The reasons due to which there is great need of management of hospitals waste are as follows:
1. Injuries from sharps leading to infection to all categories of hospital personnel and waste handler.
2. Nosocomial infections in patients from poor infection control practices and poor waste management.
3. Risk of infection outside hospital for waste handlers and scavengers and at time general public living in the vicinity of hospitals.
4. Risk associated with hazardous chemicals, drugs to persons handling wastes at all levels.
5. "Disposable" being repacked and sold by unscrupulous elements without even being washed.
6. Drugs which have been disposed of, being repacked and sold off to unsuspecting buyers.
7. Risk of air, water and soil pollution directly due to waste, or due to defective incineration emissions and ash.

Biomedical waste treatment and disposal: Healthcare waste is a heterogeneous mixture, which is very difficult to manage as such. But the problem can be simplified and its dimension reduced considerably if a proper management system is planned.

Incineration technology: This is a high-temperature thermal process employing combustion of the waste under controlled condition for converting them into inert material and gases. Incinerators can be oil fired or electrically powered or a combination thereof. Broadly, three types of incinerators are used for hospital waste: Multiple hearth type, rotary kiln and controlled air types. All the types can have primary and secondary combustion chambers to ensure optimal combustion. These are refractory lined.

Nonincineration technology: Nonincineration treatment includes four basic processes: Thermal, chemical, irradiative, and biological. The majority of nonincineration technologies employ the thermal and chemical processes. The main purpose of the treatment technology is to decontaminate waste by destroying pathogens. Facilities should make certain that the technology could meet state criteria for disinfection.

Autoclaving
1. The autoclave operates on the principle of the standard pressure cooker.
2. The process involves using steam at high temperatures.
3. The steam generated at high temperature penetrates waste material and kills all the micro-organism.
4. These are also of three types: Gravity type, prevacuum type and retort type.

Microwave Irradiation
1. The microwave is based on the principle of generation of high-frequency waves.
2. These waves cause the particles within the waste material to vibrate, generating heat.
3. This heat generated from within kills all pathogens.

Chemical method: 1% hypochlorite solution can be used for chemical disinfection.

Plasma pyrolysis: Plasma pyrolysis is a state-of-the-art technology for safe disposal of medical waste. It is an environment-friendly technology which converts organic waste into commercially useful byproducts. The intense heat generated by the plasma enables it to dispose all types of waste including municipal solid waste, biomedical waste and hazardous waste in a safe and reliable manner. Medical waste is pyrolyzed into CO, H_2, and hydrocarbons when it comes in contact with the plasma-arc. These gases are burned and produce a high temperature (around 1,200°C).

11. Explain the current schedule of short course chemotherapy for tuberculosis.

Tuberculosis (TB), an infectious disease primarily affecting the lung parenchyma, is most often caused by *Mycobacterium tuberculosis*. It may spread to almost any part of the body including the meninges, kidney, bones, and lymph nodes. The initial infection usually occurs 2–10 weeks after exposure. The patient may then develop active disease because of a compromised or inadequate immune system response. The active process may be prolonged and characterized by long remissions when the disease is arrested, only to be followed by periods of renewed activity. TB is a worldwide public health problem that is closely associated with poverty, malnutrition, overcrowding, substandard housing, and inadequate health care. Mortality and morbidity rates continue to rise.

Medical management: Pulmonary TB is treated primarily with antituberculosis agents for 6–12 months. A prolonged treatment duration is necessary to ensure eradication of the organisms and to prevent relapse.

Pharmacologic therapy:
- First-line medications: Isoniazid or INH (Nydrazid), rifampin (Rifadin), pyrazinamide, and ethambutol (Myambutol) daily for 8 weeks and continuing for up to 4–7 months
- Second-line medications: Capreomycin (Capastat), ethionamide (Trecator), para-aminosalicylate sodium, and cycloserine (Seromycin)
- Vitamin B (pyridoxine) usually administered with INH.

12. Explain about prevention of transmission of HIV infection among adults.

India has the third largest HIV epidemic in the world. In 2013, HIV prevalence in India was an estimated 0.3%. This figure is small compared to most other middle-income countries but because of India's huge population (1.2 billion) this equates to 2.1 million people living with HIV. In the same year, an estimated 1,30,000 people died from AIDS-related illnesses. Overall, India's HIV epidemic is slowing down, with a 19% decline in new HIV infections (1,30,000 in

2013), and a 38% decline in AIDS-related deaths between 2005 and 2013. Despite this, 51% of deaths in Asia are in India. HIV prevalence in India varies geographically. The five states with the highest HIV prevalence (Nagaland, Mizoram, Manipur, Andhra Pradesh and Karnataka) are in the south or east of the country. Some states in the north and northeast of the country, report rising HIV prevalence.

Effective strategies to prevent sexual transmission of HIV are easy to define but difficult to implement. Abstinence and well-defined safe-sex practices, particularly condom use, could reduce the HIV epidemic if they are widely used. The challenge is to implement strategies that are practical and realistic. Although efforts to improve safe-sex practices deserve to remain a cornerstone of infection control, other initiatives are appropriate to fill gaps anticipated by the difficulties in ensuring universal compliance with safe-sex practices and the limitations in dictating human behavior.

Safe sex is defined by practices that limit contact between bodily fluids of sexual partners, particularly blood and semen. When used consistently, male condoms, commonly used barriers to reduce the exchange of fluids, offer a degree of protection comparable to their ability to prevent pregnancy. Variability in correct use relative to consistent use may explain the wide CIs in the estimated rates of protection afforded by this practice. Although all individuals at risk should be encouraged to use condoms to reduce the risk of HIV infection, it should also be emphasized that correct use has not been demonstrated to provide complete protection from HIV and that a substantial proportion of persons who consistently use condoms during sex do not use condoms correctly.

Antiretroviral therapy has been associated with reductions in infectivity. These reductions are likely a product of the suppression of HIV RNA in the genital tract. In observational studies of HIV-serodiscordant couples, the rate of seroconversion among couples receiving antiviral therapy was 80% less than the rate among couples who received counseling on safe sex but no antiretroviral therapy. One important limitation of antiretroviral therapy as an infection-control strategy is that the peak period of infectivity occurs during the acute stage of infection which typically precedes treatment. However, prophylaxis for patients at risk for infection, treatment during acute infection, and postexposure prophylaxis are all potential strategies to circumvent this limitation.

SHORT ANSWERS

13. Write about any two specific noninvasive diagnostic procedures done in cardiac diseases.

Cardiac testing is used to help stratify patients thought to be at risk for symptomatic coronary artery disease (CAD), specifically for short-term complications, such as myocardial infarction (MI) or sudden cardiac death.

Electrocardiogram (ECG): An ECG records these electrical signals and can help your doctor detect irregularities in your heart's rhythm and structure. You may have an ECG while you are at rest or while exercising (stress electrocardiogram).

Holter monitoring: A Holter monitor is a portable device you wear to record a continuous ECG, usually for 24–72 hours. Holter monitoring is used to detect heart rhythm irregularities that are not found during a regular ECG exam.

Echocardiogram: This noninvasive test which includes an ultrasound of your chest shows detailed images of your heart's structure and function.

Cardiac computerized tomography (CT) scans: This test is often used to check for heart problems. In a cardiac CT scan, you lie on a table inside a doughnut-shaped machine. An X-ray tube inside the machine rotates around your body and collects images of your heart and chest.

Cardiac magnetic resonance imaging: For this test, you lie on a table inside a long tube-like machine that produces a magnetic field. The magnetic field produces pictures to help your doctor evaluate your heart.

14. Indicate two reasons to follow rotation of site for insulin administration.

Injecting in the same place much of the time can **cause** hard lumps or extra fat deposits to develop. These lumps are not only unsightly; they can also change the way **insulin** is absorbed, making it more difficult to keep your blood glucose on target.

Rotate within an injection site: To avoid developing hard lumps and fat deposits, it is important to inject in different spots within a general part of the body.
1. Change sides within an area. For example, if you inject your evening insulin in the thigh, try using the right thigh one evening, and the left thigh the next evening.
2. You might find it useful to picture the face of a clock on your abdomen. That helps you to keep each of your injections at least one finger's width from the last injection.
3. Lets say that you inject four times a day, and all of the injections are in your abdomen. Look down at your abdomen and picture "Noon" below your belly button. Place your first injection at Noon, your second injection at 1 o'clock, the third injection at 2 o'clock, and the fourth injection at 3 o'clock. You will not come back to the "Noon" spot again until day 4, which gives that spot a chance to rest.

15. Name two opportunistic infections among AIDS patients.

Pneumocystis infections are some of the most serious opportunistic infections (OIs) for people with HIV. According to AIDS.gov, pneumocystis pneumonia (PCP) is a leading cause of death among HIV patients. The good news is that the **infection** can be treated with antibiotics. When someone living with HIV has a weakened immune system (shown by a low CD4 count), they are at risk of other illnesses. These are known as 'opportunistic infections' because they take the opportunity of the immune system being weak.

Opportunistic infections include:
1. Cryptococcal meningitis.
2. Toxoplasmosis.
3. PCP, a type of pneumonia.
4. Esophageal candidiasis.
5. Certain cancers, including Kaposi's sarcoma.

16. Classify hemophilia.

Hemophilia is a blood clotting disorder that arises with a mutation or deletion of the gene that controls blood clotting. It is the most common congenital blood clotting disorder. There are two common types of hemophilia—A and B. Hemophilia A is the more common type and is due to a deficiency of Factor VIII while hemophilia B is due to a deficiency of Factor IX. A rare type of hemophilia involves Factor XI and is known as hemophilia C. These clotting factors are necessary in the series of steps known as the coagulation cascade, that eventually leads to the formation of a blood clot. When this process is disrupted the body cannot adequately prevent blood loss.

Classification of hemophilia: Hemophilia may be classified as severe, moderate or mild. This is based on the levels of Factor VIII or Factor IX depending on the type of hemophilia. The clinical presentation is also an indication of the severity of hemophilia.

Severe hemophilia:
1. Clotting factor levels less than 1% (<0.01 IU/mL)
2. Spontaneous bleeding: Hemarthroses (joint bleeding) and muscle hematomas.

Moderate hemophilia:
1. Clotting factor levels between 1 and 5% (0.01–0.05 IU/mL)
2. Bleeding with mild trauma or minor surgery.

Mild hemophilia:
1. Clotting factor levels between 5 and 40% (0.05–0.4 IU/mL)
2. Excessive bleeding with severe trauma or major surgery.

17. List two suture materials and its uses.

Sutures are classified as absorbable or nonabsorbable, natural or synthetic, and braided or monofilament. Numerous companies manufacture sutures; however, Ethicon, Syneture (United States Surgical/Davis and Geck suture division of Tyco Healthcare), and Look (Surgical Specialties Corporation) manufacture most of the sutures used in wound closure. Most sutures are available in standard 18 and 27-inch lengths. Several manufacturers (e.g. Delasco, Look) provide sutures in 8, 9, and 10 inch lengths. These shorter sutures are less expensive and are used primarily for biopsy wounds or small wound closures.

Surgical gut or catgut was the first absorbable suture material available. Despite its name, catgut has never been made from cat intestines. It is actually made by twisted fiber formed from the collagen of the intestines of sheep, cattle, or goats. Surgical gut is packaged in alcohol to prevent it from drying and breaking. The three forms available are plain, chromic, and fast-absorbing (Ethicon). Plain gut elicits a marked inflammatory reaction in tissue and maintain its tensile strength for only 7–10 days after implantation. Generally, it is completely absorbed by 70 days; however, loss of strength and absorption vary greatly.

Chromic gut is plain gut treated with chromium salts to slow absorption and decrease tissue reactivity by cross-linking the collagen. Its tensile strength is maintained for as long as 10–21 days and complete absorption does not occur until at least day 90. Plain and chromic gut have decreased use in modern surgery owing to the development of synthetic sutures that are hydrolyzed and therefore less inflammatory. This material is used in the closure of mucosal surfaces or as ligatures for blood vessels, among other uses.

Fast-absorbing gut is plain gut treated with heat to facilitate more rapid absorption. It was designed for percutaneous suturing and maintain its tensile strength for only 5–7 days. It is completely absorbed within 2–4 weeks. Fast-absorbing gut is useful for the percutaneous closure of facial wounds under low tension and for securing both split and full-thickness skin grafts.

18. List four major duties of scrub nurse.

The scrub nurse performs a vital role in an operating room (OR). The room is prepared with sterile drapes, sterile instruments, sterile fluids, multiple monitoring machines, and other supplies. The doctors and nurses in the room scrub their hands, making sure they are as clean as possible.

Scrub nurses, also called perioperative nurses, are registered nurses who assist in surgical procedures by setting up the room before the operation, working with the doctor during surgery and preparing the patient for the move to the recovery room. The website Nurses for a Healthier Tomorrow notes that scrub nurses work in various clinical settings, including hospital surgical departments, private physicians' offices, clinics and ambulatory (also called "day surgery") centers.

Before surgery: The scrub nurse's duties begin far before the start of the operation. He ensures the operating room is clean and ready to be set up, then prepares the instruments and equipment needed for the surgery. He counts all sponges, instruments, needles and other tools and preserves the sterile environment by "scrubbing in," which requires washing his hands with special soaps and putting on sterile garments, including a gown, gloves and face mask. When the surgeon arrives, the nurse helps her with her gown and gloves before preparing the patient for surgery.

During surgery: During the operation, one of the scrub nurse's primary duties is selecting and passing instruments to the surgeon. University of Colorado Health describes the scrub nurse's role as supporting the surgeon "while also maintaining patient safety." The nurse must know which instruments are used for specific procedures and when they are needed, so she can quickly hand them to the surgeon. The scrub nurse must also watch for hand signals to know when the surgeon is ready for the next tool or when he is done using a tool and is ready to hand it back to the scrub nurse, who cleans the tools after use and places each tool back in its place on the table. She also monitors the surgery to ensure everything remains sterile.

After surgery: After the operation, the scrub nurse again counts all instruments, sponges and other tools and informs the surgeon of the count. He removes tools and equipment from the operating area, helps apply dressing to the surgical site and transports the patient to the recovery area. He also completes any necessary documentation regarding the surgery or the patient's transfer to recovery.

Working conditions and challenges: Because scrub nurses are so vital to surgical procedures, they may work long hours, even for a single operation, and may be called in at all hours to assist in emergency operations. They must have a thorough knowledge of operating room procedures, including the tools needed for specific surgeries, and must be able to stay calm and clearheaded even under pressure. They must also have excellent communication skills, because one of their primary duties is working with the surgeon and assisting her with anything she needs during the operation.

19. Specify the incubation period for poliomyelitis.

Polio is usually spread via the fecal-oral route (i.e. the virus is transmitted from the stool of an infected person to the mouth of another person from contaminated hands or such objects as eating utensils). Some cases may be spread directly via an oral to oral route.

For the onset of paralysis in paralytic poliomyelitis, the incubation period usually is 7–21 days. The response to poliovirus infection is highly variable and has been categorized on the basis of the severity of clinical presentation.

Surprisingly, 95% of all individuals infected with polio have no apparent symptoms. Another 4–8% of infected individuals have symptoms of a minor, non-specific nature, such as sore throat and fever, nausea, vomiting, and other common symptoms of any viral illness. About 1–2% of infected individuals develop nonparalytic aseptic (viral) meningitis, with temporary stiffness of the neck, back, and/or legs. Less than 1% of all polio infections result in the classic "flaccid paralysis," where the patient is left with permanent weakness or paralysis of legs, arms, or both.

20. Write two important clinical manifestations of left ventricular failure.

Left-sided heart failure is a life-threatening condition in which the left side of the heart cannot pump enough blood to the body.

Symptoms
1. Cough (produces frothy or blood-tinged mucus)
2. Decreased urine production
3. Difficulty lying down; need to sleep with the head elevated to avoid shortness of breath
4. Fatigue, weakness, faintness
5. Irregular or rapid pulse
6. Sensation of feeling the heartbeat (palpitations)
7. Shortness of breath
8. Waking up due to shortness of breath (paroxysmal nocturnal dyspnea)
9. Weight gain from fluid retention.

Symptoms in infants may include:
1. Failure to thrive
2. Poor feeding
3. Weight loss.

21. What is DASH diet?

DASH stands for dietary approaches to stop hypertension. The DASH diet is a lifelong approach to healthy eating that is designed to help treat or prevent high blood pressure (hypertension). The DASH diet encourages you to reduce the sodium in your diet and eat a variety of foods rich in nutrients that help lower blood pressure, such as potassium, calcium and magnesium. By following the DASH diet, you may be able to reduce your blood pressure by a few points in just two weeks. Over time, your systolic blood pressure could drop by 8–14 points, which can make a significant difference in your health risks. Because the DASH diet is a healthy way of eating, it offers health benefits besides just lowering blood pressure. The DASH diet is also in line with dietary recommendations to prevent osteoporosis, cancer, heart disease, stroke and diabetes.

22. List two complications of tracheostomy.

As with any surgery, there are some risks associated with tracheostomies. However, serious infections are rare. **Early complications** that may arise during the tracheostomy procedure or soon thereafter include:
1. Bleeding
2. Air trapped around the lungs (pneumothorax)
3. Air trapped in the deeper layers of the chest (pneumomediastinum)
4. Air trapped underneath the skin around the tracheostomy (subcutaneous emphysema)
5. Damage to the swallowing tube (esophagus)
6. Injury to the nerve that moves the vocal cords (recurrent laryngeal nerve)
7. Tracheostomy tube can be blocked by blood clots, mucus or pressure of the airway walls. Blockages can be prevented by suctioning, humidifying the air, and selecting the appropriate tracheostomy tube.

Many of these early complications can be avoided or dealt with appropriately with our experienced surgeons in a hospital setting.

Over time, other complications may arise from the surgery:

Later complications that may occur while the tracheostomy tube is in place include:
1. Accidental removal of the tracheostomy tube (accidental decannulation).
2. Infection in the trachea and around the tracheostomy tube.
3. Windpipe itself may become damaged for a number of reasons, including pressure from the tube; bacteria that cause infections and form scar tissue; or friction from a tube that moves too much.

These complications can usually be prevented or quickly dealt with if the caregiver has proper knowledge of how to care for the tracheostomy site.

Delayed complications that may result after longer-term presence of a tracheostomy include:
1. Thinning (erosion) of the trachea from the tube rubbing against it (tracheomalacia).
2. Development of a small connection from the trachea (windpipe) to the esophagus (swallowing tube) which is called a tracheoesophageal fistula.
3. Development of bumps (granulation tissue) that may need to be surgically removed before decannulation (removal of trach tube) can occur.
4. Narrowing or collapse of the airway above the site of the tracheostomy, possibly requiring an additional surgical procedure to repair it.
5. Once the tracheostomy tube is removed, the opening may not close on its own. Tubes remaining in place for 16 weeks or longer are more at risk for needing surgical closure.

2015

Medical-Surgical Nursing-I

LONG ESSAYS

1. Define osteomyelitis. Discuss the pathophysiology of osteomyelitis. Explain the treatment modalities.
2. Mrs Laxmi, a 55-year-old woman is admitted to the hospital with the diagnosis of diabetes mellitus: Define diabetes mellitus. List the complications of diabetes mellitus. Explain the nursing management of a patient with diabetes mellitus.
3. Differentiate between gastric and duodental ulcer. Discuss the medical, surgical and nursing management of a patient with peptic ulcer.

SHORT ESSAYS

4. Surgical approaches of Benign prostate hypertrophy.
5. Process of inflammation.
6. Nursing care of unconscious patient.
7. Lung abscess.
8. Colostomy care.
9. Antihypertensive drugs.
10. Cardiopulmonary resuscitation.
11. Nephrotic syndrome.
12. Psoriasis.

SHORT ANSWERS

13. Pleural effusion.
14. Types of anemia.
15. Complications of AIDS.
16. Raynaud's disease.
17. Etiology of renal calculi.
18. Defibrillation.
19. Portal hypertension.
20. Antitubercular drugs.
21. Urinary incontinence.
22. Types of anesthesia and methods of administration.

LONG ESSAYS

1. Define osteomyelitis. Discuss the pathophysiology of osteomyelitis. Explain the treatment modalities.

Osteomyelitis is an infection of the bone. It may occur by extension of soft tissue infections, direct bone contamination (egg, bone surgery, gunshot wound), or hematogenous (blood-borne spread from other foci of infection. *Staphylococcus aureus* causes more than 50% of bone infections. Other pathogenic organisms frequently found include gram-positive organisms that include streptococci and enterococci, followed by gram-negative bacteria that include *Pseudomonas* species. Patients at risk include poorly nourished, elderly, and patients who are obese; those with impaired immune systems and chronic illness (e.g. diabetes); and those on long-term corticosteroid therapy or immunosuppressive agents. The condition may be prevented by prompt treatment and management of focal and soft tissue infections.

Clinical Manifestations
- When the infection is blood-borne, onset is sudden, occurring with clinical manifestations of sepsis (e.g. chills, high fever, rapid pulse, and general malaise).
- Extremity becomes painful, swollen, warm, and tender.
- Patient may describe a constant pulsating pain that intensifies with movement (due to the pressure of collecting pus).
- When osteomyelitis is caused by adjacent infection or direct contamination, there are no symptoms of sepsis; the area is swollen, warm, painful, and tender to touch.
- Chronic osteomyelitis presents with a nonhealing ulcer that overlies the infected bone with a connecting sinus that will intermittently and spontaneously drain pus.

Assessment and Diagnostic Findings
- Acute osteomyelitis: Early X-ray films show only soft tissue swelling.
- Chronic osteomyelitis: X-ray shows large, irregular cavities, a raised periosteum, sequestra, or dense bone formations.
- Radioisotope bone scans and magnetic resonance imaging (MRI).
- Blood studies and blood cultures.

Medical Management
Initial goal is to control and arrest the infective process.
- General supportive measures (e.g. hydration, diet high in vitamins and protein, correction of anemia) should be instituted; affected area is immobilized.
- Blood and wound cultures are performed to identify organisms and select the antibiotic.
- Intravenous antibiotic therapy is given around-the-clock; continues for 3–6 weeks.
- Antibiotic medication is administered orally (on empty stomach) when infection appears to be controlled; the medication regimen is continued for up to 3 months.
- Surgical debridement of bone is performed with irrigation; adjunctive antibiotic therapy is maintained.

Nursing Diagnoses
- Acute pain related to inflammation and swelling.
- Impaired physical mobility associated with pain, immobilization devices, and weight-bearing limitations.
- Risk for extension of infection: Bone abscess formation.
- Deficient knowledge about treatment regimen.

Planning and goals: Major goals may include relief of pain, improved physical mobility within therapeutic limitations, control and eradication of infection, and knowledge of the treatment regimen.

Nursing Interventions

Relieving Pain

- Immobilize affected part with splint to decrease pain and muscle spasm.
- Monitor neurovascular status of affected extremity.
- Handle affected part with great care to avoid pain.
- Elevate affected part to reduce swelling and discomfort.
- Administer prescribed analgesic agents and use other techniques to reduce pain.

Improving Physical Mobility

- Teach the rationale for activity restrictions (bone is weakened by the infective process).
- Gently move the joints above and below the affected part through their range of motion.
- Encourage activities of daily living within physical limitations.

Controlling Infectious Process

- Monitor response to antibiotic therapy. Observe intravenous sites for evidence of phlebitis or infiltration.
- Monitor for signs of superinfection with long-term, intensive antibiotic therapy (e.g. oral or vaginal candidiasis; loose or foul-smelling stools).
- If surgery was necessary, ensure adequate circulation (wound suction, elevation of area, avoidance of pressure on grafted area); maintain immobility as needed; comply with weight-bearing restrictions. Change dressings using aseptic technique to promote healing and prevent cross contamination.
- Monitor general health and nutrition of patient.
- Provide a balanced diet high in protein to ensure positive nitrogen balance and promote healing; encourage adequate hydration.

2. Mrs Laxmi, a 55-year-old woman is admitted to the hospital with the diagnosis of diabetes mellitus: Define diabetes mellitus. List the complications of diabetes mellitus. Explain the nursing management of a patient with diabetes mellitus.

Diabetes mellitus is a group of metabolic disorders characterized by elevated levels of blood glucose (hyperglycemia) resulting from defects in insulin production and secretion, decreased cellular response to insulin, or both. Hyperglycemia may lead to acute metabolic complications, such as diabetic ketoacidosis (DKA), and hyperglycemic hyperosmolar nonketotic syndrome (HHNS). Long-term hyperglycemia may contribute to chronic microvascular complications (kidney and eye disease) and neuropathic complications. Diabetes is also associated with an increased occurrence of macrovascular diseases, including coronary artery disease (myocardial infarction), cerebrovascular disease (stroke), and peripheral vascular disease.

Complications of Diabetes

Complications associated with both types of diabetes are classified as acute or chronic. Acute complications occur from short-term imbalances in blood glucose and include:
- Hypoglycemia

- Diabetic ketoacidosis
- Hyperglycemic hyperosmolar nonketotic syndrome.

Chronic complications generally occur 10–15 years after the onset of diabetes mellitus. They complications include:
1. **Macrovascular (large vessel) disease** affects coronary, peripheral vascular, and cerebral vascular circulations
2. **Microvascular (small vessel) disease** affects the eyes (retinopathy) and kidneys (nephropathy); control blood glucose levels to delay or avoid onset of both microvascular and macrovascular complications.
3. **Neuropathic disease** affects sensory motor and autonomic nerves and contributes to such problems as impotence and foot ulcers.

Collaborative Problems/Potential Complications
1. Fluid overload, pulmonary edema, congestive heart failure.
2. Hypokalemia.
3. **Hyperglycemia and DKA:** It monitor blood glucose levels and urine ketones; administer medications (insulin, oral hypoglycemic agents); monitor for signs and symptoms of impending hyperglycemia and DKA, administering insulin and intravenous fluids to correct.
4. **Hypoglycemia:** It treat with juice or glucose tablets; encourage patient to eat full meals or snacks as prescribed; review signs and symptoms, possible causes, and measures to prevent or treat.
5. **Cerebral edema:** It prevent by gradual reduction in blood glucose level; monitor blood glucose level, serum electrolyte levels, urine output, mental status, and neurological signs; minimize activities that increase intracranial pressure.

Diabetes and Foot Complications

Diabetes can lead to many different types of foot complications, including athlete's foot (a fungal infection), calluses, bunions and other foot deformities, or ulcers that can range from a surface wound to a deep infection.

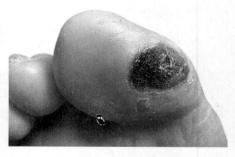

Poor circulation: Longstanding high blood sugar can damage blood vessels, decreasing blood flow to the foot. This poor circulation can weaken the skin, contribute to the formation of ulcers, and impair wound healing. Some bacteria and fungi thrive on high levels of sugar in the bloodstream, and bacterial and fungal infections can break down the skin and complicate ulcers.

More serious complications include deep skin and bone infections. Gangrene (death and decay of tissue) is a very serious complication that may include infection; widespread gangrene may require foot amputation. Approximately, 5% of men and women with diabetes eventually require amputation of a toe or foot. This tragic consequence can be prevented in most patients by managing blood sugar levels and daily foot care.

Nerve damage (neuropathy): Elevated blood glucose levels over time can damage the nerves of the foot, decreasing a person's ability to notice pain and pressure. Without these sensations, it is easy to develop callused pressure spots and accidentally injure the skin, soft tissue, bones, and joints. Over time, bone and joint damage can dramatically alter the shape of the foot. Nerve damage, also called neuropathy, can also weaken certain foot muscles, further contributing to foot deformities.

Preventing Foot Problems in Diabetes

Controlling blood sugar levels can reduce the blood vessel and nerve damage that often lead to diabetic foot complications. If a foot wound or ulcer does occur, blood sugar control reduces the risk of requiring amputation. Foot care is important, although patients should also continue to follow other general guidelines for managing diabetes.

The following strategies can reduce the chances of developing foot problems.

Quit smoking: Smoking can worsen heart and vascular problems and reduce circulation to the feet.

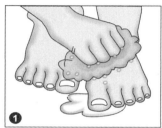
❶ Wash your feet daily with lukewarm water and soap, just as you wash your hands

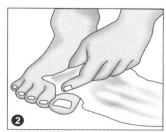
❷ Dry your feet well, also between the toes

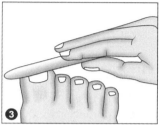
❸ Use emery board to shape to nails even with ends of your toes

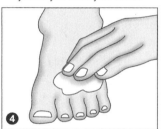
❹ Keep the skin supple with a moisturing lotion, but do not apply it between the toes

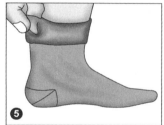
❺ Change daily into clean, soft socks or stockings which must neither too big nor too small

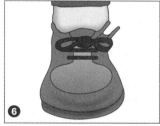
❻ Keep your feet warm and dry. Preferably wear special padded socks and shoes of leather

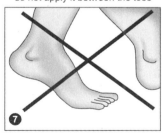
❼ Never walk barefoot. Neither indoors nor outdoors

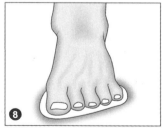
❽ Always wear shoes that fit. This applies also to sandals

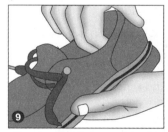
❾ Examine your shoes everyday for cracks, pebbles, nails and other irregularities which may irritate the skin

Avoid activities that can injure the feet: Some activities increase the risk of foot injury and are not recommended including walking barefoot, using a heating pad or hot water bottle on the feet, and stepping into the bathtub before testing the temperature.

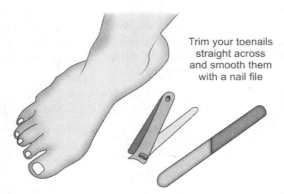

Trim your toenails straight across and smooth them with a nail file

Use care when trimming the nails: Trim the toenails along the shape of the toe and file the nails to remove any sharp edges. Never cut (or allow a manicurist to cut) the cuticles. Do not open blisters, try to free ingrown toenails, or otherwise break the skin on the feet. See a healthcare provider or podiatrist for even minor procedures.

Wash and check the feet daily: Use lukewarm water and mild soap to clean the feet. Gently pat your feet dry and apply a moisturizing cream or lotion. Check the entire surface of both feet for skin breaks, blisters, swelling, or redness, including between and underneath the toes where damage may be hidden. Use a mirror if it is difficult to see all parts of the feet or ask a family member or caregiver to help.

Choose socks and shoes carefully: Select cotton socks that fit loosely, and change the socks everyday. Select shoes that are snug but not tight, and break new shoes in slowly to prevent any blisters. Ask about customized shoes if the feet are misshapen or have ulcers; specialized shoes can reduce the chances of developing foot ulcers in the future. Shoe inserts may also help cushion the step and decrease pressure on the soles of the feet.

Ask for foot exams: Screening for foot complications should be a routine part of most medical visits, but is sometimes overlooked. Do not hesitate to ask the healthcare provider for a foot check at least once a year, and more frequently if there are foot changes.

Nursing Management

Nursing management of patients with diabetes can involve treatment of a wide variety of physiologic disorders, depending on the patient's health status and whether the patient is newly diagnosed or seeking care for an unrelated health problem. Because all patients with diabetes must master the concepts and skills necessary for long-term management and avoidance of potential complications of diabetes, a solid educational foundation is necessary for competent self-care and is an ongoing focus of nursing care.

Providing Patient Education

Diabetes mellitus is a chronic illness that requires a lifetime of special self-management behaviors. Nurses play a vital role in identifying patients with diabetes, assessing self-care skills, providing basic education, reinforcing the teaching provided by the specialist, and referring patients for follow-up care after discharge.

Developing a Diabetic Teaching Plan

- Determine how to organize and prioritize the vast amount of information that must be taught to patients with diabetes. Many hospitals and outpatient diabetes centers have devised

written guidelines, care plans, and documentation forms that may be used to document and evaluate teaching.
- The American Association of Diabetes Educators recommends organizing education using the following seven tips for managing diabetes: healthy eating, being active, monitoring, taking medication, problem solving, healthy coping, and reducing risks.
- Another general approach is to organize information and skills into two main types: Basic, initial ("survival") skills and information, and in-depth (advanced) or continuing education.
    1. Basic information is literally what patients must know to survive (e.g. to avoid severe hypoglycemic or acute hyperglycemic complications after discharge) and includes simple pathophysiology; treatment modalities; recognition, treatment, and prevention of acute complications; and other pragmatic information (e.g. where to buy and store insulin, how to contact physician).
    2. In-depth and continuing education involves teaching more detailed information related to survival skills as well as teaching preventive measures for avoiding long-term diabetic complications, such as foot care, eye care, general hygiene, and risk factor management (e.g. blood pressure control and blood glucose normalization). More advanced continuing education may include alternative methods for insulin delivery.

3. Differentiate between gastric and duodental ulcer. Discuss the medical, surgical and nursing management of a patient with peptic ulcer.

Due to a lot of circumstances and environmental factors, we cannot help or avoid having gastrointestinal problems. Millions of people suffer from this kind of problem every year from a variety of gastrointestinal disturbances. Some of the most common gastrointestinal problems are duodenal and gastric ulcers. Duodenal ulcers are different from gastric ulcers. First, the anatomy of both diseases is different. In a duodenal ulcer, ulceration occurs at the duodenum. The duodenum is part of the small intestine. The small intestine comprises the duodenum, ileum, and jejunum. While in a gastric ulcer, ulceration occurs in the stomach.
1. Gastric ulcers occur in the stomach while duodenal ulcers occur in the duodenum.
2. Gastric ulcers cause stomach pain 1–2 hours after eating. Duodenal ulcers cause pain 3–4 hours later.
3. Gastric ulcer pain cannot be relieved by eating. Stomach pain in duodenal ulcers can be relieved by eating.
4. Gastric ulcers cause hematemesis or vomiting of blood while duodenal ulcers cause melena or blood in the stool.
5. A gastric ulcer has a special diet while duodenal ulcers do not.

   A peptic ulcer is an excavation formed in the mucosal wall of the stomach, pylorus, duodenum, or esophagus. A peptic ulcer is frequently referred to as a gastric, duodenal, or esophageal ulcer depending on its location. It is caused by the erosion of a circumscribed area of mucous membrane. This erosion may extend as deeply as the muscle layers or through the muscle to the peritoneum. Peptic ulcers are more apt to be in the duodenum than in the stomach. As a rule, they occur singly, but there may be a number of them present at one time. Chronic gastric ulcers tend to occur in the lesser curvature of the stomach near the pylorus.

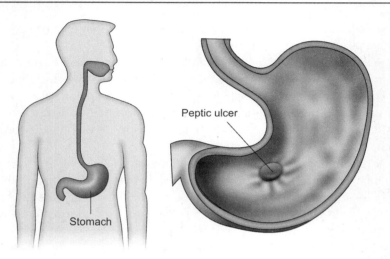

Etiology and Predisposition

The etiology of peptic ulcer is poorly understood. It is known that peptic ulcers occur only in the areas of the gastrointestinal tract that are exposed to hydrochloric acid and pepsin. The disease occurs with the greatest frequency between the ages of 20 and 60, but is relatively uncommon in women of child-bearing age, although it has been observed in childhood, and even in infancy. More men than women are affected, although there is some evidence that the incidence in women is increasing.

After menopause, the incidence of peptic ulcer in women is almost equal to that in men. Since, peptic ulcers in the body of the stomach occur without excessive acid secretion, an attempt should be made to differentiate gastric from duodenal ulcers.

Predisposition: Attempts continue to be made to delineate the ulcer personality: Psychoanalysts claim that an ulcer results from repression of strong dependency needs. Others claim that occupational stress, with no opportunity to express hostility, is another strong factor. It seems to develop in persons, who are emotionally tense, but whether this is the cause or the effect of the condition is uncertain. Familial tendency also appears as a significant predisposing factor, revealing that 3 times as many ulcer patients have relatives with the same diagnosis. A further hereditary link is noted in the finding that individuals in blood-group 0 are 35% more susceptible than persons in groups A, B, and AB. Other predisposing factors associated with peptic ulcer include emotional stress, eating hurriedly and irregularly, and smoking excessively. Rarely, ulcers are due to excessive amounts of the hormone gastrin, produced by tumors (gastrinomas-Zollinger—Ellison syndrome).

Clinical Manifestations

1. Symptoms of duodenal ulcer (most common peptic ulcer) may last days, weeks, or months and may subside only to reappear without cause. Many patients have asymptomatic ulcers.
2. Dull, gnawing pain and a burning sensation in the midepigastrium or in the back is characteristic.
3. Pain is relieved by eating or taking alkali; once the stomach has emptied or the alkali wears off, the pain returns.
4. Sharply localized tenderness is elicited by gentle pressure on the epigastrium or slightly right of the midline; some relief is obtained with local pressure to the epigastrium.

5. Other symptoms include pyrosis (heartburn) and a burning sensation in the esophagus and stomach, which moves up to the mouth, occasionally with sour eructation (burping). Vomiting is rare in uncomplicated duodenal ulcer; it may or may not be preceded by nausea and usually follows a bout of severe pain and bloating; it is relieved by ejection of the acid gastric contents.
6. Constipation or diarrhea may result from diet and medications.
7. Bleeding (15% of patients with gastric ulcers) and tarry stools may occur; a small portion of patients who bleed from an acute ulcer have no previous digestive complaints but develop symptoms later.

Assessment and Diagnostic Methods

1. **Physical examination** (epigastric tenderness, abdominal distention).
2. **Endoscopy** (preferred, but upper gastrointestinal barium study may be done).
3. **Diagnostic tests** include analysis of stool specimens for occult blood, gastric secretory studies, and biopsy and histology with culture to detect *H. pylori* (a breath test may also detect *H. pylori*).

Medical Management

Lifestyle changes: The goals of treatment are to eradicate *H. pylori* and management of gastric acidity

1. **Stress reduction and rest** are priority interventions. The patient needs to identify situations that are stressful or exhausting (e.g. rushed lifestyle and irregular schedules) and implement changes, such as establishing regular rest periods during the day in the acute phase of the disease. "Biofeedback, hypnosis, or behavioral modification may also be useful".
2. **Smoking cessation** is strongly encouraged because smoking raises duodenal acidity and significantly inhibits ulcer repair. Support groups maybe helpful.
3. **Dietary modification** may be helpful. Patients should eat whatever agrees with them; small, frequent meals are not necessary if antacids or histamine blockers are part of therapy. Oversecretion and hypermotility of the gastrointestinal tract can be minimized by avoiding extremes of temperature and over stimulation by meat extracts. Alcohol and caffeinated beverages, such as coffee (including decaffeinated coffee which stimulates acid secretion) should be avoided. Diets rich in milk and cream should be avoided also because they are potent acid stimulators. The patient is encouraged to eat three regular meals a day.

Sl. No.	Operation	Description	Comments
1.	Vagotomy	Severing of the vagus nerves which decreases gastric acid by diminishing cholinergic stimulation to the parietal cells making them less responsive to gastric	May be performed to reduce gastric acid secretion. A drainage type of procedure is performed to assist with gastric emptying. Some patients experience problems with feeling of fullness, dumping syndrome, diarrhea and gastritis

Contd...

Contd...

Sl. No.	Operation	Description	Comments
2.	Truncal vagotomy	Severing of the right and left vagus nerves as they enter the stomach at the distal part of the esophagus	This is used to decrease acid secretions and reduce gastric and intestinal motility. Ulcer recurrence rate is 10–15%.
3.	Selective vagotomy	Severing vagal innervation to the maintaining the innervation to the rest of the abdomen	
4.	Pyloroplasty	A drainage operation in which the longitudinal incision is made into the pylorus and transversely suture closed to enlarge the outlet and relax the muscle	Usually accompanies truncal and selective vagotomies which produce, delayed gastric employing due to decreased innervation
5.	Proximal (parietal cell) gastric vagotomy without poloroplasty	Denervation of acid-secreting parietal cells but preserves vagal innervation to the gastric antrum and pylorus	No dumping syndrome needs long-term follow-up ulcer recurrence is 10 to 15%
6.	Antrectomy Billroth I (gastroduodenostomy)/ Billroth II (gastrojejunostomy)	Removal of the lower portion of the antral portion of the stomach (which contains the cells that secrete gastrin) as well as a small portion of the duodenum and pylorus. The remaining segment is anastomozed to the duodenum (Billroth I) or the jejunum (Billroth II)	May be performed in conjunction with a truncal vagotomy. The patient may experience problem with feeling of fullness, dumping syndrome and diarrhea, ulcer recurrence rate is less 1%
7.	Subtotal gastrectomy with Billroth I and II anastomosis	Removal of distal third of stomach anastomosis with duodenum of jejunum (removes gastrin-producing cells in the antrum and part of the parietal cells)	Patient experiences dumping syndrome, anemia, malabsorption and weight loss, ulcer recurrence rate is 10–15%

Surgical Management

1. With the advent of H_2-receptor antagonists, surgical intervention is less common.
2. If recommended, surgery is usually for intractable ulcers (particularly with Zollinger-Ellison syndrome), life-threatening hemorrhage, perforation, or obstruction. Surgical procedures include vagotomy, vagotomy with pyloroplasty, or Billroth I or II.

Pharmacologic Therapy

1. **Antibiotics** combined with proton pump inhibitors and bismuth salts to suppress *H. pylori*.
2. **H_2-receptor antagonists** to decrease stomach acid secretion; maintenance doses of H_2-receptor antagonists are usually recommended for 1 year. Proton pump inhibitors (in high doses in patients with Zollinger-Ellison syndrome) may also be prescribed.
3. **Cytoprotective agents** (protect mucosal cells from acid or NSAIDs).
4. **Antacids in combination with cimetidine** (Tagamet) or ranitidine (Zantac) for treatment of stress ulcer and for prophylactic use.
5. **Anticholinergics** (inhibit acid secretion).
6. Patient should adhere to the prescribed medication program to ensure complete healing of the ulcer.

Nursing Management

Assessment

1. Assess pain and methods used to relieve it; take a thorough history, including a 72-hour food intake history.
2. If patient has vomited, determine whether emesis is bright red or coffee ground in appearance. This helps identify source of the blood.
3. Assess for blood in the stools with an occult blood test.
4. Ask patient about usual food habits, alcohol, smoking, medication use (NSAIDs), and level of tension or nervousness.
5. Ask how patient expresses anger (especially at work and with family), and determine whether patient is experiencing occupational stress or family problems.
6. Obtain a family history of ulcer disease.
7. Assess vital signs for indicators of anemia (tachycardia, hypotension).
8. Palpate abdomen for localized tenderness.
9. Assess for malnutrition and weight loss.

Nursing Diagnoses

1. Acute pain related to the effect of gastric acid secretion on damaged tissue.
2. Imbalanced nutrition: Less than body requirements related to changes in diet.
3. Anxiety related to coping with an acute disease.
4. Deficient knowledge about preventing symptoms and managing the condition.

Collaborative Problems/Potential Complications

1. Hemorrhage: Upper gastrointestinal
2. Perforation
3. Penetration
4. Pyloric obstruction (gastric outlet obstruction).

Planning and Goals

The major goals of the patient may include relief of pain, reduced anxiety, maintenance of nutritional requirements, knowledge about management and prevention of ulcer recurrence, and absence of complications.

Nursing Interventions

I. Relieving Pain and Improving Nutrition

1. Administer prescribed medications.
2. Avoid aspirin which is an anticoagulant, and foods and beverages that contain acid-enhancing caffeine (colas, tea, coffee, chocolate).

3. Encourage patient to eat regularly spaced meals in a relaxed atmosphere; obtain regular weights and encourage dietary modifications.
4. Encourage relaxation techniques, and assist patient to cope with stress and pain and to stop smoking.

II. Reducing Anxiety
1. Assess what patient wants to know about the disease, and evaluate level of anxiety; encourage patient to express fears openly and without criticism.
2. Explain diagnostic tests; administer medications on schedule.
3. Reassure patient that nurses are always available to help with problems.
4. Interact in a relaxing manner, help in identifying stressors, and explain effective coping techniques and relaxation methods.
5. Encourage family to participate in care, and give emotional support.

III. Monitoring and Managing Complications

If hemorrhage is a concern:
1. **Assess for faintness or dizziness** and nausea, before or with bleeding; test stool for occult or gross blood; monitor vital signs frequently (tachycardia, hypotension, and tachypnea).
2. **Monitor intake and output**; insert and maintain an intravenous line for infusing fluid and blood. Monitor laboratory values (hemoglobin and hematocrit). Insert and maintain a nasogastric tube and monitor drainage; provide lavage as ordered.
3. **Treat hypovolemic shock** as indicated.

If perforation and penetration are concerns:
1. Note and report symptoms of penetration (back and epigastric pain not relieved by medications that were effective in the past).
2. Note and report symptoms of perforation (sudden abdominal pain, referred pain to shoulders, vomiting and collapse, extremely tender and ripid abdomen, hypotension and tachycardia, or other signs of shock).

SHORT ESSAYS

4. Surgical approaches of Benign prostate hypertrophy.

Transurethral resection of the prostate (TURP) is the most common surgery for benign prostatic hypertrophy (BPH). In the United States, about 150,000 men have TURPs each year. TURP uses electric current or laser light. After anesthesia, the surgeon inserts a resectoscope through the tip of the penis into the urethra. The resectoscope has a light, valves for irrigating fluid, and an electrical loop. The loop cuts tissue and seals blood vessels. The removed tissue flushes into the bladder and out of the body. A catheter is placed in the bladder through the penis.

Transurethral incision of the prostate is used if you have a smaller prostate gland but major blockage. Instead of cutting and removing tissue, this procedure widens the urethra. The surgeon makes small cuts in the bladder neck, where the urethra joins the bladder, and in the prostate. This reduces the pressure of the prostate on the urethra. It makes urination easier. The hospital stay is one to three days. A catheter is left in your bladder for one to three days after surgery.

Transurethral resection of the prostate is the gold standard to which other surgeries for BPH are compared. This procedure is performed under general or regional anesthesia and takes less than 90 minutes. The surgeon inserts an instrument called a resectoscope into the penis through the urethra. The resectoscope is about 12 inches long and 3/8 of an inch in diameter. It contains a light, valves for controlling irrigating fluid, and an electrical loop to remove the obstructing tissue and seal blood vessels. The surgeon removes the obstructing tissue and the irrigating fluids carry the tissue to the bladder. This debris is removed by irrigation and any remaining debris is eliminated in the urine over time.

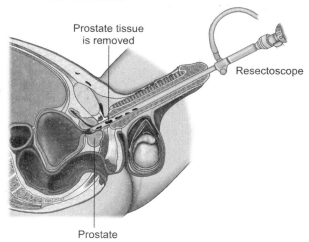

Patients usually stay in the hospital for about 3 days during which time a catheter is used to drain urine. Most men are able to return to work within a month. During the recovery period, patients are advised to:
1. Avoid heavy lifting, driving, or operating machinery.
2. Drink plenty of water to flush the bladder.
3. Eat a balanced diet.
4. Use a laxative if necessary to prevent constipation and straining during bowel movements.

Complications of TURP: Blood in the urine (hematuria) is common after TURP surgery and usually resolves by the time the patient is discharged. Bleeding also may result from straining or activity. Postsurgical bleeding should be reported to the urologist immediately. Some patients have initial discomfort, a sense of urgency to urinate, or short-term difficulty controlling urination. These conditions slowly improve as recovery progresses, but it is important to remember that the longer the urinary problems existed before surgery, the longer it takes to regain full and normal bladder function after surgery.

5. Process of inflammation.

Step 1: Invasion of the tissue by an organism—the organisms invade the healthy tissue and infect its cells. The organisms cause damage to the tissue those results in the release of chemical substances that attract the local immune cells to the site of inflammation.

Step 2: Activation of local histiocytes in the tissues—the first cells of the immune system to respond to the infections are the tissue histiocytes (macrophages). They start to fight back the invading organisms until the tactical support comes from the white blood cells in the bloodstream.

Step 3: Biochemical messages and body response—when the fight between the local immune cells and the invading organisms reach its height, they release secret chemical substances that leads to widening of the local blood vessels to bring more blood to the site of infection. The wide blood vessels allow the white blood cells to reach the site of inflammation to give support to the local immune cells. The increased blood flow to the site of inflammation leads to characteristic signs; swelling, redness, warmness and pain.

Step 4: Dendritic cells; better espionage, better response—these cells bring information and samples from the invading organisms. They process them and send the information in the form of chemical signals to the upcoming immune support from the blood (*white blood cells*). This is very important because if these cells detected that the invading organism is virus, they would send a signal to the CD8 T lymphocytes to come to fight, as they are specialized in viral attacks. If they detected that the invading organism is pyogenic bacteria, they would send signals to the neutrophils to come to the fight, because they are specialized in bacterial attacks. Another function of these cells is to instruct certain types of cells called memory cells, which is responsible for longlasting immunity after attacks by some virus, e.g. measles and mumps.

Step 5: The arrival of the main fighting force—the rescue cells coming from the tissue under attack reach the white blood cells. They arrive in forces to give tactical support against the invading organisms.

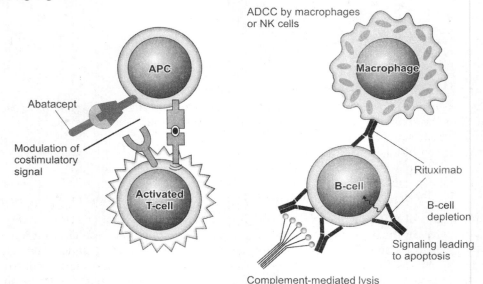

The arriving forces may be by neutrophils if it is bacterial attack, or they may be CD8 T lymphocytes if it is viral attack. These cells start to give tactical support to the fighting local immune cells leading to elimination of the invading organism, either by phagocytosis (*eating up the enemy*) or cell-mediated cytotoxicity (*injecting lethal chemicals into the invading enemy*).

Step 6: Return to normal—after elimination of the invading organism, the fighting white blood cells start to get out of the site of the infection and return back to the bloodstream. Dead cells are taken away by phagocytosis.

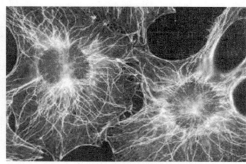

Fibroblasts (tissue engineers) start to repair the damage at the site of inflammation. After a period of time, the site returns to normal like it was before the inflammation.

6. Nursing care of unconscious patient

I. Maintaining patent airway
1. Elevating the head end of the bed to 30° prevents aspiration.
2. Positioning the patient in lateral or semiprone position.
3. Suctioning.
4. Chest physiotherapy.
5. Auscultate in every 8 hours.
6. Endotracheal tube or tracheostomy.

II. Protecting the client
1. Padded side rails.
2. Restrains.
3. Take care to avoid any injury.
4. Talk with the client in-between the procedures.
5. Speak positively to enhance the self-esteem and confidence of the patient.

III. Maintaining fluid balance and managing nutritional needs
1. Assess the hydration status.
2. More amount of liquid.
3. Start intravenous line.
4. Liquid diet.
5. Nasogastric tube.

IV. Maintaining skin integrity
1. Regular changing in position.
2. Passive exercises.
3. Back massage.
4. Use splints or foam boots to prevent foot drop.
5. Special beds to prevent pressure on bony prominences.

V. Preventing urinary retention
1. Palpate for a full bladder.
2. Insert an indwelling catheter.
3. Condom catheter for male and absorbent pads for females in case of incontinence.
4. Inducing stimulation to urinate.

VI. Providing sensory stimulation
1. Provided at proper time to avoid sensory deprivation.
2. Effort are made to maintain the sense of daily rhythm by keeping the usual day and night patterns for activity and sleep.
3. Maintain the same schedule each day.
4. Orient the client to the day, date, and time accordingly.
5. Touch and talk.
6. Proper communication.
7. Always address the client by name, and explain the procedure each time.

VII. Family needs
1. Family support.
2. Educate the needs of client.
3. Care to be provided.

VIII. Potential complications
1. Respiratory distress.
2. Pneumonia.
3. Aspiration.
4. Pressure ulcer.

7. Lung abscess.

Lung abscess is a type of liquefactive necrosis of the **lung** tissue and formation of cavities (more than 2 cm) containing necrotic debris or fluid caused by microbial infection. This pus-filled cavity is often caused by aspiration, which may occur during altered consciousness. Lung abscess is defined as necrosis of the pulmonary tissue and formation of cavities containing necrotic debris or fluid caused by microbial infection. The formation of multiple small (<2 cm) abscesses is occasionally referred to as necrotizing pneumonia or lung gangrene. Both lung abscess and necrotizing pneumonia are manifestations of a similar pathologic process. Failure to recognize and treat lung abscess is associated with poor clinical outcome.

Types of Lung Abscesses
1. Primary abscess—occurs in previously normal lungs and may follow aspiration.
2. Secondary abscess—occurs in patients with an underlying lung abnormality.

Causative organisms: Common pathogens causing lung abscess include anaerobes, *Staphylococcus aureus* and enteric gram-negative rods like *Klebsiella pneumoniae*.

Anaerobes
- *Peptostreptococcus species*
- *Bacteroides species*
- *Fusobacterium species*
- Microaerophilic streptococci.

Aerobes
- *Streptococcus aureus*
- *Streptococcus pyogenes*
- *Haemophilus influenza*
- *Pseudomonas aeruginosa*
- *Klebsiella pneumoniae*—becoming more prevalent
- *Burkholderia cepacia*—particularly associated with cystic fibrosis.

Risk Factors
- Alcoholism or drug misuse.
- Following general anesthesia.
- Diabetes mellitus.
- Severe periodontal disease.
- Stroke/cerebral palsy/cognitive impairment/impaired consciousness leading to increased risk of aspiration.

- Immunosuppression, particularly chronic granulomatous disease in children.
- Congenital heart disease.
- Chronic lung disease, particularly cystic fibrosis.

Symptoms
- Onset of symptoms is often insidious (more acute if following pneumonia).
- Spiking temperature with rigors and night sweats.
- Cough ± phlegm production (frequently foul-tasting and foul-smelling and often blood-stained).
- Pleuritic chest pain.
- Breathlessness.

Signs
- Tachypnea
- Tachycardia
- Finger clubbing in chronic cases
- Dehydration
- High temperature
- Localized dullness to percussion (if consolidation is also present or effusion)
- Bronchial breathing and/or crepitations (if consolidation is present).

Management
Supportive measures:
- Analgesia.
- Oxygen if required.
- Rehydration if indicated.
- Postural drainage with chest physiotherapy.

Antibiotics
Most lung abscesses (80–90%) are now successfully treated with antibiotics.
1. Begin with intravenous treatment, usually for about 2–3 weeks, and follow with oral antibiotics for a further 4–8 weeks.
2. Recommended first-line therapy includes beta-lactam/beta-lactamase inhibitor or cephalosporin (second or third generation) plus clindamycin.
3. Previously, therapy with a broad-spectrum penicillin and clindamycin was used. Clindamycin had also been used alone (covers *S. aureus* and anaerobes and both oral and intravenous preparations exist); however, in the 1990s it was discovered that some anaerobes were resistant to both penicillin and clindamycin.
4. An alternative regimen is to begin with a broad-spectrum cephalosporin and flucloxacillin.
5. Regimen should be altered once the organism is known.

Surgery
1. If the condition fails to resolve with conservative measures, bronchoscopy, CT-guided percutaneous drainage or cardiothoracic surgical intervention may be required.
2. Surgery is associated with a number of complications, such as empyema and bronchoalveolar air leak especially so in children.

8. Colostomy care.

There are two main ways a colostomy can be formed:

1. **A loop colostomy**—where a loop of colon is pulled out through a hole in your abdomen, before being opened up and stitched to the skin.

2. **An end colostomy**—where one end of the colon is pulled out through a hole in your abdomen and stitched to the skin.

Loop colostomies tend to be temporary and require a further operation at a later date to reverse the procedure. It is also possible to reverse an end colostomy, but this is less common. Patient will usually have to stay in hospital for 3–10 days after a colostomy or colostomy reversal.

Follow these steps to prevent infection:
1. Wash your hands with soap and water. Be sure to wash between your fingers and under your fingernails. Dry with a clean towel or paper towels.
2. If you have a 2-piece pouch, press gently on the skin around your stoma with 1 hand, and remove the seal with your other hand. (If it is hard to remove the seal, you can use special pads. Ask your nurse about these.)
3. Remove the pouch.
4. Keep the clip. Put the old ostomy pouch in a bag and then place the bag in the trash.
5. Clean the skin around your stoma with warm soap and water and a clean washcloth or paper towels. Dry with a clean towel.

Check and seal your skin:
1. Check your skin. A little bleeding is normal. Your skin should be pink or red. Call your doctor if it is purple, black, or blue.
2. Wipe around the stoma with the special skin wipe. If your skin is a little wet, sprinkle some of the stoma powder on just the wet or open part.
3. Lightly pat the special wipe on top of the powder and your skin again.
4. Let the area air-dry for 1–2 minutes.

Measure your stoma
1. Use your measuring card to find the circle size that matches the size of your stoma. Do not touch the card to your skin.
2. If you have a 2-piece system, trace the circle size onto the back of the ring seal and cut out this size. Make sure the cut edges are smooth.

Attach the pouch
1. Attach the pouch to the ring seal if you have a 2-piece ostomy system.
2. Peel the paper off the ring seal.
3. Squirt stoma paste around the hole in the seal, or place the special stoma ring around the opening.
4. Place the seal evenly around the stoma. Hold it in place for a few minutes. Try holding a warm washcloth over the seal to help make it stick to your skin.
5. If you need them, put cotton balls or special gel packs in your pouch to keep it from leaking.
6. Attach the pouch clip or use Velcro to close the pouch.
7. Wash your hands with warm soap and water.

9. Antihypertensive drugs.

Many therapeutic agents can be used for the pharmacologic management of hypertension. The general recommendation established by JNC-7 is to initiate a thiazide-type diuretic initially for stage 1 hypertensives without compelling indications for other therapies. Drugs such as angiotensin converting enzyme (ACE) inhibitors, calcium channel blockers (CCBs), angiotensin receptor blockers (ARBs), beta-blockers, and diuretics are all considered acceptable alternative therapies in patients with hypertension. The available antihypertensive agents are generally equally effective in lowering blood pressure however; there may be interpatient variability that can affect the way a patient will respond to one treatment over another.

10. Cardiopulmonary resuscitation.

Cardiopulmonary resuscitation, commonly known as CPR, is an emergency procedure that combines chest compression often with artificial ventilation in an effort to manually preserve intact brain function until further measures are taken to restore spontaneous blood circulation and breathing in a person who is in cardiac arrest. It is indicated in those who are unresponsive with no breathing or abnormal breathing, e.g. agonal respiration.

Causes of cardiac arrest:
A cardiac arrest can be caused by many things and causes tend to differ from adults to children.

For adults, they may include:
1. Heart disease—the most common cause of reversible adult cardiac arrest (70%).
2. Trauma.
3. Respiratory illness.
4. Hanging.

For children, they may include:
1. Sudden infant death syndrome (SIDS)—this is the leading cause of reversible cardiac arrest in children.
2. Cardiac disease (usually congenital).
3. Trauma.
4. Respiratory illness.

CPR can be life-saving first aid: CPR can be life-saving first aid and increases the person's chances of survival if started soon after the heart has stopped beating. If no CPR is performed, it only takes 3–4 minutes for the person to become brain dead due to a lack of oxygen. By performing CPR, you circulate the blood so it can provide oxygen to the body, and the brain and other organs stay alive while you wait for the ambulance. There is usually enough oxygen still in the blood to keep the brain and other organs alive for a number of minutes, but it is not circulating unless someone does CPR. CPR does not guarantee that the person will survive, but it does give that person a chance when otherwise there would have been none. If you are not sure whether a person is in cardiac arrest or not, you should start CPR. If a person does not require CPR, they will probably respond to your attempts. By performing CPR, you are unlikely to cause any harm to the person if they are not actually in cardiac arrest.

The basic steps of CPR: CPR is most successful when administered as quickly as possible. It should only be performed when a person shows no signs of life or when they are:
1. Unconscious
2. Unresponsive

3. Not breathing or not breathing normally (in cardiac arrest, some people will take occasional gasping breaths—they still need CPR at this point. Do not wait until they are not breathing at all).

It is not essential to search for a pulse when a person is found with no signs of life. It can be difficult to find a person's pulse sometimes and time can be wasted searching. If CPR is necessary, it must be started without delay. The basic steps for performing CPR can be used for adults, children and infants. They are based on guidelines updated in 2010 that are easy to follow and remember. This information is only a guide and not a substitute for attending a CPR course.

The basic steps are:
D – Dangers
R – Response
S – Send for help
A – Open airway
B – Normal breathing
C – Start CPR
D – Attach defibrillator (AED).

1. **Dangers:** Check for dangers. Consider why the person appears to be in trouble—is there gas present or have they been electrocuted? Might they be drunk or drug-affected and consequently a hazard to you? Approach with care and do not put yourself in danger. If the person is in a hazardous area (such as on a road), it is okay to move them as gently as possible to protect both your and their safety.

2. **Response:** Look for a response. Is the victim conscious? Gently shake them and shout at them, as if you are trying to wake them up. If there is no response, get help.

3. **Send for help:** Dial triple zero (000) – ask for an ambulance.

4. **Open airway:** Check the airway. It is reasonable to gently roll the person on their back if you need to. Gently tilt their head back, open their mouth and look inside. If fluid and foreign matter is present, gently roll them onto their side. Tilt their head back, open their mouth and very quickly remove any foreign matter (for example, chewing gum, false teeth, vomit). It is important not to spend much time doing this, as performing CPR is the priority. Chest compressions can help to push foreign material back out of the upper airway.

5. **Normal breathing:** Check for breathing—look, listen and feel for signs of breathing. If the person is breathing normally, roll them onto their side. If they are not breathing, or not breathing normally. The person in cardiac arrest may make occasional grunting or snoring attempts to breathe and this is not normal breathing. If unsure of whether a person is breathing normally, start CPR as per step six.

6. **Start CPR:**
   Cardiac compressions:
   - Place the heel of one hand on the lower half of the person's breastbone.
   - Place the other hand on top of your first hand and either grasp your own wrist or interlock your fingers, depending on what is comfortable for you.
   - The depth of compression should be one-third of the chest depth of the person.
   - The rate is either:
     - 30 compressions to two breaths (mouth-to-mouth as per step 7) aiming for 100 compressions and no more than eight breaths per minute, **OR**

- If unwilling to do mouth-to-mouth, perform continuous compressions at a rate of approximately 100 per minute.
- Thinking of the music 'Staying alive' by the Bee Gees and performing compressions on the beat can assist to keep the correct rhythm.
- Sometimes, people will have their ribs broken by chest compressions. This is still better than the alternative of not receiving CPR. If it occurs, pause and reposition your hands before continuing. Chest compressions are tiring and fatigue will affect the quality. If any other rescuers are available and willing to assist, rotate the person performing compressions every two minutes, even if you do not feel tired yet.

7. **Mouth-to-mouth**: If the person is not breathing normally, make sure they are lying on their back on a firm surface and:
   - Open the airway by tilting the head back and lifting their chin.
   - Close their nostrils with your finger and thumb.
   - Put your mouth over the person's mouth and blow into their mouth.
   - Give 2 full breaths to the person (this is called 'rescue breathing'). Make sure there is no air leak and the chest is rising and falling. If their chest does not rise and fall, check that you are tilting their head back, pinching their nostrils tightly and sealing your mouth to theirs. If still no luck, check their airway again for any obstruction.
   - If you cannot get air into their lungs, go back to chest compressions. If there is an airway obstruction, compressions may help shift the object.

Continue CPR, repeating the cycle of 30 compressions then 2 breaths until professional help arrives. Chest compressions are tiring and fatigue will affect the quality. If any other rescuers are available and willing to assist, rotate the person performing compressions every 2 minutes, even if you do not feel tired yet.

8. **Attach automated external defibrillator (AED)** as soon as one becomes available.
   - Only use an adult AED on any person over the age of 8 years who is unresponsive and not breathing normally. For children under the age of 8, ideally, a pediatric AED and pads should be used. Devices differ and instructions should be followed in each instance.
   - CPR must be continued until the AED is turned on and the pads are attached.
   - Place pads following the diagram instructions on the pads. Pad-to-skin contact is important for successful defibrillation. Remove any medication pads, excess moisture or excessive chest hair (if this can be done with minimum delay).
   - It is important to follow the prompts on the AED. Do not touch the victim during analysis or shock delivery.

CPR techniques for young children and infants: CPR steps for children aged 8 years or younger are the same as for adults and older children, but the technique is slightly different.

CPR for children aged 1–8 years
To perform CPR on children (aged 1–8 years):
1. Use the heel of **one** hand only for compressions, compressing to one-third of chest depth.
2. Follow the basic steps for performing CPR described above.

CPR for infants (up to 12 months of age)
To perform CPR on infants (up to 12 months of age):
1. Place the infant on their back. Do not tilt their head back or lift their chin (this is not necessary as their heads are still large in comparison to their bodies).

2. Perform mouth-to-mouth by covering the infant's nose and mouth with your mouth—remember to use only a small breath.
3. Do chest compressions, using two fingers of one hand, to about one-third of chest depth.
4. Follow the basic steps for performing CPR described above.

What to do if the person recovers during CPR?
CPR may revive the person before the ambulance arrives. If they do revive:
1. Review the person's condition if signs of life return (coughing, movement or normal breathing). If the person is breathing on their own, stop CPR and place them on their side with their head tilted back.
2. If the person is not breathing, continue full CPR until the ambulance arrives.
3. Be ready to recommence CPR if the person stops breathing or becomes unresponsive or unconscious again. Stay by their side until medical help arrives. Talk reassuringly to them.

It is important not to interrupt chest compressions or stop CPR prematurely to check for signs of life—if in doubt, continue full CPR until help arrives. It is unlikely you will do harm if you give chest compressions to someone with a beating heart. Regular recovery (pulse) checks are not recommended as they may interrupt chest compressions and delay resuscitation.

Stopping CPR
Generally, CPR is stopped when:
1. The person is revived and starts breathing on their own.
2. Medical help, such as ambulance paramedics arrive to take over.
3. The person performing the CPR is forced to stop from physical exhaustion.

11. Nephrotic syndrome.

Nephrotic syndrome is a condition of the kidneys. It is usually caused by one of the diseases that damage the kidneys' filtering system. This allows a protein called albumin to be filtered out into the urine (albuminuria). When the protein level in the blood drops, liquid seeps out of the smallest blood vessels (capillaries) all over the body and settles into the surrounding tissue, causing fluid swelling (edema). Treatment includes medications and dietary changes.

Symptoms of Nephrotic Syndrome
The symptoms of nephrotic syndrome include:
1. Foamy and frothy urine
2. Unexplained weight loss
3. General malaise (feeling unwell)
4. Edema (fluid retention or swelling), particularly around the abdomen (belly area), legs and eyes.
5. Muscle wasting.
6. Stomach pain.
7. Dizziness when standing up from a lying or sitting position (orthostatic hypotension).

Causes of Nephrotic Syndrome
Some of the causes of nephrotic syndrome include:
1. **Changes to the immune system (minimal change or lipoid nephrosis):** This type is most common in children. It is called 'minimal change' because the kidney filters appear normal under a microscope. The cause is thought to be changes in certain cells of the immune system. The function of the kidneys is normal and the outlook for recovery is usually excellent.

2. **Inflammation:** Local inflammation or swelling damages and scars the kidney filters. Examples of this are focal glomerulosclerosis and membranous nephropathy. Treatment may not resolve the condition, and the kidneys may gradually lose their ability to filter wastes and excess water from the blood.
3. **Secondary nephrotic syndrome:** This can be caused by certain conditions including diabetes, drugs, cancer and systemic lupus erythematosus (SLE).

Complications of Nephrotic Syndrome
Complications of nephrotic syndrome can include:
1. **Dehydration**—low protein levels may lead to a reduction in blood volume. In severe cases, intravenous fluids may be given to boost the body's water content.
2. **Blood clots**—these occur in the leg veins and occasionally in the kidney veins. Blood clots can also go into the lungs and cause chest pain, breathlessness or coughing up of blood.
3. **Infection**—infection and inflammation (peritonitis) of the peritoneal cavity. This is the thin elastic lining that contains the pancreas, stomach, intestines, liver, gallbladder and other organs. A fever may indicate infection.
4. **Kidney failure**—without treatment, the kidneys may fail in extreme cases.

Diagnosis of Nephrotic Syndrome
Diagnosing nephrotic syndrome involves a number of tests including:
1. **Urine tests**—excessive protein makes the urine appear frothy and foamy. A test for albumin/creatinine ratio may be done to measure the amount of albumin in the urine in relation to the amount of creatinine.
2. **Blood tests**—these estimate the glomerular filtration rate (eGFR) which shows how well the kidneys are working
3. **Biopsy**—a small sample of kidney tissue is taken and examined in a laboratory.

Further Tests for Nephrotic Syndrome
Sometimes, further tests may be required. These may include:
1. **Ultrasound**—an examination of the kidneys using sound waves to outline the structure of organs.
2. **Computed tomography (CT) scan or magnetic resonance imaging (MRI)**—use radio-frequency wavelengths or a strong magnetic field to provide clear and detailed pictures of internal organs and tissues.

Treatment for Nephrotic Syndrome
'Minimal change' nephrotic syndrome fixes itself in around 40% of cases. Other causes of nephrotic syndrome are also often treatable. It is essential to consult a kidney specialist (nephrologist) who can develop a management plan for your condition. Treatment depends on the severity of the condition, but may include:
1. Specific medication for some causes (for example, steroids for minimal change, immunosuppressant for membranous nephropathy or focal sclerosis)—this may lead to complete or partial remissions of the nephrotic syndrome.
2. Diuretics to control the swelling tendency.
3. Medication to control high blood pressure. People with persisting nephrotic syndrome should be treated with:
    - Angiotensin active agents (ACE inhibitors or angiotensin blockers) to reduce the amount of albuminuria and to reduce blood pressure.

- Several other blood pressure medications that work in different ways are available, if necessary.
- A diuretic (fluid pill) is often prescribed as well.

12. Psoriasis.

(See. Q. 18, 2017)

SHORT ANSWERS

13. Pleural effusion.

Each of our lungs is wrapped in a thin membrane called the visceral pleura. Our chest wall is similarly lined (parietal pleura). These two membranes touch and slide across each other while we breathe, lubricated by a slick of fluid. Pleurisy is inflammation of these membranes commonly caused by an infection of our upper respiratory tract. The activity of viruses or bacteria irritates the pleura in much the same way as it irritates the inside of the nose. The inflammation makes the pleura rub and grate against each other, rather than gliding smoothly. This causes pain which is made worse by deep breathing and coughing. Sometimes, the inflammation can cause a build-up of fluid between the two membranes. This is known as pleural effusion. Treatment options for pleurisy include addressing the underlying cause, and medications (such as antibiotics, painkillers and anti-inflammatory medications).

Symptoms of pleurisy: The symptoms of pleurisy include:
1. Prior infection of the upper respiratory tract.
2. Pain in the chest.
3. Pain in the muscles of the chest.
4. Persistent cough.
5. Fever.
6. General malaise.
7. Pain is exacerbated by deep breathing or coughing.

Causes of pleurisy: Causes of pleurisy include:
1. Viral infection.
2. Bacterial infection.
3. Pneumonia.
4. Tuberculosis.
5. Rheumatoid conditions, such as lupus erythematosus.
6. Pulmonary embolus (blood clot).

Diagnosis of pleurisy: Diagnosing pleurisy involves a number of tests including:
1. Physical examination—using a stethoscope, the doctor can hear the pleura scraping against each other. Other breath sound abnormalities that suggest pleurisy include rattling or crackling.
2. Blood tests—to determine whether the cause is viral or bacterial.
3. Chest X-rays and other imaging—including CT scans or ultrasound scans.
4. Thoracocentesis—doctors remove and examine a small sample of pleural fluid.
5. Bronchoscopy—doctors insert a thin tube with a camera down the person's windpipe to examine their airways.

Treatment for pleurisy: Treatment for pleurisy may include:
1. Treating the underlying cause—for example, treatment for tuberculosis.
2. Medications, such as antibiotics and anti-inflammatory medications.
3. Pain-killing medication.
4. Draining off the excess fluid—in the case of pleural effusion.
5. Medications to stop the fluid from building up again.

14. Types of anemia.

Causes of decreased production include iron deficiency, a lack of vitamin B_{12}, thalassemia, and a number of neoplasms of the bone marrow. Causes of increased breakdown include a number of genetic conditions, such as sickle cell anemia, infections like malaria, and certain autoimmune diseases.

The most common types of anemia are:
- Iron deficiency anemia
- Thalassemia
- Aplastic anemia
- Hemolytic anemia
- Sickle cell anemia
- Pernicious anemia
- Fanconi anemia.

15. Complications of AIDS.

Infections Common to HIV/AIDS
Tuberculosis (TB): In resource-poor nations, TB is the most common opportunistic infection associated with HIV and a leading cause of death among people with AIDS.
1. Cytomegalovirus
2. Candidiasis
3. Cryptococcal meningitis
4. Toxoplasmosis
5. Cryptosporidiosis.

16. Raynaud's disease.

Raynaud's (ray-NOHZ) disease causes some areas of your body, such as your fingers and toes—to feel numb and cold in response to cold temperatures or stress. In Raynaud's disease, smaller arteries that supply blood to your skin narrow, limiting blood circulation to affected areas (vasospasm). Women are more likely than men to have Raynaud's disease, also known as Raynaud or Raynaud's phenomenon or syndrome. It appears to be more common in people who live in colder climates. Treatment of Raynaud's disease depends on its severity and whether you have other health conditions. For most people, Raynaud's disease is not disabling, but can affect quality of life.

17. Etiology of renal calculi.

Kidney stones usually comprised of a compound called calcium oxalate, are the result of an accumulation of dissolved minerals on the inner lining of the kidneys. These deposits can grow to the size of a golf ball while maintaining a sharp, crystalline structure. The kidney stones may be small and pass unnoticed out of the urinary tract, but they may also cause extreme pain upon exiting. Kidney stones that remain inside the body can lead to many conditions including severe pain and ureter (the tube connecting the kidney and bladder) blockage that obstructs the path urine uses to leave the body.

The leading cause of kidney stones is a lack of water. Stones commonly have been found in those that drink less than the recommended 8–10 glasses of water a day. When there is not enough water to dilute the uric acid (component of urine), the pH level within the kidneys drops and becomes more acidic. An excessively acidic environment in the kidneys is conducive to the formation of kidney stones.

18. Defibrillation.

Defibrillation is a common treatment for life-threatening cardiac dysrhythmias and ventricular fibrillation. Defibrillation consists of delivering a therapeutic dose of electrical current to the heart with a device called a defibrillator. Defibrillators are the devices used to deliver shocks to the heart in cases of life-threatening cardiac disorders. Electrodes that are connected to the machine are usually held in place over the chest of a patient while one or more shocks are delivered. Defibrillators are used to re-establish a normal heart rhythm in cases of cardiac arrhythmia, ventricular fibrillation and pulseless ventricular tachycardia.

Procedure: The chest of the patient is cleared of any clothing or jewelery and adhesive or metal electrodes are applied to the chest. These electrodes are connected to the defibrillator. Adhesive gel electrodes are commonly used with the automated and semiautomated units used in ambulance or nonhospital settings due to their ease of application. These adhesive gel electrodes are available in solid-gel and wet-gel forms, with solid-gel electrodes the easier to use of the two, as there is no need to clean the patient's skin after removing the electrodes. These electrodes, however, may burn the skin, whereas wet-gel electrodes can spread the current more uniformly. The adhesive patches are also safer for healthcare personnel to use due to the very low-risk of the operator coming into contact with the electrode. The operator can stand several feet away from the patient. Furthermore, the adhesive patches require no force of application, while approximately 25 lbs of force is required to apply the metal electrodes. After application of the electrodes (metal or adhesive), the machine is charged and the shock is delivered. The electrodes are placed in one of two schemes:
1. **The anterior-posterior scheme:** This is preferred in cases of long-term electrode placement. One of the electrodes is placed over the lower part of the chest, in front of the heart, while the other is placed on the back behind the heart and in between the scapula bones.
2. **The anterior-apex scheme:** This is useful in cases where the anterior-posterior scheme is unnecessary or not practicable. The first electrode is placed on the right, below the collar bone and the other is placed over the apex of the heart, on the left side just below and to the left of the chest muscle. This is useful in defibrillation and cardioversion.

19. Portal hypertension.

Portal hypertension is abnormally high blood pressure in the portal vein (the large vein that brings blood from the intestine to the liver) and its branches.
1. Cirrhosis (scarring that distorts the structure of the liver and impairs its function) is the most common cause in Western countries.
2. Doctors base the diagnosis on symptoms and results of a physical examination, sometimes with ultrasonographer, CT, MRI, or liver biopsy.

3. Drugs can reduce blood pressure in the portal vein, but if bleeding in the digestive tract occurs, emergency treatment is required.
4. Treatment sometimes includes liver transplantation or creation of a tract through which blood can bypass the liver (portosystemic shunt).

The portal vein receives blood from the entire intestine and from the spleen, pancreas, and gallbladder and carries that blood to the liver. After entering the liver, the vein divides into right and left branches and then into tiny channels that run through the liver. When blood leaves the liver, it flows back into the general circulation through the hepatic vein.

20. Antitubercular drugs.

The main objectives of tuberculosis therapy are to cure the patients and to minimize the possibility of transmission of the bacillus to healthy subjects. Adverse effects of antituberculosis drugs or drug interactions (among antituberculosis drugs or between antituberculosis drugs and other drugs) can make it necessary to modify or discontinue treatment. We briefly review the new guidelines for the pharmacological treatment of tuberculosis, introduced by the Brazilian National Ministry of Health in 2009, and describe the general mechanism of action, absorption, metabolization, and excretion of the first-line drugs used in the basic regimen. We describe adverse drug reactions and interactions (with other drugs, food, and antacids), as well as the most appropriate approach to special situations, such as pregnancy, breastfeeding, liver failure, and kidney failure. We also describe the mechanisms by which the interactions among the antituberculosis drugs used in the basic regimen can cause drug induced hepatitis, and we discuss the alternatives in this situation.

All first-line antituberculous drug names have a standard three-letter and a single-letter abbreviation:
1. Ethambutol is EMB or E
2. Ionized is INH or H
3. Pyrazinamide is PZA or Z
4. Rifampicin is RMP or R
5. Streptomycin is SM or S.

21. Urinary incontinence.

The loss of bladder control is a common and often embarrassing problem. The severity ranges from occasionally leaking **urine** when you cough or sneeze to having an urge to **urinate** that is so sudden and strong you do not get to a toilet in time. Urinary incontinence (UI) is loss of bladder control. Symptoms can range from mild leaking to uncontrollable wetting. It can happen to anyone, but it becomes more common with age. Women experience UI twice as often as men. Most bladder control problems happen when muscles are too weak or too active. If the muscles that keep your bladder closed are weak, you may have accidents when you sneeze, laugh or lift a heavy object. This is stress incontinence. If bladder muscles become too active, you may feel a strong urge to go to the bathroom when you have little urine in your bladder. This is urge incontinence or overactive bladder. There are other causes of incontinence, such as prostate problems and nerve damage. Treatment depends on the type of problem you have and what best fits your lifestyle. It may include simple exercises, medicines, special devices or procedures prescribed by your doctor, or surgery.

22. Types of anesthesia and methods of administration.

There are three main types:
1. Local—numbs one small area of the body. You stay awake and alert.
2. Regional—blocks pain in an area of the body, such as an arm or leg. A common type is epidural anesthesia which is often used during childbirth.
3. General—makes you unconscious.

A route of administration in pharmacology and toxicology is the path by which a drug, fluid, poison, or other substance is taken into the body. Routes of administration are generally classified by the location at which the substance is applied. Common examples include oral and intravenous administration.

2014

Medical-Surgical Nursing-I

LONG ESSAYS
1. Mr Manoj an industrial worker sustained fracture of shaft of left femur after a fall from the height: Discuss the types and the clinical manifestations of fracture, explain the surgical and nursing management of Mr Manoj.
2. Mr Ram admitted to the surgical ward and is diagnosed to have peptic ulcer: Discuss the clinical manifestation, medical and surgical management of peptric ulcer, explain the postoperative nursing management of Mr Ram based on nursing process.
3. Mrs Shantha a 60-year-old lady is admitted in the dialysis unit with chronic renal failure: Discuss the clinical manifestations, drug therapy and nutritional therapy of CRF, draw a nursing care plan for Mrs Santha giving special attention to the discharge plan.

SHORT ESSAYS
4. Care of patient with intercostal drainage.
5. Standard safety precautions in acquired immunodeficiency syndrome.
6. Hernias.
7. Cardiac catheterization.
8. Care of tracheostomy.
9. Appendicitis.
10. Electrocardiogram.
11. Peritoneal dialysis.
12. Thrombolytic therapy.

SHORT ANSWERS
13. Acne vulgaris.
14. Inflammation.
15. Barium meal.
16. Atelectasis.
17. Cystotherapy.
18. Polycythemia.
19. Atherosclerosis.
20. Empyema.
21. Osteoporosis.
22. Cardioversion.

LONG ESSAYS

1. Mr Manoj, an industrial worker sustained fracture of shaft of left femur after a fall from the height: Discuss the types and the clinical manifestations of fracture, explain the surgical and nursing management of Mr Manoj.

A fracture is a break in the continuity of bone. It is defined according to type and extent. Fractures occur when the bone is subjected to stress greater than it can absorb. Fractures can be caused by a direct blow, crushing force, sudden twisting motion, or even extreme muscle contraction, When the bone is broken, adjacent structures are also affected, resulting in soft tissue edema, hemorrhage into the muscles and joints, joint dislocations, ruptured tendons, severed nerves, and damaged blood vessels. Body organs may be injured by the force that caused the fracture or by the fracture fragments.

Types of Fractures
1. Complete fracture: A break across the entire cross-section of the bone which is frequently displaced.
2. Incomplete fracture also called greenstick fracture: Break occurs through only part of the cross-section of the bone.
3. Comminuted fractures: A break with several bone fragments.
4. Closed fracture, or simple fracture: Does not produce a break in the skin.
5. Open fracture, or compound or complex fracture: A break in which the skin or mucous membrane wound extends to the fractured bone. Open fractures are classified as follows:

Grade I: A clean wound less than 1 cm long.

Grade II: Wound is highly contaminated and has extensive soft tissue damage (most severe type).

Fractures may also be described according to anatomic placement of fragments, particularly if they are displaced or nondisplaced.

Early complications of fracture include shock, fat embolism, compartment syndrome, thromboembolism (pulmonary embolism), disseminated intravascular coagulopathy (DIC), and infection. Delayed complications include delayed union and nonunion, avascular necrosis of bone, reaction to internal-fixation devices, complex regional pain syndrome, and heterotopic ossification.

Clinical manifestations: Not all of the clinical manifestations are present in every fracture.
1. The patient experiences muscle spasm and continuous pain that increases in severity until bone fragments are immobilized.
2. Loss of function, deformity, abnormal movement, and shortening of the extremity may be noted.
3. Crepitus, local swelling, and discoloration may be seen.

Medical Management

Emergency Management
1. Immediately after injury, immobilize the body part before the patient is moved. If an injured patient must be moved before splints can be applied, support the extremity above and below the fracture site to prevent rotation or angular motion.
2. Splint the fracture including joints adjacent to the fracture, to prevent damage to the soft tissue.

3. Apply temporary, well-padded splints, firmly bandaged over clothing, to immobilize the fracture.
4. Assess neurovascular status distal to the injury to determine adequacy of peripheral tissue perfusion and nerve function. Be alert for paresthesia or paralysis (compartment syndrome).
5. Cover the wound of an open fracture with a clean (sterile) dressing to prevent contamination of deeper tissues.

Reduction of Fractures

The principles of fracture treatment include reduction, immobilization, and regaining of normal function and strength through rehabilitation.
1. The fracture is reduced ('setting" the bone) using a closed method (manipulation and manual traction leg, splint or caste) or an open method (surgical placement of internal fixation devices leg, pins, wires, screws, plates, nails) to restore the fracture fragments to anatomic alignment and rotation. The specific method depends on the nature of the fracture.
2. After the fracture has been reduced, immobilization holds the bone in correct position and alignment until union occurs. Immobilization is accomplished by external or internal fixation.
3. Function is maintained and restored by controlling swelling by elevating the injured extremity and applying ice as prescribed. Restlessness, anxiety, and discomfort are controlled using a variety of approaches (e.g. reassurance, position changes, pain relief strategies including analgesic agents). Isometric and muscle-setting exercises are done to minimize disuse atrophy and to promote circulation. With internal fixation, the surgeon determines the amount of movement and weight-bearing stress the extremity can withstand and prescribes the level of activity.

Management of Complications

1. **Treatment of shock** consists of restoring blood volume and circulation, relieving pain, providing adequate splinting, and protecting the patient from further injury and other complications.
2. **Prevention and management of fat embolism** includes immediate immobilization of fractures and adequate support for fractured bones during turning and positioning. Prompt initiation of respiratory support with prevention of respiratory and metabolic acidosis and correction of homeostatic disturbances is essential. Corticosteroids may be given as well as vasoactive medications, fluid replacement therapy, and morphine for pain and anxiety. Compartment syndrome is managed by controlling swelling by elevating the extremity to heart level or by releasing restrictive devices (dressings or cast). A fasciotomy (surgical decompression with excision of the fibrous membrane covering and separating muscles) may be needed to relieve the constrictive muscle fascia. The wound remains open and covered with moist sterile saline dressings for 3–5 days. The limb is splinted and elevated. Range of motion exercises may be performed every 4–6 hours.
3. **Nonunion** (failure of the ends of a fractured bone to unite) is treated with internal fixation, bone grafting (osteogenesis, osteoconduction, and osteoinduction), electronic bone stimulation, or a combination of these.
4. **Management of reaction** to internal fixation devices involves protection from osteoporosis, altered bone structure, and trauma.

5. **Management of complex regional pain** syndrome involves elevation of the extremity, pain relief, range-of-motion exercises, and helping patients with chronic pain, disuse atrophy, and osteoporosis. Avoid taking blood pressure or performing venipuncture in the affected extremity.

2. Mr Ram admitted to the surgical ward and is diagnosed to have peptic ulcer: Discuss the clinical manifestation, medical and surgical management of peptic ulcer, explain the postoperative nursing management of Mr Ram based on nursing process.

(See Q. 3, 2015)

3. Mrs Shantha, a 60-year-old lady is admitted in the dialysis unit with chronic renal failure: Discuss the clinical manifestations, drug therapy and nutritional therapy of CRF, draw a nursing care plan for Mrs Santha giving special attention to the discharge plan.

When a patient has sustained enough kidney damage to require renal replacement therapy on a permanent basis, the patient has moved into the final stage of chronic kidney disease, also referred to as chronic renal failure (CRF) or end stage renal disease (ESRD). The rate of decline in renal function and progression of ESRD is related to the underlying disorder, the urinary excretion of protein, and the presence of hypertension. The disease tends to progress more rapidly in patients who excrete significant amounts of protein or have elevated blood pressure than in those without these conditions.

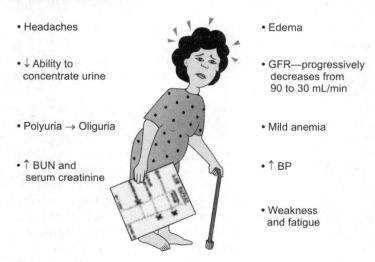

- Headaches
- ↓ Ability to concentrate urine
- Polyuria → Oliguria
- ↑ BUN and serum creatinine
- Edema
- GFR—progressively decreases from 90 to 30 mL/min
- Mild anemia
- ↑ BP
- Weakness and fatigue

Definition: Chronic or irreversible, renal failure is progressive reduction of functioning renal tissue such that the remaining kidney mass can no longer maintain the body's internal environment.

Risk Factors

1. Glomerulonephritis

2. Acute renal failure
3. Obstructions
4. Hypertension
5. Diabetes mellitus.

Causes

1. Congenital or developmental disorders
2. Golmerulonephritis
3. Tubular disorders
4. Renal multiple myelomas, neoplasm
5. Infectious renal disease
6. Obstructive renal disorders
7. Renal and systemic disorders
8. Renal problems in pregnancy
9. Diabetic retinopathy
10. UT of autoimmune disease

Pathophysiology

There is deterioration and distraction of neurons with progressive loss of renal function. As the total glomerular filtration rate falls, the serum urea, nitrogen and creatinine clearance levels rise. Remaining functioning nephritis hypertrophy and finally kidney losses the ability to concentrate urine adequately. Large volume of diluted urine is passed and salt wasting occurs glomerlar filtration rate further falls and kidney unable to filter water, salt and other wastes and body becomes intoxicated.

Clinical Manifestations

1. Cardiovascular: Hypertension, pitting edema (feet, hands, sacrum), periorbital edema, pericardial friction rub, engorged neck veins, pericarditis, pericardial effusion, pericardial tamponade, hyperkalemia, hyperlipidemia.
2. Integumentary: Gray-bronze skin color, dry flaky skin, severe pruritus, ecchymosis, purpura, thin brittle nails, coarse thinning hair.
3. Pulmonary: Crackles, thick, tenacious sputum, depressed cough reflex, pleuritic pain, shortness of breath, tachypnea, Kussmaul-type respirations, uremic pneumonitis.
4. GI: Ammonia odor to breath, metallic taste, mouth ulcerations and bleeding, anorexia, nausea and vomiting, hiccups, constipation or diarrhea, bleeding from GI tract.
5. Neurologic: Weakness and fatigue, confusion, inability to concentrate, disorientation, tremors, seizures, asterixis, restlessness of legs, burning of soles of feet, behavior changes.
6. Musculoskeletal: Muscle cramps, loss of muscle strength, renal osteodystrophy, bone pain, fractures, foot drop.
7. Reproductive: Amenorrhea, testicular atrophy, infertility, decreased libido.
8. Hematologic: Anemia, thrombocytopenia.

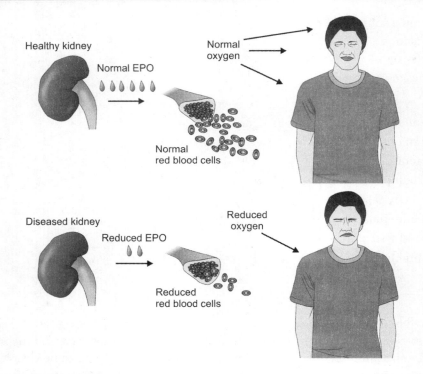

Diagnostic Evaluation

Noninvasive

1. History collection
2. Physical examination
3. Urine analysis
4. Kidney, ureter and bladder film (KUB)
5. Ultrasound
6. Computerized tomography.

Invasive:

Blood analysis test: Serum creatinine, elderly, BUN, blood chemistry, sodium, potassium, calcium, total ionized, phosphorus, magnesium, serum pH, Serum bicarbonates.

Complete Blood Count

1. Hemoglobin
2. Hematocrit
3. Creatinine clearance
4. Uric acid (serum).

Medical Management

Goals of management are to retain kidney function and maintain homeostasis for as long as possible. All factors that contribute to ESRD and those that are reversible (e.g. obstruction) are identified and treated.

Goals
1. To preserve renal function.
2. To delay the need for dialysis or transplantation as long as feasible.
3. To alleviate extra renal manifestations as much as possible.
4. To improve body chemistry values.
5. To provide an optimal quality of life for the client and significant others.

Fluid control: Fluid imbalance are identified and an intake of sodium and water equivalent to the amount of these substances excreted in a 24-hour period is prescribed.

Electrolyte control: Hyperkalemia—controlled by decrease in dietary intake of foods high in potassium. Hemodialysis with a zero potassium dialysate bath rapidly remover potassium from the body and may be used in severe situations Exchange resins, such as sodium polystyrene sulfonate are also effective in removing potassium from the body.

Hypocalcemia/Hyperphosphatemia: Hyperphosphatemia is reduced by restricting dietary phosphorus intake (eliminating dairy products and restricting protein) and using phosphate binders. Intestinal phosphate binding include the aluminum containing gels, calcium carbonate and calcium acetate. Calcium carbonate 4–12 g daily.

Pharmacologic Management
Complications can be prevented or delayed by administering prescribed phosphate-binding agents, calcium supplements, antihypertensive and cardiac medications, antiseizure medications, and erythropoietin (Epogen).
1. Hyperphosphatemia and hypocalcemia are treated with medications that bind dietary phosphorus in the GI tract (e.g. calcium carbonate, calcium acetate, sevelamer hydrochloride); all binding agents must be administered with food.
2. Hypertension is managed by intravascular volume control and antihypertensive medication.
3. Heart failure and pulmonary edema are treated with fluid restriction, low-sodium diet, diuretics, inotropic agents (e.g. digoxin or dobutamine), and dialysis.
4. Metabolic acidosis is treated, if necessary, with sodium bicarbonate supplements or dialysis.
5. Patient is observed for early evidence of neurologic abnormalities (e.g. slight twitching, headache, delirium, or seizure activity); IV diazepam (Valium) or phenytoin (Dilantin) is administered to control seizures.
6. Anemia is treated with recombinant human erythropoietin (Epogen); hemoglobin and hematocrit are monitored frequently.
7. Heparin is adjusted as necessary to prevent clotting of dialysis lines during treatments.
8. Supplementary iron may be prescribed.
9. Blood pressure and serum potassium levels are monitored.

Nutritional Therapy
1. Dietary intervention is needed with careful regulation of protein intake, fluid intake to balance fluid losses, and sodium intake, and with some restriction of potassium.
2. Adequate intake of calories and vitamins is ensured. Calories are supplied with carbohydrates and fats to prevent wasting.
3. Protein is restricted; allowed protein must be of high biologic value (dairy products, eggs, meats).
4. Fluid allowance is 500–600 mL of fluid or more than the previous day's 24-hour urine output.
5. Vitamin supplementation.

Dialysis: The patient with increasing symptoms of renal failure is referred to a dialysis and transplantation center early in the course of progressive renal disease. Dialysis is usually initiated when the patient cannot maintain a reasonable lifestyle with conservative treatment.

Nursing Management
1. Assess fluid status and identify potential sources of imbalance.
2. Implement a dietary program to ensure proper nutritional intake within the limits of the treatment regimen.
3. Promote positive feelings by encouraging increased self-care and greater independence.
4. Provide explanations and information to the patient and family concerning ESRD, treatment options, and potential complications.
5. Provide emotional support.

SHORT ESSAYS

4. Care of patient with intercostal drainage.

A chest drain involves inserting a small tube in your pleural space (the space between your lungs and ribcage) to drain air or fluid. A collection of air (pneumothorax) happens if your lung is punctured. It can cause pain and shortness of breath. A collection of fluid (pleural effusion) can make it difficult for you to breathe.

Complications
1. Pain
2. Shortness of breath, tight chest or worsening cough
3. Allergic reaction
4. Bleeding
5. Continued pneumothorax
6. Damage to structures in your chest or abdomen
7. Developing a blockage in the drain
8. Infection where the drain is inserted
9. Infection in your pleural space.

Insertion: The drain site is determined by whether air or fluid is to be cleared from the pleural space. Air tends to rise to the apex of the lung and is therefore most efficiently removed when the tip of the drain is anterior and apical to the chest cavity. Conversely, fluid tends to collect at the base of the lung and is most efficiently removed when the drain is posterior and basal to the chest cavity (Graham, 1996). Nurses are usually responsible for assembling the necessary equipment and explaining the procedure to patients, preparing them and providing them with constant reassurance, particularly during insertion of the drain.

Positioning the patient: Chest drains are inserted by medical staff under aseptic conditions while the patient is in an upright position. Patients can be made reasonably comfortable sitting on the edge of a bed with their arms crossed and raised to chin level, their head and arms resting on a pillow placed on a bedside table. Alternatively, they can sit upright in bed, resting back on the pillows with the appropriate arm raised above the head.

Insertion procedure: The proposed site is cleaned with an iodine-based antiseptic solution before the surrounding area is covered with sterile drapes, leaving only the insertion site exposed. Local anesthetic is then injected around the insertion site. When it has taken effect, a 2–3 cm incision is made in the skin. Forceps are then used to penetrate through the intercostal muscle and into the pleural space. The proximal end of the drainage tube is clamped with the forceps and inserted into the pleural space. The chest drain can then be connected to the drainage tubing and bottle.

An anchor suture is inserted to secure the drain and a purse-string suture should be placed at the incision site, with the ends left loose so that they can be tied when the drain is removed (McMahon-Parkes, 1997). A dry, nonadherent dressing with an adhesive border is applied over the site and the chest-drain connection is secured with tape.

Observations: A chest X-ray must be performed after the insertion of a chest drain to confirm that it has been placed correctly.

Routine observations—blood pressure, pulse, respiration rate and oxygen saturation—should be carried out before and after the procedure so that they can be compared. They should also be monitored at regular frequent intervals if the patient's condition is unstable.

Pain control: The insertion of a chest drain is a painful procedure. Tomlinson and Treasure (1997) recommend that 10 mL of 2% lignocaine should be used as a local anesthetic, remembering that it takes from two to five minutes to take effect.

Securing the chest drain: Current recommendations on taping the connection between the chest and drainage tubes conflict. Some practitioners tape the connection to secure it and avoid inadvertent disconnection, while others say taped connections that become disconnected are not always visible, allowing air to enter unnoticed (Godden and Hiley, 1998). Neither opinion is evidence-based, so it is advisable to secure the connection with impermeable adhesive plastic tape while maintaining visibility. A strip of tape can also be used to support the tubing against the patient's side. This reduces movement at the site and prevents pulling, which can cause pain.

Position and fluid level: Underwater sealed drainage operates as a one-way valve—air can bubble out through the water during expiration or coughing but cannot be drawn back into the chest during inspiration. The fluid level should be checked regularly and the amount, color and consistency of any drainage noted. The drainage bottle must be kept below chest level to prevent fluid re-entering the pleural space. There must also be enough water in the bottle to ensure that the end of the tubing is never exposed to air as this could then enter the pleural space. The level of water in the tubing will fluctuate as the patient breathes. A gradual decrease in fluctuation may indicate lung re-expansion but a rapid decrease suggests that the tube is blocked, perhaps with fibrous tissue from the chest cavity.

Patients with a chest drain should be encouraged to maintain an upright position and to mobilize as this increases the use of their lungs, enhancing chest expansion. Deep breathing and coughing raise intrathoracic pressure and promote pleural drainage (Erickson, 1989).

Recording drainage: Drainage bottles must be clearly labelled and the amount of fluid they contain should be noted on the patient's fluid-balance chart. How often the drainage needs to be recorded varies, depending on each patient and the amount of fluid he or she can be expected to lose? The frequency of recordings can usually be determined according to the patient's diagnosis. For example, the fluid drained from a patient with a pneumothorax may need to be measured and recorded only every four hours, as a relatively small loss can be expected. But medical staff should be present to monitor fluid loss in patients with a pleural effusion as it is usually rapid and can lead to complications. Maintaining a 24-hour record of drainage will also help to determine when a chest drain may be removed.

Suction: Low-grade suction can be used to aid the removal of air or fluid from the chest cavity. Applying suction to remove intrapleural air can resolve a pneumothorax more quickly, reducing the length of time the drain has to remain in place and therefore the patient's hospital stay.

There is no consensus on how much suction should be applied, although the most commonly used pressure is about 5kPa.

Too little suction will prevent lung expansion, increasing the risk of a tension pneumothorax, fluid accumulation and infection. Too much can perpetuate an air leak and cause air stealing, where the flow of air through the lung and into the drainage system is too rapid for adequate oxygenation to occur. This can lead to hypoxia and result in portions of lung becoming trapped in the drain (Tang et al, 1999).

Regular inspection is vital to ensure that the suction tubing is patent and set at the correct pressure. The tube should be long enough to allow the patient as much mobility as possible.

Changing dressings and bottles: If a chest drain has been sutured in place correctly air should not leak from the site and an airtight dressing will not be necessary. A small, dry nonadherent surgical dressing with an adhesive border should be sufficient and heavy strapping should be avoided as it restricts chest expansion (Welch, 1993). The site should be checked everyday, and if the dressing is clean and dry it will need to be changed only every 48–72 hours.

Removal: Chest drains are removed when drainage and fluid fluctuations have stopped, breath sounds have returned to normal and a chest X-ray shows that there is no air or fluid in the intrapleural space. The removal of a drain requires two members of staff: One to remove the drain quickly while the other ties the purse-string suture. Removing a chest drain can be a painful procedure which is often described as a stinging or burning sensation, so analgesia should be administered beforehand and given time to take effect. The type of analgesia required should be determined after careful assessment by nursing and medical staff and in accordance with the patient's tolerance of pain while the drain has been in situ. One of the main complications associated with the removal of a drain is recurrent pneumothorax. This is more likely if the patient breathes in while the drain is being removed.

To prevent this, patients should be told to take a deep breath and hold it while the drain is being removed (Gallon, 1998). Alternatively, they may be asked to perform the Valsalva maneuver—increasing their intrathoracic pressure by holding their breath while trying to breathe out against a closed glottis—as recommended by McMahon–Parkes (1997).

Patients can breathe normally once the purse-string suture has been tightened and should then be asked to cough so that the nurse can ensure that air cannot be heard escaping from the site.

A suture that has been well sited and safely tied should seal the wound and require only a simple, dry dressing. If air is heard escaping from the site, adhesive skin closure strips should be applied to seal it. Chest drain sutures may be removed five days later.

A chest X-ray should be taken after the drain has been removed and the patient's respiration rate should be recorded to ensure that a pneumothorax has not recurred. The site should be checked daily and observed for signs of bleeding, infection or necrosis, which could result if the suture is too tight.

5. Standard safety precautions in acquired immunodeficiency syndrome.

Acquired immune deficiency syndrome (AIDS) is a major public health problem in the United States and throughout the world. The spread of AIDS has raised many workplace issues of concern to union leaders and members as well as employers. As reported by the US Centers for Disease Control and Prevention (CDC), more than 1,100,000 cases of AIDS have been reported in the United States since 1981 (when the first case of the disease was reported within the US). Further, experts believe that more than one million Americans may be infected with AIDS. Moreover, according to the World Health Organization (WHO), worldwide in 2007 there were 33 million individuals living with HIV/AIDS, 2.5 million had become newly infected, and

2.1 million had died of HIV/AIDS. AIDS is a bloodborne disease for which there is no known cure that is caused by the human immunodeficiency virus (HIV). HIV progressively destroys the body's ability to fight infections and certain cancers by damaging or killing cells within the body's immune system. HIV infection can be by transmitted by the following body fluids:
1. Blood
2. Blood products, like plasma
3. Fluid around joints, the heart, lungs, the chest, and abdomen
4. Vaginal secretions
5. Fluids in childbirth
6. Fluid in the brain and spinal column
7. Semen
8. Certain other body fluids (especially those containing visible blood).

Workplace issues and policies: In 1992, OSHA established the Bloodborne Pathogens Standard, 29 CFR 1910.1030. Intended to provide necessary protection to affected workers, particularly those workers who are employed within the health care industry and some service occupations, the standard includes coverage of the following topics:
1. Exposure control plan: Covered employers must develop a written exposure control plan to prevent and reduce the amount of contact that workers have with blood. The plan should include a listing of all occupations and tasks that involve contact with blood. The exposure control plan must be provided by the employer to requesting workers and their representatives.
2. Universal precautions: Universal protections must be practiced in the workplace. This means that workers are trained to and treat all blood and certain body fluids as potentially infectious for bloodborne pathogens, such as HIV, HBV, and HCV.
3. Engineering and work practice controls: Engineering and work practice controls, i.e. work equipment and tools and design methods and procedures that prevent exposure to workplace bloodborne pathogens, must be used to eliminate or minimize worker exposure. Examples would include needles that recap themselves; IV line connections that do not use needles; needle and "sharps," i.e. other sharp tools or items like scalpel blades; containers; ventilation systems; leak-proof storage bags; as well as isolation and equipment inspection methods and procedures.
4. Hand washing: Employers must train workers in proper hand-washing procedures as well as provide the appropriate (hand washing) sinks.
5. Personal protective equipment: Employers must provide affected workers with the appropriate personal protective equipment including gloves, goggles, masks, and gowns at no cost. It should be remembered that personal protective equipment is the least preferred method of protecting workers from harmful workplace exposures.
6. Hepatitis B vaccine: Employers must provide covered workers with the hepatitis B vaccine within ten (10) working days of starting the job. The vaccine must be made available at no cost and at a reasonable time and place to the affected workers. Workers can choose not to take the vaccine. However, if later they change their minds, the employer must still provide the vaccine at no charge.
7. Postexposure evaluation and follow-up: The employer must develop and implement a written postexposure evaluation and follow-up plan that spells out how to care for workers after they have suffered a needle stick or been splashed with blood.
8. Communication and training: Employers must develop and provide communication, information, and training on the OSHA Bloodborne Pathogens Standard to all affected workers. Communication methods include warning labels that must be placed upon containers of regulated waste; refrigerators and freezers containing blood or other potentially

hazardous material; other containers used to store, transport, or ship blood or other potentially hazardous materials; and warning signs posted at the entrance to HIV and HBV research laboratory and production facilities.

6. Hernias.

A hernia is the protrusion of organs, such as intestines, through a weakened section of the abdominal wall. If left untreated, the split in the muscle widens and greater amounts of tissue or organs are pushed through the opening, forming a sac. This visible lump or bulge is one of the key characteristics of a hernia. The weakened abdominal wall can be present at birth or may develop later in life. The most common site is the groin, but hernias can also form in other areas, such as the navel. If the lump can be gently pushed back through the abdominal wall, it is known as a reducible hernia. If the lump resists manual pressure, it is a nonreducible hernia, which can mean serious complications. Both forms of hernia require surgical repair. Approximately 40,000 Australians have their hernias surgically repaired every year, making this one of the most common operations.

Symptoms of a Hernia

The symptoms of a hernia can vary depending on the location and severity, but may include:
1. A visible lump or a swollen area.
2. A heavy or uncomfortable feeling in the gut, particularly when bending over.
3. Pain or aching, particularly on exertion (such as lifting or carrying heavy objects).
4. Digestive upsets, such as constipation.
5. The lump disappears when the person is lying down.
6. The lump enlarges upon coughing, straining or standing up.

Different Types of Hernias

The abdominal wall is not a solid sheet of muscle; it is made up of different layers. Certain areas are structurally weaker than others and therefore more likely to develop hernias. The different types of hernia include:

Inguinal—occurring in the groin. This is the most common form, accounting for more than nine out of 10 hernias. A loop of intestine pushes against the small ring of muscle in the groin, eventually splitting the muscle fibers apart. Inguinal hernias affect more men than women and are particularly common in middle age.

Femoral—occurring high on the thigh, where the leg joins the body. Similar to the events that cause an inguinal hernia, intestines force their way through the weak muscle ring at the femoral canal until they protrude. This herniated section of bowel is at risk of strangulation, which is a serious complication requiring urgent medical attention. Femoral hernias are more common in women.

Umbilical—a portion of the gut pushes through a muscular weakness near the navel, or belly button. This type of hernia is more common in newborns. Overweight women, or those who have had several pregnancies, are also at increased risk

Incisional—after abdominal surgery, the site of repair will always be structurally weaker. Sometimes, the intestines can push through the closed incision causing a hernia.

Surgical procedures for a hernia: Both reducible and nonreducible hernias need to be surgically repaired. The various procedures used depend on the location of the hernia, but may include opening the abdomen and using stitches and nylon meshes to close and reinforce the weakened section of muscle. Inguinal hernias can be repaired using laparoscopic surgery. A slender instrument known as a laparoscope is inserted and the hernia repaired from the inside. This eliminates the need for large abdominal incisions. Other factors that may have been contributing to the hernia, such as obesity and flabby muscle tone, also need to be addressed. However, the hernia returns in around one out of 10 cases, requiring subsequent surgery.

7. Cardiac catheterization.

Cardiac catheterization is a procedure used to diagnose and treat cardiovascular conditions. During cardiac catheterization, a long thin tube called a catheter is inserted in an artery or vein in your groin, neck or arm and threaded through your blood vessels to your heart. Cardiac catheterization (kath-uh-tur-ih-ZAY-shun) is a procedure used to diagnose and treat cardiovascular conditions. During cardiac catheterization, a long thin tube called a catheter is inserted in an artery or vein in your groin, neck or arm and threaded through your blood vessels to your heart. Using this catheter, doctors can then do diagnostic tests as part of a cardiac catheterization. Some heart disease treatments, such as coronary angioplasty, also are done using cardiac catheterization.

8. Care of tracheostomy.

A tracheostomy is a surgical procedure to cut an opening into the trachea (windpipe) so that a tube can be inserted into the opening to assist breathing. A tracheostomy may be temporary or permanent, depending on the reason for its use. For example, if the tracheostomy tube is inserted to bypass a trachea that is blocked by blood or swelling, it will be removed once regular breathing is once again possible. A person with permanent damage or loss of function around the larynx or swallowing area may need a permanent tracheostomy tube to help them breathe at night. Speech, eating and drinking gets affected.

Medical reasons for tracheostomy: Tracheostomy may be performed as an emergency procedure to provide relief of blockage of airways above the trachea. This is called an emergency tracheostomy. It involves making a cut in the thin part of the trachea just below the larynx (voice box) and inserting a tube that is connected to a supply of oxygen or air, often using a ventilator (breathing machine). A nonemergency tracheostomy may be performed for a variety of reasons: For example, before surgery to the throat or mouth so the patient can breathe after the surgery or to make the prolonged use of ventilators more comfortable and safe.

Operation Procedure
The surgical technique depends on whether or not the tracheostomy is being performed as a medical emergency. When possible and safe, the procedure is done under general anesthesia.

Emergency tracheostomy—patient is positioned on his/her back, and a rolled-up towel (or equivalent) is placed under his/her shoulders to help stretch out his/her neck. Local anesthesia is injected into the target area, and a skin incision (cut) is made. The surgeon will then open either the trachea (this is called a 'tracheostomy') or the cricothyroid membrane—the thinnest part of the airway below the larynx (this is called a 'cricothyroidotomy'). The airway tube is inserted into the trachea and patient is connected to the oxygen supply. The entire procedure is done as quickly as possible.

Nonemergency tracheostomy—the operation is usually performed under general anesthesia in an operating room. Patient is positioned on his/her, and your neck and chest are swabbed with antiseptic. The cut is made in the lower half of the neck, between the larynx and the sternum (breastbone). First, the skin on your throat is cut horizontally. The underlying muscles are parted, then the thyroid gland may need to be cut or pulled back to expose the trachea. A cut is made through the wall of the trachea. The tracheostomy tube is then placed into the opening. Stitches are needed to hold the tube in place.

Immediately After the Operation

After the operation, you can expect the following:
1. A chest X-ray may be taken to check that the tube is correctly in place and there are no complications.
2. Antibiotics may be prescribed to reduce the risk of infection.
3. Later, you and your carers are shown how to care for the tracheostomy tube (for example, how to clean around and in the tube).
4. It takes a few days to get used to breathing through the tracheostomy tube and it will be difficult to make sounds at first. If the tube allows some air to escape and pass over the vocal cords, it may be possible to speak by holding a finger over the tube.
5. Unless there are complications, you will stay in hospital for between 3 and 5 days.

Possible Complications

Certain groups, including babies, smokers and the elderly, are more vulnerable to complications. Some of the possible risks and complications of tracheostomy include:
1. Severe bleeding
2. Damage to the larynx
3. Damage to the esophagus (rare)
4. Trapped air in the surrounding tissues
5. Lung collapse
6. Blockage of the tracheostomy tube by blood clots, mucus or the pressure of the airway walls
7. Failure of the opening to close once the tracheostomy tube is removed
8. The tube may come out of the trachea.

9. Appendicitis.

The appendix is a thin tail, tube or appendage growing out of the cecum, which is part of the large intestine located on the lower right side of the abdomen. The precise function of the appendix in the human body is something of a mystery, although it clearly plays a role in digestion for other animal species.

Appendicitis means inflammation of the appendix. Food or fecal matter can sometimes lodge in the narrow tube of the appendix, and the blockage becomes infected with bacteria. This is a medical emergency. If the appendix bursts, its infected contents will spread throughout the abdominal cavity. Infection of the lining of the abdominal cavity (peritonitis) can be life-threatening without prompt treatment. Anyone of any age can be struck by appendicitis, but it seems to be more common during childhood and adolescence. It is less common for anyone over the age of 30 years to develop appendicitis. Treatment options include surgery.

Symptoms of Appendicitis

Symptoms of Appendicitis Include:
1. Dull pain centred around the navel, which progresses to a sharp pain in the lower right side of the abdomen
2. Pain in the lower back, hamstring or rectum (less commonly)
3. Fever
4. Vomiting

5. Diarrhea or constipation
6. Loss of appetite.

Diagnosis of appendicitis: Appendicitis can mimic the symptoms of other disorders, such as gastroenteritis, ectopic pregnancy and various infections (including those of the kidney and chest). Diagnosis may include a thorough physical examination and careful consideration of the symptoms. If the diagnosis is not clear, then laboratory tests and ultrasound or CT scans may be needed. Since appendicitis is potentially life threatening if left untreated, doctors will err on the side of caution and operate, even if there is no firm diagnosis.

Treatment for appendicitis: Treatment includes an operation to remove the appendix completely. This procedure is known as an appendicectomy or appendectomy. The appendix can often be removed using laparoscopic (keyhole) surgery. The surgeon will use a slender instrument (laparoscope) which is inserted through tiny incisions (cuts) in the abdomen. This eliminates the need for an abdominal incision.

If this is not possible, a small incision is made in the lower abdomen. The appendix is cut away and the wound on the large intestine stitched. If the appendix has burst, the surgeon will insert a tube and drain the abdominal cavity of pus. Antibiotics are given to the patient intravenously to reduce the possibility of peritonitis.

The typical hospital stay for an appendicectomy is between 3 and 5 days. Removing the appendix appears to have no effect on the workings of the digestive system, in either the short- or long-term.

An alternative to surgery is antibiotic therapy. Studies that have compared the outcome of surgery to the outcome of antibiotics show that about 70% of cases may resolve with antibiotic therapy and not require surgery. However, the factors leading to failure of antibiotic therapy are not known, so antibiotic therapy alone is usually reserved for patients too frail to undergo surgery.

10. Electrocardiogram.

An electrocardiogram (ECG or EKG) records the electrical activity of the heart. The heart produces tiny electrical impulses which spread through the heart muscle to make the heart contract. These impulses can be detected by the ECG machine. You may have an ECG to help find the cause of symptoms, such as the feeling of a 'thumping heart' (palpitations) or chest pain. Sometimes, it is done as part of routine tests—for example, before you have an operation.

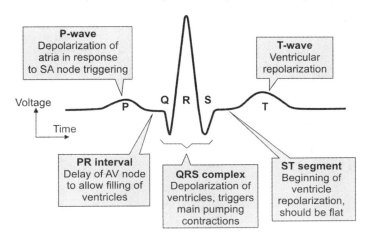

An ECG is used to monitor your heart. Each beat of your heart is triggered by an electrical impulse normally generated from special cells in the upper right chamber of your heart. An ECG records these electrical signals as they travel through your heart. Doctor can use an ECG to look for patterns among heartbeats and rhythms to diagnose various heart conditions. An ECG is a noninvasive, painless test with quick results. Doctor may discuss results with patient the same day the ECG is done, or at the next appointment.

11. Peritoneal dialysis.

During **peritoneal dialysis**, a cleansing fluid (dialysate) is circulated through a tube (catheter) inside part of patient's abdominal cavity (**peritoneal** cavity). The dialysate absorbs waste products from blood vessels in patient's abdominal lining (**peritoneum**) and then is drawn back out of his/her body and discarded. Peritoneal dialysis is a way to remove waste products from patient's blood when your kidneys can no longer do the job adequately. A cleansing fluid flows through a tube (catheter) into part of patient's abdomen and filters waste products from his/her blood. After a prescribed period of time, the fluid with filtered waste products flows out of abdomen and is discarded. Peritoneal dialysis differs from hemodialysis, a more commonly used blood-filtering procedure. With peritoneal dialysis, patient can give himself/herself treatments at home, at work or while traveling. Peritoneal dialysis is not an option for everyone with kidney failure. Patient need manual dexterity and the ability to care for himself/herself at home, or a reliable caregiver.

The benefits of peritoneal dialysis compared with hemodialysis can include:
1. **Greater lifestyle flexibility and independence:** These can be especially important if you work, travel or live far from a hemodialysis center.
2. **More flexible dietary guidelines:** Peritoneal dialysis is done more continuously than hemodialysis, resulting in less accumulation of potassium, sodium and fluid.
3. **More stable blood chemistry and body hydration:** Peritoneal dialysis does not require intravenous (IV) access which can disrupt your circulation and fluid levels.
4. **Longer lasting residual kidney function:** People who use peritoneal dialysis might retain kidney function slightly longer than people who use hemodialysis.

12. Thrombolytic therapy.

Thrombolytics restore cerebral blood flow in some patients with acute ischemic stroke and may lead to improvement or resolution of neurologic deficits. Thrombolytic therapy is of proven and substantial benefit for selected patients with acute cerebral ischemia. The evidence base for thrombolysis in stroke includes 21 completed randomized controlled clinical trials enrolling 7,152 patients, using various agents, doses, time windows, and intravenous or intra-arterial modes of administration.

Streptokinase (SK)—derived from group C, β-hemolytic streptococci. Not fibrin specific. Activates adjacent plasminogen by forming a non-covalent SK-plasminogen activator complex. Plasma half-life 30 minutes. Stimulates antibody production making retreatment difficult.

Urokinase (UK)—derived from cultured human cells. Not fibrin specific. Activates plasminogen directly by enzymatic action. Plasma half-life 20 minutes.

Tissue plasminogen activator—derived by recombinant genetics from human DNA. Fibrin specific. Activates plasminogen associated with fibrin directly by enzymatic action. Short plasma half-life.

Three preparations of tPA:
1. Alteplase (tPA) is the glycosylated protein of 527 amino acids produced by recombinant DNA technology.
2. Reteplase (sometimes called rPA) is the 39,571 molecular weight nonglycosylated deletion mutein of tPA. It contains 355 of the 527 amino acids of native tPA and includes the kringle 2 and the protease domains of the parent molecule.
3. Tenecteplase is the 527 amino acid protein produced by recombinant DNA technology. It differs from alteplase by 6 amino acids.

Indications
1. Acute myocardial infarction—streptokinase, tPA (alteplase, reteplase and tenecteplase)
2. Acute ischemic stroke—tPA (alteplase)
3. Acute pulmonary embolism—SK, UK, tPA (alteplase)
4. Acute deep venous thrombosis—SK
5. Clotted AV fistula and shunts—UK.

Precautions
1. Bleeding is the major complication of thrombolytic therapy. Consequently, **absolute** contraindications include dissecting aortic aneurysm, pericarditis, stroke, or neurosurgical procedures within 6 months or known intracranial neoplasm. **Relative** contraindications include major surgery or bleeding within 6 weeks known as bleeding diathesis, and severe uncontrolled hypertension.
2. Allergic reactions: SK and anistreplase are potentially allergenic. Patients are usually pretreated with intravenous hydrocortisone 100 mg.
3. Antibody production: SK and anistreplase induce antibody production which makes retreatment with either of these agents less effective.

SHORT ANSWERS

13. Acne vulgaris.

Acne, medically known as **acne vulgaris**, is a skin disease that involves the oil glands at the base of hair follicles. It commonly occurs during puberty when the sebaceous (oil) glands come to life—the glands are stimulated by male hormones produced by the adrenal glands of both males and females.

Acne vulgaris is characterized by noninflammatory, open or closed comedones and by inflammatory papules, pustules, and nodules. It typically affects the areas of skin with the densest population of sebaceous follicles (e.g. face, upper chest, back). Its local symptoms may include pain, tenderness, or erythema. Systemic symptoms are most often absent in acne vulgaris. Severe acne with associated systemic signs and symptoms, such as fever is referred to as acne fulminans. Severe acne characterized by multiple comedones without the presence of systemic symptoms is known as acne conglobata. This severe form of acne frequently heals with disfiguring scars. Additionally, acne vulgaris may have a psychological impact on any patient regardless of the severity or the grade of the disease.

14. Inflammation.

Inflammation does not mean infection, even when an infection causes inflammation. Infection is caused by a bacterium, virus or fungus, while inflammation is the body's response to it. Inflammation is a vital part of the body's immune response. It is the body's attempt to heal itself after an injury; defend itself against foreign invaders, such as viruses and bacteria; and repair damaged tissue. Without inflammation, wounds would fester and infections could become deadly. Inflammation can also be problematic, though, and it plays a role in some chronic diseases. Inflammation is often characterized by redness, swelling, warmth, and sometimes pain and some immobility.

15. Barium meal.

A barium meal is a diagnostic test used to detect abnormalities of the esophagus, stomach and small bowel using X-ray imaging. X-rays can only highlight bone and other radio-opaque tissues and would not usually enable visualization of soft tissue. However, infusion of the contrast medium barium sulfate, a radioopaque salt, coats the lining of the digestive tract, allowing accurate X-ray imaging of this part of the abdomen.

16. Atelectasis.

Atelectasis is a condition where a portion of the lung has collapsed or is not able to completely expand. Normally, oxygen enters the body through the lungs. Carbon dioxide is released through the lungs. The lungs expand and contract to create the exchange of these gases. Atelectasis is not a disease, but a condition or sign that results from disease or abnormalities in the body.

17. Cystotherapy.

Cytotherapy is an essential global resource for clinical researchers, oncologists, hematologists, physicians, and regulatory experts involved in cell processing and therapy.

18. Polycythemia.

An abnormally increased concentration of hemoglobin in the blood, either through reduction of plasma volume or increase in red cell numbers. It may be a primary disease of unknown cause, or a secondary condition linked to respiratory or circulatory disorder or cancer.

19. Atherosclerosis.

Atherosclerosis is a disease in which plaque builds up inside arteries. Arteries are blood vessels that carry oxygen-rich blood to heart and other parts of body. Plaque is made up of fat, cholesterol, calcium, and other substances found in the blood. Over time, plaque hardens and narrows the arteries. This limits the flow of oxygen-rich blood to organs and other parts of body.

Atherosclerosis is a slow, progressive disease that may begin as early as childhood. Although the exact cause is unknown, atherosclerosis may start with damage or injury to the inner layer of an artery. The damage may be caused by:
1. High blood pressure
2. High cholesterol
3. High triglycerides, a type of fat (lipid) in the blood
4. Smoking and other sources of tobacco
5. Insulin resistance, obesity or diabetes

Inflammation from diseases, such as arthritis, lupus or infections, or inflammation of unknown cause.

20. Empyema.

Pus is a fluid filled with immune cells, dead cells, and bacteria. Empyema is a condition in which pus accumulates in the area between the lungs and the inner surface of the chest wall. This area is known as the pleural space. Empyema, also called pyothorax or purulent pleuritis, usually develops after pneumonia, which is an infection of the lung tissue. Pus in the pleural space cannot be coughed out. Instead, it needs to be drained by a needle or surgery. Empyema usually develops after you have pneumonia. Many different types of bacteria may cause pneumonia, but the two most common bacterial causes of empyema are *Streptococcus pneumoniae* and *Staphylococcus aureus*. Clear fluid builds up in the pleural space. The fluid becomes infected with the bacteria that caused the pneumonia. The infected fluid thickens and can cause the lining of lungs and chest cavity to stick together and form pockets. This is called an empyema. Lungs may not be able to inflate completely. This can lead to breathing difficulties. Occasionally, empyema may happen after patient has the had surgery on the chest. Medical instruments can transfer bacteria into pleural cavity.

21. Osteoporosis.

Osteoporosis, or thinning bones, can result in painful fractures. Risk factors for osteoporosis include aging, being female, low body weight, low sex hormones or menopause, smoking, and some medications. Prevention and treatment include calcium and vitamin D, exercise, and osteoporosis medications.

22. Cardioversion.

Cardioversion is a procedure that can restore a fast or irregular heartbeat to a normal rhythm. A fast or irregular heartbeat is called arrhythmia. Arrhythmias can prevent your heart from pumping enough blood to the body.

Communication and Educational Technology

2019

Communication and Educational Technology

LONG ESSAYS

1. a. Define education. b. What are the aims and functions of education?
2. a. Define educational objectives. b. Explain blooms taxonomy of educational objectives.
3. a. Classify audio-visual aids. b. Overhead projector as an audio-visual aid in nursing.

SHORT ESSAYS

4. Explain the communication process.
5. Bedside clinic.
6. Explain the criteria for selection of assessment techniques and methods.
7. Multiple choice questions.
8. Any two philosophy of education.
9. Purposes and steps of lesson plan.
10. Qualities of a good teacher.
11. Maxims of teaching.
12. Preparation and uses of charts.

SHORT ANSWERS

13. Bulletin board.
14. Objective structure clinical examination.
15. Teamwork.
16. Guidance and counseling.
17. Advantages and disadvantages of role play.
18. Enlist any four principles of health education.
19. Components of unit plan.
20. Advantages of clinical teaching.
21. Barriers of effective interpersonal relationship.
22. Attitude scale.

LONG ESSAYS

1. a. Define education (*See* Q. 2, 2015). b. What are the aims (*See* Q. 2, 2016) and functions of education.

2. a. Define educational objectives. b. Explain blooms taxonomy of educational objectives. (*See* Q. 9, 2018)

3. a. Classify audio-visual aids. b. Overhead projector as an audio-visual aid in nursing.

Audio-visual aids are also called instructional material. Audio literally means "hearing" and "visual" means that which is found by seeing. So all such aids which endeavor to make the knowledge clear to us through our sense are called audio-visual aids or instructional material. All these learning material make the learning situations as real as possible and give us firsthand knowledge through the organs of hearing and seeing. Therefore, any device which can be used to make the learning experience more concrete and effective, more realistic and dynamic can be considered audio visual material.

Audio-visual Aids Definition
According to Burton, these are sensory objectives and impages which stimulate and emphasis on learning process. Carter V Good. It is a trainable (motivation, classification and stimulation) process of learning.

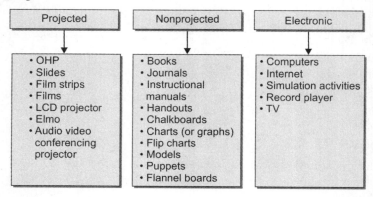

Types
It can be classified simply on the bases of sensory experience. Because human beings derive their experiences mainly through direct sensory contact. Keeping this in view, it can be classified into three main groups:
1. **Audio aids:** Examples are radio, tape-recorder, gramophone, linguaphone, audio cassette player, language laboratory
2. **Visual aids:** Examples are chart, black and while board, maps, pictures, models, text-books, slide projector, transparency, flash-cards, print materials, etc.
3. **Audio-visual aids:** Examples are LCD project, film projector, TV, computer, VCD player, virtual classroom, multimedia, etc.

Overhead projector as an audio-visual aid in nursing.

Overhead projector (OHP) is one of the most frequently used visual aid in nursing education which has replaced the blackboard in most of the classrooms. As the name indicates, it is a projecting device that is made of a lamp, lens and mirror arrangement which projects material, which is written or drawn on a transparent plastic sheet (transparency) on a screen.

Guidelines for Overhead Projector

1. Make sure that every student in the class can see the screen easily without any obstacle. The OHP should be set up for optimum image size and focused before the class starts.
2. The stage of OHP where the transparency is placed should be clean so that it will not obscure the images of the transparency.
3. Follow the general rule of one idea-one transparency.
4. The transparency must be covered with a opaque sheet while putting it on the OHP stage then progressively disclose one point at a time.
5. While using a transparency do not talk to the screen, but talk to the students and use a pointer on the OHP stage to point out on the transparency.
6. Be creative while preparing a transparency; for example, to build up complex diagram three or four transparencies can be used as overlays on the original transparency or you may employ cutouts to build visuals in stages.
7. Radiographs can be projected successfully with the overhead projector. For this purpose, the classroom must be darkened.
8. Switch off the projector light when you are not using the OHP because the bright screen will distract the students and also it is not good for the health of the OHP (projector may overheat).
9. Black, blue and green colors are considered good for transparency preparation. Avoid yellow, orange and red (not projected well by OHP).
10. Not necessary to write text content in running CAPITAL LETTERS.
11. Write in legible letters.
12. While preparing transparencies, follow the rule of seven or eight lines per transparency and seven or eight words per line.

Advantages of the Transparency

1. Transparencies can be prepared well in advance and can be stored and reused whenever required.
2. Progressive disclosure of a transparency is helpful to gradually build up the concept under study.
3. Material can be prepared by the teachers themselves.
4. It is a time-saving and cost-effective visual aid.

Disadvantages of the Transparency

1. Novice teachers may feel difficulty in proper use of transparency.
2. Creativity and imagination is required to make good transparency.
3. Students may read on the transparency if the teacher exposed it entirely in the beginning, creating disharmony in what the teacher is teaching and what the student is reading.
4. Difficult to handle and preserve the transparency.
5. Electricity is a must for its use.
6. Teachers usually tend to talk to the screen instead of students.
7. Inappropriate teacher's position may cause difficulty in watching the transparency.

8. Printed transparencies which teachers use because of lack of time to prepare a transparency cannot be considered as good approach.
9. Students require notes or handouts if class is taken with the help of transparency because most of their time is spent in reading the transparency.
10. Not useful for students with visual impairment and dyslexia.

SHORT ESSAYS

4. Explain the communication process. *(See Q. 8, 2016)*

5. Bedside clinic.

Bedside clinic is a process in which a clinical teacher and a group of learners sees a patient, elicits or verifies physical signs, discusses provisional diagnosis, therapeutic options in clinical settings.

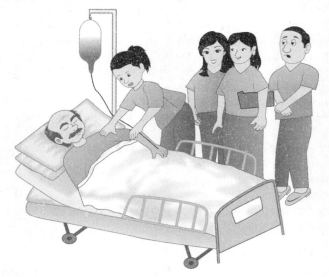

1. A process in which a clinical teacher and a group of learners sees as patients, elicits or verifies physical signs, discusses provisional diagnosis, diagnostic or therapeutic options in the clinical settings.
2. It is also the time in which the medical practitioner can say or explain something about the patient's concern regarding on his/her health if possible.
3. Bedside clinic always helps to study the problems typically associated with a particular disease or disorder, and to give a clear picture of the related nursing care by associating it with a specific individual.
4. It always ensures the presence of the patient. Either the group visits the patient or the patient is brought to the conference room.
5. Nursing clinic maybe conducted by the head nurse or the clinical instructor.
6. The patient should be the center of attention and nothing should be done to embarrass or upset him.
7. Willingness of the patient to participate in the teaching program is needed for the bedside clinic.

Purposes

1. To portray nursing problem and to provide a complete picture of the related nursing care by associating with a specific individual.
2. To improve the quality of nursing care.
3. To improve the student's ability to solve nursing problems by detailed study and analysis of nursing situation.
4. Helps the students to sharpen their observation skill in a systematic and organized manner.
5. To realize the need for understanding every patient as an individual and appreciate their problems and outlook.
6. Provides a learning experience for nursing students to collect information about the patient.
7. To plan and execute nursing care plan according to the needs and problems of the patient.

Advantages

1. Bedside clinic allows the students to prepare extensively in advance to participate effectively in patient care.
2. It helps the students to develop autonomy.
3. It allows students to select patients with disease conditions of common interest.
4. It helps the students to ably review and investigate the quality of clinical practice.
5. Bedside clinic allows the students to develop and maintain professional competence.
6. It promotes a better understanding among the students in terms of health, illness and healthcare system.
7. Bedside clinic promotes clinical competencies like reasoning, psychomotor and communication skills among students.
8. It develops the ability of the students to evaluate critically and improve own performance.

Disadvantages

1. Bedside clinics may be an encumbrance to the patients.
2. Its narrowness limits the utilization of the process.
3. Bedside clinic is an expensive procedure.
4. It may disturb the privacy of the patient.
5. Results in poor standardization.

6. Explain the criteria for selection of assessment techniques and methods.

Assessment methods are the strategies, techniques, tools and instruments for collecting information to determine the extent to which students demonstrate desired learning outcomes. Several methods should be used to assess student learning outcomes.

Direct and indirect methods of assessment: Direct methods of assessment ask students to demonstrate their learning while indirect methods ask students to reflect on their learning. Tests, essays, presentations, etc. are generally direct methods of assessment, and indirect methods include surveys and interviews.

Examples of assessment criteria: Constructively aligned assessment criteria begin with a noun that complements the verb in the assessment tasks objective. For example, if the objective is for students to "explain how concepts in the subject interrelate" one of the criteria might be "Clarity of explanation". That is, the criterion describes the quality in the assessment task that will be judged during marking.

Other commonly used quality words used in criteria include:
1. Accuracy
2. Currency
3. Depth
4. Impact
5. Legibility
6. Originality
7. Succinctness
8. Relevance.

Guidelines to follow when selecting assessment methods:
1. Collect information that will answer the program's questions
2. Use multiple methods to assess each student learning outcome
3. Include both indirect and direct assessment methods
4. Include both qualitative and quantitative methods
5. Choose methods that allow the assessment of both strengths and weaknesses
6. Utilize capstone courses or "second-year" projects/assignments to directly assess student learning outcomes
7. Use established accreditation criteria/standards when developing the assessment plan.

7. Multiple choice questions.

A multiple choice question is a question type where the respondent is asked to choose one or more items from a limited list of choices. A multiple choice question consists of a stem, the correct answer, and distractors. The stem is the beginning part of the item that presents the item as a problem to be solved, a question, or an incomplete statement to be completed. The options are the possible answers you can choose from, with the correct answer called the key and the incorrect answers called distractors.

Multiple choice question tips:
1. Use simple sentence structure and precise wording
2. Make all options plausible
3. Keep all answer choices the same length
4. Avoid double negatives
5. Mix up the order of the correct answers (when testing knowledge)
6. Keep the number of options consistent
7. Avoid tricking test-takers; you should test their knowledge, not their reading skills.

Multiple Choice Examples
The capital of India is:
Mumbai, Delhi, Bangaluru, Hyderabad

Advantages of Multiple Choice Questions:
1. They have fast processing times
2. There is no room for subjectivity
3. You can ask more questions, it takes less to time to complete a multiple choice question compared to an open question
4. Respondents do not have to formulate an answer but can focus on the content.

Disadvantages of Multiple Choice Questions
1. While they are fast processed, they are time-consuming to create: They require time to draw up effective stem questions and corresponding choices

2. They do not produce any qualitative data, solely quantitative
3. They limit the respondent in his answers, that is why it is important to provide an "other" option with a textbox.

8. Any two philosophy of education.

A philosophy of education is a statement (or set of statements) that identifies and clarifies the beliefs, values and understandings of an individual or group with respect to education. Defined in this sense, it may be thought of as a more-or-less organized body of knowledge and opinion on education, both as it is conceptualized and as it is practiced. A philosophy of this sort is critical in defining and directing the purposes, objectives and focus of a school. It should also serve to inspire and direct educational planning, programs and processes in any given setting.

Perennialism

1. For Perennialists, the aim of education is to ensure that students acquire understandings about the great ideas of Western civilization.
2. These ideas have the potential for solving problems in any era.
3. The focus is to teach ideas that are everlasting, to seek enduring truths which are constant, not changing, as the natural and human worlds at their most essential level, do not change.
4. Teaching these unchanging principles is critical.
5. Humans are rational beings, and their minds need to be developed. Thus, cultivation of the intellect is the highest priority in a worthwhile education.
6. The demanding curriculum focuses on attaining cultural literacy, stressing students' growth in enduring disciplines.
7. The loftiest accomplishments of humankind are emphasized—the great works of literature and art, the laws or principles of science.

Essentialism

1. Essentialists believe that there is a common core of knowledge that needs to be transmitted to students in a systematic, disciplined way.
2. The emphasis in this conservative perspective is on intellectual and moral standards that schools should teach.
3. The core of the curriculum is essential knowledge and skills and academic rigor. Although this educational philosophy is similar in some ways to Perennialism, Essentialists accept the idea that this core curriculum may change.
4. Schooling should be practical, preparing students to become valuable members of society.
5. It should focus on facts-the objective reality out there--and "the basics," training students to read, write, speak, and compute clearly and logically.
6. Schools should not try to set or influence policies. Students should be taught hard work, respect for authority, and discipline.
7. Teachers are to help students keep their nonproductive instincts in check, such as aggression or mindlessness.

9. Purposes and steps of lesson plan.

Purposes of lesson plan:

1. Helps to review the subject and gives up to date knowledge
2. Enables to evaluate the teaching sessions
3. Helps to choose effective method of teaching

4. Ensures selection, presentation and interpretation of subject matter
5. Keeps the teacher on track
6. Ensures definite objective for the day's work
7. Facilitates microteaching
8. Develops reasoning, imagination and decision making ability of the teacher
9. Enables teacher to organize classroom teaching activities
10. It stimulates the teacher to think of related material, illustrations and audio-visual aids.
11. Gives the teacher greater confidence
12. Helps to clarify the ideas.

Steps of lesson plan

Seven steps to prepare an exciting and effective lesson plan:
Step 1: Choose realistic learning goals
Step 2: Pick exciting topics or learning contexts
Step 3: Know your students' needs and talents
Step 4: Use a range of teaching approaches and methods
Step 5: Select appealing resources
Step 6: Fair assessment
Step 7: Evaluation

10. Qualities of a good teacher.

A good teacher is accountable.
Accountable: Holding yourself to the same expectations and standards as you hold your students.
 A teacher cannot have double standards. For example, if you do not allow your students to chew gum in your class, then you should not chew gum either.

A good teacher is adaptable.
Adaptable: Making changes to lessons or activities on the fly because of an unforeseen situation or problem.
 A teacher must be willing to change. If half the class does not understand a particular concept, then you cannot move on and must quickly come up with a better way to teach that concept.

A good teacher is caring.
Caring: Going the extra mile to ensure that every student is successful no matter what.
 A teacher must figure out the personalities and interest of each student and incorporate components that connect with each individual.

A good teacher is compassionate.
Compassionate: Recognizing that your students have problems outside of school, and making the necessary adjustment to help them through those issues.
 A teacher must take outside factors into consideration. For example, if a student has just lost a loved one, the teacher should be sensitive to that and adjust accordingly.

A good teacher is cooperative.
Cooperative: The ability to work effectively with administrators, other teachers, and parents for the good of your students.
 A teacher must be able to build cooperative relationships with others around them even if they do not necessarily like them.

A good teacher is creative.
Creative: Taking a concept and shaping a lesson that is unique, engaging, and dynamic.
 A teacher must be able to create lessons that grab their students' attention and make them want to keep coming back for more.

A good teacher is dedicated.
Dedicated: Showing up everyday and spending the necessary time to provide your students with the best education.
 Teachers often arrive early and stay late. They work parts of weekends and summer to ensure that they are prepared.

A good teacher is determined.
Determined: Finding any means necessary to reach all students no matter the challenge.
 Teachers must be willing to do anything to ensure that all students receive the education they need.

A good teacher is empathetic.
Empathetic: Being sensitive to a student's struggles even though you may not personally be able to relate to them.
 A teacher must put themselves in the student's shoes and see it from their perspective. This approach is often transcending in how to help the child succeed.

A good teacher is engaging.
Engaging: The ability to grab the attention of a classroom full of students and to maintain their attention throughout the entirety of class.
 A teacher must create lessons that are fun, fresh, and energetic. You want your student to walk out of your class each day looking forward to the next.

A good teacher is evolving.
Evolving: A continuous process of year over year improvement and growth.
 A teacher must continuously look for ways to improve themselves as well as individual lessons or components of lessons.

A good teacher is fearless.
Fearless: Trying a new approach that may be outside the norm and may receive criticism or scrutiny.
 A teacher must be willing to try anything within the parameters of school policy to reach their students. They must also be ready to defend their approach to criticism.

A good teacher is forgiving.
Forgiving: Quickly putting incidents with student, parents, or other teachers behind you so that it does not impact your teaching.
 Teachers must be able to get past hurtful actions or accusations quickly. They must not hold it against any student or let it impact how they teach in the classroom.

A good teacher is generous.
Generous: Volunteering for extra assignments and/or giving money out of your own pocket for classroom needs or individual student needs.
 Teachers do not make enough money, but most teachers are willing to donate time and/or money to help out in areas where a need is recognized.

A good teacher has grit.
Grit: The determination to overcome any obstacle in the way of obtaining a long-term goal.

A teacher must possess the grit necessary to make the personal sacrifices necessary to ensure that every goal is reached every year.

A good teacher is inspirational.
Inspirational: The ability of a teacher to get their students to buy into, believe in, and to be motivated to become lifelong learners.

A teacher should make a lasting inspirational impact that follows a student throughout their life.

A good teacher is joyful.
Joyful: Coming to class each day in a good mood, excited, and enthusiastic about doing your job.

If the teacher has a lousy attitude, the students are going to have lousy attitudes. If the teacher is joyful, the students are going to be joyful.

A good teacher is kind.
Kind: The ability of a teacher to say and do things that uplifts, motivates, and inspires.

Kindness should be innate in all teachers. A mean spirit will turn students off, but a kind spirit is invaluable.

A good teacher is organized.
Organized: The ability to keep things neat and in order allowing teachers to access materials quickly and to make efficient transitions.

Organization is a necessary quality for every teacher. Teaching encompasses so much that those who are unorganized will be overwhelmed and swallowed up.

A good teacher is passionate.
Passionate: Teaching with enthusiasm and exuberance on a daily basis because you love the content and your students.

A passionate teacher connects with their curriculum and their students which maximizes learning.

A good teacher is patient.
Patient: The ability to see the whole picture and to understand that the school year is a marathon, not a sprint.

A teacher must never give up on a student. They should continuously try new strategies understanding that eventually something will work.

A good teacher is resilient.
Resilient: Not allowing adversity to stop you from accomplishing your goals.

A teacher must be resilient in overcoming the many obstacles that will present themselves over the course of a year.

A good teacher is resourceful.
Resourceful: Finding a way to make things happen.

A teacher must be able to figure out how to get supplies and materials for their classroom when the funding is not available and to reach a student who has no interest in learning.

A good teacher is trustworthy.
Trustworthy: The ability to get others around you to believe in you and what you are doing.

A teacher must gain the trust of both their students and parents. Any distrust will negatively impact the classroom.

A good teacher is vulnerable.
Vulnerable: Allowing your students to gain insight into your life without revealing a lot.
   Vulnerability allows students to relate to their teachers as they share in common interests such as sports, television, etc.

11. Maxims of teaching. (See Q. 9, 2016)

12. Preparation and uses of charts.

Charts are often used to ease understanding of large quantities of data and the relationships between parts of the data. Charts can usually be read more quickly than the raw data. They are used in a wide variety of fields, and can be created by hand (often on graph paper) or by computer using a charting application.

Vertical bar charts: Vertical bar charts are best for comparing data that is grouped by discrete categories. Vertical bar charts are best when you do not have too many groups (less than 10 is usually good). Each bar is separated by blank space which indicates that there is no inherent order to your groups.

Stacked bar charts: Stacked bar charts are a great choice if you not only want to convey the size of a group relative to other groups, but also illustrate the parts that make up the whole group.

Histogram: A histogram is visually interesting combination of a vertical bar chart and a line chart. The continuous variable shown on the x-axis is broken into discrete intervals and the number of data you have in that discrete interval determines the height of the bar. Histograms are great for illustrating distributions of your data.

Horizontal bar: The horizontal bar chart is similar to a vertical bar chart but is typically used when the number of categories is large (greater than 10 or so) or you have long labels that you would like to display for each category. It is much easier to read the labels when they are displayed in proper orientation.

Pie charts: Pie charts are easy to read and fun to look at making them a great choice if you want to understand the parts of a whole. It is a good practice to order the pieces of your pie according to size an always ensure the total of all the pieces add up to 100%.

Line charts: Line charts are used to show resulting data relative to a continuous variable—most commonly time or money. They are great for projections of performance beyond your data. If you plot your sales vs. month on a line chart over the past 2 years, it is easy for the reader to identify any trends that may be useful as you plan for the upcoming year.

Area charts: An area chart is similar to a line chart, but the space between the x-axis and the line is filled with a color or pattern. It is useful for showing part-to-whole relations, such as showing individual sales reps' contribution to total sales for a year. It helps you analyze both overall and individual trend information.

Scatter plot: A scatter plot chart will show the relationship between two different variables. Scatter plots are useful for quickly understanding if there is a relationship between two variables. If the data forms a band extending from lower left to upper right, there most likely a positive correlation between the two variables. If the band runs from upper left to lower right, a negative correlation is probable. If it is hard to see a pattern, there is probably no correlation.

Funnel chart: Funnel charts are most often used to represent how something moves through different stages in a process. A funnel chart displays values as progressively decreasing proportions amounting to 100% in total. Funnel charts start at 100% and ends with a lower percentage indicating how something drops out of the process at each step or stage. A very common use of a funnel chart is to track sales conversions in a sales pipeline.

Bullet chart: Used typically to display performance data relative to a goal. A bullet graph reveals progress toward a goal, compares this to another measure, and provides context in the form of a rating or performance.

SHORT ANSWERS

13. Bulletin board.

A bulletin board (pin board, pin board, notice board, or notice board in British English) is a surface intended for the posting of public messages, for example, to advertise items wanted or for sale, announce events, or provide information. Bulletin boards are often made of a material, such as cork to facilitate addition and removal of messages, as well as a writing surface, such as blackboard or white board. A bulletin board which combines a pin board (corkboard) and writing surface is known as a combination bulletin board.

14. Objective structured clinical examination.

The objective structured clinical examination (OSCE) is a versatile multipurpose evaluative tool that can be utilized to assess healthcare professionals in a clinical setting. It assesses competency, based on objective testing through direct observation. It is precise, objective, and reproducible allowing uniform testing of students for a wide range of clinical skills. Unlike the traditional clinical exam, the OSCE could evaluate areas most critical to performance of healthcare professionals, such as communication skills and ability to handle unpredictable patient behavior.

15. Teamwork.

Teamwork means that people will try to cooperate, using their individual skills and providing constructive feedback, despite any personal conflict between individuals. Teamwork is generally understood as the willingness of a group of people to work together to achieve a common aim. For example, we often use the phrase: "He or she is a good team player". This means someone has the interests of the team at heart, working for the good of the team.

16. Guidance and counseling.

Basis for comparison	Guidance	Counseling
Meaning	Guidance refers to an advice or a relevant piece of information provided by a superior, to resolve a problem or overcome from difficulty	Counseling refers to a professional advice given by a counselor to an individual to help him in overcoming from personal or psychological problems
Nature	Preventive	Remedial and curative
Approach	Comprehensive and extroverted	In-depth and introverted
What it does?	It assists the person in choosing the best alternative	It tends to change the perspective, to help him get the solution by himself or herself

Contd...

Contd...

Basis for comparison	Guidance	Counseling
Deals with	Education and career related issues	Personal and sociopsychological issues
Provided by	Any person superior or expert	A person who possesses high level of skill and professional training
Privacy	Open and less private	Confidential
Mode	One to one or one to many	One to one
Decision-making	By guide	By the client

17. Advantages and disadvantages of role play.

Using role playing in the classroom can help teach children in the class about certain situations in a relatable and dramatic fashion. This will cause the children to better remember the situations, making role playing a good teaching method for new hypothetical theories. It allows the students to play the roles of certain characters in these situations so they are able to see things from a new perspective. Empathy for others in their class may increase when children are given an opportunity to look at a situation from another's person's vantage point. Through role play, they may better understand why people often strongly disagree on a particular topic when their personal values, beliefs and social or cultural backgrounds differ.

Role play in the classroom is forms of instruction in which you have students take the part of someone else so that they can understand a situation from a different perspective than they normally would. However, it is not a perfect form of instruction, as it has both advantages and disadvantages to its use.

18. Enlist any four principles of health education.

Interest: It is a psychological principle that pupils do not listen to those things which are not to their interest. That is why health teaching should relate to the interests of the pupils. The pupils are not interested in health slogans, such as 'take care of your health' or 'be healthy'. Health educators must find out the real health needs of the pupils.

Participation: Participation is based on the psychological principle of active learning and group discussion, panel discussion, workshop—all provide opportunities for active learning. Health education must include not only the personal element but also social. However the personal and community health are closely interlinked and interdependent. 'To live must and to live best' may be a very desirable motto for health education.

Comprehension: In health education one must know the level of understanding for which the teaching is directed. One barrier to communication is the use of words which cannot be understood. Especially in the lower grades children do not understand the meaning of health. They are not interested in it as adults are.

Reinforcement: Few children can learn all that is new in a single period. Repetition at intervals is extremely useful. It assists comprehension and understanding so health instruction needs reinforcement which the doctors call booster dose.

Motivation: In every person there is a fundamental desire to learn. Awakening of this desire is called motivation. There are two types of motives—primary and secondary. Primary motives are sex, hunger, survival which initiate people into action. These motives are inborn desires! But secondary motives are based on desires created by the outside forces or incentive.

19. Components of unit plan.

1. **Set goals and objectives for students:** Using content standards, teachers can begin to create a unit plan by identifying what they want students to accomplish. This plan should include identifying goals in the form of what students should know or be able to accomplish upon completion of the unit. An example of a science goal might be that students will be able to identify and state the purpose of all the major organelles of a cell.
2. **Choose content:** Working within a unit, teachers must identify all of the content that needs to be taught. For example, a unit on decimals might include adding, subtracting, multiplying, and dividing numbers that contain decimals.
3. **Choose instruction methods:** Here the teacher will address the teaching methods that he or she will be use. This is an opportune moment to consider the special needs of students in the classroom. Will instruction include direct instruction, cooperative learning experiences, or the reteaching of content to a peer? Some students with writing difficulties might require the additional assistance of peer help or partially completed notes. By planning ahead, teachers can include strategies to help ensure the success of all students.
4. **Connect learning activities to experiences:** Students need to learn the required content by the end of the unit. Learning activities should be designed to utilize the strengths of the students. Determine in what circumstances concrete models and examples could be included to help facilitate understanding.
5. **Choose and list resources:** Be sure to list all of the materials necessary to complete the unit. By planning ahead, teachers will help themselves avoid a last-minute rush to find the materials they will need to complete specific activities.
6. **Choose assessment methods:** Use assessments that determine whether students have met unit objectives. Select a variety of assessments, such as multiple-choice tests, individual or group projects, or research papers.

20. Advantages of clinical teaching. (*See* Q. 3, 2015)

21. Barriers of effective interpersonal relationship.

Psychological barriers: Psychological barriers may include shyness or embarrassment. Sometimes, a person may present herself as being abrupt or difficult when she may actually be nervous.

Cultural barriers: Acceptable styles of communication vary between cultures. In some societies physical gestures are extravagant, and touch is more acceptable. In these societies, it is generally acceptable to hug and touch a person's arm when you are speaking to him.

Language barriers: A communication barrier may be present because the parties do not share a common language. Interpreters and translators may be used to good effect in these circumstances. If a person is deaf or visually impaired, this presents an obvious barrier that needs to be addressed prior to the meeting

Environmental barriers: Environmental barriers to communication can include noise and lack of privacy. An environment which is too hot or cold will not be conducive to effective communication. Some places of business are busy with many distractions, such as constantly ringing telephones and other messaging systems.

22. Attitude scale. (*See* Q. 11, 2016)

2018

Communication and Educational Technology

LONG ESSAYS
1. a. List the clinical teaching methods. b. Explain briefly any two of the clinical teaching methods.
2. a. Define lesson plan. b. Discuss the purposes and steps of lesson planning.
3. a. Define guidance and counseling. b. Explain the importance of guidance and counseling in nursing.

SHORT ESSAYS
4. Advantages of group discussion.
5. Explain the relationship between philosophy and education.
6. Overhead projector.
7. Advantages and disadvantages of objective structured clinical examination.
8. Phases of demonstration.
9. Classification of educational objectives.
10. Principles of teaching.
11. Microteaching and its steps.
12. Purposes of interpersonal relations.

SHORT ANSWERS
13. Nursing care plan.
14. Elements of communication.
15. Any four functions of education.
16. Workshop.
17. Write on principles of audio-visual aids.
18. Essay type questions.
19. Teaching skills.
20. Domains of learning in nursing.
21. Types of assessment.
22. Principles of preparing transparencies.

LONG ESSAYS

1. a. List the clinical teaching methods. b. Explain briefly any two of the clinical teaching methods.

Clinical practice provides an opportunity for students to gain knowledge and skills needed to care for patients. Case method is one of the effective way to develop the learning among nursing students. Case method, case study describes a clinical situation developed around an actual or hypothetical patient for student review and critique. In case method, the case provided for analysis is generally shorter and more specific than in case study. Case studies are more comprehensive in nature, thereby presenting a complete picture of the patient and clinical situation. With case method, student apply concepts and theories to practice situations, identify actual and potential problems and proposed varied approaches to solve them, weigh different decisions possible and arrive at the judgment as to the effectiveness of interventions.

When using case method in teaching situation, problem solving is emphasized and taught in order to acquire the skills and later be able to apply them in new situation. The case method is a student active teaching form that assists students to develop, discuss and test their train of thought regarding problematic situation.

Some cases are designed with the problems readily apparent. With these cases the problem is described clearly and sufficient information is included to guide decisions on how to intervene. Nitko (1996) called these cases well structured, providing an opportunity for students to apply concepts to a patient situation and develop an understanding of how they are used in clinical practice cases of these type, link knowledge presented in class and through reading to practice situation.

2. a. Define lesson plan. b. Discuss the purposes and steps of lesson planning.

Definition

"Lesson plan is actually a plan of action" which includes the working philosophy of the teacher, his knowledge of philosophy, his information about his understanding of his pupil, comprehension of the objectives of education, his knowledge of the material to be taught and his ability to utilize effective method". LB Sands.

Lesson plan is a comprehensive chart of classroom teaching-learning activities. An elastic but systematic approach of the teaching of concepts, skills and attitudes.

Importance of Lesson Planning

1. It makes teaching systematic, orderly and economical.
2. It delimits the field of work of the teacher as well as of the students.
3. It helps to stick on to what is necessary to teach within the stipulated time. Prevents going away from the topic, thus prevents wastage of time and energy of the teacher.
4. Prevents unnecessary repetition.
5. Planning helps the teacher to overcome the feeling of nervousness and insecurity. It gives confidence to the teacher.
6. It gives opportunities to the teacher to think out new ways and means of making the class interesting.
7. Lesson plan helps to link the new knowledge with the previous lesson.
8. It helps the teacher to prepare questions, illustrations, teaching learning aids and activities.
9. Lesson plan enables the teacher to provide for suitable summaries.
10. Lesson plan provides periodical evaluation.

Steps involved in planning a lesson: There are few steps which should be followed while making a lesson plan. These are:
1. **Preparation/introduction:** This in fact, is a means of exploration of the student's knowledge which helps to lead them on to the lesson. The teacher needs to prepare the students to receive new knowledge. She can introduce the lesson by testing the previous knowledge of the student by asking questions. This in turn may reveal their, ignorance; arouse interest and curiosity to learn new matter. Charts, maps, diagrams, pictures also can be used.
2. **Presentation:** The aim of lesson plan should clearly state before the presentation of the subject matter, which helps both the teacher and the student to have a common pursuit.
3. **During presentation:** In this stage both the teacher and the student must actively participate in the teaching learning process. The students must get some new ideas and knowledge.
4. **Questioning**, discussion, appropriate examples from real life situations should feature in presentation to make the presentation interesting and to motivate the students to learn.
    a. Teaching aids: Teaching aids should be used to make the lessons meaningful, clear, explanatory and comprehensive.
    b. Blackboard summary can be developed side-by-side.
5. **Comparison or association:** This step is important where the students are given examples and they are asked to observe carefully and compare them with other set of examples and facts. These will enable the student to deduce definitions and arrive at generalizations on their own.
6. **Generalization:** This step involves reflective thinking. The knowledge presented through the lesson should be thought provoking, innovating and stimulating to assist the students to generalize and untested formula, etc.
7. **Application:** The students make use of the knowledge acquire in familiar and unfamiliar situations and at the same time it tests the validity of the generalizations arrived at by the students. The students of nursing especially need to develop the skill of learning to apply the knowledge and skills gained in the classroom in their day-to-day nursing practice in the wards, clinic and home situations. This makes learning more permanent and worthwhile.
8. **Recapitulation:** This being the last step in the planning of a lesson, understanding and comprehension of the subject matter taught by the teacher can be tested by asking suitable, stimulating and pivotal questions to be students on the topic. This also gives a feedback to the teacher regarding the efficacy of the methods of teaching adopted by her. It tells whether further explanation, clarifications, etc. are needed or not, as well.

3. a. Define guidance and counseling. b. Explain the importance of guidance and counseling in nursing.

1. Guidance refers to an advice and a relevant piece of information provided by a superior, to resolve a problem or overcome from difficulty.
2. Counseling refers to a professional advice given by a counselor and an individual to help him in overcoming from personal or psychological problems. The counseling situation arises when a needy person is face to face with expert who makes available his assistance to the needy individual to fulfill his needs.

Organizing Guidance and Counseling Program in Nursing Educational Institutions

Purposes of Organizing Counseling Services

1. To help adolescents with normal developmental problems.
2. To help individuals through temporary crisis.
3. To identify signs of disturbed/problem behavior at the earliest.
4. To refer cases needing specialist treatment.
5. To facilitate communication within and between the nursing schools, home, the communities and the resources.
6. To support tutors who are helping individuals but who themselves want guidance and reassurance.

Guidance and counseling has made an integral part of higher education to make it meaningful and purposeful for the students.

The kind of guidance and counseling programs can be

1. Inherent (unintentional and unorganized).
2. Informal (intentional but not coordinated).
3. Professional (well-organized).

A well-organized structure covering the three major functions of the program, e.g. adjustmental, oriental, and developmental.

The Organizational Setup

I. **For constituent colleges on the campus:** If 1,000 students on rolls—
1. A counseling officer assisted by guidance committee can plan the program according to their needs and implement the same with the cooperation of deputy chief and academic adviser.
2. If less than 1,000 students, a liaison officer will look after.
3. If more than 1,000 students an assistant counseling officer (lecture scale) may be appointed to assist the counseling officer (reader scale).

II. **For affiliated college at a distance**
1. If 1000 students: Counseling officer assisted by guidance committee implement the activities with the help of vocational guidance officer.
2. If less than 1,000 students, liaison officer will look after.

III. **At universities:** Deans are assisted by HOD of psychology and education—guidance committee, counseling officer can plan the program and implement the activities.

Essential Activities

1. Formation of guidance and counseling committee.
2. To serve in an advisory capacity or a policy making body for the program.
3. The committee can list out problems requiring group solution.
4. It should plan, monthly, quarterly and yearly program.
5. Coordinate guidance activities and assess the work done.

Members in the Committee

1. Dean
2. Counseling/liaison officer
3. Teachers from different specialties and academic disciplines
4. Student representatives

5. Parents
6. Deputy chief
7. Vocational guidance officer
8. Peer group
9. Librarian
10. Warden
11. Medical staff.

The principal has to specify the roles of each faculty member. Clerical assistance will be provided for liaison officer.

Counseling center: Every university and a large college should have a counseling center headed by a (trained professional) counseling officer with PhD or Master's degree in psychology and counseling with considerable experience.

Functions: Gives assistance either or individuals, small groups of students, staff members with special educational, vocational and personal problem. Develops counseling programs and consultation especially on psychological problems.
- Provides psychological testing facility both for individuals and groups.
- Carryout research activities on testing procedures and experimental programs.
- Helps in the training of PG students in counseling and testing.
- Conducts special clinics for developing study skills and reading improvement.

Maintains integrity and confidentiality of the students and groups, faculty will refer the students to it and students too would like to visit and get help from center.

Orientation talks to students and parents to give information regarding:
- The courses of studies.
- Facilities available in the institution like library, workshops, laboratory, playgrounds, fee concessions, etc.

Career talks: Information about a particular job, e.g. themes avenues open to graduates, PG, self-employment schemes, government jobs, abroad jobs.

Career conferences: Providing occupational information for the group of students.

Plan tours: For example, visits to research institutions, professional colleges, etc. provide the students with direct and firsthand experience of the work done and the physical, social environment in which it is done. Starting the cumulative record of students. Identification of students with problems. Arranging personality counseling for low achievers and students with other problems or sending them to specialists.

Tools for Collecting Information

The information collected through the use of these tools should be cumulative; about the individual as a whole based on a variety of sources and tools.

They provide a set of tools for individual assessment without the use of psychological tests. These tools are generally developed by the counselors and teachers themselves.

1. **Interview** is basic tools of counseling. It is described as a conversation with a definite purpose. Information with the help of interview can be collected from the individual student (counselee) herself or from her family members, friends or teachers. Interview permits flexibility, clarity and an opportunity for observation to the counselor. It also provides the counselor with an opportunity to understand the counselee better. At later stages, the understanding forms the basis of therapeutic interview in the process of counseling. Structuring of these interviews helps in making the information more reliable and valid.

2. **Observation** is a careful study of counselee with a specific purpose. Counselor makes the observations either by participating observations, i.e. as a member of the group of counselee—participative or as an outsider—nonparticipative observations. Nonparticipative observations can be made interview or testing or in the classroom, or in the community/ward. Sometimes one-way screens are used to make these observations. By structuring and using rating scale/checklist. These observations can be made more reliable and valid.
3. **Anecdotal records** consists recording important incidents. It is a verbal snapshot of an incident. Case should be taken to record the incident as it has happened. Tutors should be encouraged to participate in it. Decisions should not be made on the basis of a single anecdote.
4. **Cumulative record card** is a method of recording and providing meaningful, significant and comprehensive information about the individual over the years. It is useful in organizing and integrating information collected through the use of different tools. Besides recording attendance and achievement and also it registers pupil's social adjustment in the school, her behavior with other pupils, attitude towards school and teachers. It also contains the counselor's estimate of qualities like hard work, perseverance, tolerance, sociability and such other attributes which make a portrayal of the pupil more complete. Cumulative record card can be maintained either in folder form or file form or card form.

SHORT ESSAYS

4. Advantages of group discussion.

1. **More information:** A group is better equipped as far as information is concerned. An individual cannot have all the information that is available to a group as it consists of several individuals.
2. **Diversity of views:** A group always has the advantage of varied views. This is because a group always has more than one member, and since every member is unique, there is bound to be a variety in their views also. This is also the reason why there are varied approaches to solving a problem. As group decisions tend to cover a greater area, they provide a better insight for decision-making.
3. **Greater acceptability:** The views expressed by a group have more acceptance than those from an individual. This is because the decisions are not imposed, but are part of a larger consensus (general agreement). A group decision is automatically assumed to be more democratic, and the decision of an individual can be perceived as being autocratic (dictatorial).
4. **Expert opinions:** There may be some group decisions that require expert opinion. The group can either include experts or can call them from outside to form a separate group to take a decision on a particular issue.
5. **Degree of involvement:** The members of a group feel involved with a given problem. This minimizes their resistance. It strengthens an organization and facilitates decision-making.
6. **Encourages people's participation:** A group usually provides a platform for people to present their ideas. Group dynamics is more likely to draw out participation from people who may otherwise be hesitant to talk or interact. It encourages people to take an initiative as they feel part of the decision-making process.

5. Explain the relationship between philosophy and education.

Education is the deliberate and systematic influence exerted by the mature person upon the immature through instruction, discipline and the harmonious development of all the powers of the human being, physical, social, intellectual, esthetic, and spiritual, according to their essential hierarchy, by and for their individual and social use, and directed toward the union of the educand with his creator as the final end.

Philosophy and education are so closely connected that one without the other is meaningless. Many bonds unite education with philosophy. A brief discussion of some of these bonds will help to point out the close relationship between philosophy and education.

1. **Natural bonds:** A natural bond signifies an association between two or more things or processes that is rooted in their very nature. There is a natural association between spiritual life and education, as well as the ideals and the cultural standards of the adult generation.
2. **Logical bonds:** The core or heart of any given system of education is found in the ideals it sets out to attain. These ideals are determined through the philosophy. Once ideals have been established, it may be said to follow logically that a system of education must be set up in order to perpetuate them.
3. **Social bonds:** Education aims at the perpetuation of social institutions which are based on a philosophy of the life and the process of society. History is the authentic method of recording in the interests of posterity, human's activities and the progress of human society.
4. **Cultural bonds:** Culture embraces not only the sum total of people's accomplishments, but the ideals and the virtues after which they strive. Therefore, there is a cultural bond between philosophy and education.
5. **Human bonds:** Psychology, or the dealing in human relationship, is the basis for education. A recognized aim of education is to develop the personality of the student. This is done by knowing the individual student and the ideal that will best serve as a model for his education.
6. **Religious bonds:** Philosophy and education are joined by religious bonds in addition to those bonds already mentioned, for education realizes its finest expression in religion.

6. Overhead projector.

The overhead projector is a device for projecting matter written (or drawn) on a transparent plastic sheet (25 x 20 cm) on to a screen. It uses a lamp, lens and mirror arrangement. The versatility of the overhead projector has made it a powerful teaching tool and it has largely replaced the blackboard in the classrooms of affluent countries.

Benefits: Although overhead projectors seem outdated in more technologically advanced classrooms, they provide a valuable backup if the Internet or another technological tool fails to work, and the teacher needs to share visuals with the whole class. Teachers can keep salient information on a transparency to continue with an alternate lesson.

Teachers trying to use more modern ways to communicate information and develop understanding might not consider overhead projectors as their first choice. When overused, they bore students and lose their efficacy. However, they can still prove extremely beneficial when used appropriately.

It has several advantages over the blackboard:
1. The surface area is limitless.
2. Material (including illustrations) can be prepared well in advance.

3. The teacher faces the class all the time and eye-to-eye contact is not lost.
4. The prepared transparencies can be preserved for future use.

The overhead projector also has several advantages over slides:
1. There is no need to darken the room (the students may stay awake!!)
2. Progressive disclosure is very easy.
3. The services of a projectionist are not required.
4. Material can be prepared at short notice by the speaker himself.
5. The material on the stage of the overhead projector can be manipulated, added to, or altered in a way that is not possible with slides.

7. Advantages and disadvantages of objective structured clinical examination.

Objective structured clinical examination (OSCE) was introduced by Harden and his colleagues in 1975. In an objective structured clinical assessment, a series of stations in an examination room is set up to examine students. At each station, students may be asked to carry out a procedure, which may involve taking history, performing preset clinical tasks and diagnosing patients' problems. When performing the clinical tasks, students may often interact with 'patients', who may be healthy volunteers or mock patients. Students also have to answer questions based on their findings and their interpretation. Students are observed and scored at some stations by examiners with checklists.

Advantages of Objective Structured Clinical Examinations
1. Provides a uniform marking scheme for examiners and consistent examination scenarios for students.
2. It provides an authentic way to assess medical students including pressure from patients.
3. Generates formative feedback for both the learners and the teaching program. Immediate feedback collected may improve students' competency at subsequent stations and even enhance the quality of the learning experience.
4. Minimizes the effect of cueing: When students go to a station, they will need to diagnose patients' problems or carry out some clinical procedures. When they go to a subsequent station, they have to answer some questions relevant to their diagnosis or clinical tasks. However, students cannot go back to correct any mistakes or omissions on what they did in the previous station.
5. More students can be examined at any one time. When a student is carrying out a procedure, another student who has already completed that stage is answering the question at another station.
6. In the objective structured clinical examination, the setting is more controlled (only two variables exist: The patient and the examiner) and a more objective assessment of the student's clinical competency can be made.
7. Provides more insights about students' clinical and interactive competencies.
8. It can objectively assess other important aspects of clinical expertise, such as physical examination skills, interpersonal skills, technical skills, problem-solving abilities, decision-making abilities, and patient treatment skills.

Disadvantages of Objective Structured Clinical Examinations

1. It requires an extensive amount of organizing.
2. It is expensive in terms of manpower, resources and time (such as number of examiners, patients, and even space of examination room).
3. It may discourage students from looking at the patient as a whole because the students' knowledge and skills are being put into compartments.
4. The assessment examines a narrow range of knowledge and skills and does not test for history-taking competency properly. Students only examine a number of different patients in isolation at each station instead of comprehensively examining a single patient.

8. Phases of demonstration.

Entire demonstration can be divided into three phases namely, the planning and preparation phase, performance phase and evaluation phase.

1. **Planning and preparation phase:** In this phase, the teacher prepares herself, procures and arranges article and creates a conducive environment suitable to the group. Well set objectives, content may be prepared. It is ideal to use a procedure manual prepared by the faculty. If a mock patient is required, plan for their comfort and safely. Ensure adequacy and good working condition of equipments, and assemble equipment in a convenient order plan for return demonstration by the students which help to gain skill, clarify their doubts and gain confident in performing the procedure independently. This is to prepare students, so that they can perform the procedure in the real situation, i.e. on a patient in the hospital or in a family in the community, etc.
2. **Performance phase:** In this phase, the teacher performs the demonstration. She performs the steps in sequence with appropriate explanation. Explain the name and use of articles kept ready. Explain the purposes and scientific principles and give appropriate rationale for the steps. Whenever possible encourage students to seek clarification on replace equipment and explain the after care of equipment. Explain how to record the procedure. Performance phase may be concluded with a discussion.
3. **Evaluation phase:** This phase is mainly through return demonstration.

9. Classification of educational objectives.

The objectives of a curriculum must be decided after considering various sources of information that provide a basis for wise and comprehensive decisions about the objectives. A comprehensive philosophy of education is necessary guide in making the decisions.

Purposes of Educational Objectives

1. To prepare the nurses for rendering (provide) community services through primary health.
2. To prepare nurses for providing education at institutional level.
3. To prepare nurse education to handle teaching learning situation in all the clinical areas.

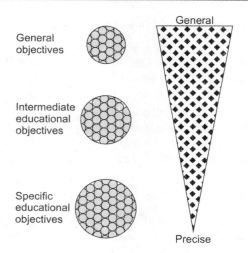

Definitions
1. Objectives are the behaviors to be displayed by a learner, aims are for the teacher and objectives are for the learners to achieve through the support and guidance of the teacher.
2. Objectives are the statement of those changes in behavior which are desired as a result of specific learner and teacher activity which is a two-way process.

Classifications of Objectives

I. **General objectives:** General objectives corresponding to the function of the learner after completion of the education objectives or the program of school, e.g.
1. Providing preventing and curative care to individual and the community in health and sickness.
2. Health education of the public will depend on the population's general level of education.
3. Obtain health histories and make general health assessments.
4. Provide safe and competence care in emergency situation and acute illness.
5. Provide supportive care to person with chronic terminal health problems.
6. Provide health teaching, guidance and counseling.
7. Assist persons to maintain optimal health status.
8. Provide leadership responsibility for planning and evaluating nursing care.
9. Work effectively with all persons concerned with healthcare problem.

II. **Intermediate objectives:** One arrived at by breaking down the professional functions into component activities which together indicate the nature of those functions. For example, planning and carrying out blood sampling session for a group of adults in the community.

These components are professional activities which in twin can be broken down into more specific act that one called, Professional tasks as long as they can be measure against given criteria. Sometime, there can be several intermediate levels rather than a single one.
1. Intermediate objectives reflect the health needs of a population living in a given context.
2. Objectives act only a means or working instrument and not an end itself.
3. Objects were drawn up as a basis for choosing instruments of evaluation for measuring the skills of students.

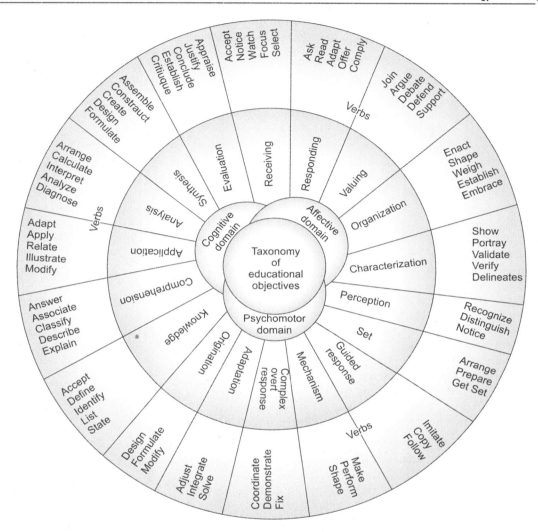

III. Specific or instructional objectives (professional tasks):

Definition: Instructional objectives are descriptions of performance the instruction is expected to produce:

1. Defining objectives help to identify the terminal outcomes of instruction in terms of observable performance of learners.
2. These outcomes are to be presented in behavioral terms.

Steps in formulating cognitive domain: McGuire (1963) described the levels in cognitive domain:

Recall of facts: Remembering the fact, principles, processes, patterns, methods necessary for efficient performance of a professional task.

Interpretation of data: The process of application or use of ideas, principles, methods to deal with a new phenomenon or situation.

Problem-solving: Relating to diagnosis, treatment, organization and so on. It includes finding solutions for problem arising from new situations. It will serve as a guide.

Bloom's categories in cognitive domain:

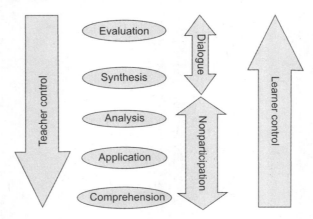

Bloom's taxonomy refers to a classification of the different objectives that educators set for students (learning objectives). The taxonomy was first presented in 1956 through the publication 'The Taxonomy of Educational Objectives' by Benjamin Bloom, an educational psychologist at the University of Chicago.

1. **Evaluation:** Ability to judge the value.
2. **Synthesis:** Ability to put parts together.
3. **Analysis:** Break apart material.
4. **Application:** Ability to put to use.
5. **Comprehension:** Understanding ability to grasp meaning.

I. Knowledge: Exhibit memory of previously-learned materials by recalling facts, terms, basic concepts and answers. Knowledge is (here) defined as the remembering (recalling) of appropriate, previously learned information.

1. **Knowledge of specifics-recall** of specific and isolable bits of information. This emphasis is on symbols with concrete referents.
    a. Knowledge of terminology-knowledge of the referents for specific symbols—verbal and nonverbal.
    b. Knowledge of specific facts—knowledge of dates, events, person, places, etc.
2. **Knowledge of ways and means** of dealing with specific—knowledge of the ways of organizing, studying, judging and criticizing.
    a. **Knowledge of conventions:** Knowledge of characteristic ways of treating and presenting ideas and phenomena.
    b. **Knowledge of trends and sequences:** Knowledge of the processes, directions and movements of phenomena with respect to time.
    c. **Knowledge of classifications and categories:** Knowledge of the classes, sets, divisions and arrangements which are regarded as fundamental for a given subject field, purpose, argument or problem.
    d. **Knowledge of criteria:** Knowledge of criteria by which facts, principles, opinions and conduct are tested or judged.
    e. **Knowledge of methodology:** Knowledge of scientific methods for evaluating health concepts.

3. **Knowledge of the universals and abstractions in a field:** Knowledge of major schemes and patterns by which phenomena and idea are organized.
    a. **Knowledge of principles and generalizations:** Knowledge of particular abstractions which summarize observations of phenomena.
    b. **Knowledge of theories and structures:** Knowledge of body of principles and generalizations together with their interrelations which present a clear, rounded and systematic view of a complex phenomena, problem or field.

II. **Comprehension:** Demonstrative understanding of facts and ideas by organizing, comparing, translating, interpreting, giving descriptions, and stating main ideas:
1. **Translation:** Comprehension as evidenced by the care and accuracy with which the communication is paraphrased or rendered from one language or form of communication to another. Translation is judged on the basis of faithfulness and accuracy, that is, on the extent to which the material in the original communication is preserved although the form of communication has been altered.
2. **Interpretation:** The explanation or summarization of a communication. Whereas translation involves an objective part-for-part rendering of a communication, interpretation involves a reordering, rearrangement or new view of a material.
3. **Extrapolation:** The extension of trends or tendencies beyond the given data to determine implications, consequences, corollaries, effects, etc. which are in accordance with the conditions described in the original communication.

III. **Application:** Using new knowledge. Solve problems to new situations by applying acquired knowledge, facts, techniques and rules in a different way. The use of previously learned information in new and concrete situations to solve problems that have single or best answers. Application is the use of abstractions in particular and concrete situations. The abstractions may also be technical principles, ideas and theories which must be remembered and applied.

IV. **Analysis:** Examine and break information into parts by identifying motives or causes. The breakdown of a communication into its constituent elements or parts such that the relative hierarchy of ideas is made clear and/or the relations between the ideas expressed are made explicit. Such analyses are intended to clarify the communication is organized and the way in which it manages to convey its effects, as well as its basis and arrangement.
1. **Analysis of elements:** Identification of the elements included in a communication.
2. **Analysis of relationships:** The connections and interactions between element and parts of a communication.
3. **Analysis of organizational principles:** The organization, systematic arrangement and structure which hold the communication together. This includes 'explicit' as well as 'implicit' structure. It includes the bases, necessary arrangement and mechanics which make the communication a unit.

V. **Synthesis:** Creatively or divergently applying prior knowledge and skills to produce a new or original whole. Compile information together in a different way by combining elements in a new pattern or proposing alternative solutions.
1. **Production of a unique communication:** The development of a communication in which the writer or speaker attempts to convey ideas, feelings and/or experiences to others.
2. **Production of a plan or proposed set of operations:** The development of a plan of work or the proposal of a plan of operations. The plan should satisfy requirements of the task which may be given to the student or which he may develop for himself.
3. **Derivation of a set of abstract relations:** The development of a set of abstract relations either to classify or explain particular data or phenomena or the deduction of propositions and relations from a set of basic propositions or symbolic representations.

VI. **Evaluation:** Judging the value of material based on personal values/opinions resulting in an end product with a given purpose without real right or wrong answers. Present and defend opinions by making judgments about information, validity of ideas or quality of work based on a set of criteria.
1. Judgments in terms of internal evidence: evaluation of the accuracy of a communication from such evidence as logical accuracy, consistency and other internal criteria.
2. Judgments in terms of external criteria: evaluation of material with reference to selected or remembered criteria.

10. Principles of teaching.

Principle of motivation: It creates curiosity among students to learn new things.

Principle of activity (learning by doing): Froebel's Kindergarten (KG) system is based on this principle. It includes both physical and mental activities. For example, students are asked to make charts and models.

Principle of interest: By generating genuine interest among the learner's community, the effectiveness of the teaching-learning process can be increased.

Principle of linking with life: Life is a continuous experience, and learning linked with life can be more enduring.

Principle of definite aim: This is important for optimum utilization of teaching resources and making learning more focused.

Principle of recognizing individual differences: Every student is unique in term of intelligence, attitude, abilities and potentialities, socioeconomic background. The teaching method should be devised in such a manner to make all the students to avail equal opportunities in life.

Principle of selection: The horizon of knowledge is expanding each day. The teacher should be able to pick contents that can be more relevant and update to the learner's objectives.

Principle of planning: Every teacher has certain time-bound objectives, and hence, teaching should be systematic to make optimum use of resources within the time limit.

Principle of division: To make learning easier, the subject matter should be divided into units, and there should be links between the units.

Principle of revision: To make learning enduring, the acquired knowledge should be revised immediately and repeatedly.

Principle of certain and recreation: This principle is a must to make classroom environment humorous and creative.

Principle of democratic dealing: It entails students in planning and executing different activities; It helps in developing self-confidence and self-respect among the learner's.

11. Microteaching and its steps. (*See* Q. 3, 2016)

12. Purposes of interpersonal relations.

Interpersonal relationship skills refer to the ability to build rapport with individuals having similar interests and goals as we do. In a workplace, interpersonal relationship skills allow us to share a special bond with our coworkers such that trust and positive feelings for one another are maintained.

Interpersonal relationship skills at workplace allow a better understanding among employees as well as more effective communication. For individuals spending, on average, seven to eight hours of their day at work, it is irrational to believe they can work all by themselves. So we all ought to have healthy interpersonal relationships at work in order to be able to have a friendly ambience.
1. To enhance your speaking skills
2. To boost your confidence
3. To groom your personality
4. With interpersonal communication we try to interact with others and hence we get to know others.

In our life interpersonal relationship is more important. It is the communication where the people exchange information, feelings. Actually it is face-face communication. Being able to communicate well with others is often essential to solving problems that unavoidably occur both in our private and profession. The purpose of an interpersonal relationship is to actively and continually facilitate the personal growth and development of each other as individuals, to enjoy the process together as it unfolds, to maximize ease, and to have fun doing it.

SHORT ANSWERS

13. Nursing care plan.

A nursing care plan (NCP) is a formal process that includes correctly identifying existing needs, as well as recognizing potential needs or risks. Care plans also provide a means of communication among nurses, their patients, and other healthcare providers to achieve health care outcomes. Without the nursing care planning process, quality and consistency in patient care would be lost.

Objectives: The following are the goals and objectives of writing a nursing care plan:
1. Promote evidence-based nursing care and to render pleasant and familiar conditions in hospitals or health centers.
2. Support holistic care which involves the whole person including physical, psychological, social and spiritual in relation to management and prevention of the disease.
3. Establish programs, such as care pathways and care bundles. Care pathways involve a team effort in order to come to a consensus with regards to standards of care and expected outcomes, while care bundles are related to best practice with regards to care given for a specific disease.
4. Identify and distinguish goals and expected outcome.
5. Review communication and documentation of the care plan.
6. Measure nursing care.

14. Elements of communication.   (*See* Q. 13, 2016)

15. Any four functions of education.

1. Development of inborn potentialities—education helps the child to develop the inborn potentialities of child providing scope to develop.
2. Modifying behavior—education helps to modify the past behavior through learning and through different agencies of education.
3. All-round development—education aims at the all-round development of child—physical, mental, social, emotional, and spiritual.

4. Preparing for the future—after completion of education the child can earn its livelihood getting proper education, which has productivity. The education should be imparted according to the own interest of the child.
5. Developing personality—the whole personality of the child is developed physically, intellectually, morally, socially, aesthetically and spiritually. He is recognized in the society.
6. Helping for adjustability—man differs from beast. Man has reasoning and thinking power. Man tries his best to adjust with his own environment through education.

16. Workshop.

A workshop is an instructional situation which is used for the following purposes: 1. It is used to realize the higher cognitive and psychomotor objectives. 2. It is a technique which can be effectively used for developing understanding and proficiency for the approaches and practice in education.

Functions of Workshop

1. The workshop method is used to seek, explore and identify the solutions to a problem; to permit the extensive study of a situation, its background and its social and philosophical implications.
2. It is used for teachers for giving awareness and training of new practices and innovation in education.
3. It provides an opportunity to prepare specific professional, vocational or community, service functions. A high degree of individual participation is encouraged. It permits group determination of goal and method.

17. Write on principles of audio-visual aids.

They should have in the realization of desired learning objectives. They should be the true representatives of the real things. It should be interesting and motivating. They should suit the age level, grade level, and other characteristics of the learners:

1. **Principles of selection:** Students may be associated in the preparation of aids. The teachers themselves should prepare some of the aids. The teachers should receive some training in the preparation of aids. As far as possible locally available material should be used.
2. **Principles of preparation:** Arrangement of keeping aids safely and also to facilitate their lending to the teachers for use.
3. **Principles of handling:** The aid should be displayed properly so that all the students are able to see it, observe it and derive maximum benefit out of it. Adequate care should be taken to handle an aid in such a way as no damage is done it. They should fully familiar themselves with the use and manipulation of the aids. Teachers should carefully visualize the use of teaching aids before their actual presentation.
4. **Principles of presentation:** Continuous evaluation is necessary. Teachers guide the students to respond activity to the AV stimuli.

18. Essay type questions.

An essay test may give full freedom to the students to write any number of pages. The required response may vary in length. An essay type question requires the pupil to plan his own answer and to explain it in his own words. The pupil exercises considerable freedom to select, organize and present his ideas. Essay type tests provide a better indication of pupil's real achievement in learning. The answers provide a clue to nature and quality of the pupil's thought process.

Advantages of the Essay Tests

1. It is relatively easier to prepare and administer a six-question extended- response essay test than to prepare and administer a comparable 60-item multiple-choice test items.
2. It is the only means that can assess an examinee's ability to organize and present his ideas in a logical and coherent fashion.
3. It can be successfully employed for practically all the school subjects.
4. Some of the objectives, such as ability to organize idea effectively, ability to criticise or justify a statement, ability to interpret, etc. can be best measured by this type of test.
5. Logical thinking and critical reasoning, systematic presentation, etc. can be best developed by this type of test.
6. It helps to induce good study habits, such as making outlines and summaries, organizing the arguments for and against, etc.
7. The students can show their initiative, the originality of their thought and the fertility of their imagination as they are permitted freedom of response.
8. The responses of the students need not be completely right or wrong. All degrees of comprehensiveness and accuracy are possible.
9. It largely eliminates guessing.
10. They are valuable in testing the functional knowledge and power of expression of the pupil.

Limitations of Essay Tests

1. One of the serious limitations of the essay tests is that these tests do not give scope for larger sampling of the content. You cannot sample the course content so well with six lengthy essay questions as you can with 60 multiple-choice test items.
2. Such tests encourage selective reading and emphasise cramming.
3. Moreover, scoring may be affected by spelling, good handwriting, colored ink, neatness, grammar, length of the answer, etc.
4. The long-answer type questions are less valid and less reliable, and as such they have little predictive value.
5. It requires an excessive time on the part of students to write; while assessing, reading essays is very time-consuming and laborious.
6. It can be assessed only by a teacher or competent professionals.
7. Improper and ambiguous wording handicaps both the students and valuers.
8. Mood of the examiner affects the scoring of answer scripts.
9. There is halo effect-biased judgement by previous impressions.
10. The scores may be affected by his personal bias or partiality for a particular point of view, his way of understanding the question, his weightage to different aspect of the answer, favoritism and nepotism, etc.

19. Teaching skills.

There are a number of teaching skills that all educators should have. While some teaching skills may vary from teacher to teacher, there are still a few personal skills that are important for all teachers to possess. In addition to being knowledgeable in your area of expertise and having the ability to plan and execute lesson plans, successful teachers also need to possess a few "Extra" personal skills. These specialized teaching skills will not only help you be an effective teacher, but a successful one as well. If you do not already have, the following are, essential skills:

1. **Patience teaching skills:** One of the most important qualities a teacher can have is patience. Without patience, you are going to have a really hard time being an effective teacher. Children tend to like to test their teachers' patience, so if you tend to lose your

patience easily, and get angry quickly, then being an educator is not a job for you. Patience is a quality that will help you be successful in the classroom.
2. **Creativity:** Successful teachers are creative in many ways. They have the ability to think outside of the box, use the resources that they have to create amazing lessons and activities, and come up with creative ways to handle discipline in the classroom.
3. **Communication and collaboration:** Having the skill set to be able to communicate and collaborate with others is an extremely important personal skill to have as an educator. Whether you are communicating with students, parents or colleagues, teachers need this skill in order to be successful at their job. Teachers need the ability to communicate important information, as well as understand different perspectives.
4. **Likeable personality:** Another personal skill all teachers should foster is an engaging and likeable personality. Even if you may be an introvert (which many teachers usually are NOT), you can still cultivate a likeable personality in the classroom. This does not mean that you have to be a comedian and make your students laugh every chance that you get, it only means that a teacher who has the ability to engage their students and have a relationship with them will only make the class more interesting and fun to be in.
5. **Self-discipline:** In order to discipline your students, you need to have self-discipline. Having self-discipline means that you have the willpower and the control to not be affected when your students are misbehaving. You are firm and fair with your discipline techniques, and have the ability to not let your students walk all over you. This is an essential personal trait that teachers need to have in order to be successful in their classroom.

20. Domains of learning in nursing.

Cognitive domain: The cognitive domain involves the development of our mental skills and the acquisition of knowledge. The six categories under this domain are: Knowledge, comprehension, application, analysis, synthesis and evaluation.

Affective domain: The affective domain involves our feelings, emotions and attitudes. This domain is categorized into five subdomains which include: Receiving phenomena, responding to phenomena, valuing, organization and characterization.

Psychomotor domain: The psychomotor domain is comprised of utilizing motor skills and coordinating them. The seven categories under this include: Perception, set, guided response, mechanism, complex overt response, adaptation and origination.

21. Types of assessment

1. Formative assessment: Formative assessment is an integral part of teaching and learning
2. Summative assessment.
3. Authentic' or work-integrated assessment
4. Diagnostic assessment
5. Dynamic assessment
6. Synoptic assessment
7. Criterion referenced assessment
8. Ipsative assessment.

22. Principles of preparing transparencies.

1. Prepare a rough design.
2. Drawing, lettering should be restricted to a rectangular message area of about 6" x 9".

3. Visual ideas, such as charts, graphs, pictures, maps, etc. in addition to keypoints can be drawn and written.
4. Have one basic idea in each transparency.
5. Use simple lettering. Have letter size of ¼" height with sufficient spacing.
6. Use underlines to draw attention.
7. Avoid vertical composition.
8. Minimum verbiage.
9. The three 8 principle viz. 8 lines per transparency, 8 words per line and not less than 8 mm letter height shall be followed in writing/typing the transparency.
10. Sufficient line space(1½ letter height between lines) should be given.
11. Use ruled paper backing while writing sentences.
12. Use 2–3 colors.
13. Transparencies should be serially mounted and numbered.

2017

Communication and Educational Technology

LONG ESSAYS
1. Define communication; explain the steps in communication process.
2. What is the role of counselor in nursing education. Explain the organization of counseling services in nursing educational institutions.
3. Describe aims, functions and principles of nursing education.

SHORT ESSAYS
4. Different phases of interpersonal relationships.
5. Importance of teamwork in nursing education.
6. Maxims of teaching.
7. Characteristics of an educational objectives.
8. Process recording.
9. Managing disciplinary problems.
10. Philosophy of idealism.
11. Microteaching.
12. Describe the characteristics of learning.

SHORT ANSWERS
13. List four 3-dimensional aids.
14. Advantages of field trip.
15. Use of pamphlets in education.
16. List four issues for counseling in nursing students.
17. Advantages of multiple choice questions.
18. Uses of slides.
19. Define health education and health behavior.
20. Types of chalkboard.
21. List down the purposes of evaluation.
22. Barriers in effective group discussion.

LONG ESSAYS

1. Define communication. Explain the steps in communication process
(*See* Q. 2, 2014)

2. What is the role of counselor in nursing education. Explain the organization of counseling services in nursing educational institutions.

Everyone in this universe come across some problem or other irrespective of their age, sex, and occupation or profession, for which from time immemorial man has been talking help of elders, parents, friends and teachers in solving their problem. In the field of education, most teachers provide a high standard of pupil care but it is fact that they have little talent and attitude of counsellor. It requires special knowledge and attitudes to recognize the problem and help an individual's pupils.

Role of counselor in nursing education: Counselors provide support to people experiencing emotional difficulties by helping them to identify and work through their issues. A Counselor uses techniques, such as talking therapy to assist people to reach their own resolutions or develop strategies to address and remedy their concerns.
1. Pupil appraisal---using appropriate test and nontesting devices.
2. Pupil orientation---involving tutors, wardens, librarians, doctors, and other resources.
3. Helping emotionally disturbed pupil-using counseling techniques.
4. Helping pupil overcome academic and social deficiencies.
5. Helping pupil overcome their financial, health, sex, residential and messing problems.
6. Gaining cooperation from other tutors and helping them in gaining understanding of the pupils.
7. Gaining cooperation from parents and other personnel of the counseling process.
8. Maintaining up-to-date records of pupils concerning counseling.
9. Arranging for referral services for those who need them.
10. Evaluating and doing the follow-up work.
11. Giving career talks to potential entrants to the nursing profession.
12. Disseminating information relating to employment, recreational and professional opportunities.

Organization of counseling services in nursing educational institutions:
Types or forms of the organization of counseling services in educational institutions are:
1. Centralization counseling services: The entire responsibilities of the guidance and counseling services is vested upon a group of trained personnel of the department of guidance and counseling services.
2. Decentralization counseling services: The responsibilities of the counseling services are vested upon teachers.
3. Combination of centralized and decentralized counseling services: In this mixed form, guidance and counseling services are provided by teachers and expert collectively.

Purposes of organization counseling services:
1. To help individuals with normal development problems.
2. To help individuals through a temporary crisis during the different stages of life.
3. To identify signs of disturbed behavior at early stage, so manage it.
4. To refer critical cases to specialists for best possible management.

5. To facilitate communication within and between nursing institutions and homes.
6. To support not only the tutors/nursing faculty who are helping individuals but also who themselves want guidance and reassurance at times.

Ingredients of guidance and counseling services:
1. The admission service ---admitting the right candidates for the right course, selecting those candidates most likely.
2. The orientation service ---a "welcome service" as it is concerned with welcoming fresher's to the world of nursing.
3. The student information service ---assist the student to obtain a realistic picture of his abilities, interests, personality characteristics, achievements, levels of aspiration, state of health, etc.
4. The information service-- information provide usually related to education, occupational and personal-social.
5. The counseling service ---understand what he can do and what he should do, handle his difficulties in a rational way, make his own decision, etc.
6. The placement service--- help students to be in proper scholastic track, to realize their career expectations, organize campus selection interviews, provide information regarding current trends, etc.
7. The remedial service--- it is mainly oriented towards helping students to improve their study habits, improve their adjustment in the clinical area, reducing stress, etc.
8. The follow-up service-- it is that review or systematic evaluation which is carried out to find out whether guidance services in particular and educational program in general satisfies the needs of the students.

3. Describe aims (*See* Q. 2, 2016), functions and principles of nursing education.

Functions of Nursing Education

Nursing education must supply the nation with RNs prepared for a wide range of roles and responsibilities: Providing direct care to patients in hospitals, nursing homes, and patients' homes; helping to safeguard the health of community and school populations; assisting with ambulatory care of individuals and families; performing clinical nurse specialist services; administering nursing services at both middle and top management levels; conducting nursing research; and providing professional and educational leadership to the profession.

Principles of Nursing Education

1. Entry gates the nursing profession must control entry to the profession.
2. Level of award the level of award on completion of nursing education programs should be at the level of a first degree.
3. Accountability at the point of registration: At the point of registration nurses are accountable for their own practice.
4. Knowledge development: The creation of knowledge for the discipline of nursing and its application to the needs of society is as integral to nursing education as the communication of knowledge.
5. Practice experience: Appropriate high quality practice experience delivered in partnership with practice is an essential element of nursing educational programs with a practice component.

6. **Teaching nursing:** Nursing must be taught by expert nurses who will be supported, where appropriate, by contributions from other academic and professional colleagues and users of nursing services.
7. **Continuing professional development (CPD) and lifelong learning (LLL):** All nurses must embrace and engage in the principles of continuing professional development.
8. **Support for students:** Nursing students at all levels require adequate financial and pastoral support in order to complete their courses successfully.
9. **Workforce planning:** A rigorous system of workforce planning is essential in order to underpin educational commissioning.
10. **Free movement of labor:** It is essential that the nursing strategies to ensure free movement across the countries.
11. **Multiprofessional education:** Professions who work together should learn together.
12. **Nursing in higher education:** Nursing must be treated equitably alongside other disciplines in higher education.

SHORT ESSAYS

4. Different phases of interpersonal relationships.

Dr Hildegard Peplau, in her book, Interpersonal Relations in Nursing, presented a thorough analysis of Harry Stack Sullivan's interpersonal theory in psychiatry and gave nursing a sound conceptual model for practice. Although, other nurse scholars have developed other models and changed forms of the interpersonal model, Peplau's contribution regarding the phases of the nurse-client relationship remains applicable. Following is a brief summary of the phases and their purposes, with associated functions of the nurse in each phase.

I. **Orientation phase:** The purposes of the orientation phase include:
   1. Introduction of nurse and client.
   2. Elaboration of the client's need to recognize and understand both his difficulty and the extent of his need for help.
   3. Acceptance of the client's need for assistance in recognizing and planning to use services that professional personnel can offer.
   4. Agreement that the client will direct energies toward the mutual responsibility for defining, understanding, and meeting productively the problem at hand.
   5. Clarification of limitations and responsibilities in the delivery system environment.

   When the nurse and the client validate understanding of the client's need for help and acceptance of resources to meet those needs, and they do so with feelings of shared responsibility and a sense of trust, they move into a new phase of the relationship.

II. **Identification phase:** The purposes of the identification phase include:
   1. Provision of the opportunity for the client to respond to the helpers offer to assist.
   2. Encouragement for the client to express what he feels to reorient his feelings and strengthen positive forces.
   3. Provision of the opportunity for the nurse and the client to clearly understand each other's preconceptions and expectations.

III. **Exploitation phase:** The purposes of the exploitation phase include:
   1. Full utilization of the nurse-client relationship to mutually work on the solution to problems and the changes needed to improve health.
   2. Provision of opportunities for the client to explore earlier experiences and behaviors and to have emerging needs met.

IV. **Resolution phase:** The purposes of the resolution phase include:
1. Provision of opportunity to formulate new goals.
2. Encouragement of gradual freeing of the client from identifying with the nurse.
3. Promotion of the client's ability to act more independently.

Overlapping in various stages, the following roles of the professional nurse tend to emerge as the nurse promotes growth (change) in the client:
I. **Orientation phase:** Stranger
II. **Identification phase:**
   1. Unconditional mother surrogate
   2. Resource person
   3. Teacher
   4. Leader
   5. Counselor
   6. Surrogate
III. **Exploitation phase:** The adult support person in new enactment of the aforementioned roles.
IV. **Resolution phase:** Same adult roles.

It should be noted that the nurse moves back and forth in some of these roles in the various phases. Essentially, however, as the client's needs are met, more mature needs arise; thus the need for more mature roles.

5. Importance of teamwork in nursing education.

1. **Improved patient satisfaction and outcome:** Healthcare professionals serve patients not as individual providers, but as multidisciplinary teams. These teams include nurses, primary care physicians, and specialists. Ideally, every individual on the team works together toward the common goal of enhancing the patient's health and providing the highest possible level of care.
2. **Higher job satisfaction:** Nursing careers may present possible challenges, from long hours to high-stress situations. It is crucial for professionals in this field to maintain a high level of job satisfaction to avoid potential burnout.
3. **Increased professional accountability:** Teamwork contributes directly to accountability in nursing. Daily huddles enhance this by keeping nurses in the loop and reinforce changes to policies and procedures.
4. **Lower rates of job turnover:** Employee turnover is a major problem for hospitals. Nursing Solutions, Inc.'s National Health Care Retention and RN Staffing Report revealed that employee turnover in hospitals was 16.2% in 2016. The turnover rate for RNs was slightly lower at 14.6%, but certified nursing assistants had the highest turnover rate of all the reported occupations, at 24.6%. RNs in surgical services, women's health, and pediatrics had the lowest rates of turnover, while those in behavior health and emergency care had the highest turnover.
5. **Improved engagement in the workplace:** Employee engagement is closely linked to workplace relationships. In a research report by the Society for Human Resource Management, 77 percent of employees said that relationships with their coworkers contributed to their engagement. Sixty-four percent felt that engagement was improved when they knew the people in their work group would not give up in the face of difficulties, and 65% were more engaged when their colleagues could quickly adapt to challenges or crises.

6. Maxims of teaching. *(See Q. 2, 2015)*

7. Characteristics of educational objectives.

1. **Institutional objectives:** When the objectives describe the broad over all aspects of an organization or institution or school, they are called institutional objectives. e.g. providing curative care to the individual in sickness.
2. **Intermediate objectives:** These are developed from the institutional objectives. They are broader than the specific objectives. For example, they are prepared at the level of departments in an institution, planning and carrying out a blood sampling session for a group of adults in the community.
3. **Instructional objectives:** They are specific, precise and narrow at the level of a short learning period. They are also called as specific objectives.

8. Process recording.

Process recording is a form of recording used frequently by the caseworker. In this type, the process of interview is reported and is a rather detailed description of what transpired with considerable paraphrasing. It preserves a sequence in which the various matters were discussed. It includes not only what both the worker and the client said but also significant reaction of the client and changes in mood and response. In this the interview and observation go hand-in-hand. It may be verbatim or nonverbatim reproduction.

Purposes
- To modify subsequent behavior, resulting in improved quality of therapeutic communication and nursing care.
- To critically analyze communication and its effects on behavior of the individual.
- To know about the patients illness and to understand the psychodynamics of illness.
- To establish rapport with the patient.
- To gain the patients confidence and get his co-operation.
- Assists the nurse to plan, structure and evaluate the interaction on a conscious level rather than an intuitive level.

Advantages
- Process recording helps in differentiating thoughts and feelings.
- Helps to clarify the purpose of the interview or intervention.
- Helps to improve written expression.
- Helps in identifying strengths and weakness.
- Helps to improve self awareness.
- Helps to separate facts from judgments.
- Helps to explore the interplay of values operating between the student and the patient system through an analysis of the filtering process used in recording the session.

Disadvantages
- It is more time-consuming as the clinical instructor may take more time to make an evaluation about an individual student.
- Technical problems are frequent and become a source of frustration.
- The process is laborious because it requires actual observation and subsequent participation by the clinical instructor during student–patient interviews.

9. Managing disciplinary problems.

The term discipline refers to the orderly activities by a person in their progress towards the attainment of some goal which either they themselves desire or which someone desires for them.

How to Prevent Discipline Problems
1. Be organized
2. Deal with **problems** while they are still small
3. Have good control procedures
4. Teach your procedures well
5. Keep your students engaged
6. Move around the classroom
7. Develop a rapport with your students
9. Be professional.

Help students to develop self discipline.
1. Use discipline to strengthen the students self control, self direction and sense of responsibility
2. Do not use discipline for self revenge
3. Disciplinary talks should be made in private/confidentially.

Principles/ general guidelines for managing disciplinary problems
1. Give students good standards of conduct, instead of rules
2. Use a positive approach, not a negative approach.
3. Offer a challenge. Most students respond whole heartedly to a challenge, if it is within the scope of their abilities.
4. Definitely relate act of misconduct to the act of correction, otherwise it is not educative
5. Do not punish the whole group for the mistake done by one or two individuals
6. Do not let disciplinary measures interfere with other educative activities.

10. Philosophy of idealism.

Idealism is the metaphysical and epistemological doctrine that ideas or thoughts make up fundamental reality. Essentially it is any philosophy which argues that the only thing actually knowable is consciousness, whereas we never can be sure that matter or anything in the outside world really exists thus the only the real things are mental entities not physical things which exist only in the sense that they are perceived. A broad definition of idealism could include many religious viewpoints although an idealistic viewpoint need not necessarily include God, supernatural beings or existences after death. In general parlance, "idealism" is also used to describe a person's high ideals (principles or values actively pursued as a goal) the word "ideal" is also commonly used as an adjective to designate qualities of perfection, desirability and excellence.

Definition: "Idealistic philosophy takes many and varied forms but the postulate underlying all this is that mind or spirit is the essential world stuff, that the rule reality is a material character".

Idealism in education: Idealism pervades all the creation and it is an underlying, unlimited and ultimate force which regions supreme overall mind and matter. They all advocate its great importance in education and lay more emphasis on aims and principles of education than on models, aids and devices.

Idealism and aims of education: The following are the aims of education according to the philosophy of idealism:

Self-realization or exhalation of personality: According to the idealism man is the most creation of God. Self-realization involves full of knowledge of the self and it is the first aim of education. "The aim of education especially associated with idealism is the exhalation of personality or self-realization it is the making actual or real personalities of the self."

To ensure spiritual development: Idealistic give greater importance to spiritual values in comparison with material attainments. The second aim of education is to develop the child mentally, morally and above all spiritually. "Education must enable mankind through its culture to enter more and more fully into the spiritual realm".

Development of intelligences and rationality: "In all things their regions an external law this all pervading energetic, self conscious and hence eternal law this all pervading energetic. This unity is God. Education should lead and guide man to face with nature and to unity and God".

Idealism and curriculum: Idealists give more importance to thoughts, feelings ideals and values than to the child and his activities. They firmly hold that curriculum should be concerned with the whole humanity and its experience.

11. Microteaching. *(See* Q. 3, 2016)

12. Describe the characteristics of learning. *(See* Q. 2, 2015)

SHORT ANSWERS

13. List four 3-dimensional aids.

Three-dimensional aids: All the AV materials, three-dimensional aids are nearest to living experiences. This side, such as models and Mock-ups are replies or reconstructions of the real thing. They are contrived experiences where reality is altered or simplified for teaching purposes.

Models: Recognizable three-dimensional representation of real things.

Objects: Real things which have been removed as units from their natural setting.

Specimens: Objects which are incomplete or which are representative of a group or class of similar objects.

Mock up: Devices which are imitations of real things without involving similarity of appearance, the nonfunctioning parts that are unnecessary for understanding operational functions being omitted.

Dioramas: Three-dimensional scenes incorporating miniature objects and backgrounds in perspective.

Advantages
1. To recreate things from the past or the future.
2. To reduce the size of things.
3. To make model of things too small to examine.
4. To made model of things from faraway places.
5. To explain difficult concepts.
6. To show working parts.
7. To attract interests attention.
8. To promote increased learner participation.

9. To show some selected aspect of the whole in a simple elemental way.
10. To present an immediate sensation.

14. Advantages of field trip.

A field trip is a visit to a place outside the regular classroom which is designed to achieve certain objectives which cannot be achieved as well by using other means.

Advantages of field trip:
1. On a field trip, students are more likely to retain information. Being immersed in information and being involved in visual and practical experiences will help students remember, learn and understand subjects.
2. Field trips will help reinforce classroom materials bringing lessons to life. School trips give students the opportunity to visualize, experience and discuss information on a subject.
3. Going on field trips offers students a unique cultural learning experience. It allows students to be involved in new environments, key to encouraging curiosity about a given subject. It is also valuable as an exercise in broadening a student's understanding of the world and their place in it.
4. Educational trips encourage the development of social, personal and study skills. It has been observed that students appear to come out of their shell on field trips, becoming creative and displaying leadership qualities

15. Use of pamphlets in education.

Pamphlets can be folded in a variety of ways, such as in half, in thirds, or in fourths. ... While a brochure is used to advertize a company and its products or services, a pamphlet provides educational information on one topic.

Pamphlets are used for noncommercial promotion, while brochures are used to advertize products and services. Brochures also typically have more pages and images. Pamphlets can have multiple pages, but are generally contain fewer pages and more words than images to inform the reader.

16. List four issues for counseling in nursing students.

1. Inadequate knowledge: Many **students** did not have sufficient knowledge to care at the bedside when dealing with clinical learning environment and providing care to the patients was challenging for them
2. Deficient practical skills
3. Insufficiently developed communication skills
4. Behavioral problems.

17. Advantages of multiple choice questions.

Advantages of Multiple Choice Questions
1. They have fast processing times
2. There is no room for subjectivity
3. You can ask more questions, it takes less to time to complete a multiple choice question compared to an open question
4. Respondents do not have to formulate an answer but can focus on the content.

18. Uses of slides. *(See Q. 4, 2015)*

19. Define health education and health behavior.

Health education is any combination of learning experiences designed to help individuals and communities improve their health, by increasing their knowledge or influencing their attitudes.

Behavior, health-related: Health-related behavior is one of the most important elements in people's health and well-being. Its importance has grown as sanitation has improved and medicine has advanced. Diseases that were once incurable or fatal can now be prevented or successfully treated, and health-related behavior has become an important component of public health.

20. Types of chalkboard.

A **chalkboard** is a slightly abrasive writing surface made of wood, ply, hardboard, cement, ground glass, asbestos, slate, plastic, etc. with green or bluish green paint on it.

    Black ceramic unbreakable board: It is framed with aluminum or teak wood frame. Useful for chalk piece writing.

    Black or green glass chalkboard: It is framed with teak wood. Available in black or green color. Useful for chalk piece writing.

    The ordinary chalkboard held by easel: A portable and adjustable blackboard put on a wooden easel, used to take open classes.

    The roller type chalkboard with a mat surface: Made of thick canvas wrapped on a roller.

21. List down the purposes of evaluation.

Evaluation is a broader term than the Measurement. It is more comprehensive than mere inclusive than the term measurement. It goes ahead of measurement which simply indicates the numerical value. It gives the value judgement to the numerical value. It includes both tangible and intangible qualities.

The purpose of the evaluation is five-fold:
- To inform the ongoing work of the Alliance so that year-to-year improvements can be made and to support the development of model programs for adoption by other higher education institutions
- To determine the extent to which the short and long-term goals of the Alliance's four main interventions have been achieved
- To establish short- and long-term tracking of student outcomes (completion of CS undergraduate and graduate degrees, tracking of students throughout intervention courses and experiences, commitment to research careers)
- To provide an evaluation model which can be used by other institutions who adopt these interventions in the future and
- To provide information that supports the success of the Alliance as a partnership.

22. Barriers in effective group discussion.

Several common barriers get in the way of effective group communication:
1. Lack of clear goals. A lack of shared goals in a work team can lead to conflict in communication
2. Facts vs feelings
3. Fighting fair
4. Misunderstandings and misconceptions.

2016

Communication and Educational Technology

LONG ESSAYS
1. Define evaluation. What are the criteria for assessment of tools? Prepare an observational checklist to assess surgical wound dressing.
2. What are the aims of nursing education? Prepare a lesson plan on prevention of dental caries to a group of high school children.
3. Discuss the steps and observations to be made in microteaching.

SHORT ESSAYS
4. Explain the steps of demonstration.
5. Explain about Johari window.
6. Steps of group dynamics.
7. Media used to transmit health education to a community.
8. Describe communication process.
9. Maxims of teaching.
10. Phases of counseling process.
11. Write briefly on attitude scales.
12. What are the skills and importance of human relations?

SHORT ANSWERS
13. List down the elements of communication.
14. Social behavior.
15. Characteristics of counseling.
16. Idealism.
17. Three main domains of an objective.
18. Guidelines for preparing power point slides.
19. Essentials of lecture method.
20. Benefits of computer-aided learning and teaching.
21. Advantages of audiovisual aids.
22. Checklist.

LONG ESSAYS

1. Define evaluation. What are the criteria for assessment of tools? Prepare an observational checklist to assess surgical wound dressing.

The term evaluation is derived from the word valoir means to be worth. To evaluate means to ascertain the value or amount or appraise carefully. Hence, evaluation is judging is the worth or value of something that represents the satisfaction of human need, such as an object, event or activity.

Definitions
1. Evaluation is a relatively new technical term introduced to designate a more comprehensive concept of measurement than is implied in conventional tests and examination (ringtone).
2. Evaluation is essential in the never ending cycle of formulating goals, measuring progress towards then and determining the new goals which emerge as a result of new warnings (Clara M Brown).
3. Evaluation in education is a process of judging the effectiveness of educational experiences through careful appraisal (LE Hidgerken).

What are the criteria for assessment of tools?
Major criteria used in selecting and developing evaluation tools are:
1. Sample of objectives.
2. Sampling of the content.
3. Checking validity, reliability, practicability and usefulness.

Evaluation methodology: There is certain methodology for evaluation. The educational spinal illustrated by Gilberto is given below. It has 4 steps—
1. Defining objectives
2. Planning evaluation system
3. Preparing
4. Implementing evaluation.

The processes are repeated giving feedback and re-examining the objectives, and making necessary changes in the education system (program). Evaluation is continuous process and the results are used for the educational spiral—by Guilbert.

Qualities of Good Assessment Tools
1. Congruent with educational objectives.
2. Objectivity of assessment techniques/methods.
3. Practicability of measuring techniques/methods.
4. Evaluation tools constructed on wide curricular content.
5. Clear and comprehensive.
6. Concise and precise.
7. Relevance.
8. Adequate and appropriate.
9. Understandability.
10. The power of discrimination.
11. Validity of assessment tools.
12. Reliability of assessment tool.

Checklist

Checklist is a prepared list of statements relating of behavior traits, performance in some area or practical work or a product of some performance list an art work.

Definition: A checklist is a simple instrument consisting prepared list of expected items of performance or attributes, which are checked by a evaluator for their presence or absence.

Characteristics of Checklist

1. Observe one respondent at one time.
2. Clearly specify the characteristics of the behavior to be observed.
3. Use only carefully prepared checklists to avoid more complex traits.
4. The observer should be trained.
5. Use checklist only when you are interested in calculating a particular characteristics.

Steps of Checklist (by Groulund)

1. Identify and describe clearly each of the specific desired actions in the performance.
2. Add to the list those actions which represent common error if they are limited in number and can be clearly identified.
3. Arrange the desired actions and likely errors in the approximate order in which they are expected to occur.
4. Provide a simple procedure for numbering the actions in sequenance or checking each action as it occurs.

Advantages
1. Easy to evaluate
2. Easy for scoring
3. Better content validity.

Disadvantages
1. Takes a lot of time
2. Observed must be trained
3. Individual check list needed for each candidate.

2. What are the aims of nursing education? Prepare a lesson plan on prevention of dental caries to a group of high school children.

Nursing education is a professional education which is consciously and systematically planned and implemented through instruction and discipline and aims the harmonious development of the physical, intellectual, social, emotional, spiritual and aesthetic powers or abilities of the student in order to render professional nursing care to people of all ages, in all phases of health and illness, in a variety of settings, in the best or highest possible manner.

Aims of Nursing Education

1. **Harmonious development:** Nursing education aims the harmonious development of the physical, intellectual, emotional, social, spiritual and aesthetic powers or abilities of the student. Harmonious development is essential for achieving the qualities required for leading a successful professional and personal life. In short, nursing education aims to prepare students as good human beings with qualities of a professional nurse.

2. **Inculcating the right attitude:** Right attitude towards nursing forms the basis of nursing career. Right attitude helps to adjust with the student life and motivate to achieve excellence in the upcoming professional life. Nursing education offers a variety of learning experiences with an aim to inculcate proper attitude among students.
3. **Knowledge and skill aim:** Nursing education provides the much needed knowledge and skill required to practice the profession in a successful manner. Technological advancements in the field of education helps nurse educators to fulfill, this aim in a meticulous way.
4. **Emphasis on high-tech-high-touch approach:** High-tech-high-touch approach in nursing care was devised to preserve the human component of nursing care without undermining the advantages of the technological advancements in the field of patient care. Nurse educators have to motivate the students to maintain the human element of nursing while rendering care with the help of sophisticated gadgets.
5. **Prepare students to take up a proactive role in learning:** The model of teacher as the pivotal and dominant figure in education, presenting a variety of information to pupils has practically disappeared. To a certain extent, this is applicable to nursing education also. Nurse educator of today is considered as a facilitator of learning, whose main duty is to prepare students to adopt a proactive role in learning, so that they will actively participate in the teaching-learning process.
6. **Professional development:** Nursing education prepares the student to render professional nursing care in the best or highest possible manner. Nurse educators can fulfill the professional aspirations of the students by way of providing guidance, arranging adequate learning experiences and serving as role models. The need of professional development in this era of competition and knowledge explosion should be explained properly to the students. Easy access to information, availability of staff development programs and increased opportunities for higher education will help nurses to maintain the professional development.
7. **Assist to build a promising career:** Nursing profession offers a variety of career opportunities. Helping students to realize their potentials and interests will enable them to build a promising career.
8. **Social aim:** Nursing education prepares the student to become a useful member in the society. This will in turn help them to interact effectively with the people and render dedicated care without any discrimination.
9. **Citizenship:** Nursing education should motivate the student to perform his/her duties as a citizen for the welfare of the fellow human beings.
10. **To prepare global nurses:** Globalization and liberalization has created worldwide opportunities for professional nurses ever than before.

Lesson plan: Lesson plan is a plan prepared by a teacher to teach a lesson in an organized manner. It is a plan of action and calls for an understanding on the teacher's part, about the students, knowledge and experience about the topic being taught and her/his ability to use effective methods.

Advantages of Planning a Lesson
1. It helps the teacher to be systematic, orderly in the treatment of the subject matter.
2. It provides confidence and self-reliance to the teacher. She set fourth some definite aims that she is to develop in students through certain activities or some other means.
3. It encourages the continuity in the teaching process and unnecessary repetition is avoided.
4. The interest of the students can be maintained throughout the lesson when it is well-planned.

Steps involved in planning a lesson: There are few steps which should be followed while making a lesson plan. These are:
1. **Preparation/introduction:** This in fact, is a means of exploration of the student's knowledge which helps to lead them on to the lesson. The teacher needs to prepare the students to receive new knowledge. She can introduce the lesson by testing the previous knowledge of the student by asking questions. This in turn may reveal their, ignorance; arouse interest and curiosity to learn new matter. Charts, maps, diagrams, pictures also can be used.
2. **Presentation:** The aim of lesson plan should clearly state before the presentation of the subject matter, which helps both the teacher and the student to have a common pursuit.
3. **During presentation:** In this stage both the teacher and the student must actively participate in the teaching learning process. The students must get some new ideas and knowledge.
4. **Questioning**, discussion, appropriate examples from real life situations should feature in presentation to make the presentation interesting and to motivate the students to learn.
    a. Teaching aids: Teaching aids should be used to make the lessons meaningful, clear, explanatory and comprehensive.
    b. Blackboard summary can be developed side-by-side.
5. **Comparison or association:** This step is important where the students are given examples and they are asked to observe carefully and compare them with other set of examples and facts. These will enable the student to deduce definitions and arrive at generalizations on their own.
6. **Generalization:** This step involves reflective thinking. The knowledge presented through the lesson should be thought provoking, innovating and stimulating to assist the students to generalize and untested formula, etc.
7. **Application:** The students make use of the knowledge acquire in familiar and unfamiliar situations and at the same time it tests the validity of the generalizations arrived at by the students. The students of nursing especially need to develop the skill of learning to apply the knowledge and skills gained in the classroom in their day-to-day nursing practice in the wards, clinic and home situations. This makes learning more permanent and worthwhile.
8. **Recapitulation:** This being the last step in the planning of a lesson, understanding and comprehension of the subject matter taught by the teacher can be tested by asking suitable, stimulating and pivotal questions to be students on the topic. This also gives a feedback to the teacher regarding the efficacy of the methods of teaching adopted by her. It tells whether further explanation, clarifications, etc. are needed or not, as well.

Suggested performa for a lesson plan: There are various performa which can be used as an outline for lesson plan. Whatever format is used the essential elements which should feature in a lesson plan are—
1. Statement of central and contributory objectives.
2. Relationship of the present lesson with the previous lesson.
3. Inclusion of learning objectives (refer to student activities).
4. Inclusion of learning activities (refer to teacher activities).
5. Methods of teaching to be used.
6. Audio-visual aids to be used.
7. Summary of the lesson being taught.
8. Evaluative questions.
9. Assignments for students.
10. References on the topic of the lesson.

3. Discuss the steps and observations to be made in microteaching.

A training procedure aimed at simplifying the complexities of the regular teaching process. It is difficult for the teacher to assess all the teaching skills of a student teacher at a time and give necessary corrections. By way of scaled down teaching, teacher can easily identify the deficiencies of the student teacher in performing a particular teaching skill and help him to attain proficiency in that skill by providing assistance to rectify the identified deficiencies.

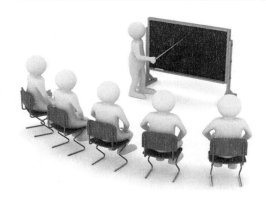

Definition
1. According to Allen "Microteaching as a scaled down teaching encounter in class size and class time". The number of students is from 5–10 and the duration of period ranges from 5–20 minutes.
2. DW Allen (1966): Microteaching is a scaled down teaching encounter in class size and time.
3. Allen and Eve (1968): Microteaching is defined as a system of controlled practice that makes it possible to concentrate on specific teaching behavior and to practice teaching under controlled conditions.
4. RN Bush (1968): Microteaching is a teacher education technique which allows teachers to apply clearly defined teaching skills in carefully prepared lessons in a planned series of 5–10 minute encounters with a small group of real students, often with an opportunity to observe the result on video tape.

Characteristics of Microteaching
1. It is relatively a new experience or innovation in the field of teacher education, more specifically in student teaching.
2. It is a training technique and not a teaching technique. In other words, it is a technique or design used for the training of teachers (or makes them learn the art of teaching). It is not a method of classroom instruction or teaching like inductive-deductive, demonstration or question-answer method.

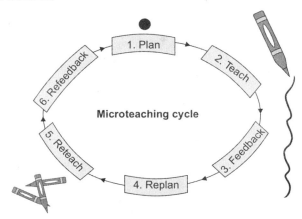

3. It is micro- or miniaturized teaching in the sense that it scales down the complexities of real teaching with the provisions, such as:
   a. Practicing one skill at a time.
   b. Reducing the class size to 5–10 pupils.
   c. Reducing duration of the lesson to 5–10 minutes.
   d. Limiting the content to a single concept.
4. There is provision of adequate feedback in microteaching as it provides trainees due information about their performances immediately after the completion of their lesson.
5. Teaching is said to be composed of very specific skills. These skills cannot be mastered through the traditional approach to teacher training. Microteaching provides opportunity to select one skill at a time and practice it through its scaled down encounter and then take other in a similar way.
6. Microteaching is a highly individualized training device permitting the imposition of a high degree of control in practicing a particular skill.

Looking at the above characteristics and features, the term microteaching may be defined appropriately as a technique or device of imparting training to the inexperienced or experienced teachers for learning the art of teaching by practicing specific skills through a "scaled down teaching encounter", i.e. reducing the complexities of real normal teaching in terms of size of the class, time and content.

Phases of Microteaching

1. **Orientation:** In the beginning, the student teacher should be given necessary theoretical background about microteaching by having a free and fair discussion of the following aspects:
   a. Concept
   b. Significance or rationale of using microteaching
   c. Procedure
   d. Requirements and setting for adopting microteaching technique.
2. **Discussion of teaching skills:** Under this step, the knowledge and understanding about the following aspects is to be developed:
   a. Analysis of teaching into component teaching skills.
   b. Discussion of the rationale and role of teaching skills in teaching.
   c. Discussion about the component teaching behavior comprising various teaching skills.

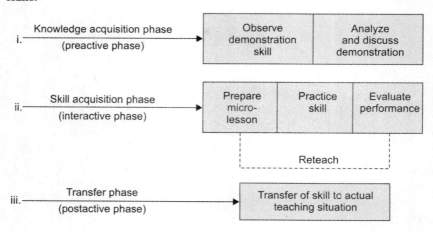

3. **Selection of a particular teaching skill:** The teaching skills are to be practiced by taking them one at a time. Therefore, the student teachers are persuaded to select a particular skill for practice. They are also provided with necessary orientation and processing material for the practice. Most of such material may be found in the literature available with NCERT. The student/teacher may be given a necessary background for the observation of a model or demonstration lesson on the selected teaching skill.
4. **Presentation of a model demonstration lesson:** Here, a demonstration or model lesson for the use of the selected teaching skill is presented before the trainees. This is also termed as "modeling", i.e. demonstration of the desired behaviors in relation to a skill for imitation by the observer. Depending on the availability of the resources and the type of skill involved, demonstration or model lesson can be given in a number of ways:
    a. Providing written material such as handbook, guides, illustrations, and video tape.
    b. Exhibiting a film or videotape.
    c. Making the trainees listen to an audiotape.
    d. Arranging a demonstration from a live model, i.e. a teacher educator or an expert demonstrating the use of the skill.
5. **Observation of the model lesson and criticism:** What is read, viewed, listened and observed through a modeling source here is carefully analyzed by the trainee. In a demonstration given by an expert or teacher educator, the student teachers are expected to note down their observations. An observation schedule especially designed for the observation of the specific skill is distributed among the trainees and they are also trained in its use beforehand. Such an observation of the model lesson and its relevant criticism provide desired feedback to the person giving the model lesson.
6. **Preparation of microlesson plan**: Under this step, the student/teachers are required to prepare microlesson plans by selecting proper concept for the practice of demonstrated skill. For their preparation, help may be taken from the teacher educators and the sample lessons available in NCERT.
7. **Creation of microteaching setting:** The following is the standard setting for a microclass:
    a. Number of pupils: 5–10.
    b. Types of pupils: Real pupils or preferably peers.
    c. Types of supervisor: Teacher educators and peers.
    d. Time duration of a microlesson: 6 minutes.
    e. Time duration of a microteaching cycle: 36 minutes.
8. **Practice of the skill (teaching session):** Here, the student/teacher teaches his prepared microlesson for 6 minutes (prescribed time schedule for teach-session) a microclass consisting of 5–10 real pupils or peers (Student teachers). It is supervised by the teacher educator and peers both with the help of appropriate observation schedule. Where possible, the student/teacher may also have his lesson taped on a video- or audiotape.
9. **Providing feedback:** The greatest advantage of microteaching lies in providing immediate feedback to the student teacher on his teaching performance demonstrated in his micro-lesson. The feedback is provided in terms of his use of component teaching behaviors emphasizing the skill under practice, so that he may be able to modify them in the desired direction. This feedback in the Indian situation may be properly provided by the peers and teacher educators observing microlesson. Where possible, help may be taken from the mechanical gadgets like videotape, audiotape, and closed circuit television.
10. **Replanning (replan session):** In view of the feedback received from the different sources, the student/teacher tries to replan his micro-lesson. He is provided 12 minutes time for this purpose.

11. **Reteaching (reteach session):** In this session of 6 minutes, the student teacher re-teaches his microlesson on the basis of the prepared plan and rearranged setting.
12. **Providing refeedback (refeedback session):** On the basis of his performance in the retaught microlesson, the student teacher is provided refeedback in the way outlined earlier.
13. **Repetition of the microteaching cycle:** A microteaching cycle used to practice a teaching skill consists of planning, teaching, feedback, replanning, and refeedback operations. The microteaching cycle is repeated and the student/teacher is required to replan and reteach his lesson till he attains mastery over the skill under practice.
14. **Integration of teaching skills:** The last step is concerned with the task of integrating various teaching skills individually mastered by a student teacher. This helps in bridging a gap between training in isolated teaching skills and the real teaching situation faced by a student teacher.

Advantages of Microteaching

In the Indian context, microteaching has the following advantages over the traditional methods of learning the art of teaching:
1. In our traditional mode of teacher training, a great dependence is observed on the availability of pupils, classrooms and cooperation from the staff of the practicing schools. The microteaching approach incorporating simulating technique helps a training institution in overcoming the hardships faced in the task of organizing students teaching.
2. The global concept of teaching is replaced by the analytical concept in microteaching approach. Here, complex task of teaching is looked upon as a set of simpler skills comprising specific classroom behaviors. This helps in the proper understanding of the meaning and concept of the term teaching.
3. Microteaching helps in reducing the complexities of the normal classroom teaching. It is a scaled down or miniaturized classroom teaching as it reduces the size of the class and duration of the lesson and provides proper opportunities for practicing one component teaching skill at a time by using single concept of the content.
4. In microteaching, the student teacher concentrates on practicing a specific and well-defined teaching skill consisting of a set of teacher behaviors that are observable, controllable and practicable. Consequently, it provides a more appropriate technique of learning the art of teaching (although mastering one teaching skill at a time) than the traditional program.
5. Microteaching helps in the systematic and objective observation by providing a specific observation schedule.
6. Microteaching works as a laboratory exercise to focus training on the acquisition of teaching skills and instructional techniques. Here, a trainee can experiment with several alternatives in a limited time and resources. It is just like learning the art of operating human body parts in a medical laboratory by a student doctor before actually operating a patient.
7. Microteaching provides economy in mastering the teaching skills. It saves the time and energy of the student teacher as well as of the pupils. It is not only easy for a student teacher to handle a microgroup (5–10 pupils) but it is also safe because they will have less problems of classroom discipline and subsequent mental tension as faced commonly in the traditional practice teaching program. It also saves the pupils from being unnecessarily used as guinea pigs for training student teachers.

Disadvantages
1. It is skill-oriented and not content-oriented.
2. Teacher educator requires adequate training before it is implemented.

3. It disturbs normal class time table.
4. The question of integrating the skill is quite challenging.

SHORT ESSAYS

4. Explain the steps of demonstration.

Demonstration method is very important in teaching of nursing then in any other fields. It is very instructional method that is chosen depends on the learning needs of the student's time available to teach. The setting the resources and the teacher own comfort. An experienced and skilled teacher uses a variety of a techniques depends on the subject on the topic.

Objectives
1. To give a vivid picture of the related nursing care.
2. To make specific observation by the student.
3. To provide a deal situation to learn the particular procedure thoroughly.
4. To get a realistic idea about the procedure.
5. To stimulate and encourage for the development of initiation among the students.
6. To obtain active participation among the students.

Important steps in good demonstration
1. Preliminary assessment.
2. Preparation of the patient unit and articles.
3. Procedure.
4. After the procedure care of the patient and articles.
5. Recording and reporting.
6. Know the students well; whom do you wish to teach. What is the level of the knowledge and literacy and their sphere of influence.
7. Keep ready the resources.
8. Remember that changing people's practices is a more delicate than surgery.

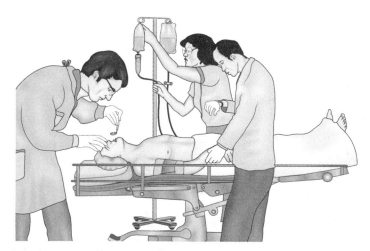

9. Check whether there is sufficient staff equipment, transport, inputs, etc. before carrying over the demonstration.
10. Ask oneself can freely provide knowledge inputs when needed.

11. Do not try to show too much one or two variables are usually can be demonstrate at one time.
12. Keep watch and demonstrate their interaction of the variable.
13. Maintain proper checks to illustrate efficiency of the practice.
14. Plan and inform campaign to ensure contact with the target students.
15. Choose your cooperator carefully; be sure the cooperator cooperates with you.
16. Get them involved and keep them informed.
17. Consider location and accessibility both for the lay formers and VIPs.
18. Involve the agencies, individuals and others in all the operations. This lens creditability to the demonstration.
19. Organize field day trips and visits of people, who may be potential user of the demonstration and its results.
20. Keep records prepare talks, charts, photo's, slides, news, stories, technical bulletins and other aids, frequently use them.

Advantages of demonstration method
1. Activates several senses.
2. Uses all the teaching approaches like telling, participating, interesting and reinforcing.
3. Motivation to learn.
4. Improves physical and cognitive level.

5. Explain about Johari window.

A Johari window is a cognitive psychological tool created by Joseph cuft and Harry Ingham in 1955 in United States, used to help people better understand their interpersonal communication and relationships. It is used primarily in self-help groups and corporate settings as a heuristic exercise. When performing the exercise, the subject is given a list of 55 adjectives and she picks five or six adjectives that they feel describe their own personality. Peers of the subject are then given the same list, and each pick five or six adjectives that describe the subject. These adjectives are then mapped on to a grid. Charles Handly calls this concept the Johari window. House with four rooms Or quadrants.

	Known to self	Not known to self
Know to other	Open	Blind
Not known to others	Hidden	Unknown

Johari window

- Room 1 is the part of ourselves that we see and others see
- Room 2 is the aspect that others see but we are not aware of
- Room 3 is the most mysterious room in that the unconscious or subconscious bit of us is seen by neither ourselves nor others
- Room 4 is our private space which we know but keep from others.

6. Steps of group dynamics.

Group dynamics is concerned with the interactions and forces between group members in a social situation. When the concept is applied to the study of organizational behavior, the focus is on the dynamics of members of formal or informal groups in the organization, i.e. it is concerned with the gaining knowledge of groups, how they develop, and their effect on individual members and the organizations in which they function.

Definition: Group dynamics is the interactions that influence the attitude and behavior of people when they are grouped with others through each choice or accidental circumstances.

Meaning of group dynamics: The term "group dynamics" refers to the interactions between people who are talking together in a group setting. Group dynamics can be studied in business settings, in volunteer settings, in classroom settings, and in social settings. Any time there are three or more individuals interacting or talking together, there are group dynamics.
1. A branch of social psychology which studies problems involving the structure of a group.
2. The interactions that influence the attitudes and behavior of people when they are grouped with others through either choice or accidental circumstances.
3. A field of social psychology concerned with the nature of human groups, their development, and their interactions with individuals, other groups, and larger organizations.

Objective of group dynamics
1. To identify and analyze the social processes that impact on group development and performance.
2. To acquire the skills necessary to intervene and improve individual and group performance in an organizational context.
3. To build more successful organizations by applying techniques that provide positive impact on goal achievement.

Principles of group dynamics
1. The members of the group must have a strong sense of belonging to the group.
2. Changes in one part of the group may produce stress in other person, which can be reduced only by eliminating or allowing the change by bringing about readjustment in the related parts.
3. The group arises and functions owing to common motives.
4. Groups survive by placing the members into functional hierarchy and facilitating the action towards the goals.
5. The intergroup relations, group organization and member participation is essential for effectiveness of a group.
6. Information relating to needs for change, plans for change and consequences of changes must be shared by members of a group.

7. Media used to transmit health education to a community.

A health education program requires four kinds of planning:
1. **Diagnosing the health problems:** Before designing and implementing a health education program, the health worker must understand as much as possible about:
    a. General socioeconomic situation.
    b. Patterns of illness.
    c. Target group in the population.
    d. Health needs.
    e. Attitudes, customs, feelings and ideas that can be changed by education.
    f. Identification of communicators.
2. **Design appropriate educational content:** The messages of the program must be clear, understandable and acceptable.
3. **Plan for appropriate setting:** The health education program should be conducted at a time and place most suitable for the people. This may include:
    1. At home
    2. Clinics

3. Hospitals
4. Community meeting places
5. Anganwadi and schools.
4. **Use appropriate teaching methods/aid:** The health educators must learn to use appropriate audio-visual aids.

8. Describe communication process.

Face-to-face communication involves a sender, a message, a receiver and a response or feedback. In its simplest form, communication is a two-way process involving the sending and the receiving of a message. Because the intent of communication is to elicit a response, the process is ongoing, the receiver of the message then becomes the sender of a response, and the original sender then becomes the receiver.

Sender: The sender, a person or group who wishes to convey a message to another, can be considered the source-encoder. This term suggests that the person or group sending the message must have an idea or reason for communicating. Source must put the idea or feeling into a form that can be transmitted. Encoding involves the selection of specific signs and symbols to transmit the message, such as which language and words to use, how to arrange the words, and what tone of voice and gestures to use.

The sender's message acts as a referent for the receiver, who is responsible for attending to, translating and responding to the sender's message.

Message: The second component of the communication process is the message itself. He what is actually said or written, the body language that accompanies the words, and how the message is transmitted. Message may contain verbal, nonverbal and symbolic language. The medium used to convey the message is the channel, and it can target any of the receivers, senses. It is important for the channel to be appropriate for the message and it should help make the intent of the message clearer.

Talking face-to-face with a person may be more effective in some instances than telephoning or writing a message. Recording message on tape or communicating by radio or TV may be more appropriate for larger audiences. Written communication is also appropriate for long explanations and the nonverbal channel of touch is often highly effective.

Receiver: The receiver, the third component of the communication process, is the listener, who must listen, observer and attend. This person is the decoder, who must perceive what the sender intended. Perception uses all of the senses to receive verbal and nonverbal messages. To decoder means to relate the message perceived to the receiver's storehouse of knowledge and experience and to sort out the meaning of the message. Whether the message is decoded accurately by the receiver, according to the sender's intent, depends largely on their similarities in knowledge and experience and sociocultural background.

Channels: Channels are means of conveying and receiving messages through visual, auditory and tactile senses. Facial expressions send visual messages, spoken words travel through auditory channels, and touch uses tactile channels. The more channels the sender uses to convey a message, the more clearly, it is usually understood. Nurses use verbal, nonverbal, and mediated communication channels.

Response or feedback: The fourth component of the communication process, the response, is the message that the receiver returns to the sender. It is also called as feedback. Feedback can be either verbal, nonverbal or both. Feedback indicates whether the meaning of the sender's message was understood. Sender need to seek verbal and nonverbal feedback to ensure that good communication has occurred. To be effective, the sender and receiver must be sensitive and open to each other's messages, clarify the messages and modify behavior accordingly. In a social relationship, both persons assume equal responsibility for seeking openness and clarification, but the nurse assumes primary responsibility in the nurse-client relationship.

9. Maxims of teaching.

Importance of maxims of teaching: The maxims of teaching are very helpful in allowing active participation of learners in the teaching learning process. They increase the interest and motivate the students. They make learning effective, inspirational, interesting and meaningful.

The maxims of teaching are as follows:
1. **Proceed from the known to unknown:** A simple way of teaching is to proceed from what the students already know to what they do not know. Since they are familiar with known things, they develop interest in knowing more. As the teacher proceeds, she arouses interest and curiosity in the student. The teacher should proceed step by step from known things to unknown things.
2. **Proceed from simple to complex:** The simple topics must be discussed first and then deal with the complex topics. A complex topic may contain a number of simple topics put together which makes it complex. So when a child learns simple ones, he tries to solve the complex problems also. So one should precede form simple to complex.
3. **Proceed from easy to difficult:** Proceed from easier tasks. Once the child is able to successfully complete easy task, he develops self-confidence which further motivates him to deal with difficult tasks. The child feels comfortable to solve easy tasks first and later the difficult task. The individual interest of the child should be considered.
4. **Proceed for the concrete to the abstract:** It is easy for the child to learn about what he is able to see than what he is unable to see (abstract), for example, children can see the moon so teach about the sun, moon, stars and then the planetary system.
5. **Proceed from particular to general:** A study of particular facts should lead the children themselves to frame general rules. The rules of arithmetic, grammar, physical geography, science are based on the principle of proceeding from particular instance to general rules.
6. **Proceed from indefinite to definite:** Ideas in children are indefinite incoherent and vague. They must be making definite, clear and systematic.
7. **Proceed from empirical to relational:** Observation and experience are the basis of empirical knowledge. Rational knowledge gives reasoning. They general feeling is that the child experiences the rational basis.
8. **Proceed from psychological to logical:** Logical approach deals with arranging the subject matter wherever psychological approach deals with the child's interests, needs, mental make-up, etc. In psychological approach, we proceed from concrete to abstract, simple the complex, etc.
9. **Proceed from whole to part:** Whole is more interesting to the child than a part. For example, A flower is more attractive than a petal. About 50% proceed from whole to part. The "whole" makes more sense to the child than the part.
10. **Proceed from near to far:** A child learns well from the environment which is nearer to him. Gradually, he learns about far off places.
11. **Proceed from analysis to synthesis:** Analysis is breaking down into simpler parts and synthesis is grouping of these separated parts into one unit.
12. **Proceed from actual to representative:** When actual objects are shown to children they remember for a long time. Representative objects like models, pictures can be shown to elder children.

13. **Proceed from inductively:** Proceed from making simple tasks gather all such tasks and make whole. In the inductive approach, we start from particular examples and establish general rules through the active participation of the learners. This goes on from specific to general. In deductive approach are assuming a definition, a general rule or formula and apply it to particular examples. This goes on from general to specific.

All the maxims are interrelated. Different maxims suit different situations and different children. The teacher has to judiciously select appropriate maxims.

10. Phases of counseling process.

The counselor through his warm and friendly behavior, must create a cordial atmosphere for the counseling session, through a process involving the personal talk in the form of discussion, the counselor must attempt to understand the various aspects of the problem. The counselor gives his advice as to how to hope with the problems. He suggests number of solutions and asks the counselee to choose the appropriate one. The session is terminated when the counselee is convinced about his future plan of action. The final step in counseling is follow-up. The effectiveness of the prescription given by the counselor to the student must be seen in practice. The counselor keeps a watch over the students behavior. The counselor sees that the problem does not recur.

Principles of counseling:

1. **Acceptance:** The client must be accepted as a whole person, as a human being.
2. **Respect for the individual:** Importance is attached to respect for individual.
3. **Permissiveness:** All schools of counseling would accept relative permissiveness of counseling relationship.
4. **Learning:** All schools of counseling should accept the learning element in counseling.
5. **Thinking with rather than for the client:** It is another basic principle of counseling.

Types of counseling

There are two major types of counseling namely: Individual counseling and group counseling.
1. **Individual counseling:** This is referred to as one-to-one counseling. It occurs between the professionally trained counselor (Therapist) and his client (Counselee). The goal of this is to help the client to understand himself, clarify and direct his thought, in order to make a worthwhile decision. Through this, clients' problems are alleviated. Frumboltz and Thoreson (1967) as cited in Ojo (2005) remarked that it is mainly to bring about change in the client either by altering maladaptive behavior, learning the decision making process or preventing problems.
2. **Group counseling:** This is a counseling session that takes place between the professionally trained counselor and a group of people. Number of this group should not be more than seven, or at least ten, in order to have a cohesive group and an effective well-controlled counseling session. Members of the groups are clients/counselees whose tasks or problems that are meant for resolution are similar.

11. Write briefly on attitude scales.

Assessment of attitude, evaluation must be translated into some number system. For some purpose, it is adequate to assess attitude with two categories favorable and unfavorable. By far the most common method of measuring attitudes is the self-report method, in which people are asked to respond to questions by expressing their personal evaluation. Unfortunately, informal procedures suffer from several serious drawbacks. People are always concerned with looking good to others, so their statements may reflect what they think will put them in a favorable light rather than their actual views. To avoid these and related problems, social psychologists measures or assessment of attitudes by more formal means, generally involving the use of scales or questionnaires.

Attitude scales: The attitude scales are used for measuring the social attitudes.

Types of attitude scales:
1. Point scale
2. Differential scale (LL Thurstone scale)
3. Likert scale (Summated scale)

- **Point scale:**
    - Select the word which will give the opinion.
    - Ask the responded to cross out every word that is more annoying to him.
    - The attitude of a respondent is calculated by the number of words crossed out or not crossed out. The words selected should be suggestive of an attitude.
    - One point is given to each agreement or disagreement whichever is to be chosen.

    Two set of words in dictating both favorable and unfavorable opinions are given. The unfavorable items may be crossed and favorable items may be left unscored.

- **Differential scale (LL Thurstone scale):** These scales are used to measure the social phenomenon.

    Thurstone's adaptation of psychophysical methods to the quantification of judgment data represented an important milestone in attitude scale construction. Thurstone and his co-workers prepared about 20 scales for measuring attitudes towards war, capital punishment, patriotism, etc.

    Thurstone scale begins with the assembling of many statements expressing a wide range of attitudes toward the object under consideration. A large number of judges are asked individually to sort the statement into piles for degree of favorableness.

- **Likert scale (summated scale):** Respondents completing scales indicate the extent to which they agree or disagree with strong positive and negative statement about the attitude, e.g. BSc Nursing students have positive attitude towards their profession.

Strongly disagree	Disagree	Neutral	Agree	Strongly disagree
1	2	3	4	5

The items on attitude scales can be presented to respondents in many different formats, but one important approach involves what is known as Likert scale. On such scale, the times are statements either highly favorable or unfavorable towards the attitude object, and respondents indicate the extent to which they agree or disagree with each of these statement. People with positive attitudes are earning confident, patience and humble. Positive attitude foster teamwork solves problems, reduce stress and make the person an asset to his society. Negative attitude leads to bitterness, or a purposeless life, ill health and high level of stress in themselves and others.

12. What are the skills and importance of human relations?

Nurse is a member of the healthcare team: The health team in a healthcare system may be as simple as consisting only of three members, the doctor, the nurse and the patient or it may be a large team consisting of members of many other specialized fields of care like physical therapists and the occupational therapists, the dieticians and people who look into the spiritual and social needs of the patient.

Each member of the team possesses unique knowledge and skill which he/she contributes to the total healthcare system. There are also many areas of shared knowledge and skill, e.g. communication skills, physiology, psychology and sociology. The essence of the team concept is that all members work cooperatively for individual family or a community towards their common goal of attaining the highest level of health possible.

Establishing interpersonal relationship

Interpersonal communication is both a science and an art. As a science, it requires a disciplined study of concepts and practice of techniques to gain certain skills. As an art, it requires the fusion of the nurse herself with creativity, insight and practice to achieve style. Human communication is a complex process in which two or more persons exchange message and derive meaning.

Effective communication occurs when persons exchange message and derive a mutual understanding of intended meaning. A general classic principle of communication is applicable to nurse-client interactions as well as to all other interactions, both people are perceived by another. The community health nurse is an important member of the healthcare teamwork in cooperation and harmony for the care of the individual, family and community.

Nurse plays several roles in human relation:
1. **Caregiver:** The caregiver role traditionally included those activities that assist the patient physically and psychologically while preserving the patient's dignity.
2. **Caregiving encompasses** the physical, psychological, developmental, cultural and spiritual levels.
3. **Communicator:** In the role of communicator, nurses identify patient's problems and then communicate these verbally or in writing to other members of the health team. The nurse must be able to communicate clearly and accurately in order for a client's healthcare needs to be met.
4. **Teacher:** As a teacher, the nurse helps the client learn about their health and the healthcare procedures they need to perform to restore or maintain their health. The nurse assesses the client's learning needs and readiness to learn.
5. **Client advocate:** A client advocate acts to protect the client. In this role, the nurse may represent the client's needs and wishes to other health professionals, such as relaying the client's wishes for information to the physician.
6. **Counselor:** The nurse counsel's primarily healthy individual with normal adjustments difficulties and focuses on helping the person develop new attitudes, feelings and behaviors by encouraging the client to look at alternative behaviors, recognize the choices, and develop a sense of control.
7. **Change agent:** The nurse acts as a change agent when assisting others, that is clients, to make modifications in their own behavior, nurses also often act to make changes in a system, such as clinical care, if it is not helping a client return to health. Nurses are continually dealing with change in the healthcare system.
8. **Leader:** The leader role can be employed at different levels individual client, family, groups of clients, colleagues or the community.
9. **Manager:** The nurse manager also delegates nursing activities to ancillary workers and other nurses, and supervises and evaluates their performance.
10. **Case manager:** Nurse case managers work with the multidisciplinary healthcare team to measure the effectiveness of the case management plan and to monitor outcomes. Each agency or unit specifies the role of the nurse case manager.

11. **Research consumer:** Nurses often use research to improve client care. In a clinical area, nurses need to (a) have some awareness of the process and language of research, (b) be sensitive to issues related to protecting the rights of human subjects, (c) participate in the identification of significant researchable problems, and (d) be a discriminating consumer of research findings.
12. **Expanded career roles:** Nurses are fulfilling expanded career roles, such as those of nurse practitioner, clinical nurse specialist, nurse midwife, nurse educator, nurse researcher and nurse anesthetist.

SHORT ANSWERS

13. List down the elements of communication.

1. **Source idea:** The source idea is the process by which one formulates an idea to communicate to another party. This process can be influenced by external stimuli, such as books or radio, or it can come about internally by thinking about a particular subject. The source idea is the basis for the communication.
2. **Message:** The message is what will be communicated to another party. It is based on the source idea, but the message is crafted to meet the needs of the audience. For example, if the message is between two friends, the message will take a different form than if communicating with a superior.

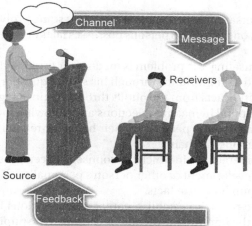

3. **Encoding:** Encoding is how the message is transmitted to another party. The message is converted into a suitable form for transmission. The medium of transmission will determine the form of the communication. For example, the message will take a different form if the communication will be spoken or written.
4. **Channel:** The channel is the medium of the communication. The channel must be able to transmit the message from one party to another without changing the content of the message. The channel can be a piece of paper, a communications medium, such as radio, or it can be an email. The channel is the path of the communication from sender to receiver. An email can use the internet as a channel.
5. **Receiver:** The receiver is the party receiving the communication. The party uses the channel to get the communication from the transmitter. A receiver can be a television set, a computer, or a piece of paper depending on the channel used for the communication.

6. **Decoding:** Decoding is the process where the message is interpreted for its content. It also means the receiver thinks about the message's content and internalizes the message. This step of the process is where the receiver compares the message to prior experiences or external stimuli.
7. **Feedback:** Feedback is the final step in the communications process. This step conveys to the transmitter that the message is understood by the receiver. The receiver formats an appropriate reply to the first communication based on the channel and sends it to the transmitter of the original message.

14. Social behavior.

Social behavior is behavior among two or more organisms, typically from the same species. Social behavior is exhibited by a wide range of organisms including social bacteria, slime moulds, social insects, social shrimp, naked mole-rats, and humans. Social behavior is defined as interactions among individuals, normally within the same species, that are usually beneficial to one or more of the individuals. It is believed that social behavior evolved because it was beneficial to those who engaged in it, which means that these individuals were more likely to survive and reproduce.

15. Characteristics of counseling.

The following facts become distinct about counseling after studying and analyzing the above mentioned definitions:
1. Counseling is a conversation with someone regarding some problem.
2. Normally, not always, one of the two persons possesses facts or experiences or abilities which the other lacks.

In the process of counseling, the problem is made clear through discussion. The counselor explores the problem and its importance through his skillful questioning.
- Counselor draws out the facts from the pupils through counseling process.
- Counseling helps the pupil in making selections and following those selections.
- Counseling is assistance to the persons in their behavior-related problems in which their emotions and motivations are main.
- Counseling involves interactions in which the counselor accepts the responsibility of positive contribution in the development of other person's personality.
- He also informs the pupils certain facts.
- Counselor guides the pupils to establish contacts with various factors in the counseling process. He explains the importance of those facts which the pupils consider unimportant.
- Counseling is a vital part of the entire guidance program.
- Counseling is only one aspect of guidance.
- Counseling is a learning-oriented process.
- Counseling is a face-to-face relationship with a person. This relationship is between a counselor and a client.
- Counseling is democratic. It lays down the democratic system. The client can behave as he wishes.
- Counseling is a professional service.
- Counseling is problem-oriented.
- Counseling is based on the appropriateness of counselor's prediction.
- Best counseling is in the form of the decision made by the counselee.
- Counseling is possible in humorous and cooperative environment only.
- Counseling is completely based on self-guidance.

16. Idealism.

Idealism is a very old philosophical thought and it was exercised a great and potent influence on man and his mind. Even today, idealism has certain attracting and we Indian have cherished those and a living with those ideas.

If we look into history, it was found that right advocate like Socrates froebel and WE Hocking, then in India idealism was reached by Gurdev and Rabindarnath Tagore which has something meaning and associated with other currents. Man is also spirit or mind, he is more important in the world. Idealism drives the importance of matter and mechanism. The idealist does not accept the biological account man in terms of his evolution. Idealism entirely different from naturalism because it denies the existence of the nature and accepts of existence of existence of conscious.

Meanings of idealism
1. One who accepts and lives by lofty moral, esthetic and religious standards.
2. Who is able to visualize and who advocates some play or program that yet does not exist, e.g. social reforms.
3. Who is a dreamer ignores practical conditions of a situation?
4. Who can give this as a compliment? For example Mr and Mrs So and so is an idealist that refers to one's attitude.

Philosophical meaning if idealism: According to Mahathma Gandhi, idealism does from the core of Gandhi philosophy in his education. It is not found reflected in his ultimate aim of education which is nothing but self-realization.

According to Titus, it has been derived from the world "idea" then ideal. Idealism has come from the fact of ideas, which originate from the mind or idealism, is in brief, assets that reality consists of ideas, thoughts, minds or selves and no different from material forces.

Assumption of idealism
1. **Ideas are final:** Ideas or spirits or thoughts or ideals are the final reality. Idealism emphasize mind as is some senses—prior to matter. Mind and ideas are real. Matter is subordinate.
2. **Belief in universal mind:** It means God and his presence everywhere, human an individual's mind. The environment of the universal spirit in their kinds: (a) intellectual, (b) feeling, and (c) willing.
3. **Concept of man:** The concept of man according to idealist is entirely different that man is not a animal, but may live or die, yet the body may perish but believe that body is underlying spirit.
4. **Idealism and knowledge:** It is a secondary phase; knowledge is gained through the senses.

17. Three main domains of an objective.

Humans are lifelong learners: From birth onward, we learn and assimilate what we have just learned into what we already know. Learning in the geosciences, like all learning, can be categorized into the domains of concept knowledge, how we view ourselves as learners and the skills we need to engage in the activities of geoscientists. As early as 1956 Educational Psychologist Benjamin Bloom divided what and how we learn into three separate domains of learning.

There are three main domains of learning and all teachers should know about them and use them to construct lessons. These domains are cognitive (thinking), affective (emotion/feeling), and psychomotor (physical/kinesthetic). Each domain on this page has a taxonomy associated with it. Taxonomy is simply a word for a classification. All of the taxonomies below are arranged, so that they proceed from the simplest to more complex levels.

1. **Cognitive domain**—this domain includes content knowledge and the development of intellectual skills. This includes the recall or recognition of specific facts and concepts that serve developing intellectual abilities and skills. There are six major categories, starting from the simplest behavior (recalling facts) to the most complex (evaluation).
2. **Affective domain**—how does one approach learning? With confidence, I can do attitude. The affective domain includes feelings, values, appreciation, enthusiasms, motivations, and attitudes.
3. **Psychomotor domain**—the psychomotor domain includes physical movement, coordination, and use of the motor-skill areas. Development of these skills requires practice and is measured in terms of speed, precision, distance, procedures, or techniques in execution.

18. Guidelines for preparing powerpoint slides.

These tips apply regardless of whether the time for the presentations is short (less than 30 minutes) or long. Complaints about poor presentations have been received for decades and continue to be received.

Preparation

I. Content organization

1. Make sure the audience walks away understanding the five things any listener to a presentation really cares about:
   a. What is the problem and why?
   b. What has been done about it?
   c. What is the presenter doing (or has done) about it?
   d. What additional value does the presenter's approach provide?
   e. Where do we go from here?
2. Carefully budget your time, especially for short (e.g. 15 minutes) presentations.
3. Allow time to describe the problem clearly enough for the audience to appreciate the value of your contribution. This usually will take more than 30 seconds.
4. Leave enough time to present your own contribution clearly. This almost never will require all of the allotted time.
5. Put your material in a context that the audience can relate to. It is a good idea to aim your presentation to an audience of colleagues who are not familiar with your research area. Your objective is to communicate an appreciation of the importance of your work, not just to lay the results out.
6. Give references and a way to contact you so those interested in the theoretical details can follow-up.

II. Preparing effective displays

Here are some suggestions that will make your displays more effective:
1. Keep it simple. The fact that you can include all kinds of cute decorations, artistic effects, and logos does not mean that you should. Fancy designs or color shifts can make the important material hard to read. Less is more.
2. Use at least a 24-point font so everyone in the room can read your material. Unreadable material is worse than useless—it inspires a negative attitude by the audience to your work and, ultimately, to you. Never use a photocopy of a standard printed page as a display—it is difficult to overstate how annoying this is to an audience.
3. Try to limit the material to eight lines per slide, and keep the number of words to a minimum. Summarize the main points—do not include every detail of what you plan to say. Keep it simple.

4. Limit the tables to four rows/columns for readability. Sacrifice content for legibility—unreadable content is worse than useless. Many large tables can be displayed more effectively as a graph than as a table.
5. Do not put a lot of curves on a graphical display—busy graphical displays are hard to read. Also, label your graphs clearly with big, readable type.
6. Use easily read fonts. Simple fonts like Sans Serif and Arial are easier to read than fancier ones like Times Roman or Monotype Corsiva. Do not use Italic fonts.
7. Light letters (yellow or white) on a dark background (e.g. dark blue) often will be easier to read when the material is displayed on LCD projectors.
8. Use equations sparingly if at all—audience members not working in the research area can find them difficult to follow as part of a rapidly delivered presentation. Avoid derivations and concentrate on presenting what your results mean. The audience will concede the proof and those who really are interested can follow-up with you, which they are more likely to do if they understand your results.
9. Do not fill up the slide—the peripheral material may not make it onto the display screen—especially the material on the bottom of a portrait-oriented transparency.
10. Identify the journal when you give references: The reader that the article is in a 1996 issue of biometrics, and is much more useful than just Smith 1996.
11. Finally, and this is critical, your presentation. You will look foolish if symbols and Greek letters that looked OK in a Word document did not translate into anything readable in powerpoint—and it happens.

III. Timing your talk

Do not deliver a 30 minutes talk in 15 minutes. Nothing irritates an audience more than a rushed presentation. Your objective is to engage the audience and have them understand your message. Do not flood them with more than they can absorb. Think in terms of what it would take if you were giving (or, better, listening to) the last paper in the last contributed paper session of the last day. This means:

1. Present only as much material as can reasonably fit into the time period allotted. Generally that means 1 slide per minute, or less.
2. Talk at a pace that everybody in the audience can understand. Speak slowly, clearly, and loudly, especially if your English is heavily accented.
3. Ask a colleague to judge your presentation, delivery, clarity of language, and use of time.
4. Balance the amount of material you present with a reasonable pace of presentation. If you feel rushed when you practice, then you have too much material. Budget your time to take a minute or two less than your maximum allotment. Again, less is more.

19. Essentials of lecture method.

The lecture method has been the earliest known method of instruction. At present, the method is used to a greater extent in colleges only. Many peoples, young people cannot stand sustained narration since their span of attention is limited. The lecture method is a one-way communication system and in a classroom, only the teacher remains active and the students passive. Yet this method has following advantages as well as disadvantages.

Often the cornerstone of university teaching, a lecture can be an effective method for communicating theories, ideas and facts to students. The lecture method is extensively used to present appreciation and to integrate ideas. The range of subjects that can be covered by this method is unlimited. But the speakers at a given meeting present a specific subject to a particular audience number of persons in a short period of time. —**A Adivi Reddy.**

Purposes of Lecture Method

1. Lecture method is only appropriate method for making available to a large class.
2. It draws the attention of the student in its vital elements and bring students abstract of development in the forefront of research.
3. It helps to promote the students with factual basis from which to build concepts by concrete examples.
4. Students can feasible involving in arriving at the general information like formulation of laws.

Principles of Lecture Method

1. **Principle of aim:** Lecture is based on aim, nobody likes aimless lecture. Even the best teacher will fail if his lecture is not based on some objectives.
2. **Principles of activity:** If you want to learn a thing you have to actively participate.
3. **Principle of correlation:** The lecture is not effective lecture is scientific planning. The subject matter of the topic which is sort to be taught should be well planned.
4. **Principles of looking ahead:** Good lecture is always prognostic on the basis of the past experiences of a teacher; certain predictors are made about the future of the child.
5. **Good lecture needs effective preparation:** The lecture has to be prepared physically, socially, emotionally and spiritually to enable him to take the lecture.

20. Benefits of computer-aided learning and teaching.

Computer-assisted instruction (CAI), as the name suggests, stands for the type of instruction aided or carried out with the help of a computer as a machine. It is just one step ahead of the use of teaching machine and, probably, two of the use of programed textbook in making the instructional process as self-directed and individualized as possible. Computer influence every sphere of human activity and bring many changes in education, healthcare scientific research, social sciences, etc. usage of computers in healthcare system will save the time, economizes energy and help the nurses to provide quality nursing.

Advantages of Computer-assisted Learning

1. It saves time in learning.
2. It performs miracles in processing the performance data.
3. It helps to determine subsequent activities in the learning situation.
4. The large amount of information stored in the computer is made available to the learner more rapidly.
5. The dynamic interaction between the student and instructional program is possible.

21. Advantages of audio-visual aids.

Audio-visual aids or devices or technological media or learning devices are added devices that help the teacher to clarify, establish, corelate accurate concepts, interpretations and appreciations and enable him to make learning more concrete, effective, interesting, inspirational, meaningful, and vivid. They help in completing the triangular process of learning viz, motivation, clarification, stimulation. The aim of teaching with technological media is clearing the channel between the learning and the things that are worth learning. The basic assumption underlying audiovisual aids is that learning—clear understanding stems from sense experience. The teacher must show as well as tell. Audiovisual aids provide significant gains in informational learning, retention and recall, thinking and reasoning, activity, interest, imagination, better assimilation and personal growth and development. The aids are the stimuli for learning why, how, when, and where. The

hard to understand principles are usually made clear by the intelligent use of skillfully designed instructional aids.
1. **Best motivators:** They are the best motivators. Students work with more interest and zeal. They are more attentive.
2. **Fundamental to verbal instructions:** They help to reduce verbalism which is a major weakness of our schools. They convey the same meaning as words mean. They give clear concepts and thus help to bring accuracy in learning.
3. **Clear images:** Clear images are formed when we see, hear, touch, taste and smell as our experiences are direct, concrete and more or less permanent. Learning through the senses becomes the most natural and consequently the easiest.
4. **Vicarious experience:** Everyone agrees to the fact that the first-hand experience is the best type of educative experience but such an experience cannot always be provided to the pupils an so in some situations certain substitutes have to be provided. For this, we find a large number of inaccessible objects and phenomenon. For example, all the students in India, cannot possibly be shown Taj Mahal, etc. In all such cases, audiovisual aids provide us the best substitutes.
5. **Variety:** Audio-visual aids provide variety and provide different tools in the hands of the teacher.
6. **Freedom:** The use of audiovisual aids provide various occasions for the pupil to move about, talk, laugh and comment upon. Under such an atmosphere the students work because they want to work and not because the teacher wants them to work.
7. **Opportunities to handle and manipulate:** The use of audiovisual aids provides immense opportunities to the pupils to see, handle and manipulate things.

22. Checklist.

A checklist is a type of informational job aid used to reduce failure by compensating for potential limits of human memory and attention. It helps to ensure consistency and completeness in carrying out a task. A basic example is the "to do list."

2015

Communication and Educational Technology

LONG ESSAYS

1. Explain the steps in communication process. Explain the different barriers in communication.
2. Define education. What are the characteristics of learning? Explain the maxims of teaching.
3. List the various teaching methods used in clinical area. Explain in detail about the case method.

SHORT ESSAYS

4. Principles of preparing slides.
5. Discussion method.
6. Basic principles in counseling.
7. Programmed instructions.
8. Types of counseling approaches.
9. Mention the types of audio-visual aids. Write briefly on printed aids.
10. Factors to improve good human relations.
11. Scope of guidance and counseling in nursing education.
12. Barriers in interpersonal relations.

SHORT ANSWERS

13. Define evaluation.
14. Principles of teaching.
15. List the different types of projected aids.
16. Purpose of interpersonal relationship.
17. Self-instructional module.
18. Symposium.
19. Disadvantages of essay question.
20. Process recording.
21. Nursing rounds.
22. List two specific objectives for a lesson plan on anemia.

LONG ESSAYS

1. Explain the steps in communication process. Explain the different barriers in communication.

The communication has been derived from Latin word communis, which implies common. Communication is an exchange of facts, ideas, opinions or emotions by two or more persons. Communication is much more than simply transmission of information. It also involves interpretation and understanding of the message. It is an interchange of thoughts and informational intercourse through words, letters, symbols or message. Communication is the basic element of human interactions. It is one of the most vital components of all nursing practice.

Communication Process Steps

Communication is the two-way process involving the sending and receiving of a message. Since, the purpose of communication is to elicit a response the response the process in ongoing. The receiver of the message becomes the sender of the response and the original sender becomes the receiver.

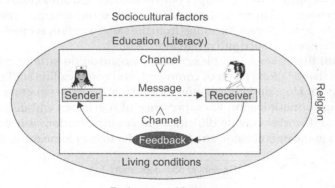

The basic elements of communication are:
1. **The sender:** The sender is on the individual or group who wishes to convey the message to another. He is the initiator of the communication process and is sometimes called the source encoder. The individual or group sending the message must have a reason for communicating and must put it in a form that can be transmitted. Encoding means translating the thoughts into specific signs and symbols. Effective encoding depends on a clear message delivered at a right place at right time and phrased in such a way as to attract the receiver's attention.
2. **The message:** It is the information that is selected and conveyed by the sender. It requires the sender's decision's about what will be side, how, when and where it will be said and the selection of words in a language that can be understood by the receiver.
3. **The channel:** It is the means by which the message is transmitted. For example, through the visual, auditory and tactile senses. It is important that the channel be appropriate for the message to make the infant of the message clear. Talking face to face with person may be more effective in some instances than telephoning or writing the message. Recording message on tapes or communicating by radio or television may be appropriate for larger audiences.

4. **Receiver:** The receiver is the individual to whom the message is transmitted. This individual is sometimes called the decoder. He interprets and decodes the sender's message into information that has meaning. Understanding is the key to the decoding process. The intended meaning will be communicated when the sender and the receiver have common knowledge and experience.
5. **The feedback:** It is the message that the receiver returns to the sender. It is also called feedback. The receiver's verbal and nonverbal responses to the sender reveal the receiver understands of the message. It helps the sender to recognize whether the meaning of his message has been received as intended. Communication is not successful until the message received has been understood and acted upon it appropriately.

Barriers of Communication

Though communication is essential, perfect communication is rarely achieved in practice. There are obstacles which continuously block and distort the flow of ideas and information. Some of these barriers to communication are given below:

1. **Badly expressed messages:** Very often the message is expressed in poorly chosen words or empty phrases, lack of coherence, poor organization of ideas, awkward sentence structure. There is use of inappropriate language, poor vocabulary and ambiguous words. The lack of clarity and precision lead to misunderstanding, costly errors and unnecessary clarification. Different people drive different meanings from the same words or symbols due to difference in their education, experience and orientation.
2. **Organizational distance:** A complex of faulty organization structure involving several layers of supervision, a long chain of command, and complex line staff relations impedes the interchange of ideas and information. At every layer of the structure the message gets distorted. Long communication lines, presence of specialties and distance between top management and workers create difficulties in communication. It is necessary to make improvements in the organization structure in order to overcome these difficulties.

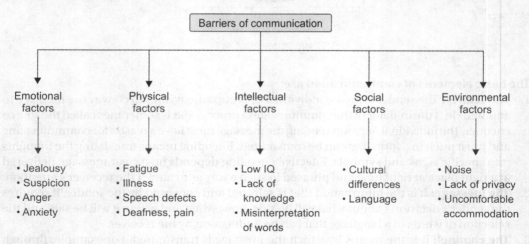

3. **Status and position:** Vertical communication is hampered by difference in the status and position of the superior and subordinate. Status refers to the regard and attitude of member of the organization towards a position and its occupant. Status arises on account of formal position in the hierarchy, job title, salary and other privileges. Supervisors tend to keep information to themselves and they do not want to listen to subordinates. Subordinates are

reluctant to seek clarification for fear of loss of prestige. Effective communication becomes difficult when people become strong conscious of status and position. Subordinate tend to tell the boss what is pleasant and withhold unpleasant information.

4. **Inattention:** Many people simply do not pay adequate attention to the message. They do not listen the spoken words attentively or they fail to read the message carefully. Generally, people pay attention to the information which confirms their beliefs and ignore those conflicts with what they believe. Such selective listening hampers effective communication. Sometimes people pay perfunctory attention because they are victims of communication overload or because the information is solicited. Communication overload arises when people posses more information than they can assimilate or cannot adequately responds to the messages directed to them. Inattention also arises due to lack of interest, over stimulation, tendency to criticize the mode of delivery or noting everything. The source of communication and the way in which it is presented also determine the degree of attention paid to it. Listening is the most neglected skill of communication.

5. **Poor retention (screening or filtering):** Successive transmissions of the same message are decreasingly accurate. At each level, the message is screened by receiver and only such information is passed further which gives a favorable impression of the sender. Such filtering arises due to the fact that no one likes to show his mistakes to others. Noise can distort communication at every step in the communication process. In order to overcome the barrier of filtering, it is necessary to develop a well-designed feedback system and rapport with subordinates. The manager should listen to subordinate with an understanding attitude.

6. **Perception:** When people with different perceptions communicate, they have trouble in getting the meaning across. Every one perceives the message from his own angle or viewpoint. Perceptions of people differ due to differences in their needs, education, social back ground, interest etc. in the absence of an open mind and willingness to see things through the eyes of others; people perceive the same information differently. When the communicator does not enjoy trust and credibility, he fails to convey his ideas to others. Differences in value judgments and references frames also inhibit communication.

7. **Resistance to change:** Human being by nature prefers to maintain status and generally resist new ideas. When the communication contains a new idea, the receiver may not take it seriously or may receive it according to his own convenience. Everyone likes to receive the information which confirms his present belief and tends to ignore anything that is contrary to such belief. A manager should provide sufficient time and assistance to make subordinates receptive to change.

2. Define education. What are the characteristics of learning? Explain the maxims of teaching.

In literary sense, education owes its origin to the two Latin words: 'Educare' and 'Educe'. 'Educare' means 'to nourish', 'to bring up', 'to raise'; 'Educe' means to bring forth', 'to lead out', 'to draw out'. 'Educatum' means' the act of teaching and training'. The word education is derived from the Latin word educare which means to lead out. This derivation connotes growth from the within. Thus, the root meaning of education can be given as manifestation of the inherent potentials in child. The idea of education is not merely to impart knowledge to the pupil in some subjects but to develop in him those habits and attitudes with which he may successfully face the future. Education is the process of helping the child to adjust with this changing world. By means of education, the child is subjected to certain experiences that are intended to modify his behavior in order to bring about proper adjustment with the changing environment. In fact, education is the basis of life, for leading a purposeful and ideal life.

Definitions

1. Swami Vivekananda viewed education as, 'the manifestation of divine perfection already existing in man. Education means the exposition of man's complete individuality'.
2. According to John Dewey, 'Education is development of all those capabilities in the individual, which will help him to control his environment and fulfill his possibilities'.

Characteristics of Learning

1. **Learning is growth:** The individual grows as he lives. This growth implies in both physical as well as mental development of the learner. The individual gains experiences through various activities. These are all sources of learning. The individual grows through living and learning. Thus, growth and learning are inter-related and even synonymous.
2. **Learning is adjustment:** Learning enables the individual to adjust himself properly, with the new situations. The individual faces new problems and new situations throughout his life and learning helps him to solve the problems encountered by him. That is why; many psychologists describe learning as "a process of progressive adjustment to the ever changing conditions which one encounters." The society in which we live is so complex and so dynamic that any one type of adjustment will not be suitable for all or many situations and problems. It is through learning that one could achieve the ability to adjust adequately to all situations of life.
3. **Learning is purposeful:** All kinds of learning is goal-oriented. The individual acts with some purpose. He learns through activities. He gets himself interested when he is aware of his objectives to be realized through these activities. Therefore, all learning is purposive in nature.
4. **Learning is experience:** The individual learns through experiences. Human life is fall of experiences. All these experiences provide new knowledge, understanding, skills and attitudes. Learning is not mere acquisition of the knowledge, skills and attitudes. It is also the reorganization of experiences or the synthesis of the old experiences with the new.
5. **Learning is intelligent:** Mere cramming without proper understanding does not make learning. Thus, meaningless efforts do not produce permanent results. Any work done mechanically cannot yield satisfactory learning outcomes. Learning therefore, must be intelligent.
6. **Learning is active:** Learning is given more importance than teaching. It implies self-activity of the learning. Without adequate motivation he cannot work whole-heartedly and motivation is, therefore, at the root of self-activity. Learning by doing is thus an important principle of education, and the basis of all progressive methods of education like the project, the Dalton, the Montessori and basic system.
7. **Learning is both individual and social:** Although, learning is an individual activity, it is social also. Individual mind is consciously or unconsciously affected by the group activities. Individual is influenced by his peers, friends, relatives, parents and classmates and learns their ideas, feelings and attitudes in some way or others. The social agencies like family, church, markets, and clubs exert immense influence on the individual minds. As such, learning becomes both individual as well as social.
8. **Learning is the product of the environment:** The individual lives in interaction with the society. Particularly, environment plays an important part in the growth and development of the individual. The physical, social, intellectual and emotional development of the child is moulded and remoulded by the objects and individuals in his environment. Therefore, it is emphasized that child's environment should be made free from unhealthy and vicious matters to make it more effective for learning.

9. **Learning affects the conduct of the learner:** Learning is called the modification of behavior. It affects the learner's behavior and conduct. Every learning experience brings about changes in the mental structure of the learner. Therefore, attempts are made to provide such learning experiences which can mould the desired conduct and habits in the learners.

Maxims of Learning

The maxims of teaching are very helpful in obtaining the active involvement and participation of the learners in the teaching learning process. They quicken the interest of the learner and motivate them to learn. They make learning effective, inspirational, interesting and meaningful. They keep the students attentive to the teaching-learning process. A good teacher should be quite familiar with them. Now we proceed to discuss them.

1. **Proceed from the known to the unknown:** The most natural and simple way of teaching a lesson is to be proceed from something that the students already know to those facts which they do not know. What is already known to the students is of great use to the students? This means that the teacher should arouse the interest in a lesson by putting questions on the subject matter already known to the pupils. The teacher is to proceed step by step to connect the new matter to the old one. New knowledge cannot be grasped in a vacuum.

2. **Proceed from simple to complex:** The simple task or topic must be taught first and the complex one can follow later on. The word simple and complex are to be seen from the point of view of the child and not that of an adult. We would be curbing the interest and initiative of the children by presenting them complex problems before the simpler ones are presented.

3. **Proceed from easy to difficult:** We must graduate our lessons in order of ease of undertaking them. Student's standards must be kept in view. This will help in sustaining the interest of the students. In determining what is easy and what is difficult we have to take into account the psychological make-up of the child. Logically viewed one skill may be easy but psychologically it may be difficult. There are many things which look easy to us but are in fact difficult for children. The interest of the children has also to be taken into account.

4. **Proceed from the concrete to the abstract:** A child's imagination is greatly aided by a concrete material. Things first and words after is the common saying. Children in the beginning cannot think in abstracts. Small children learn first from things which they can see and handle. Very young pupils learn counting with the help of pebbles, etc. a child understands is aeroplane with the help of a model. Actual visits to canals and rivers provide a clear idea of them. A lesson in geography can be made interesting with the help of models, pictures and illustrations of bridges, rivers and mountains, etc. Care must be taken exercised to ensure that the students do not remain at the concrete stage all the times. This is only the initial step for children with a view to reach the higher stage of abstraction as they advance in age.

5. **Proceed from particular to general:** Before giving principles and rules, particular examples should be presented. As a matter of fact a study of particular facts should lead the children themselves to frame general rules. The rules of arithmetic, of grammar, of physical geography and almost of all sciences are based on the principle of proceeding from particular instances to general rules.

6. **Proceed from indefinite to definite:** Ideas of children in the initial stages are indefinite, incoherent and very vague. These ideas are to be made definite, clear, precise and systematic. Effective teaching necessitates that every word and idea presented should stand out clearly in the child's mind as a picture. For classifying ideas, adequate use must are made of actual objectives, diagrams and pictures. Every possible effort should be make the children interested in the lesson.

7. **Proceed from empirical to rational:** Observation and experience are the basis of empirical knowledge. Rational knowledge implies a bit of abstraction and arguments approach. The general feeling is that the child first of all experiences knowledge in his day-to-day life and after that he feels the rational basis. For instance, plane geometry makes better sense when taught in the context of everyday life instead of in the format of a highly abstract theory. It is always better to begin with what the children see, feel and experience than arguing and generalizing.
8. **Proceed from psychological to logical:** Logical approach is concerned with the arrangement of the subject matter. Psychological approach looks at the child's interests, needs, mental make-up and reactions. When we treat a subject logically, we are usually thinking of it from our own point of view and not from the point of view of the child. In psychological approach, we proceed from the concrete to the abstract, from the simple to the complex and from known to unknown. We start reading by teaching the child to read a whole sentence as it is for the adult. This is psychological approach. In drawing lesson, a child has little sense in lines and curves. Logically we start with simple lines and curves but psychologically we start with drawing a whole animal.
9. **Proceed from whole to parts:** Whole is more meaningful to the child than the parts of the whole. The learner sees a relationship between the central ideas of the material to be learned. The whole unit or passage for slow learner should be smaller than the whole for the fast learners.
10. **From near to far:** A child learns well in the surroundings in which he resides. So, he should be first acquainted with his immediate environment. Gradually, he may be taught about things which are away from his immediate environment. In a geography lesson, we start from the local geography and then take up tehsil, district, state, the country and the world gradually.
11. **From analysis to synthesis:** Analysis means breaking a problem into convenient parts and synthesis means grouping of these separated parts into one complete whole. Complex problems can be made simple and easy by dividing it into units.
12. **From actual to representative:** When actual objectives are shown to children, they learn easily and retain them in their minds for a longer time. This is especially suitable for younger children. Representative objectives in the form of pictures, models, etc., should be used for the grown-ups.
13. **Proceed inductively:** This maxim include almost all the maxims stated above. In the inductive approach, we start from particular examples and establish general rules through the active participation of the learners. In the deductive approach, we assume a definition, a general rule or formula and apply it to particular examples. An example will make this distinction very clear. The 'farmers in India are very poor' is a general statement in the deductive type of reasoning.

3. List the various teaching methods used in clinical area. Explain in detail about the case method.

Nursing is a field requiring clinical skills to care for the patients as we deal and handle with real life situations. Clinical experience in the education of nursing students is considered as lifeblood of nursing education. Nurse educators have a responsibility to provide most effective clinical instruction to facilitate best learning. The learning process in nursing is very unique because nursing student should be able to perform the activities of the profession in live situations where as in general education there is simply understanding of principles in the laboratory set-up or on nonhuman articles. Learning experiences in nursing must provide opportunities to apply theoretical principles to real time situations on a daily basis at bedside/community. In this unit we shall discuss about various clinical teaching methods.

Methods of Clinical Teaching

Methods of clinical teaching are:
- Nursing clinic/bedside clinic
- Nursing care conference
- Nursing rounds demonstration
- Nursing care study
- Clinical simulation
- Virtual learning/game-based show mastery learning.

Uses

1. It acts as a method to meet individual learner needs.
2. It creates best learning environment that facilitates learner to socialize as nurse.
3. It promotes development of the learner in improving knowledge, psychomotor skills and positive attitude.
4. It raises challenges for students to face the nursing situations.
5. It provides opportunities for real-life experiences and transfer of knowledge to practical situations.

Important Characteristics of Clinical Teacher

1. Clinical competence
2. Nonjudgmental
3. Role model
4. Enthusiasm
5. Feedback skills
6. Availability
7. Respectful of learner's autonomy.

Case Method

Nursing case study is one of the common and useful methods of teaching in clinical area. It is a form of quantitative and qualitative analysis involving a very careful and complete observation of a patient, and his situation.

Purpose of Case Study

1. It provides opportunity to the student to learn nursing skills using the problem-solving approach.
2. Students able to identify and define a patients problems.
3. It trains the students to locate, gather and process the information required to solve the patients problem.
4. To develop a sense of accomplishment from providing individualized comprehensive care.
5. It helps the student to solve the patients problems by critical and reflective thinking.
6. It accentuates the health and social aspects of nursing.
7. It emphasis the facts that the patient is an individual personality with unique problems.

Meaning

1. Case study is the intensive study of a phenomenon including subjective information and objective information.

2. Case study is an analysis of the nursing problems of an individual patient, which grow out of his diagnosis, his physical and mental condition, treatment, which are influenced by personality and socioeconomic development.
3. Case study is a close, deep, cumulative and clinical study of a patient.
4. Case study is a fairly exhaustive study of a person or group.

Criteria for a Good Case Study
1. Continuity
2. Completeness of data
3. Validity of data
4. Confidential recording
5. Analysis and scientific synthesis.

Sources of Case Data
1. Personal documental diaries, history of previous illness.
2. Health team members.
3. Related persons.
4. Official records.
5. Subject itself.

Principles
1. The students should be able to make their nursing care study on a patient for whose nursing care they are responsible.
2. The selection of patients can be done by coordination between the clinical instructor and students.
3. The case study should be emphasized on the individual needs of a patient and how they are met.
4. Special emphasis should be made on patient learning.
5. Case study should serve as an excellent tool to demonstrate nursing skills, scientific knowledge and sociological and psychological insight into the problems of the patient.
6. The case study should encourage critical evaluation of solutions presented by others. The student is presented with the whole situation so that she may visualize it completely.

Steps in Nursing Case Study
1. **Selection of the case:** The level of knowledge of the students is taken into considerations while assigning patients. Selection of cases should be based on the level of care needed, e.g. wholly independent patient is not assigned for case study.
2. **Collection of data:** Collection of data is divided into two aspects:
   a. **Subjective data:** All the information, the patient himself gives.
   b. **Objective data:** Data which are documents through observation, investigation or intervention.
3. **Examination:** Examination of patient includes anthropometric measures, biological measures, clinical examination and dietary examination. History relevant to present and past conditions is collected using the relevant formats.
4. **Diagnosis and identification of casual factors:** Through laboratory investigations and invasive procedures, the casual factors are identified.
5. **Nursing process:** The nursing process includes assessment of the patient, forming nursing diagnosis on the basis of assessment, planning the care and implementation.
6. **Evaluation and follow-up:** The effectiveness of care rendered is identified here.

SHORT ESSAYS

4. Principles of preparing slides.

Teaching slides, glass slides or projection slides or lantern slides carry immense value in teaching procedures. The use of single slide can visualize entire teaching session. This is a successful teaching device which helps in the retention of the material taught in the minds of the pupils. A few carefully selected slides or even one partinent slide can:
1. Attract attention.
2. Arouse interest.
3. Assist lesson development.
4. Test student understanding.
5. Review instruction.
6. Facilitate student-teacher participation.

A glass side is made up of a piece of sensitized glass, similar to the sensitized paper for use in photography. The slide may be in color or in black and white. Different forms of glass slides, phonographer etched glass slide, ink slides, etc. may be used for teaching purposes.

Using Slide in Teaching

As pointed out earlier, slides and slide-projectors are useful teaching devices which offer huge mass of usual material. Right from the lower, primary to the high school and even at the post-school level. Slides serve useful teaching purpose. Even at the program of adult education, slides can be usefully exhibition and instruction imparted. Some of the important instructional areas in which sets of slides are available and can be used are:
1. Reading.
2. Languages.
3. Science.
4. Mathematics.
5. Social studies.
6. Music.
7. Art.

Though, it is possible to have slide projectors on reasonable price in the market, yet every school cannot afford to have as slide projector. A magic lantern is a convenient device to replace the slide projector. It is not very costly. It can be conveniently improvised for classroom use.

The Filmstrip

The teaching filmstrip or the discussion filmstrip, "is a continuous strip of film consisting of individual frames or pictures arranged in sequence, usually with explanatory titles. Each strip contains from 25 to 100 or more pictures with suitable copy." A filmstrip is also a transparent projection, but differs from slides in that it is a fixed sequence of related stills on a role of 35 mm film. The filmstrip has a number of advantages, among which may be mentioned the following:
1. It is an economical visual material.
2. It is easy to make and convenient to handle and carry.
3. It takes up little space and can be easily stored.
4. It provides a logical sequence to the teaching procedure and the individual picture on the strip can be kept before the students for a length of time.
5. It is a available both in color and in black and white.

The filmstrip can be projected on the screen or wall or paper screen or the back side of a map, etc. as the convenience and the teaching situation demands. A large number of subjects come within the range of filmstrips. The teacher only needs to tap the right source and the right type of strip for his teaching purpose. History, civics, geography, science, mathematics, current affairs are some of the subjects which have been adapted to filmstrips. A number of filmstrips are available with the Central Film Library, Government of India, and New Delhi.

The following suggestions should be kept in mind while using film strip as a device:
1. For presenting filmstrips in the classroom, follow the procedure outlined for teaching slides.
2. Determine the lesson that could be effectively illustrated with a strip.
3. Use instructional materials that are well-selected and interesting. The filmstrips selected should serve for the specific lesson.
4. Never miss opportunities for using the filmstrip in a variety of curricular areas, such as science, history, geography, spelling, reading, art, and music, etc.
5. Preview filmstrips before using them.
6. Show again any part of film strip needing more specific study.
7. Use filmstrip to stimulate emotions, build attitudes, and to point up problems.
8. Use a pointer to direct attention, to specific details on the screen.

Vocabulary

Man, woman, child, mother, hands, legs, chair, table, training, leaning, lying waling, erect, practising, sitting, posture, walk, run, stomach.

5. Discussion method.

In its simple meaning, the term group discussion stands for the discussion held within a group. In this sense, group discussion as teaching strategy may be defined as some sort of discussion, i.e. interchange of ideas between students and the teacher or among a group of students, resulting into active learning for the realization of the predetermined teaching-learning objectives. This group discussion, in no way, occurs occasionally or incidentally but is planned and organized with deliberate efforts on the part of the teacher and students for achieving the set goals.

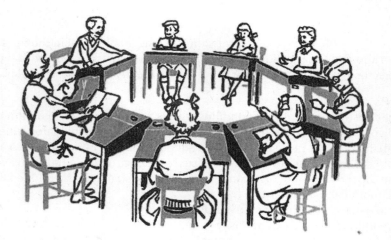

Definition

Group discussion is a cooperative, problem-solving activity which seeks a consensus regarding the solution of a problem.

Purpose of Group Discussion

1. It provides opportunity for sharing information.
2. It provides opportunity to attend group consortium.
3. It helps to gain knowledge.
4. It helps to develop skills of group development.
5. It helps to learn variety of information in short time.

Advantages of Group Discussion

Group discussion strategy has the following advantages:
1. It ensures the active participation of the students in the process of teaching-learning.
2. It trains the students for carrying out group activities and cooperative tasks. The qualities linked to proper social development and democratic living is also developed with the adoption of this strategy.
3. It provides opportunities to the students for imbibing the qualities of a good listener as well as an effective leader. When a group member speaks others listen to it with patience and try to show respect for his opinion, but at the same time they may also put up their own views in a quite democratic way.

6. Basic principles in counseling.

Listening Skills

Listen attentively to the client in an attempt to understand both the content of their problem, as they see it, and the emotions they are experiencing related to the problem. Do not make interpretations of the client's problems or offer any premature suggestions as to how to deal with, or solve the issues presented. Listen and try to understand the concerns being presented. Most people want and need to be heard and understood, not advised.

Resistance

Changing human behavior is not usually a linear, direct, and logical process. It is very emotional and many habits of behavior and thought that are dysfunctional are difficult to break. People invest a sense of security in familiar behavior, even some behavior that causes them pain. Changing this is often a difficult and tangential process. Many threads of behavior are tied to others and when one thing is changed a new balance must be established, otherwise people could not function. This means people change at different rates depending on how well they can tolerate the imbalance that comes from change. So, when people resist certain changes that one hopes will occur in therapy it is important that the therapist not take this personally and recognize the stressful nature of the process for the client. Some resistance to therapeutic change is quite natural.

Respect

No matter how peculiar, strange, disturbed, weird, or utterly different from you that the client is, they must be treated with respect! Without this basic element successful therapy is impossible. You do not have to like the client, or their values, or their behavior, but you must put your personal feelings aside and treat them with respect. In some institutional settings you made observe some slippage in this principal among staff which is both inadequately trained and overstressed and overworked, but you must try to keep this principal in mind at all times in you want to be an effective counselor or therapist.

Empathy and Positive Regard

Based in the writings of Carl Rogers, these two principles go along with respect and effective listening skills. Empathy requires you to listen and understand the feelings and perspective of the other person (in this case your client) and positive regard is an aspect of respect. While Rogers calls this "unconditional positive regard" it may be a bit too much to ask that it be "unconditional." Treating the client with respect should be sufficient.

Clarification, Confrontation, Interpretation

These are techniques of therapeutic intervention that are more advanced, although clarification is useful even at a basic level. Clarification is an attempt by the therapist to restate what the client is either saying or feeling, so the client may learn something or understand the issue better. Confrontation and interpretation are more advanced principles and we would not go into them except to mention their existence.

Transference and Countertransference

This is a process wherein the client feels things and has perceptions of the therapist that rightly belong to other people in the client's life, either past or present. It is a process somewhat related to projection. Understanding transference reactions can help the client gain understanding of important aspects of their emotional life. Countertransference refers to the emotional and perceptional reactions the therapist has towards the client that rightly belong to other significant people in the therapists life. It is important for the therapist to understand and manage their countertransference.

7. Programmed instructions.

Programmed learning or programmed instruction represents one of the effective innovations in the teaching-learning process. As a highly individualized and systematic instructional strategy, it has been found quite useful for classroom instruction as well as self-learning or auto-instruction. In our country, also there have been attempts for the use of programmed instructions especially in providing material to the students of correspondence courses. Suitable self-instructional programmed materials for different subjects and grades have been prepared and it is being used for instructional or self-instructional purposes. Programmed learning occupies a unique place in the teaching and learning of all the school subjects especially those requiring logical and systematic study coupled with independent practice and drillwork.

Definitions

Smith and Moore (1962): Programmed instruction is the process of arranging the material to be learned into a series of sequential steps, usually it moves the students from a familiar background into a complex and new set of concepts, principles and understanding.

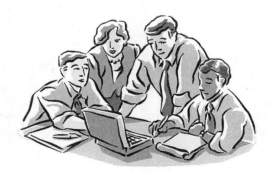

Advantages of Programmed Instruction
1. Student is kept active and alert.
2. The teacher gets relieved of doing ordinary jobs and she can play the important role of a guide, counselor, motivator, organizer.
3. Social and emotional problems can be eliminated.
4. The problems of discipline have been automatically solved by the use of self-instructional material.
5. Programmed instruction makes learning interesting.
6. Every student can work at his own place.
7. Programmed instructions is useful in situations where the human instructions are not available.
8. Intellectual and some motor skills will be taught more efficiently.
9. More complex of the concepts can be known.

Disadvantages
1. Student-teacher interaction lost.
2. It is costly when compared to traditional teaching methods.
3. It does not eliminate competition or grades as often examined.
4. No scope of providing language learning.
5. It restricts the learners freedom of choice.
6. It cramping the imagination and initiative.

8. Types of counseling approaches.

There are many approaches to counseling, but these approaches can be grouped under the following three headings:
1. **Indirect approach:** The indirect approach to counseling is also regarded as the client-centered approach. In this approach, the counselee is allowed to express self while the counselor only listen with rapt attention and intermittently, when necessary, approach rely on the tenets of the client-centered theory as their major counseling skill.
2. **Direct approach:** This is just the opposite of the indirect or client-centered approach. In this counseling approach, the talking is done by the counselor who uses questions and various counseling skills to elicit responses from the counselee about the problems at hand. Here, the counselor dictates the pace and directs the counselee based on what can be made out of the sparing responses gathered from the counselee.
3. **Eclectic approach:** This approach to counseling does not rely totally on either the indirect or direct approach. Rather it finds the two approaches named above with any other suitable one handy during counseling sessions. It thereby relies on chosen skills that suit the counseling session at hand, from all the available approaches, to resolve the counselee's problems.

9. Mention the types of audio-visual aids. Write briefly on printed aids.

Audio-visual aids or devices or technological media or learning devices are added devices that help the teacher to clarify, establish, corelate accurate concepts, interpretations and appreciations and enable him to make learning more concrete, effective, interesting, inspirational, meaningful, and vivid. They help in completing the triangular process of learning viz motivation, clarification and stimulation.

Classification 1: Projected and nonprojected aids.

Projected aids	Graphic aids	Display boards	3-dimensional aids	Audio aids	Activity aids
Films	Cartoons	Black board	Diagrams	Radio	Computer-assisted instruction
Filmstrips	Charts	Bulletin board	Models	Recordings	Demonstration
Opaque projectors	Comics	Flannel board	Mock-ups	Television	Dramatics
Overhead projectors	Diagrams	Magnetic board	Objectives		Experimentation
Slides	Flash cards Graphs Maps Photographs Pictures Postures	Peg board	Puppets Specimens		Field trips Programmed instruction Teaching machines

Classification 2: Audio materials, visual materials and audio-visual materials.

Audio materials	Visual materials	Audio-visual materials
Language laboratories	Bulletin boards	Demonstration
Radio	Chalkboards	Films
Sound distribution system sets	Charts	Printed materials with recorded sound
Tape and disco recording	Drawings, etc.	Sound filmstrips
	Exhibits	Study trips
	Filmstrips	Television
	Flash cards	Videotapes
	Flannel boards	
	Flip books	
	Illustrated books	
	Magnetic boards	
	Maps	
	Models	
	Pictures	
	Postures	
	Photographs	
	Self-instructional	
	Silent films	
	Slides	

Classification 3: Big medias and little medias:
- Big medias include: Computer, VCR, and TV.
- Little media include: Radio, filmstrips, graphic, audio cassettes and various visuals.

Classification 4: Three-dimensional aids:
1. Models.
2. Mock-ups.
3. Specimens

Three-dimensional aids are the replicas or substitutes of real objective.

Printed aids: Printed media are material used in inform, motivate or instruct learners. Kemp and Dayton (1985) classify printed media into three types:
1. Learning aids: Guide sheets, job aids, picture series.
2. Training material: Handouts, study guides, instructor's manuals.
3. Information materials: Brochures, newsletters and reports.

Lewis and Paine (1986), listed the advantages as follows:
1. Easy to use, generate, produce, modify and update.
2. Cheap, especially if the media are black and white. Color is more expensive.

Disadvantages of printed media are:
1. They may be too familiar and be ignored because they look like high school materials.
2. It may be difficult to teach skills or convey emotions and feelings through print media, they will be difficult to update if the printed materials is bound as a book.

Criteria for leaflet or pamphlet:
1. The words written should be clear, concise, understable and short.
2. The sentence formed should not be too clumsy and crowded.
3. The background color and the colors used for printing the letters should be contrast.
4. The letter style should be attractive and bright.
5. The size of the paper should be less than 20–30 cm in length, 10–20 cm in breath.
6. Both the sides can be used to print the letters.
7. The sentence used should be elicited in the form of points.
8. The letter size of the heading should be slightly bigger than the points that are included.

10. Factors to improve good human relations.

Human relations are important in everyday life, but they are essential for health staff dealing with people in pain and discomfort. Unfortunately, in the past not much importance was given to this important facet of human dealing. Stress was made on technical skills, and how good one was at diagnosing and treating illness. This highly technical orientation of health professionals lead to high level of patient dissatisfaction, and often lead to bitterness and sometimes even litigation. It was recognized that good human dealing was necessary to heal the pain and reduce dissatisfaction of the patients. Hospitals started moving towards patient centered approach and gave up the physician focused care. However, a vacuum was felt in the training and needs of the highly technical and competent staff, in areas of human relations.

Factors to Improve Good Human Relations

Organization should be viewed as a social system. Human relations in the organization are determined by the work group leader and work environment. Following factors influence the human relation in organization.

1. **Work environment:** Human relationists advocated the creation of a positive work environment where organizational goals are achieved through satisfaction of employees. In general, when employee needs are satisfied, the work environment is termed positive and when employee needs are not satisfied, the work environment is termed negative. Positive work environments are characterizing by such factors like: goals are clearly stated incentives are properly used to improve performance, feedback is available on performance decisions are timely and participative, rules are minimum conflict is confronted openly and squarely, the work is interesting and growth-oriented.
2. **Work-group:** The work-group is the center of focus of human relations studies. It has an important role in determining the attitudes and performance of individual workers. The Hawthorne studies showed that the informal groups exert tremendous influence over the behavior patterns of workers At Western Electric Co., the informal groups countermanded official orders quite frequently and played a decisive role in determining production standards. Work is a social experience and most workers find satisfaction in membership in social groups. Unless managers recognize the human relations at work productivity will not improve.
3. **Individual:** The human being is an important segment of the organization. Behavior of an individual is affected by his feelings, sentiments and attitudes. Motivation of employees should give due consideration to their economic, social and psychological needs. Thus, motivation is a complex process.
4. **Leader:** The human relationists gave great importance to leadership. The leader must ensure full and effective utilization of all organizational resources to achieve organizational goals. He must be able to adjust to various personalities and situations. He must behave in a way that generates respect. As the Hawthorne studies showed, a supervisor can contribute significantly in increasing productivity by providing a free, happy and pleasant work environment where bossism is totally absent and where members are allowed to participate in decision-making processes. Authoritative tendencies must give way to democratic values. The essence of the human relations philosophy is to cultivate and develop an environment where the employees as individuals and in groups would wish to contribute their best to the organizational goals. This environment is cultivated and developed where there is an awareness of the needs, aspirations, feelings and emotions of the employees on the part of management.

11. Scope of guidance and counseling in nursing education.

The scope of guidance is all pervading. Its scope is very vast in the light of modernization and industrialization and is ever increasing. As the life is getting complex day by day, the problems for which expert help is needed are rapidly increasing. The scope of guidance is extending horizontally to much of the social context, to matters of prestige in occupations, to the broad field of social trends and economic development. Crow and Crow have rightly quoted, " As now interpreted, guidance touches every aspect of an individual's personality-physical, mental, emotional and social. It is concerned with all aspects of an individual's attitudes and behavior patterns. It seeks to help the individual to integrate all of his activities in terms of his basic potentialities and environmental opportunities.

Kothari Commission has stressed the need of guidance services in the schools. Regarding scope of guidance Commission was of the view " Guidance services have a much wider scope and function than merely that of assisting students in making educational and vocational choices. The aims of guidance are both adjustive and developmental: it helps the student in making the best possible adjustments to the situations in the educational institutions and in the home. Guidance, therefore, should be regarded as an integral part of education."

The scope of guidance has been increasing with the advancement of science and technology, embracing all spheres of life and providing facilities for it. Therefore, it will be difficult to put a fence around it. While discussing the scope of guidance we may think of some specific or specialized areas of guidance. Even though the guidance program is addressed to the whole individuals treated as an integral unit. It is possible to classify an individual's problems broadly into educational, vocational and personal.

Counseling

Counseling refers to a progress in which the people are made to approach or an individual level. He gets help in educational, vocational or psychological field only at problem points. In counseling the subject matter would be pupil's needs, abilities, aims, aspirations, plans, decisions, actions and limitations. Counseling may be referred to a sort of specialized personalized and individualized service which makes effective use of information gathered about any individual. This information provides self-insight, self-analysis and self-direction. This self-direction helps individual to make maximum education, vocational and psychological adjustments.

Definitions

1. Crow and Crow's view, counseling or assisting an individual in the solution of his problems. The interview has an important place in guidance, but is only one stage in the whole process of counseling.
2. Bernard and fullmer's views, basically counseling involves understanding and working with the individual to discover his unique needs, motivations and potentialities and to help him appreciate them.

Characteristics of Counseling

1. Counseling is based on person-to-person relations.
2. It involves two individuals one seeking help and the other, a professionally trained who can help the first.
3. The main aim is to help the counselor to discover and solve his personal problems independently.
4. In order to help and assist properly the counselor must establish a relationship of mutual respect, cooperation and friendliness between the two individuals.
5. The counselor will try to discover the problems of the client and helps him to set up goals and guide him through difficulties and problems.
6. The main emphasis in the role of counseling process is laid on the counselor's self-direction and self-acceptance.
7. Counseling is democratic and the counselor sets up a democratic pattern and allows the counsel to do freely whatever he like while with the consultant and not under the consultant.

12. Barriers in interpersonal relations.

1. **Lack of sensitivity to receiver:** A breakdown in relationship may result when a message is not adapted to the receiver. Recognizing the receivers' needs, status, knowledge of the

subject matter and language skills, assist an individual in living a healthy relationship. If a customer is angry for instance, an effective response may be just to listen to the person's vent, for a while.

2. **Lack of basic communication skills:** The receiver is less likely to understand the message, if the sender has trouble with choosing the precise words and arranging these words in a grammatically correct sentence.

3. **Emotional distractions:** If emotions interfere with the creation and transmission of a message, they can also disrupt the reception. If you receive a report from your supervisor regarding a proposed change in work procedure and you do not particularly like your supervisor, you may have problem reaching the report objectively. You may find fault by misinterpreting words for negative compressions, consequently, they may be a strain relationship.

4. **Walls and doors:** Physical barriers such as high cubicle walls and closed office doors can hinder effective communication in the workplace, as they can make workers seem less accessible to each other. To facilitate communication, organizations can create a more open workplace layout that is free of high walls and doors where workers have close proximity to each other while still enjoying personal space. This type of layout can also help to remove the sense that some people have elevated status that can hinder communication between supervisors and their subordinates.

5. **Cultural and language differences:** In multicultural workplaces, cultural and language differences can impede communication. Cultural barriers can also take the form of a unique workplace environment where workers are expected to behave in a particular way to gain acceptance. For example, some workplaces exhibit an autocratic culture where differing points of view are not tolerated, which can limit communication. In addition, language barriers can result not only when workers have different native languages but when they use jargon, buzzwords or terminology that is unfamiliar to new workers, who may feel excluded until they can master the lexicon.

6. **Gender issues:** Differences between genders can create communication barriers in a number of ways. For instance, in a traditionally male-dominated work environment, women may have difficulty getting their ideas accepted, or they may be treated harshly or even ignored. Different communication styles can result in barriers, as men and women do not always form and express thoughts in the same manner. Some men may feel uncomfortable with or even resent working for a female supervisor, which can also get in the way of effective communication.

7. **Competition:** In a highly competitive work environment, workers may be more concerned with their own career advancement than helping or communicating effectively with their coworkers. An atmosphere of distrust can also result, making it difficult for workers to perform in a collaborative manner due to fear of "backstabbing." As a result, workers may be reluctant to share important information with one another. Competition can also result in power struggles, where certain individuals or factions within an organization fail to communicate with each other.

SHORT ANSWERS

13. Define evaluation.

Evaluation is the collection of, analysis and interpretation of information about any aspect of a program of **education** or training as part of a recognized process of judging its effectiveness, its efficiency and any other outcomes it may have.

The generic goal of most evaluations is to provide "useful feedback" to a variety of audiences including sponsors, donors, client-groups, administrators, staff, and other relevant constituencies. Most often, feedback is perceived as "useful" if it aids in decision-making. But the relationship between an evaluation and its impact is not a simple one—studies that seem critical sometimes fail to influence short-term decisions, and studies that initially seem to have no influence can have a delayed impact when more congenial conditions arise. Despite this, there is broad consensus that the major goal of evaluation should be to influence decision-making or policy formulation through the provision of empirically-driven feedback.

14. Principles of teaching.

Teaching is a complex, multifaceted activity, often requiring us as instructors to juggle multiple tasks and goals simultaneously and flexibly. The following small but powerful set of principles can make teaching both more effective and more efficient, by helping us create the conditions that support student learning and minimize the need for revising materials, content, and policies. While implementing these principles requires a commitment in time and effort, it often saves time and energy later on.

1. Effective teaching involves acquiring relevant knowledge about students and using that knowledge to inform our course design and classroom teaching.
2. Effective teaching involves aligning the three major components of instruction: Learning objectives, assessments, and instructional activities.
3. Effective teaching involves articulating explicit expectations regarding learning objectives and policies.
4. Effective teaching involves prioritizing the knowledge and skills we choose to focus on.
5. Effective teaching involves recognizing and overcoming our expert blind spots.
6. Effective teaching involves adopting appropriate teaching roles to support our learning goal.
7. Effective teaching involves progressively refining our courses based on reflection and feedback.

15. List the different types of projected aids.

Projected visual aids are pictures shown upon a screen by use of a certain type of machine such as a filmstrip projector, slide projector, overhead projector or TV/VCR.

Values of projected visuals:
1. Provides greater enjoyment in learning.
2. Stimulates more rapid learning.
3. Increases retention: Larger percentages and longer retention.
4. Makes teaching situation adaptable to wider range.

5. Compels attention.
6. Enlarges or reduces actual size of objects.
7. Brings distant past and the present into the classroom.
8. Provides an easily reproduced record of an even.
9. Influences and changes attitude.

Types of projections used most frequently in church work:
1. Video.
2. Film strips.
3. Overheads.

16. Purpose of interpersonal relationship.

Interpersonal relationship refers to a strong association among individuals working together in the same organization. Employees working together ought to share a special bond for them to deliver their level best. It is essential for individuals to be honest with each other for a healthy interpersonal relationship and eventually positive ambience at the workplace.

The purpose of an interpersonal relationship is to actively and continually facilitate the personal growth and development of each other as individuals, to enjoy the process together as it unfolds, to maximize ease, and to have fun doing it.

17. Self-instructional module.

There are many methods for teaching. Each method has its own advantages and disadvantages. Self-instructional module has become more popular throughout the past decade. These modules can be used to facilitate learning that requires knowledge acquisition and application. Modules can be developed by educators by using specific format. These modules are useful for teaching the disciplines and ideas of humankind. The method chosen will depend on the number of students to teach.

Definitions:
1. Information on one concept presented according to a few specific objectives in a format that allow skipping of a section if the student has previously mastered the content; typically includes self-checks (pretest, post-tests) of student learning throughout the self-contained packet.
2. A module is a self-contained learning activity that allows learners to progress at their own place.

Components of a module:
A well-designed learning module usually consists of the following:
1. Overall purpose of learning activity.
2. Behavioral objectives.
3. Learning resources contained within model (e.g. written content, audiovisual aids, equipment).
4. Direction for use of the module.
5. Pretest.
6. Exercise with feedback that provide for application for knowledge throughout the module.
7. Post-test with feedback.

Purposes of self-instructional module:
1. To provide students with the opportunity to learn how to develop and implement a module.
2. To allow for individual differences in motivation and interest.
3. To enable the student to progress at his/her own rate.
4. To allow the student to choose his/her own learning mode and resources.
5. To allow for increasing skills in self-evaluation and self-direction and to facilitate sharing among learners.
6. Facilitating friendships and building social network for students.
7. Person centered planning for students.
8. Instructional modifications and curricular adaptations.
9. Develop support networks.
10. Promote school wide and classroom cultures that welcome, appreciate and accommodate diversity.
11. Promote strong leadership.

18. Symposium.

Symposium is a type of socialized technique whereas each of participants is expected to present a well-reasoned argument or point at view with respect to the problem being discussed. The point of view may be presented through speakers or paper reading. Fact and feeling of each presentation vary with the speakers and with the situation. This makes symposium constant in form but flexible in method.

Meaning of symposium: Symposium is a Greek term for drinking party. Symposia were very frequent at Athens. Their enjoyment was heightened by agreeable conversation, by introduction of music and dancing, Sometimes philosophical subjects were discussed at them.

Derivation of word:
Syn—together.
Posis—a drinking.
1. A drinking parting at which there was intellectual conversation.
2. Any meeting or social gathering at which ideas are freely exchanged.
3. Conference or meeting to discuss a particular academic subjects.
4. A collection of opinion especially a published group of essay on a subject given.

Definition: Symposium is a method of group discussion in which two or more persons under the direction of chairman present separate speeches which gives several aspects of one question.

Aims and objectives of symposium:
1. To clarify thought in debatable questions.
2. To investigate a problem from several points of view.
3. To acquire increased knowledge, intellectual abilities and skills.
4. To increase interest towards the subject.
5. To change attitudes and values towards common goal.
6. For better personnel and social adjustments.
7. To get good cooperation.

Purpose of symposium:
1. To identify and understand various aspects of them and problems.
2. To encourage the students to study independently.
3. To boost students ability to speak in the group.

4. To investigate problems from several points of view.
5. To develop the ability to come to a discussion and provide judgment regarding a problem.
6. To develop values and feelings regarding a problem.
7. To enable the listeners from policies regarding a theme or problem.

Characteristics of symposium:
1. Provides broad understanding.
2. Provides opportunity to take part in discussion.
3. Used in higher classes for specific themes.
4. Develops feeling of cooperation and adjustments.
5. Provides different views on the topic of the symposium.

19. Disadvantages of essay question.

1. Require extensive time to grade.
2. Encourage use of subjective criteria when assessing answers.
3. If used in class, necessitate quick composition without time for planning or revision which can result in poor-quality writing.

20. Process recording.

The traditional process recording is a verbatim recall of the dialogue between the student and the client and a subjective commentary of the student's reactions during the course of the interview. The purpose of the process recording is to focus on the student's subjective reactions to a client session and identify areas for discussion. Process recordings can be used for assessment purposes to offer some measure an interns level of skill and knowledge. Because process recordings are very time intensive they should be used no more than three times over the course of an academic year. Process recording can offer one means of feedback to the student and FI regarding progress over the course of the placement.

21. Nursing rounds.

There are several methods that can be used effectively in clinical teaching. Nursing rounds are conducted by the head nurse/nurse teacher for the members of her staff/students. To be successful every nurse must be prepared to participate in the discussion of nursing care.

Definition: Nursing rounds are conducted by the head nurse/nurse teacher for the members of her staff/students for a clear understanding of the disease process and the effect of nursing care for each patient.

Types of ward rounds:
1. Rounds with the doctors.
2. Rounds to discuss psychological problem of patients.
3. Social service rounds.
4. Medical rounds for nurses.
5. Rounds with the physical therapists.
6. Nursing rounds.

Meaning of nursing rounds: To acquaint nurse with all patients in the ward in order that better understanding and more purposeful care may be achieved for each patient.

Purposes of nursing rounds: The purpose for ward rounds includes:
1. To observe the physical and the mental condition of the patients and the progress made day-to-day.
2. To observe the work of staff.
3. To make specific observation of the patient and to give report to doctor, e.g. wound, drainage, bleeding, etc.
4. To introduce the patients to the personnel and vice versa.
5. To carry out the plan made for the care of the patients.
6. To evaluate the results of treatment and the satisfaction of the patient with his care.
7. To ensure the safety measures employed for the patient and personnel.
8. To orient the nurse/student in handing over/taking over regarding patient's treatment, care done, care yet to be completed and condition of the patient.
9. To teach the nursing students and the hospital aids regarding specific conditions.
10. To check any preventable conditions present in the patient such as bedsore, foot drop, etc.
11. To check the emergency equipment kept near the patient and to cheek their safety and working order.
12. To compare the clinical manifestation of the patients having some disease so that the student understand in a better manner and gain better insight.
13. To prescribe any modification in nursing action.

22. List two specific objectives for a lesson plan on anemia.

The anemia chapter of this pathophysiology syllabus resource and lesson plans course is designed to help you plan and teach the types and causes of anemia in your classroom. The video lessons, quizes and transcripts can easily be adapted to provide your lesson plans with engaging and dynamic educational content. Make planning your course easier by using our syllabus as a guide.

2014

Communication and Educational Technology

LONG ESSAYS
1. Prepare a lesson plan on importance of exercise for BSC nursing 1st year students.
2. a. Define communication. b. Explain the channels of communication, c. List measures to overcome the barriers of communication.
3. a. List the different types of AV aids. b. Explain about flash card.

SHORT ESSAYS
4. Factors to improve good human relations.
5. Steps in counseling process.
6. Microteaching.
7. Role of counselor in managing stress situation.
8. Write briefly on clinical conference.
9. Importance of team method in nursing.
10. Characteristics of a good demonstration.
11. Questioning technique in classroom teaching.
12. Psychometric assessment.

SHORT ANSWERS
13. Simulation.
14. Group dynamics.
15. Explain briefly on any one of the projected aids.
16. Objective structured clinical examination.
17. Purpose of interpersonal relations.
18. Advantages of MCQs.
19. List four counseling techniques.
20. Types of assessment tools.
21. Differentiate between symposium and panel discussion.
22. Benefits of a field trip.

LONG ESSAYS

1. Prepare a lesson plan on importance of exercise for BSC nursing 1st year students.

Lesion plan is a plan prepared by a teacher to teach a lesson in an organized manner. It is a plan of action and calls for an understanding on the teacher's part, about the students, knowledge and experience about the topic being taught and her/his ability to use effective methods.

Advantages of Planning a Lesson

1. It helps the teacher to be systematic, orderly in the treatment of the subject matter.
2. It provides confidence and self-reliance to the teacher. She set fourth some definite aims that she has to develop in students through certain activities or some other means.
3. It encourages the continuity in the teaching process and unnecessary repetition is avoided.
4. The interest of the students can be maintained throughout the lesson when it is well planned.

Steps Involved in Planning a Lesson

There are few steps which should be followed while making a lesson plan. These are:

1. **Preparation/introduction:** This in fact, is a means of exploration of the student's knowledge which helps to lead them on to the lesson. The teacher needs to prepare the students to receive new knowledge. She can introduce the lesson by testing the pervious knowledge of the student by asking questions. This in turn may reveal their ignorance; arouse interest and curiosity to learn new matter. Charts, maps, diagrams, pictures also can be used.
2. **Presentation:** The aim of lesson plan should clearly state before the presentation of the subject matter, which helps both the teacher and the student to have a common pursuit.
    - During presentation: In this stage both the teacher and the student must actively participate in the teaching–learning process. The students must get some new ideas and knowledge.
    - Questioning, discussion, appropriate examples from real life situations should feature in presentation to make the presentation interesting and to motivate the students to learn.
    - Teaching aids: Teaching aids should be used to make the lessons meaningful, clear, explanatory and comprehensive.
    - Blackboard summary can be developed side by side.
3. **Comparison or association:** This step is important where the students are given examples and they are asked to observe carefully and compare them with other set of examples and facts. These will enable the student to deduce definitions and arrive at generalizations on their own.
4. **Generalization:** This step involves reflective thinking. The knowledge presented through the lesson should be thought provoking, innovative and stimulating to assist the students.
5. **Application:** The students make use of the knowledged acquired in familiar and unfamiliar situations and at the same time it tests the validity of the generalizations arrived at by the students. The students of nursing especially need to develop the skill of learning to apply the knowledge and skills gained in the classroom in their day-to-day nursing practice in the wards, clinic and home situations. This makes learning more permanent and worthwhile.
6. **Recapitulation:** This being the last step in the planning of a lesson, understanding and comprehension of the subject matter taught by the teacher can be tested by asking suitable, stimulating and questions to be students on the topic. This also gives a feedback to the teacher regarding the efficacy of the methods of teaching adopted by her. It tells whether further explanation, clarifications, etc. are needed or not as well.

Suggested Performa for a Lesson Plan

There are various performa which can be used as an outline for lesson plan. Whatever format is used the essential elements which should feature in a lesson plan are:
1. Statement of central and contributory objectives.
2. Relationship of the present lesson with the previous lesson.
3. Inclusion of learning objectives (refer to student activities).
4. Inclusion of learning activities (refer to teacher activities).
5. Methods of teaching to be used.
6. Audio-visual aids to be used.
7. Summary of the lesson being taught.
8. Evaluative questions.
9. Assignments for students.
10. References on the topic of the lesson.

2. a. Define communication. b. Explain the channels of communication. c. List measures to overcome the barriers of communication.

The communication has been derived from Latin word "communis", which implies common. Communication is an exchange of facts, ideas, opinions or emotions by two or more persons. Communication is much more than simply transmission of information. It also involves interpretation and understanding of the message. It is an interchange of thoughts and informational intercourse through words, letters, symbols or message. Communication is the basic element of human interactions. It is one of the most vital components of all nursing practice.

Definitions
1. Communication is the process of exchanging information, thought, ideas and feeling from one individual to another.
2. Communication is the process by which a message is passed from the sender to the receiver with the objective that the message sent is received and understood as intended.
3. Communication is the process of passing information and understanding from one person to another to bring about commonness of interest, efforts, purpose and attitudes.

Channels of Communication

Communication channels are the means through which people in an organization communicate. Thought must be given to what channels are used to complete various tasks, because using an inappropriate channel for a task or interaction can lead to negative consequences. Complex messages require richer channels of communication that facilitate interaction to ensure clarity.

Face-to-face: Face-to-face or personal communication is one of the richest channels of communication that can be used within an organization. Physical presence, the tone of the speaker's voice and facial expressions help recipients of a message interpret that message as the speaker intends. This is the best channel to use for complex or emotionally charged messages, because it allows for interaction between speaker and recipients to clarify ambiguity. A speaker can evaluate whether an audience has received his message as intended and ask or answer follow-up questions.

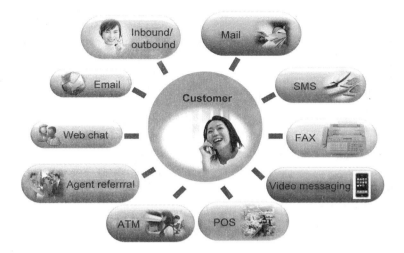

Broadcast media: TV, radio and loud speakers all fall within the broadcast media communication channel. These types of media should be used when addressing a mass audience. Businesses seeking to notify customers of a new product may advertise or do promotions using a broadcast channel. Similarly, a CEO may do a global company address by having a television feed broadcast across global sites. When a message intended for a mass audience can be enhanced by being presented in a visual or auditory format, a broadcast channel should be used.

Mobile: A mobile communication channel should be used when a private or more complex message needs to be relayed to an individual or small group. A mobile channel allows for an interactive exchange and gives the recipient the added benefit of interpreting the speaker's tone along with the message. Some within an organization may opt to use this channel versus a face-to-face channel to save on the time and effort it would take to coordinate a face-to-face meeting.

Electronic: Electronic communication channels encompass email, internet, intranet and social media platforms. This channel can be used for one-on-one, group or mass communication. It is a less personal method of communication but more efficient. When using this channel, care must be taken to craft messages with clarity and to avoid the use of sarcasm and innuendo unless the message specifically calls for it.

Written: Written communication should be used when a message that does not require interaction needs to be communicated to an employee or group. Policies, letters, memos, manuals, notices and announcements are all messages that work well for this channel. Recipients may follow up through an electronic or face-to-face channel if questions arise about a written message.

Measures to Overcome the Barriers of Communication

Effective communication is essential for successful interpersonal relationship. Breakdown in communication are not only expensive and time consuming, they are also injurious to team-work and morale. It is, therefore, necessary to take steps to ensure effective communication. Though, it may not possible to eliminate these barriers altogether, effort must be made to achieve adequate communication. The following measures can be adopted for this purpose.
1. **Clarify the idea:** The communicator must be quiet clear about what he wants to communicate. He should know the objective of his communication. Very often the communicator mistakes the form of communication for its subject matter. Too much attention is paid to media

and devices and too little to purpose and content. The mind of message should be clearly formulated in the mind of the communicator. It should be expressed in as simple and precise language as possible so that the receiver can understand it easily and quickly. The message should be concise, concrete and correct. Technical terms should be avoided and the language of the listener should be used. This obviously requires a familiarity with the language patterns of the receiver.

2. **Completeness of the message:** If the information is not supplied, people make assumptions about the message it must be complete, timely and adequate in all respects, or otherwise it is likely to be misunderstood. No important details should be omitted and underlying assumptions must be clarified. If all the information is not supplied, people make assumption about the missing information. This can distort the meaning. Incomplete communication delays action, spoils relations and increases costs. The message should be relevant to the nature and purpose of the communication.

3. **Understand the receiver:** The communicator must become aware of the total physical and human setting in which the message will be received. Before conveying the message he must find out the needs, feelings, receptivity, perceptions and understanding levels of the receiver. The message should be designed from the viewpoint of the receiver. The sender of the message must work at the problems from the receiver's point of view. This is called empathy in communications.

4. **Use appropriate channels:** The media and channels used in communication must be appropriate to the message, the receiver and the purpose of communication. A judicious combination of formal and informal channels and written and oral media will help to improve the effectiveness of communication. Use of multiple channels, certain amount of repetition and participation of subordinates is essential for an orderly flow of information.

5. **Consistency in communication:** The message should be consistent with objectives, policies and programs of the organization. This will avoid chaos and confusion in the organization. Different messages should not mutually conflict. Whatever, it is necessary to amend the old message; this fact should be started in the new message to avoid confusion and chaos. Communication should be supported by actions and behavior to ensure credibility in communications. Actions speak louder than words. If actions are contrary to communications, people do not take them seriously.

6. **Feedback:** Communication should be a two-way process. The communicator should try to know the reactions of the receiver. The use of feedback mechanism invokes effective participation of subordinates and it help to make future communications more effective. There should be continuous evaluation of the flow of communication in different directions. A feedback system helps to build up mutual understanding and distortions of message can be avoided. Feedback indicates the return flow of communication.

7. **Simplified structure:** The communication system can be strengthened by simplifying the procedure, reducing the layer, making constructive use of grapevine and regulating information flow. Lines of communication should be as short and direct as possible and the number of levels should be minimized. Regulating the flow of information eliminates communication overload and ensures an optimum flow of information to members of organization. Filtering of information should be discouraged. The communication system should be tailor made to the needs and characteristics of the enterprise.

8. **Improve listening:** The sender of the message as well as receiver must listen with attention, patience and empathy. The communicator can gather useful information for future messages by good listening. Generally, manager suffers from bad listening and

they need to avoid valve judgments. They must develop awareness of actions and their impact on others. They must develop the habit of empathic listening to secure free and frank responses.
9. **Mutual trust and confidence:** Communication is an interpersonal process. Therefore, it can be made effectively by developing mutual trust, respect and confidence among the members of the organization.

3. (a) List the different types of AV aids. (b) Explain about flash card.

As we all know that today's age is the age of science and technology. The teaching–learning programs have also been affected by it. The teaching–learning process depends upon the different type of equipment available in the classroom.

Need of Teaching Aids
1. Every individual has the tendency to forget. Proper use of teaching aids helps to retain more concept permanently.
2. Students can learn better when they are motivated properly through different teaching aids.
3. Teaching aids develop the proper image when the students see, hear, taste and smell properly.
4. Teaching aids provide complete example for conceptual thinking.
5. The teaching aids create the environment of interest for the students.
6. Teaching aids helps to increase the vocabulary of the students.
7. Teaching aids helps the teacher to get sometime and make learning permanent.
8. Teaching aids provide direct experience to the students.

Types of Teaching Aids
There are many aids available these days. We may classify these aids as follows:
1. **Visual aids:** The aids which use sense of vision are called visual aids. For example, actual objects, models, pictures, charts, maps, flash cards, flannel board, bulletin board, chalkboard, overhead projector, slides, etc. Out of these black board and chalk are the commonest ones.
2. **Audio aids:** The aids that involve the sense of hearing are called audio aids. For example, radio, tape recorder, gramophone, etc.
3. **Audio-visual aids:** The aids which involve the sense of vision as well as hearing are called audiovisual aids. For example, television, film projector, filmstrips, etc.

Importance of Teaching Aids
Teaching aids play an very important role in teaching–learning process. Importance of teaching aids are as follows:
1. Motivation teaching aids motivate the students so that they can learn better.
2. Clarification: Through teaching aids, the teacher clarify the subject matter more easily.
3. Discouragement of cramming: Teaching aids can facilitate the proper understanding to the students which discourage the act of cramming.
4. Increase the vocabulary: Teaching aids help to increase the vocabulary of the students more effectively.
5. Saves time and money.
6. Classroom live and active: Teaching aids make the classroom live and active.
7. Avoids dullness.
8. Direct experience.

Teaching aids provide direct experience to the students.

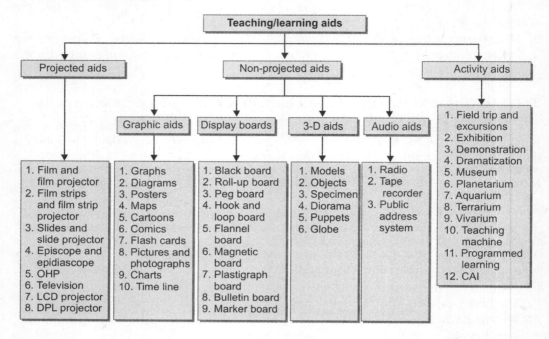

Flash card

These are the series of cards which can be presented before the audience in proper sequence, which tell a complete story; size of the flash card is 10 inch × 12 inch and it contains a picture or diagram. Each individual card is flashed before the audience accompanied by the verbal commentary, the extension worker or the student who wants to use them, holds them in hand and flashes the card one after another.

Preparation of flash cards: A brief story should be written. The story should end with suggestions or a morale that leads to action. A suitable title should be selected for the story. The story should be divided into a number of scenes which are to be presented in a number of individual cards. The cards are numbered in sequence, every set of cards should have a title. There should be a commentary written on the reverse of each cards so that the person who presents it to the audience can easily read the commentary from the reverse. Attractive lettering increases the effectiveness of the flash cards.

How to use a flash card?
1. They should be familiar to the students or person who presents the card.
2. He should use simple words and local expressions.
3. He must hold cards in a way that the audience can see clearly, better against the body and should point out the pictures on the card.
4. Some important points may be jotted down on the back side of the cards to help in telling the story.
5. The cards should be stacked in order, as one card is finished it may be slid behind the other. In this way they will remain in order for the next time.

SHORT ESSAYS

4. Factors to improve good human relations.

Human relation is an interdisciplinary field because the study of human behavior in organizational settings draws on the fields of communications, management, psychology, and sociology. It is an important field of study because all workers engage in human relation activities. Several trends have given new importance to human relations due to the changing workplace.

Relationships between employees and management are of substantial value in any workplace. Human relation is the process of training employees, addressing their needs, fostering a workplace culture and resolving conflicts between different employees or between employees and management. Understanding some of the ways that human relations can impact the costs, competitiveness and long-term economic sustainability of a business helps to underscore their importance.

Factors to Improve Good Human Relations

Good human relations are like a seedling that will later on become a tree. It needs to be grown, tended, nourished, watered and above all nurtured. But if this is not the case then human relations will be eroded through negative traits, tendencies and attitudes of mind. In a nutshell factors affecting good human relations are:
1. Tendency to boss rather than facilitate ongoing activities.
2. Making promises which are never fulfilled.
3. Being too easy going (a yes man or yes woman).
4. Tendency to despise or hate one's cultural way of doing things.
5. Boasting of one's achievements and looking down upon others.

Basics

Human relations in the workplace are a major part of what makes a business work. Employees must frequently work together on projects, communicate ideas and provide motivation to get things done. Without a stable and inviting workplace culture, difficult challenges can arise both in the logistics of managing employees and in the bottom line. Businesses with engaging workplaces and a well-trained workforce are more likely to retain and attract qualified employees, foster loyalty with customers and more quickly adapt to meet the needs of a changing marketplace.

Improving Retention

The quality of workplace relations is critical to employee retention. Employee retention may seem trivial, especially in a workplace that is used to a high turnover, but managers must remember that turnover is financially very costly. Every new employee requires a substantial investment of time and energy in their recruitment and training. In addition, severing ties with old employees can sometimes be challenging, especially if the circumstances are not particularly amicable. Making sure quality employees remain interested and engaged in the business requires patience, compassion and flexibility, but can actually make the business more financially sound.

Motivation and Productivity

Workplace relationships provide a source of employee motivation, which is important to maintaining productivity. Employees who are interested in their work and in the well-being of other employees tend to be more productive than those who are not. The productivity pays obvious financial dividends to the company, as it can get more done in less time with fewer costs. Building relationships, by both recognizing an employee's value to the company and a concern for their needs, often goes a long way.

Fostering Creativity

The modern business environment often rewards businesses that are able to quickly develop products that meet changing consumer needs. In some industries, such as technology, employees' ability to come up with effective new ideas is often the difference between the entire company's success and failure. According to Sallyport Magazine, research shows that creativity is based to large degree in social interaction. Employees' creativity is often dependent on their ability to communicate with other employees and share ideas. Without quality workplace relationships, employees are less likely to be able to develop and share the solutions that a business needs to survive.

5. Steps in counseling process.

A counseling session is therefore sometimes referred to as the 50-minute hour. It takes place in a session, depends on the client's needs and the counselor's personal approach to counseling. Although there is some variation during a session, there is a basic structure. That structure was described by Cormier and Hackney (1987) as a five-stage process: Relationship building, assessment, goal setting, interventions, and termination and follow-up. These stages have been expanded in the following six-stage model of the counseling process.

Steps in Counseling Process

1. Establish a safe, trusting environment.
2. Clarify: Help the person put their concern into words.
3. Active listening: Find out the client's agenda:
   - Paraphrase, summarize, reflect, interpret.
   - Focus on feelings, not events.
4. Transform problem statements into goal statements.
5. Explore possible approaches to goal.
6. Help person choose one way towards goal.
7. Make a contract to fulfill the plan (or to take the next step).
8. Summarize what has occurred, clarify, get verification.
9. Get feedback and confirmation.

6. Microteaching.

A training procedure aimed at simplifying the complexities of the regular teaching process. It is difficult for the teacher to assess all the teaching skills of a student teacher at a time and give necessary corrections. By way of scaled down teaching, teacher can easily identify the deficiencies of the student teacher in performing a particular teaching skill and help him to attain proficiency in that skill by providing assistance to rectify the identified deficiencies.

Definitions

1. According to Allen "Microteaching as a scaled down teaching encounter in class size and class time". The number of students is from 5 to 10 and the duration of period ranges from 5 to 20 minutes.
2. DW Allen (1966): Microteaching is a scaled down teaching encounter in class size and time.

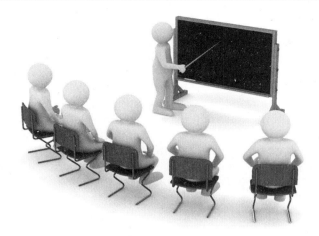

3. Allen and Eve (1968): Microteaching is defined as a system of controlled practice that makes it possible to concentrate on specific teaching behavior and to practice teaching under controlled conditions.

Characteristics of Microteaching
1. It is relatively a new experience or innovation in the field of teacher education, more specifically in student teaching.
2. It is a training technique and not a teaching technique. In other words, it is a technique or design used for the training of teachers (or makes them learn the art of teaching). It is not a method of classroom instruction or teaching like inductive-deductive, demonstration or question-answer method.
3. It is micro- or miniaturized teaching in the sense that it scales down the complexities of real teaching with the provisions, such as:
    - Practicing one skill at a time.
    - Reducing the class size to 5–10 pupils.
    - Reducing duration of the lesson to 5–10 minutes.
    - Limiting the content to a single concept.
4. There is provision of adequate feedback in microteaching as it provides trainees due information about their performances immediately after the completion of their lesson.
5. Teaching is said to be composed of very specific skills. These skills cannot be mastered through the traditional approach to teacher training. Microteaching provides opportunity to select one skill at a time and practice it through its scaled down encounter and then take other in a similar way.
6. Microteaching is a highly individualized training device permitting the imposition of a high degree of control in practicing a particular skill.

Looking at the above characteristics and features, the term microteaching may be defined appropriately as a technique or device of imparting training to the inexperienced or experienced teachers for learning the art of teaching by practicing specific skills through a "scaled down teaching encounter", i.e. reducing the complexities of real normal teaching in terms of size of the class, time and content.

7. Role of counselor in managing stress situation.

Counselors often become involved because a student's studies will be interrupted and appropriate arrangements must be negotiated with the academic staff. Study programs can be modified to make it possible for students to continue successfully but it is best to begin negotiating early. Counselors are experienced in dealing with difficult situations. They know how to listen to difficult emotional situations and provide students with an opportunity to share feelings that students are unsure about or may not want to express to those with whom students are close with. The counselor will assist students in securing the best possible support from services throughout the community while taking into consideration students' culture, religion, personal abilities and preferences. They will also assist students in negotiating study arrangements that will be realistic. Some of the topics to explore could include:
1. Discussing and assessing your level of physical and emotional distress and current safety.
2. Looking at students' available support through family, friends and community services.
3. Working out any long-term needs that require some immediate action.
4. Assisting students' to explain their circumstances to relevant academic staff and gain the special consideration that is appropriate.

Prevention Programs
At least five strategies should be used in all institutions to prevent various kinds of crises from occurring. They are discussed below:
1. **Educational workshops and program:** An educational workshop is a short intensive course of study on a topic that generates emotions and feelings. As a result, workshops emphasize on student participation and discussion. Programs such as class meetings help students to express their feelings about what is occurring around in the social environment and helps them to free from anxiety that may have occurred in the classroom.
2. **Anticipatory guidance:** It is also referred to as emotional inoculation. Offering anticipatory guidance consists of orienting a student intellectually to events that are likely to occur in future and help him/her prepare effective coping strategies.
3. **Screening programs:** It consists of designing tools such as questionnaire, rating scales of group tests to determine who is at high-risk of not coping. The follow-up intervention will be anticipatory guidance, a workshop or remediation program of preventive counseling. Consultation: Serving as a consultant is another important way that psychologists and other special services personnel can act preventively in crises.
4. **Consultation is defined** as one professional helping a second professional be more effective in his/her job (Caplan, 1970).
5. **Research:** Doing research is not usually conceived of as a preventive activity. Nevertheless, the better the phenomena are known through research the better we can predict and control the phenomena.

8. Write briefly on clinical conference.

It is same like a bedside clinic but the patient is not usually present for the class. This may be a method of choice when the entire group is acquainted with the patient. Bedside clinic and nursing care conference can be used to evaluate the students. Both should be planned earlier if it is to be made more effective. But the nurse instructor conducts it on the spot if she wishes to evaluate the students.

Definition

Nursing conference is a course of action, discussion on assessing the nursing problems and arriving at possible solutions by helping the staff to examine patient's problems from his point of view.

Types of Nursing Conference

1. **Individual conference:** It is a conversation between two persons, usually the nursing student and the clinical instructor or head nurse.
2. **Group nursing conference:** It includes the conversation between large groups of person, which may include the head nurse, physician, clinical instructor and nursing students in order to solve a nursing problem.

Uses of Nursing Conference

1. It is a method of solving the patients' problem by discussion.
2. It acts as a means of communication among the health team members.
3. It helps in all-round development of the personnel by keeping them up-to-date on knowledge.
4. It helps to pass on the skill and knowledge to nursing students.

Phases of Nursing Conference

1. **Opening phase:** The task here is to make a commitment to work on the problem of a particular patient.
2. **Working phase:** The task of the working phase is to arrive at a consensus on problem identification and solution.
3. **Closing phase:** The task here is to delegate responsibility to one or more of the staff to act on the procedure.

Advantages

1. It provides a real practical learning environment to the students.
2. It fortifies the thinking of students, thereby increasing creativity and judgment capacity.
3. It provides free opportunity to think.
4. Each member will be actively participating in the conference.

Disadvantages

1. It will be of little use if the students do not set accustomed to each solution.
2. Active participation of the student is needed.

9. Importance of team method in nursing.

Patient centered care and efficient/cost effective use of available personnel. Divides workers into teams, each containing nurses with different levels of knowledge and skill so that each member is 'used' at the level at which they are capable of performing. (Example: The RN is used to do complex skills/care and his/her time which costs the hospital more money is not "wasted" on tasks that an Aid or LVN can safely perform.)

Head nurse picks team leaders and the team members for each team. The team leader assigns patients to each team member and decides how he/she will help each team member. The team leader often gives all medications and IV therapy to all the patients being cared for by them. The team leader also helps with complex procedures, teaches staff and patients and conducts conferences to plan care. **All team members feel responsible for all patients assigned to the team.**

Impact on the unit: Efficient use of staff and reasonably efficient use of time—some might say that time is lost in the shift reports attended by the whole team and during the team conference. Staff turns over decreased due to job satisfaction in most cases.

Impact on staff: Often staffs are happy when they see themselves as growing in ability and knowledge, motivation and satisfaction is fostered, feel important in that their opinions are valued in planning effective care. RNs are responsible for safe delegation/assignment and support of LVNs and unlicensed staff members. RNs share legal responsibility for care provided by the members on their team.

Impact on client: Client can identify one RN and an additional team member (an LVN or an aid) as their nurses for the shift. All team members know about the patient and can safely answer the call light when the assigned nurse is on break.

Other features: Head nurse delegates responsibility and authority to team leader who manages the team members. 8 hours responsibility for planning care, assignments based on ability, and team members learn and grow.

10. Characteristics of a good demonstration.

Demonstration method is very important in teaching of nursing than in any other fields. It is very instructional method that is chosen, depends on the learning needs of the student's time available to teach. The setting the resources and the teacher own comfort. An experienced and skilled teacher uses a variety of a techniques depends on the subject on the topic.

The main features of demonstration-cum-discussion method are as follows:
1. The demonstration-cum-discussion method is not a single method. It is combination of two methods, more clearly a resultant method resulting from the combination of discussion method as well as demonstration method.
2. This method involves the active participation of teachers and students at the same time, which is unlikely in other methods. Say in lecture method, the teacher is active, in laboratory work and in heuristic method; students are active and so on.
3. Demonstration-cum-discussion method of teaching science encourages maximum amount of participation among students than other methods.
4. Demonstration-cum-discussion method through group participation develops keen observation power and scientific reasoning in students, which is not possible either in lecture method or in heuristic method.
5. Demonstration-cum-discussion method is the only method in which the interest and zeal of students are maintained.
6. Demonstration-cum-discussion method develops skill in scientific thinking. These are some of the main features of demonstration-cum-discussion method.

The advantages and disadvantages of the method are discussed below:
Advantages
1. This method is economic from the point of view of money and time.
2. The method obeys the rule of "learning by doing", what the students do or see they learn. So, this method is very much psychological.
3. It is useful when the apparatus required for practical work is costly. There the teacher can improvise the apparatus and demonstrate it.

4. If the teacher wants to revise some of the principles of science subject, he can do it by demonstration-cum-discussion method.
5. Through this method free discipline is maintained.
6. This method develops skill in handling apparatus, freethinking and cooperative spirit among students.

Disadvantages
1. If demonstration-cum-discussion method is not properly used, then all students do not get a chance to take part either in discussion or in experimentation. Thus, the principle of 'Learning by doing' is not abided by this method.
2. The students do not get direct experience of doing experiment. So, their skill in apparatus handling is not properly developed.
3. If the teacher does not take care, students become indiscipline through this method.

11. Questioning technique in classroom teaching.

Questioning in teaching and learning not only encourages students to think critically; it allows teachers to assess whether their students understand a particular concept. This requires the teacher to be able to come up with the right questions in order to get students to provide responses that are both relevant and of high standard.

Critical thinking means your students are able to go beyond what is on the surface and really dig deep in order to answer a given question. This means the teacher does not want to ask a basic question like, who are the main characters in the story? Instead, the teacher may ask— how are each of the main characters important to the progression of the plot? Students will not only have to be able to identify the main characters, but they will also need to understand the plot in order to provide meaningful responses to the latter question. This type of questioning, if done consistently, will develop the critical thinking skills that students need as 21st century learners.

Questioning techniques are heavily used, and thus widely researched teaching strategy. Research indicates that asking questions is second only to lecturing. Teachers typically spend anywhere from 35 to 50% of their instructional time asking questions. But are these questions effective in raising student achievement? How can teachers ask better questions to their students? How can current educational research inform practice?

Types of questions: Educators have traditionally classified questions according to Bloom's taxonomy, a hierarchy of increasingly complex intellectual skills. Bloom's Taxonomy includes six categories:
1. Knowledge—recall data or information.
2. Comprehension—understand meaning.
3. Application—use a concept in a new situation.
4. Analysis—separate concepts into parts; distinguish between facts and inferences.
5. Synthesis—combine parts to form new meaning.
6. Evaluation—make judgments about the value of ideas or products.

The Questioning Process

When teachers raise the level of their questions, they will increase the likelihood that their students will raise the level of their responses. If in doubt about the type of questions that should be used in order to encourage critical thinking skills, it may be a good idea to use Bloom's taxonomy as a guide.

Bloom's taxonomy is a systematic approach to teaching and learning that can be used as a resource for question design. Levels of teaching and learning are broken into at least six components: Evaluation, synthesis, analysis, application, comprehension and knowledge. Teachers can use the various levels to create questions based on learning objectives. If you, as the teacher, want to assess students' ability to analyze, you might ask—how would you compare the hero and the villain in this story?. If you want students to synthesize, you may ask—how would you develop the plot so that the ending of the story would not be tragic?

Characteristics of Effective Questions

1. Questions should be asked in a positive manner so that students will enjoy responding. If your students perceive your questions to be too negative or too aggressive, they will probably not want to answer them.
2. The idea of questioning is to engage students in the learning process, not put students on the spot as punishment for misbehavior. For example, if Sally is talking during instruction, you would not want to punish her by asking her a question regarding the instruction. By doing this you, as the teacher, have turned a positive learning opportunity into a negative one.
3. Questions should be clear and to the point. While your goal as the teacher is to challenge your students, you certainly do not want them to disconnect from the process because they do not understand what you are asking.
4. Ask a question and pause for a few seconds before calling on a student to answer it. This gives students a chance to think about the question and form an appropriate response.

Teachers ask questions for a variety of purposes, including:

1. To actively involve students in the lesson.
2. To increase motivation or interest.
3. To evaluate students' preparation.
4. To check on completion of work.
5. To develop critical thinking skills.
6. To review previous lessons.
7. To nurture insights.

12. Psychometric assessment.

Psychometric tests are impersonal, standardized and objective, and practice tests are readily available. The psychometric test is a level playing field. Employers value them because they are a fair way of comparing different candidates' strengths regardless of educational background.

Psychometric tests may be used at different stages of the graduate selection process:
1. After you submit your online application form.
2. Alongside a first interview.
3. At a later stage, possibly with a second interview or as part of an assessment center. You may be re-tested at this point to confirm the results of earlier tests.

Ability tests measure either general or particular skills, capability and acumen. This category of test can include:
1. **Numerical tests:** Assess how well you interpret data, graphs, charts or statistics. Can test basic arithmetic.
2. **Verbal reasoning tests:** Assess how well you understand written information and evaluate arguments and statements.
3. **Nonverbal reasoning tests:** Assess how well you follow diagrammatic information or spot patterns. Can check spatial awareness. Diagrammatic or abstract reasoning tests are sometimes described as **inductive reasoning tests**.

4. **Logical reasoning tests:** Assess how well you follow through to a conclusion given basic information, or using your current knowledge or experience.
5. **Deductive reasoning tests**, in which you are given information or rules to apply in order to arrive at an answer.

Deductive reasoning tests assess a different type of logical problem solving. Broadly speaking, inductive reasoning moves from observation of specific instances to forming a theory that can be used to make predictions. Deductive reasoning starts with a number of rules and applies them in order to work out what happens in specific cases. Inductive reasoning can arrive at new solutions rather than using what is already known to solve a problem, so you can see why employers who focus on technological innovation are interested in it. Employers may also run tests to assess your problem-solving skills or ability to identify mistakes accurately, e.g. proof-reading or basic spelling and grammar tests.

Aptitude tests examine your potential to learn a new skill that is needed to do the job you have applied for. If you are considering careers in IT, you may be asked to complete a programing aptitude test (this could take the form of a diagrammatic, abstract reasoning or inductive reasoning test). For other career areas, such as finance, you may find that numerical and verbal reasoning tests are focused on the kind of information you would come across in your daily work.

Ability and aptitude tests are usually conducted under timed, exam conditions. Most involve multiple-choice or true/false answers. They can be done on paper but increasingly employers use computer-based programs.

The results compare your ability levels to a 'normal' expectation for a demographic group chosen by the employer or test provider (this could be the results of a group of previously successful applicants, people typical of your level of education, or the general public).

Critical thinking and situational judgment tests assess candidates' natural responses to given situations. They are used in two ways:
1. To give graduates the chance to evaluate themselves. Several employers host tests in a quiz or game format on their websites to enable graduates to see if they would be a good fit. These tests are usually designed to be fun and appealing, but can be a wake-up call if you are less well suited to working for that particular organization than you think.
3. As part of the recruitment process, to gauge how a candidate operates. The test results may also help the recruiter decide which area of the business the candidate would suit best.

SHORT ANSWERS

13. Simulation.

Simulations (and models, too) are abstractions of reality. Often they deliberately emphasize one part of reality at the expense of other parts. Sometimes, this is necessary due to computer power limitations. Sometimes it is done to focus your attention on an important aspect of the simulation. Whereas models are mathematical, logical, or some other structured representation of reality, simulations are the specific application of models to arrive at some outcome (more about models are discussed below).

Three Types of Simulations

Simulations generally come in three styles: Live, virtual and constructive. A simulation also may be a combination of two or more styles. Within these styles, simulations can be *science-based* (where, for example, interactions of things are observed or measured), or involve interactions with humans. Our primary focus at IST is on the latter human-in-the-loop simulations.

1. **Live simulations** typically involve humans and/or equipment and activity in a setting where they would operate for real. Think war games with soldiers out in the field or manning command posts. Time is continuous, as in the real world. Another example of live simulation is testing a car battery using an electrical tester.
2. **Virtual simulations** typically involve humans and/or equipment in a computer-controlled setting. Time is in discrete steps, allowing users to concentrate on the important stuff, so to speak. A flight simulator falls into this category.
3. **Constructive simulations** typically do not involve humans or equipment as participants. Rather than by time, they are driven more by the proper sequencing of events. The anticipated path of a hurricane might be "constructed" through application of temperatures, pressures, wind currents and other weather factors. Science-based simulations are typically constructive in nature.

Effectiveness Instructional Simulations Require
1. **Instructor preparation:** The good news is that instructional simulations can be very effective in stimulating student understanding. The bad news is that many simulations require intensive lesson preparation.
2. **Active student participation:** The learning effectiveness of instructional simulation rests on actively engaging students in problem solving.
3. **Postsimulation discussion:** Students need sufficient time to reflect on the simulation results.

14. Group dynamics.

Group dynamics are the processes that occur between group members. These dynamics are affected by each member's internal thoughts and feelings, their expressed thoughts and feelings, their nonverbal communication, and the relationship between group members. Group dynamics helps you understand how each person's actions make sense in the context of the group.

In any group working together, influences or social forces will shape the contributions of individual members—factors, such as social norms, power relationships, and taken for granted or contested meanings. Group dynamics or group process describes the way in which any group of humans interact and develop as a group, and the relationship between the group and the individuals within it. For qualitative market researchers who work often with groups it is important to learn to maximize the beneficial aspects of group working and minimize those that are disruptive or unproductive for the purposes of the research.

15. Explain briefly on any one of the projected aids.

Projected visuals are very effective aids to classroom teaching. They have a characteristic appeal of their own, which is especially suitable for influencing learner. When combined with recorded or on the spot commentary, they prove to be useful in a large number of situations.

However, like all other visual and audiovisual aids, they are only aids and it cannot be safely assumed that they alone can do the entire gamut of teaching. Projected visuals have some specific limitations. They require special equipment for their display. This equipment is usually costly, needs meticulous care and attention and in many cases, call for special training for its handling and maintenance. There are many factors that can affect the quality of projected images. Three of these are particularly important:
1. Kind of screen.
2. The placement of audience in relation to the screen.
3. The size of image and its brightness.

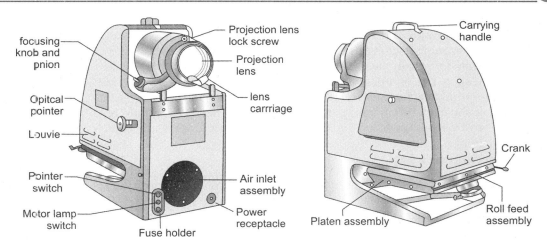

Understanding of these factors contribute to more effective preparation and use of projected aids. These limitations however, do not lessen the importance of using these visuals wherever suitable, because of their definite advantages. The important projected visual aids are slide projectors, overhead projector and opaque projector.

16. Objective structured clinical examination.

The objective structured clinical examination (OSCE) is a versatile multipurpose evaluative tool that can be utilized to assess healthcare professionals in a clinical setting. It assesses competency, based on objective testing through direct observation. It is precise, objective and reproducible allowing uniform testing of students for a wide range of clinical skills. Unlike the traditional clinical exam, the OSCE could evaluate areas most critical to performance of healthcare professionals, such as communication skills and ability to handle unpredictable patient behavior.

The OSCE is a versatile multipurpose evaluative tool that can be utilized to evaluate health care professionals in a clinical setting. It assesses competency, based on objective testing through direct observation. It is comprised of several "stations" in which examinees are expected to perform a variety of clinical tasks within a specified time period against criteria formulated to the clinical skill, thus demonstrating competency of skills and/or attitudes. The OSCE has been used to evaluate those areas most critical to performance of healthcare professionals, such as the ability to obtain/interpret data, problem-solve, teach, communicate and handle unpredictable patient behavior, which are otherwise impossible in the traditional clinical examination. Any attempt to evaluate these critical areas in the old-fashioned clinical case examination will seem to be assessing theory rather than simulating practical performance.

17. Purpose of interpersonal relations.

Close relationships are sometimes called interpersonal relationships. The closest relationships are most often found with family and a small circle of best friends. Interpersonal relationships require the most effort to nurture and maintain. These are also the relationships that give you the most joy and satisfaction. An interpersonal relationship is an association between two or more people that may range from fleeting to enduring. This association may be based on inference, love, solidarity, regular business interactions, or some other type of social commitment. Interpersonal relationships are formed in the context of social, cultural and other influences. The context can vary from family or kinship relations, friendship, marriage, relations with associates, work, clubs, neighborhoods and places of worship. They may be regulated by law, custom, or mutual agreement and are the basis of social groups and society as a whole. A relationship is normally viewed as a connection between individuals, such as a romantic or intimate relationship, or a parent–child relationship. Individuals can also have relationships with groups of people, such as the relation between a pastor and his congregation, an uncle and a family, or a mayor and a town. Finally, groups or even nations may have relations with each other. When in a healthy relationship, happiness is shown and the relationship is now a priority.

18. Advantages of MCQs.

1. Good MCQs are designed to be objective. They usually have one (or a few) definite answers that are given as choices for the students to select. Thus, there will be no ambiguity in marking due to subjective factors in the questions. Objective MCQs are easy to mark (a set of answer sheets is all that is required from the assessor) and thus do not require experienced tutor to mark them.
2. MCQs take less time to complete, with shorter assessment time required, more questions can be assessed. Feedback is fast.
3. MCQs can be administered as online assessments, such online assessments can be very effective and can prompt correct answers directly after completion with clarification and reasoning of the answers.
4. Factors irrelevant to the assessed material (such as handwriting and clarity of presentation) do not come into play in multiple choice assessments.
5. MCQs have high reliability, validity and manageability.

19. List four counseling techniques.

The **pattern of sessions** has a predictable rhythm with an introduction, information gathering, discussion and a conclusion.

Active listening happens when you "listen for meaning". The listener says very little but conveys much interest. The listener only speaks to find out if a statement (or two or twenty) has been correctly heard and understood.

Body language takes into account our facial expressions, angle of our body, proximity of ourself to another, placement of arms and legs, and so much more. Notice how much can be expressed by raising and lowering your eyebrows!

You need to **monitor the tone of your voice** in the same way that you monitor your body language. Remember, the person may not remember what was said, but they will remember how you made them feel!

An **open question** is one that is used in order to gather more information—you ask it with the intent of getting a long answer.

A **closed question** is one used to gather specific information—it can normally be answered with either a single word or a short phrase. Good counseling techniques to know!

Paraphrasing is when you restate what the speaker said. Often different words are used and the listener may be using this to draw attention to a particular concern or aspect. Sometimes paraphrasing is used to clarify.

Summarizing is focusing on the main points of a presentation or conversation in order to highlight them. At the same time you are giving the "gist", you are checking to see if you are accurate.

Note taking is the practice of writing down pieces of information, often in an shorthand and messy manner. The listener needs to be discreet and not disturb the flow of thought, speech or body language of the speaker.

20. Types of assessment tools.

Formative assessment occurs in the short-term, as learners are in the process of making meaning of new content and of integrating it into what they already know. Feedback to the learner is immediate (or nearly so), to enable the learner to change his/her behavior and understandings right away. Formative assessment also enables the teacher to "turn on a dime" and rethink instructional strategies, activities, and content based on student understanding and performance. His/her role here is comparable to that of a coach. Formative assessment can be as informal as observing the learner's work or as formal as a written test. Formative assessment is the most powerful type of assessment for improving student understanding and performance.
Examples: A very interactive class discussion; a warm-up, closure, or exit slip; a on-the-spot performance; a quiz.

Interim assessment takes place occasionally throughout a larger time period. Feedback to the learner is still quick, but may not be immediate. Interim assessments tend to be more formal, using tools such as projects, written assignments and tests. The learner should be given the opportunity to re-demonstrate his/her understanding once the feedback has been digested and acted upon. Interim assessments can help teachers identify gaps in student understanding and instruction, and ideally teachers address these before moving on or by weaving remedies into upcoming instruction and activities.
Examples: Chapter test; extended essay; a project scored with a rubric.

Summative assessment takes place at the end of a large chunk of learning, with the results being primarily for the teacher's or school's use. Results may take time to be returned to the student/parent, feedback to the student is usually very limited, and the student usually has no opportunity to be reassessed. Thus, summative assessment tends to have the least impact on improving an individual student's understanding or performance. Students/parents can use the results of summative assessments to see where the student's performance lies compared to either a standard (MEAP/MME) or to a group of students (usually a grade-level group, such as all 6th graders nationally, such as Iowa Tests or ACT). Teachers/schools can use these assessments to identify strengths and weaknesses of curriculum and instruction, with improvements affecting the next year's/term's students.
Examples: Standardized testing (MEAP, MME, ACT, Work Keys, Terra Nova, etc.); final exams; major cumulative projects, research projects, and performances.

21. Differentiate between symposium and panel discussion.

The panel discussion is held to exchange ideas and expression agreement and disagreement on points of mutual interests. The moderator guides the whole discussion and defines differences. This discussion may or may not have a general audience.

The symposium presents various insights into a subject matter by experts. The format is such that there are various speakers and a chairman. After all the speeches have been delivered the audience can ask questions from the speakers. The symposium presents various insights into a subject matter by experts. The format is such that there are various speakers and a chairman. After all the speeches have been delivered the audience can ask questions from the speakers.

22. Benefits of a field trip.

Field trips give students educational experiences away from their regular school environment. Popular field trip sites include zoos, nature centers, community agencies, such as fire stations and hospitals, government agencies, local businesses and science museums. Not only do field trips provide alternative educational opportunities for children, they can also benefit the community if they include some type of community service.

Students visiting different educational facilities learn in a more hands-on and interactive manner than they do in school. Science museums, for example, often have displays that children can touch to help them understand the material that is being covered. Zoos, nature centers and botanical gardens show kids animal and plant life up close, and often have areas where kids can touch displays, such as petting zoos and interactive computer programs.